INTERACTIVE
Electrocardiography

SECOND EDITION

CD-ROM WITH WORKBOOK

INTERACTIVE
Electrocardiography

SECOND EDITION

CD-ROM WITH WORKBOOK

Curtis M. Rimmerman, M.D., M.B.A., FACC

Medical Director, Cleveland Clinic Westlake,
  Lakewood, and Avon Pointe Family Health Centers
Gus P. Karos Chair of Clinical Cardiovascular Medicine
Associate Professor of Medicine, Cleveland Clinic Lerner
  College of Medicine of Case Western Reserve University
Department of Cardiovascular Medicine
Cleveland Clinic
Cleveland, Ohio

Anil K. Jain, M.D.

Managing Director, eResearch, eCleveland Clinic
Associate Program Director, Medicine Informatics Fellowship
Staff, General Internal Medicine
Cleveland Clinic
Cleveland, Ohio

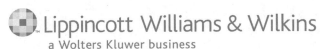 Lippincott Williams & Wilkins
a Wolters Kluwer business
Philadelphia · Baltimore · New York · London
Buenos Aires · Hong Kong · Sydney · Tokyo

Acquisitions Editor: Frances R. DeStefano
Managing Editor: Chris Potash
Project Manager: Bridgett Dougherty
Marketing Manager: Kimberly Schonberger
Design Coordinator: Stephen Druding
Production Services: Maryland Composition

Second Edition
© 2008 by Lippincott Williams & Wilkins, a Wolters Kluwer business
First Edition © 2001 by Lippincott Williams & Wilkins

Printed in the United States

ISBN-13: 978-0-7817-7863-3
ISBN-10: 0-7817-7863-8

Care has been taken to confirm the accuracy of the information presented and to describe generally accepted practices. However, the authors, editors, and publisher are not responsible for errors or omissions or for any consequences from application of the information in this book and make no warranty, expressed or implied, with respect to the currency, completeness, or accuracy of the contents of the publication. Application of this information in a particular situation remains the professional responsibility of the practitioner; the clinical treatments described and recommended may not be considered absolute and universal recommendations.

The authors, editors, and publisher have exerted every effort to ensure that drug selection and dosage set forth in this text are in accordance with current recommendations and practice at the time of publication. However, in view of ongoing research, changes in government regulations, and the constant flow of information relating to drug therapy and drug reactions, the reader is urged to check the package insert for each drug for any change in indications and dosage and for added warnings and precautions. This is particularly important when the recommended agent is a new or infrequently employed drug.

Some drugs and medical devices presented in this publication have Food and Drug Administration (FDA) clearance for limited use in restricted research settings. It is the responsibility of health care providers to ascertain the FDA status of each drug or device planned for use in their clinical practice.

The publishers have made every effort to trace copyright holders for borrowed material. If they have inadvertently overlooked any, they will be pleased to make the necessary arrangements at the first opportunity.

To purchase additional copies of this book, call our customer service department at (800) 638-3030 or fax orders to 1-301-223-2400. Lippincott Williams & Wilkins customer service representatives are available from 8:30 am to 6:00 pm, EST, Monday through Friday, for telephone access. Visit Lippincott Williams & Wilkins on the Internet: http://www.lww.com.

10 9 8 7 6 5 4 3 2 1

To my wife, Maria, and daughter, Eleanor,
who demonstrated unwavering support during this project.

C.R.

To my wife, Kamna, my daughter Nikita, and my sons,
Akshay and Vikas—without their support, this project
would not have been possible.

A.J.

CONTENTS

INTRODUCTION

Electrocardiography is a fundamental diagnostic test performed by health personnel of all medical and surgical disciplines. During the initial comprehensive evaluation of a patient, the electrocardiogram remains the key component for assessing the cardiac rhythm, for detecting the presence of chamber enlargement, conduction abnormalities and ischemic heart disease. It serves as an excellent serial diagnostic test to monitor for both occult and symptomatic cardiac pathology. In circumstances of urgent clinical decision making where prompt and accurate electrocardiogram interpretation is critical, the electrocardiogram remains important for patient evaluation, assessment and care. Thus, it is essential for health care professionals to both develop and maintain proficiency in electrocardiogram interpretation.

This computer-based interactive electrocardiogram CD-ROM with its companion workbook is aimed toward physicians, nurses, other health care professionals and students of both differing disciplines and experience. The collection is purposefully divided into three levels of electrocardiogram complexity, allowing the user to assess their individual learning curve at their own pace of interpretation. More than 630 clinical electrocardiograms are available and quickly retrievable for systematic review. It also serves as a resource library of both common and uncommon electrocardiogram examples that can be readily accessed and used for teaching and reference. Progressing through the self-study collection, the user will actively develop and expand their electrocardiogram interpretive abilities. Specific objectives upon completing this interactive electrocardiogram collection include the following:

1. The recognition and diagnosis of both normal and abnormal cardiac rhythms including complex arrhythmias.
2. The recognition and diagnosis of myocardial infarction patterns.
3. The accurate determination of the cardiac electrical axis and cardiac intervals including abnormal findings.
4. The recognition of specific cardiac chamber abnormalities.
5. The recognition of the electrocardiogram manifestations of serum electrolyte abnormalities.
6. The ability to thoughtfully reason why a specific electrocardiogram pattern is present, integrating the clinical history and electrocardiogram findings.

The CD-ROM and its companion workbook are divided into three separate levels, each categorized by increasing electrocardiogram complexity. Each electrocardiogram in the book is reproduced in the exact order as found on the CD-ROM. An area for interpretation notes accompanies each electrocardiogram. The workbook is meant to supplement the CD-ROM and allow the user to interpret the electrocardiogram in hard copy format as traditionally performed at an electrocardiography heart station. The CD-ROM provides additional clinical information, author electrocardiogram interpretation, annotations, comments, key word listings, multiple choice questions and diagnostic categories unique for each tracing.

A recommended approach to utilizing the CD-ROM with the supplemental workbook is as follows:

1. In the workbook, thoroughly read A Recommended Approach for Electrocardiogram Interpretation.
2. Initially interpret the first 20 electrocardiograms in the Level I section, utilizing the diagnostic category list found in the back of the workbook.
3. After interpretation is complete for this group of tracings, refer to the CD-ROM.
4. Open the CD-ROM and retrieve the first electrocardiogram. Enter your diagnoses under the diagnostic categories section. The program will provide answer feedback.
5. Next review the history, author interpretation and comments sections.
6. Annotated arrows will appear on the electrocardiogram under review, providing interactive interpretation feedback.
7. Multiple choice questions are available for each electrocardiogram and diagnostic key word to further test your knowledge.
8. A comprehensive glossary is also available with an individual, readily retrievable definition for each diagnostic key word.

This electrocardiography CD-ROM with its accompanying workbook is meant to provide an interactive educational experience, gradually introducing interpretation principles by utilizing a comprehensive electrocardiogram collection. Repetition is purposefully emphasized to provide concept reinforcement. Accurate clinical histories are provided for each electrocardiogram, permitting the user to correlate electrocardiogram interpretation with the patient's clinical presentation. This feature ensures the clinical relevance of this educational product with the ultimate goal of positively influencing patient care.

A RECOMMENDED APPROACH TO
Electrocardiogram Interpretation

Introduction

To assure accurate and consistent electrocardiogram interpretation, a systematic approach is required. Electrocardiogram interpretation is not an exercise in pattern recognition. Instead, it requires an interpreter with an inquisitive mind who strives to understand why the electrocardiogram demonstrates a specific morphology. This requires a thorough understanding of the cardiac conduction sequence, cardiac anatomy and cardiac physiology.

Similar cardiac pathology is manifest differently on the surface electrocardiogram depending upon the electrocardiogram lead undergoing analysis. For instance, precordial lead V_1 predominantly overlies the right ventricle. Right ventricular cardiac electrical events are often best seen in this lead. Conversely, precordial lead V_6 overlies the left ventricle and predictably best represents left ventricular cardiac electrical events. Knowledge of electrocardiogram anatomic correlates helps plan an interpretation strategy reducing the likelihood of overlooking an important finding. Additionally, oftentimes the electrocardiogram serves as the first indicator of occult cardiac pathology. Interpretation is most rewarding when the interpreter deduces a disease state and alerts the clinician to the findings. With experience, certain electrocardiogram findings are identified simultaneously, together representing a unifying cardiac diagnosis. A recommended systematic approach to electrocardiogram interpretation is outlined below.

Cardiac Rhythm Determination

The initial interpretive step for each electrocardiogram is to identify atrial activity and to determine the cardiac rhythm. If P waves are present, it is important to precisely measure the P wave to P wave interval. This determines the atrial depolarization rate. After identifying the dominant P wave morphology, the P wave frontal plane axis is ascertained. A normal P wave frontal plane axis reflects a sinus node origin, demonstrating a positive P wave vector in leads I, II, III and aVF. An abnormal P wave axis supports an ectopic, non-sinus node P wave origin. Possible atrial rhythms include the following:

1) *Normal Sinus Rhythm:* a regular atrial depolarization rate of sinus node origin between 60–100 per minute demonstrating a positive P wave vector in leads I, II, III and aVF.
2) *Sinus Bradycardia:* a regular atrial depolarization rate of sinus node origin less than 60 per minute demonstrating a positive P wave vector in leads I, II, III and aVF.
3) *Sinus Tachycardia:* a regular atrial depolarization rate of sinus node origin greater than 100 per minute demonstrating a positive P wave vector in leads I, II, III and aVF.

4) *Sinus Arrhythmia:* a normal P wave morphology and frontal plane axis of sinus node origin with an atrial depolarization rate between 60–100 per minute demonstrating a P wave to P wave cycle length variation greater than 160 msec.

5) *Atrial Fibrillation:* a rapid, irregular and disorganized atrial depolarization rate of 400–700 per minute without discrete P waves. Atrial activation is represented by fibrillatory waves. In the absence of atrioventricular block, the ventricular response is irregularly irregular. The fibrillatory waves can vary in amplitude between patients generating a subclassification of atrial fibrillation as either coarse or fine.

6) *Atrial Flutter:* a rapid regular atrial depolarization rate of 250–350 per minute felt most commonly to represent an atrial re-entrant circuit. The atrial waves are termed "F waves" and demonstrate a "saw-toothed" appearance, best seen in leads V_1, II, III and aVF. The ventricular rate is either regular or irregular depending on the atrioventricular conduction ratio.

7) *Atrial Tachycardia:* a regular automatic tachycardia from a single ectopic atrial focus demonstrating a P wave possessing an abnormal frontal plane axis. The typical atrial rate is between 180–240 per minute. The ventricular rate is either regular or irregular depending on the atrioventricular conduction ratio.

8) *Wandering Atrial Pacemaker:* the atrial depolarization rate is between 60–100 per minute. The P wave to P interval varies reflecting the different foci of atrial activation. To satisfy this diagnosis, greater than three atrial foci and P wave morphologies are present on a single 12-lead electrocardiogram.

9) *Multifocal Atrial Tachycardia:* a tachycardic heart rhythm with an atrial depolarization rate greater than 100 per minute with a P wave preceding each QRS complex. On a single 12-lead electrocardiogram, P waves of at least three different morphologies are necessary to satisfy the diagnostic criteria. The PR intervals vary and the ventricular response is irregularly irregular given the unpredictable timing of atrial depolarization. Non-conducted atrial complexes during absolute ventricular refractoriness are often present.

10) *Ectopic Atrial Rhythm:* a regular atrial depolarization rate of non-sinus node origin between 60–100 per minute. The P wave frontal plane axis is abnormal reflecting the non-sinus node single atrial focus origin.

11) *Ectopic Atrial Bradycardia:* a regular atrial depolarization rate of non-sinus node origin less than 60 per minute. The P wave frontal plane axis is abnormal reflecting the non-sinus node single atrial focus origin.

12) *Sinus Node Re-entrant Rhythm:* a re-entrant circuit involving the sinus node and peri-sinus nodal tissues. The P wave morphology and frontal plane axis is normal given the sinus node origin. Atrial depolarization is regular at a rate between 60–100 per minute. This dysrhythmia is characterized by abrupt onset and termination.

13) *Sinus Node Re-entrant Tachycardia:* a re-entrant circuit involving the sinus node and peri-sinus nodal tissues. The P wave morphology and frontal plane axis is normal given the sinus node origin. Atrial depolarization is regular at a rate greater than 100 per minute. This dysrhythmia is characterized by abrupt onset and termination.

14) *Atrioventricular Nodal Re-entrant Tachycardia:* dependant on the presence of two separate atrioventricular nodal pathways with slowed conduction in one pathway and unidirectional conduction block in

the other pathway. Electrocardiographic criteria include a ventricular rate between 140–220 per minute and a regular rhythm with abrupt onset and termination. Dysrhythmia onset is often initiated by a premature atrial complex. Inverted P waves may occur prior to the QRS complex, within the QRS complex or after the QRS complex within the ST segment. The QRS complex may be conducted normally or aberrantly.

15) *Supraventricular Tachycardia:* a global term encompassing regular tachycardic dysrhythmias originating within the atria or the atrioventricular junction. This term is best utilized in the presence of a regular narrow complex tachycardia where identifiable atrial activity is not readily identified and the exact determination of the supraventricular rhythm disturbance is not possible from the 12-lead electrocardiogram.

When electrocardiogram evidence for atrial depolarization is absent, it is important to identify a subsidiary pacemaker origin such as the atrioventricular junction. Several different types of atrioventricular junctional rhythms exist including the following:

1) *Junctional Rhythm:* this dysrhythmia commonly occurs in the setting of digitalis intoxication with suppression of sinus node activity and sinus exit block. A subsidiary pacemaker such as the junction assumes the primary pacemaker role at a regular rate between 40–60 per minute.

2) *Junctional Bradycardia:* this dysrhythmia originates within the atrioventricular node and represents a regular heart rhythm generated from a subsidiary pacemaker at a rate less than 60 per minute. Retrograde P waves representing atrial activation may be present and can occur before, within or after the QRS complexes.

3) *Junctional Tachycardia:* the ventricular rate is regular and typically between 120–200 per minute. The atrioventricular junction serves as the primary cardiac pacemaker. Retrograde P waves may precede, be superimposed or follow the QRS complexes depending on the level of junctional tachycardia origin.

4) *Accelerated Junctional Rhythm:* the rhythm is regular with a rate between 60–100 per minute. The atrioventricular junction serves as the cardiac pacemaker. Retrograde P waves may precede, be superimposed or follow the QRS complexes depending on the level of junctional rhythm origin.

5) *Junctional Escape Rhythm:* this dysrhythmia commonly occurs in the setting of digitalis intoxication with suppression of sinus node activity and sinus exit block. With depression of the sinus node, a subsidiary pacemaker such as the atrioventricular junction assumes the primary pacemaker role at a rate between 40–60 per minute.

Each electrocardiogram should also be assessed for the presence of an independent ventricular rhythm. Possible ventricular rhythm disturbances include the following:

1) *Ventricular Tachycardia:* a sustained cardiac rhythm of ventricular origin occurring at a regular rate of 140–240 per minute. Common featues include a widened QRS complex, frontal plane QRS complex left axis deviation, precordial lead QRS complex concordance, atrioventricular dissociation, capture and fusion complexes.

2) *Polymorphic Ventricular Tachycardia (Torsades de Pointes);* a paroxysmal form of ventricular tachycardia with a non-constant R to R interval, a ventricular rate of approximately 225–250 per minute, QRS

complexes of alternating polarity, prolongation of the QT interval at arrythmia onset and a changing QRS complex amplitude often resembling a sine wave pattern.

3) *Ventricular Fibrillation:* a terminal cardiac rhythm with chaotic ventricular activity without organized ventricular depolarization.

4) *Ventricular Parasystole:* an independent ventricular rhythm with regular discharge and ventricular depolarization. This is characterized by varying coupling intervals, a constant R to R interval of the interectopic complexes and the presence of fusion complexes when the parasystolic focus discharges simultaneously with the native ventricular depolarization.

5) *Idioventricular Rhythm:* a regular rhythm at a ventricular rate less than 60 per minute. Widened QRS complexes are present with the ventricular complexes commonly dissociated from the atrial activity. This rhythm disturbance is often seen in abnormalities of advanced atrioventricular conduction where the ventricle serves as a subsidiary pacemaker and escape rhythm.

6) *Accelerated Idioventricular Rhythm:* a regular rhythm at a ventricular rate of 60–100 per minute. Widened QRS complexes are present with the ventricular complexes commonly dissociated from the atrial activity. This rhythm disturbance is often seen in abnormalities of advanced atrioventricular conduction where the ventricle serves as a subsidiary pacemaker and escape rhythm.

Electrocardiogram Intervals

PR Interval: Early identification and accurate determination of the PR interval is important. A constant PR interval of normal duration (120–200 msec) reflects normal intra-atrial conduction, atrioventricular nodal conduction and atrioventricular association. A varying PR interval supports the possibilities of atrioventricular dissociation and differing types of heart block, both requiring further detailed analysis. A shortened PR interval may reflect facile intra-atrial and atrioventricular conduction or ventricular pre-excitation. A prolonged PR interval reflects delayed intra-atrial or atrioventricular conduction.

R to R interval: A precise measurement of the R wave to R wave interval determines the ventricular rate of depolarization. In the presence of normal atrioventricular conduction, the ventricular rate will equal the atrial rate. If an atrioventricular conduction abnormality exists, a determination of the atrioventricular conduction ratio (number of P waves for each QRS complex) is performed. In the presence of atrioventricular dissociation or complete heart block two independent cardiac rhythms exist originating from separate cardiac foci, each necessitating interpretation. Important forms of atrioventricular conduction abnormalities include the following:

1) Second Degree Mobitz Type I Wenckebach Atrioventricular Block
2) Second Degree Mobitz Type II Atrioventricular Block
3) Advanced Atrioventricular Block
4) Complete Heart Block
5) Variable Atrioventricular Conduction

QRS Complex Interval: The QRS complex duration is best measured in the limb leads from R wave onset (Q wave onset, if present) to S wave offset. A normal QRS complex interval is less than 100 msec. If greater than 100 msec but less than 120 msec, the QRS complex conduction delay is best classified as nonspecific. If the QRS complex duration is greater than 120 msec but without a specific ascribable morphology, it is still best classified as a nonspecific intraventricular conduction delay. If greater than 120 msec, a careful assessment of the QRS complex morphology is important as complete left or right bundle branch block may exist. Complete left bundle branch block represents a QRS complex duration greater than 120 msec, the absence of a q wave (septal depolarization) in leads I and V_{5-6}, an upright QRS complex in leads I, V_{5-6} and ST segment depression and T wave inversion in leads I and V_{5-6}. Complete right bundle branch block represents a QRS complex duration greater than 120 msec, widened terminally slowed S waves in leads I, V_{5-6}, a widened RSR' QRS complex morphology in leads V_{1-2} and ST segment depression and T wave inversion in leads V_{1-2}.

QT Interval: Unlike the other cardiac intervals, the QT interval demonstrates heart rate interdependence. The QT interval duration is inversely proportional to the R to R cycle length. The QTc interval represents the QT interval divided by the square root of the R to R interval. This adjusts the QT interval for heart rate and standardizes this measurement. This is a cumbersome manual measurement and calculation for each electrocardiogram. At present, electrocardiogram machines provide a comprehensive print-out of all cardiac intervals including the QTc interval. These values serve as a useful *reference* but are not without limitation and potential error. The interpreter is encouraged to verify the accuracy of the computer-generated intervals for each tracing. For the QT interval, a fairly accurate shortened approach involves visually assessing this interval in limb lead II. If the QT interval is less than 50 percent of the R wave to R wave interval, prolongation is not likely present. If the QT interval is greater than 50 percent of the R wave to R wave interval, this usually reflects prolongation best confirmed with a manual measurement by the interpreter. Causes of a prolonged QT interval include the following:

1) Idiopathic Long QT Interval Syndrome
2) Central Nervous System Event
3) Hypocalcemia
4) Cardiac Antiarrhythmic Medication
5) Pyschotropic Medication
6) Hypothyroidism

The presence of a shortened QT interval, which may represent an underlying electrolyte disturbance, is best done by careful interval assessment and visual inspection. It often is first suggested by a truncated ST segment. This is an easily overlooked electrocardiogram finding which reinforces the need for a consistent and diligent interpretation approach. Causes of QT interval shortening include:

1) Digitalis Administration
2) Hypercalcemia

QRS Complex Frontal Plane Axis

The QRS complex frontal plane axis is next assessed for each electrocardiogram. The QRS complex vector is carefully assessed in each limb lead. An isoelectric vector is concluded if the area of positivity (R wave) is equal to the area of negativity (Q wave plus S wave).

A simplified approach is as follows:

1) Assess the QRS complex vector in leads I and aVF. If both are positive, the QRS complex frontal plane axis is between zero and positive 90 degrees and therefore normal.
2) If the QRS complex vector is positive in lead I and negative in lead aVF, assess the QRS complex vector in lead II. If the lead II QRS complex vector is positive, the QRS complex frontal plane axis is between zero and negative 30 degrees, best classified as QRS complex frontal plane left axis deviation.
3) If the QRS complex vector is positive in lead I and negative in leads aVF and II, the QRS complex frontal plane axis is greater than negative 30 degrees reflecting left anterior hemiblock.
4) If the QRS complex vector is negative in lead I and positive in leads III and aVF, QRS complex right axis deviation is present.

Electrocardiogram Morphologies

Once the cardiac rate, rhythm, intervals and QRS complex frontal plane axis are assessed, it is appropriate to proceed with identification of specific electrocardiogram morphologic findings. The approach of addressing the P wave first, the QRS complex second and the ST-T waves last is both systematic and logical.

P Wave: Besides P wave identification and P wave frontal plane axis determination, specific P wave morphologies suggest underlying conduction and structural cardiac pathology. The P wave morphology is best assessed in leads V_1 and lead II. Important findings in these leads include left atrial abnormality and right abnormality. The electrocardiogram findings of left atrial abnormality include a prominent terminally negative or biphasic P wave in lead V_1. This reflects delayed left atrial depolarization manifest as a terminally negative P wave vector with left atrial depolarization transpiring opposite lead V_1. In lead II, the P wave duration is prolonged to greater than 110 msec with a bifid positive vector. The second or terminal component of this positive P wave vector represents delayed left atrial depolarization. The electrocardiogram finding of right atrial abnormality demonstrates a P wave amplitude of 2.5 mm or greater in lead II. Given the anterior P wave vector in the presence of right atrial abnormality, a tall P wave of 1.5mm or greater is often seen in lead V_1. *It is not possible to discern from the surface electrocardiogram if an atrial abnormality represents chamber enlargement and/or delayed conduction. The less specific term, abnormality, is therefore most appropriate.*

QRS Complex: Evaluation of the QRS complex morphology is an important individual step. It is best to precede with an initial careful evaluation for the presence or absence of Q waves. Q waves of diagnostic duration in most circumstances represent an underlying myocardial infarction. In the inferior and lateral leads, Q waves of 40 msec duration or greater represent a myocardial infarction. In leads V_{2-4}, a Q wave of diagnostic duration is 25 msec or greater. In the presence of a myocardial infarction, Q waves are most commonly grouped into electrocardiogram "regions" reflecting a specific coronary artery distribution. When a Q wave is identified, it is helpful to evaluate contiguous leads integrating a working knowledge of coronary artery anatomy. For instance, in the presence of an inferior myocardial infarction careful evaluation for the presence of a posterior, lateral and right ventricular myocardial infarction is prudent. Alternatively, when an anterior myocardial infarction is noted, lateral and apical involvement may be seen.

Q waves can also demonstrate a pseudo-infarction pattern and thus not reflect a true myocardial infarction. This is most commonly seen in the presence of the Wolff-Parkinson-White syndrome. The pseudo-infarction Q waves instead reflect ventricular pre-excitation. The delta wave possesses a negative vector indicating ventricular conduction opposite the electrocardiogram lead. This is most often seen in the inferior, lateral and high lateral leads. *A prominent R wave in lead V_1 in isolation should be interpreted with caution.* It is unusual to diagnose an isolated true posterior myocardial infarction. Other causes such as ventricular pre-excitation, counterclockwise cardiac rotation, right ventricular hypertrophy and right ventricular conduction delay should be carefully considered. QRS complex frontal plane right axis deviation and left posterior fascicular block are other causes of a pseudo-infarction pattern. In these examples, the pseudo-infarction Q waves are located inferiorly.

ST Segment: The ST segment is the segment between the terminal aspect of the QRS complex (also known as the J point) and T wave onset. As part of a complete electrocardiogram interpretation, each ST segment is assessed for deviation from the electrocardiogram baseline. The isoelectric comparative segment on the electrocardiogram is the TP segment. This is the segment between the terminal aspect of the T wave and P wave onset. Most often ST segment deviation is best termed nonspecific as the exact cause is not discernable from the electrocardiogram alone, instead requiring a complete clinical history and medication record.

Causes of ST segment elevation include the following:

1) *Acute Myocardial Injury:* convex upward (coved) ST segment elevation confined to at least two contiguous electrocardiogram leads.
2) *Pericarditis:* diffuse concave upward ST segment elevation not confined to contiguous electrocardiogram leads.
3) *Left Ventricular Aneurysm:* most commonly right precordial lead convex upward (coved) ST segment elevation overlying the infarct zone persisting for months to years.

Causes of ST segment depression include the following:

1) *Myocardial Ischemia:* most commonly exercise-induced as seen during stress testing. ST segment depression often reflects coronary artery disease and myocardial ischemia. Horizontal or down sloping ST segment depression demonstrates greater specificity.
2) *Non-Q Wave Myocardial Infarction:* horizontal or down-sloping ST segment depression with supporting clinical and laboratory markers of acute myocardial injury.
3) *Cardiomyopathy:* abnormal ST segments including ST segment depression are present in both dilated and hypertrophic cardiomyopathic forms.
4) *Ventricular Hypertrophy:* down sloping ST segment depression is commonly present in both left and right ventricular hypertrophy.
5) *Supraventricular Tachyarrhythmias:* paroxysmal ST segment depression is frequently present at high heart rates during supraventricular tachycardic rhythms. These findings may persist after arrhythmia cessation. They may or may not represent co-existent myocardial ischemia and oftentimes, further corroborative testing is necessary.

T Wave: The T wave begins at the terminal aspect of the ST segment and ends at the onset of the TP segment. Precise identification of the exact beginning and end of the T wave is often difficult. T wave abnormalities are seen in many clinical conditions and are not a specific finding. T wave abnormalities are found in the following circumstances:

1) Cardiomyopathies
2) Ventricular Hypertrophy
3) Electrolyte Disturbances
4) Valvular Heart Disease
5) Coronary Artery Disease
6) Central Nervous System Event
7) Wolff-Parkinson-White Syndrome
8) Bundle Branch Block
9) Pericarditis
10) Medication Administration
11) Hyperventilation
12) Positional Change

U Wave: The U wave is variably present on the electrocardiogram. When seen, it begins at the terminal aspect of the T wave and ends within the TP segment. Often, T wave and U wave fusion is present and therefore it is not possible to separately measure the T wave and U wave duration. Both positive and negative U waves may exist. The U wave generally does not exceed 25 percent of the T wave amplitude and is best seen in leads V_{2-3}.

Causes of a positive U wave include the following:

1) Bradycardia
2) Central Nervous System Disease
3) Cardiac Antiarrythmic Medication
4) Electrolyte Disturbances
    A) Hypokalemia
    B) Hypomagnesemia

Causes of negative U waves include the following:

1) Left Ventricular Hypertrophy
2) Coronary Artery Disease

Conclusion

To successfully interpret electrocardiograms, a deliberate, consistent and reproducible approach is essential. Through experience and repetition, the interpreter will demonstrate improved interpretive abilities and confidence rendering greater diagnostic accuracy. The once complex and intimidating electrocardiogram will now represent a routine tracing which is readily interpreted. The former student will assume the role of a knowledgeable educator.

ACKNOWLEDGMENTS

We thank our families who have demonstrated unwavering support during this extensive educational project. We also thank the late Mrs. Jeannette Goodman for her expert secretarial assistance, without whose help this project would not have been possible. We remain most appreciative of Dr. Donald Underwood's expert editorial review of the electrocardiograms.

INTERACTIVE
Electrocardiography

SECOND EDITION

CD-ROM WITH WORKBOOK

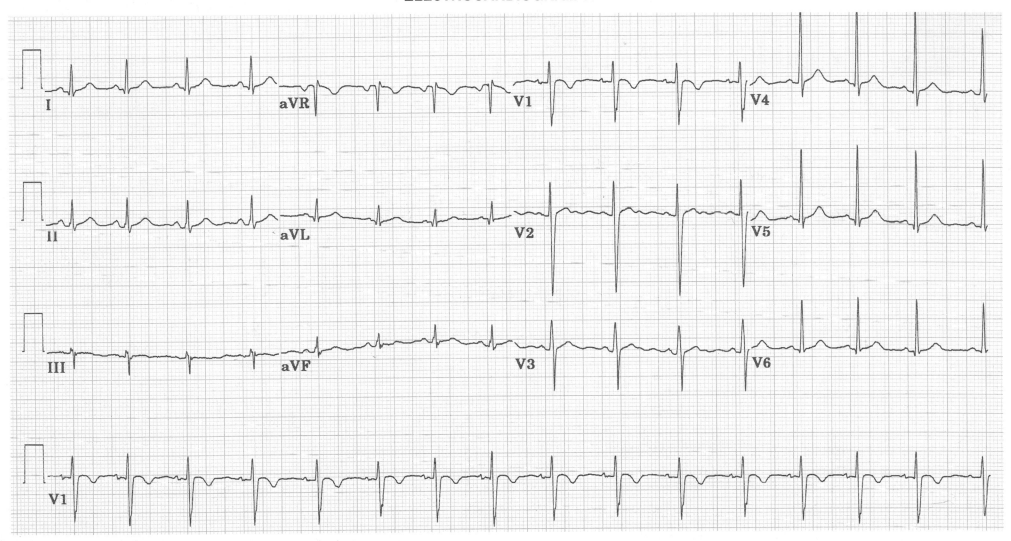

ECG 1 Eighteen year old gentleman with a seizure disorder who returns for outpatient neurology follow-up. His medications included phenytoin, carbamazepine, and diazepam.

Interpretation Notes:

LEVEL I

ELECTROCARDIOGRAM 2

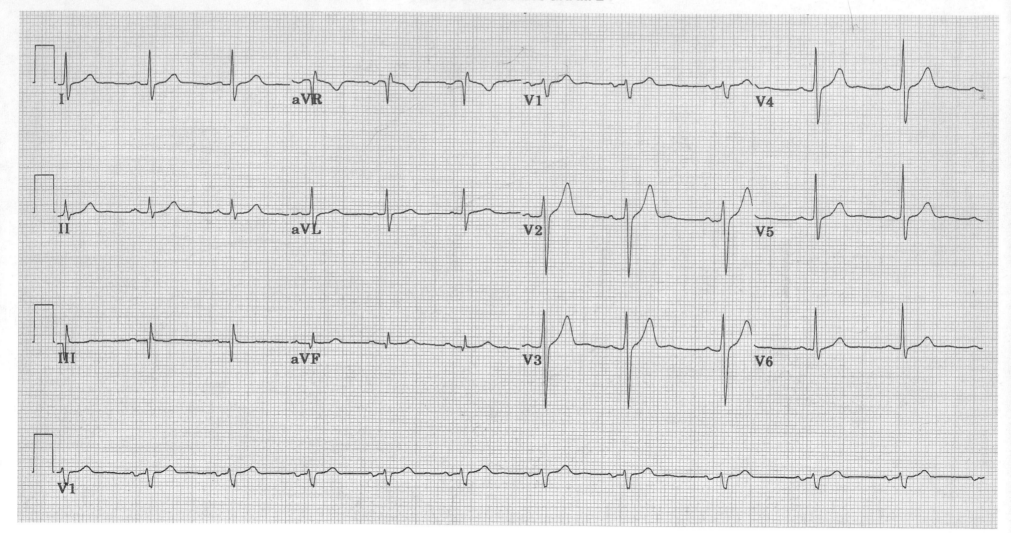

I aVR V1 V4

II aVL V2 V5

III aVF V3 V6

V1

Interpretation Notes: _____

_____

ECG 2 Fifty-two year old gentleman who presents for a routine physical examination in the preventive medicine department. His past medical history includes elevated triglycerides and a low HDL cholesterol value. He otherwise remains in good health.

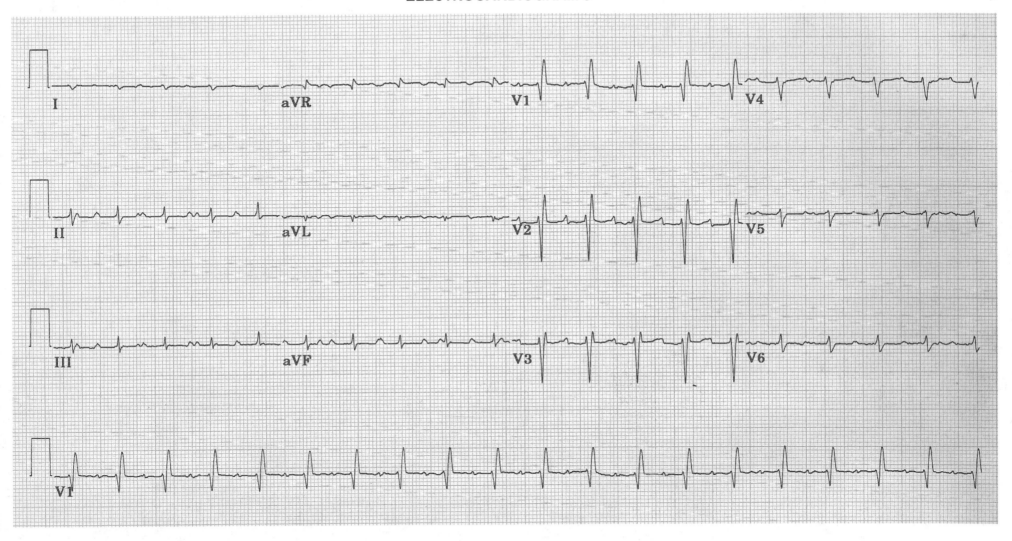

Interpretation Notes: _____

_____

ECG 3 Fifty-six year old gentleman who underwent a cardiac transplant procedure six weeks prior to this electrocardiogram secondary to an idiopathic non-ischemic dilated cardiomyopathy and recurrent ventricular tachycardia. His medications at the time of this electrocardiogram included digoxin, furosemide, lisinopril, potassium, and aspirin.

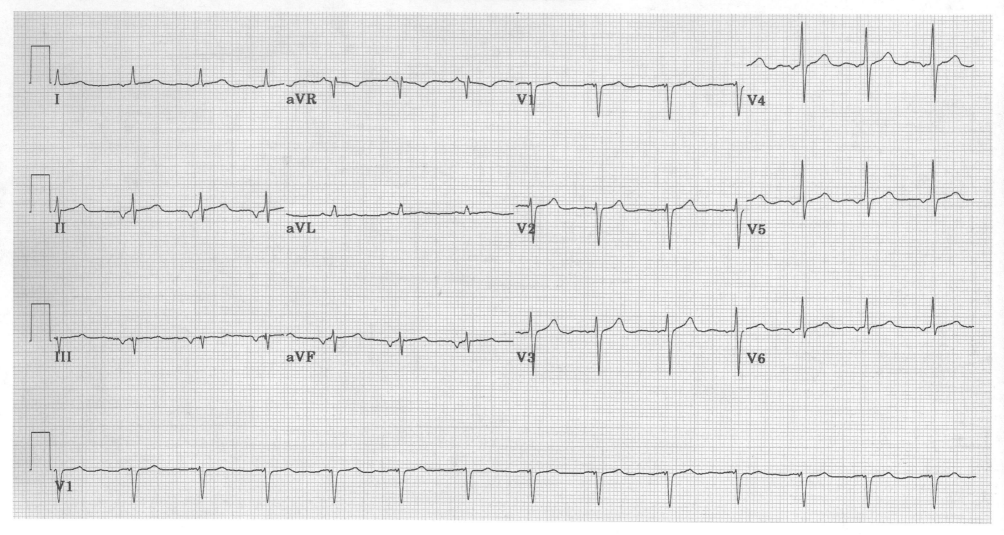

I   aVR   V1   V4

II   aVL   V2   V5

III   aVF   V3   V6

V1

Interpretation Notes: _____

_____

ECG 4 Fifty-four year old woman with a history of metastatic malignant melanoma who is being evaluated for a subsequent course of chemotherapy. Her past cardiac history includes an angioplasty to the left circumflex coronary artery eight years prior to this tracing. She is currently asymptomatic. Her cardiac medications included diltiazem and aspirin.

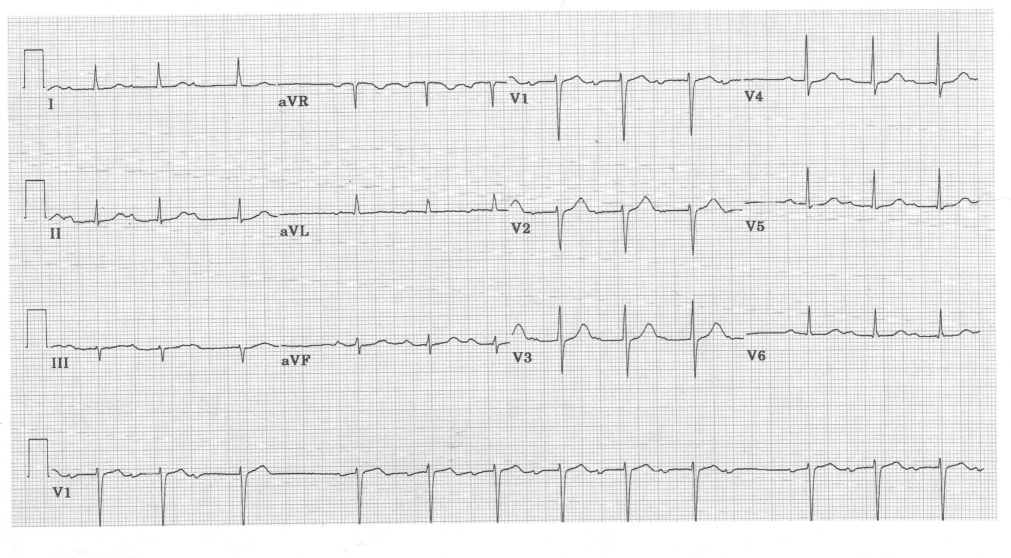

Interpretation Notes: _____

ECG 5 Seventy year old woman who presents for a general physical examination. She has a history of coronary artery obstructive disease and is status post a myocardial infarction of unknown location four years prior to this electrocardiogram. Other co-morbid conditions include extensive past tobacco use, hypertension, and gastroesophageal reflux disease. Her medications at the time of this electrocardiogram included potassium, thyroxine, triamterene/hydrochlorothiazide, and naprosyn.

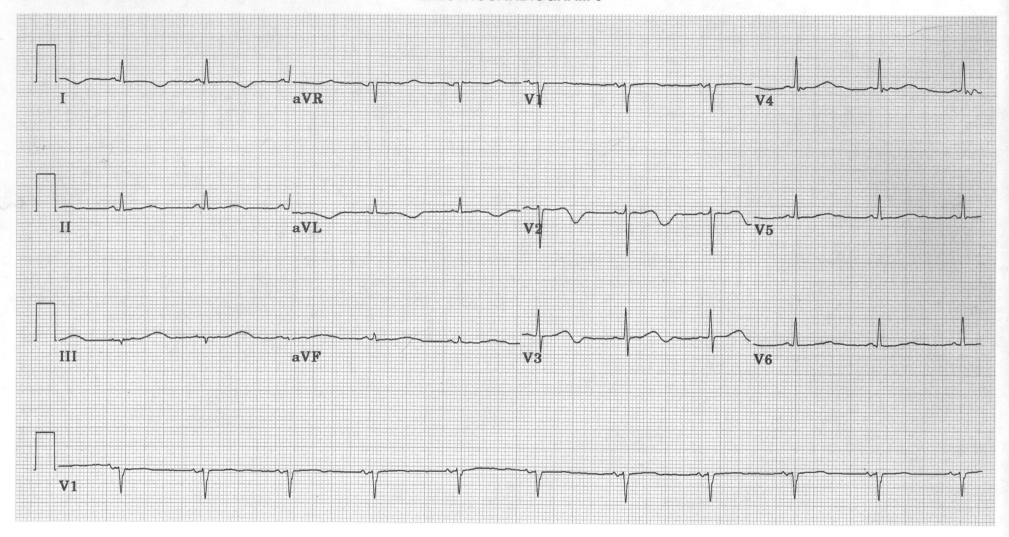

Interpretation Notes: _____

_____

_____

ECG 6 Forty-one year old gentleman with myelodysplastic syndrome and insulin requiring diabetes mellitus admitted for a bone marrow transplantation. His serum potassium at the time of this electrocardiogram was 3.4 meq/L.

LEVEL I

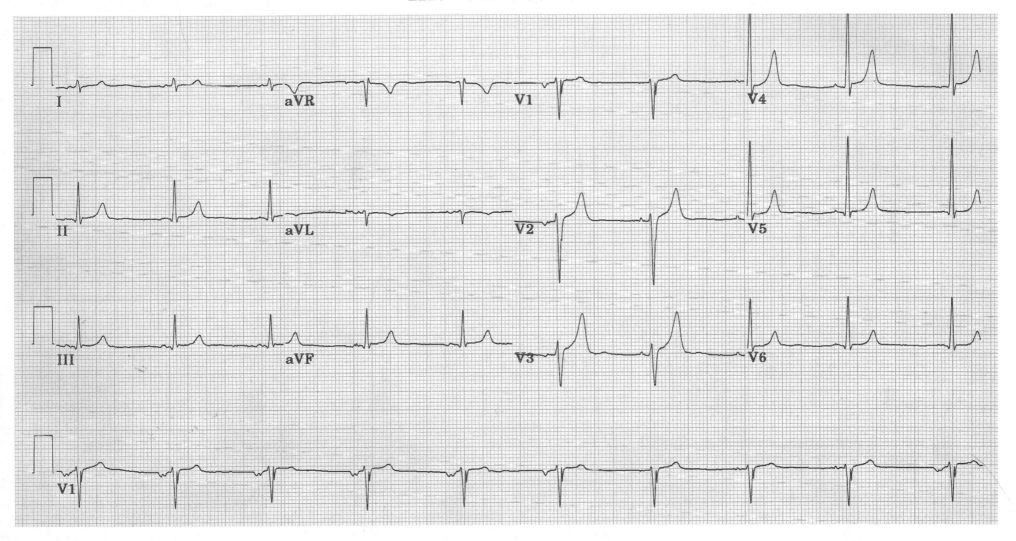

I   aVR   V1   V4

II   aVL   V2   V5

III   aVF   V3   V6

V1

Interpretation Notes: _____

_____

ECG 7 Thirty-one year old gentleman who recently underwent a right upper lung wedge resection for a necrotic granuloma. He has no known cardiac history.

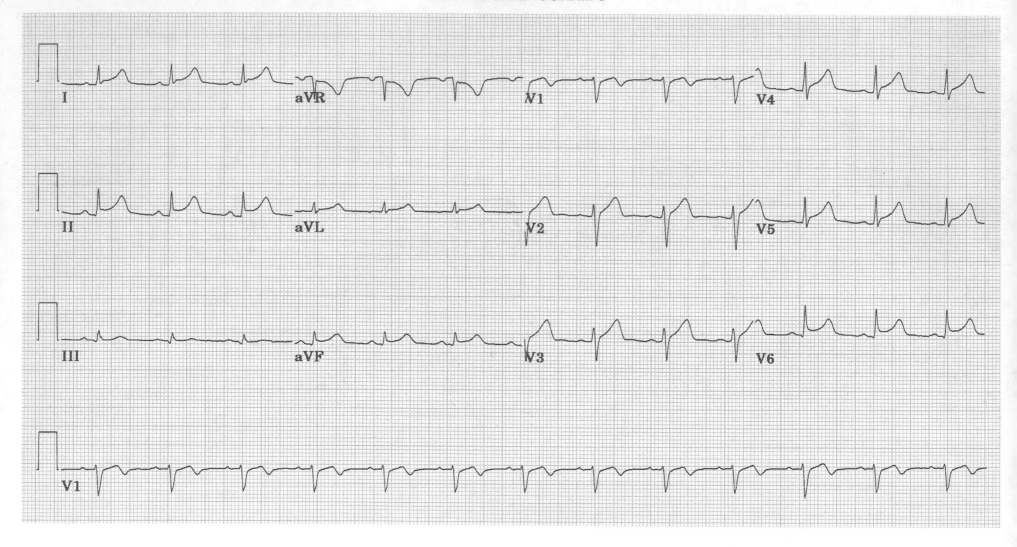

Interpretation Notes: _____

_____

_____

ECG 8 Thirty-nine year old woman, unrestrained passenger who suffered an aortic transection distal to the left subclavian artery from a motor vehicle accident. This electrocardiogram was taken postoperatively shortly after thoracic aorta repair.

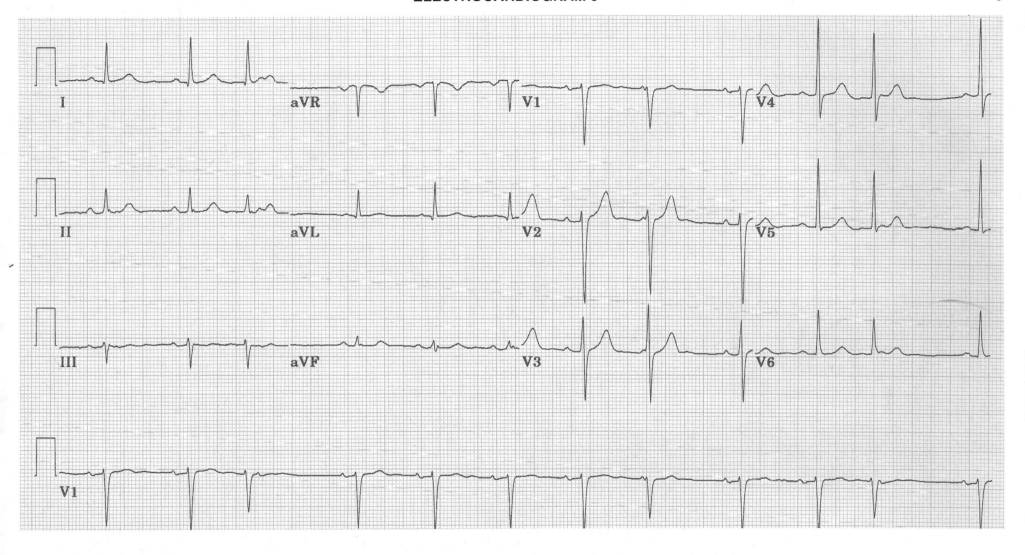

I aVR V1 V4

II aVL V2 V5

III aVF V3 V6

V1

Interpretation Notes: _____

_____

_____

ECG 9 Sixty-two year old gentleman who is undergoing preoperative anesthesia clearance prior to planned rotator cuff repair. His past medical history is notable for hypertension but no known cardiac disease. His medications included verapamil.

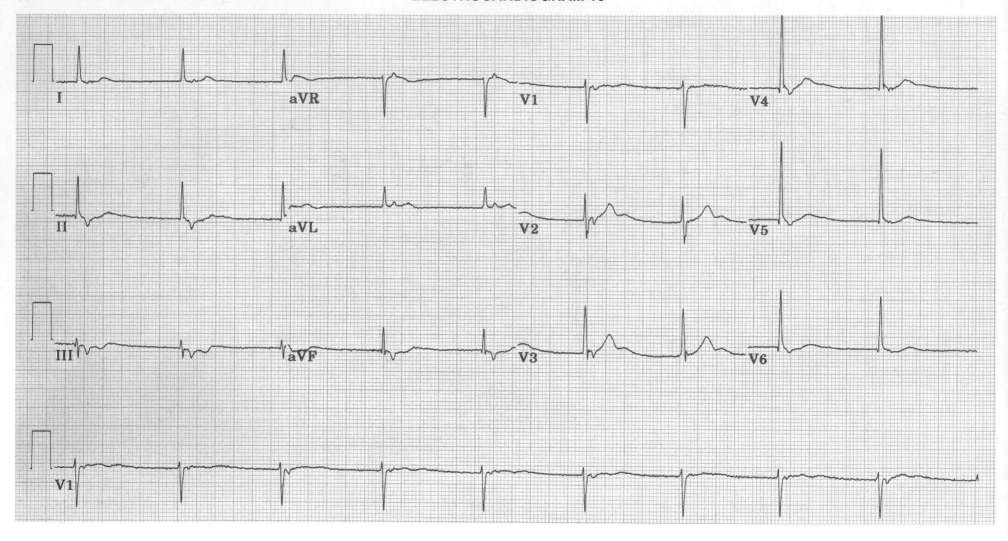

Interpretation Notes: _____

_____

_____

ECG 10 Fifty-nine year old gentleman with coronary artery disease status post remote percutaneous transluminal coronary angioplasty of the right coronary artery who re-presents with chest discomfort. A myocardial infarction was excluded by cardiac enzymes and a subsequent stress test was normal. The patient was felt to be suffering from non-cardiac musculoskeletal chest discomfort.

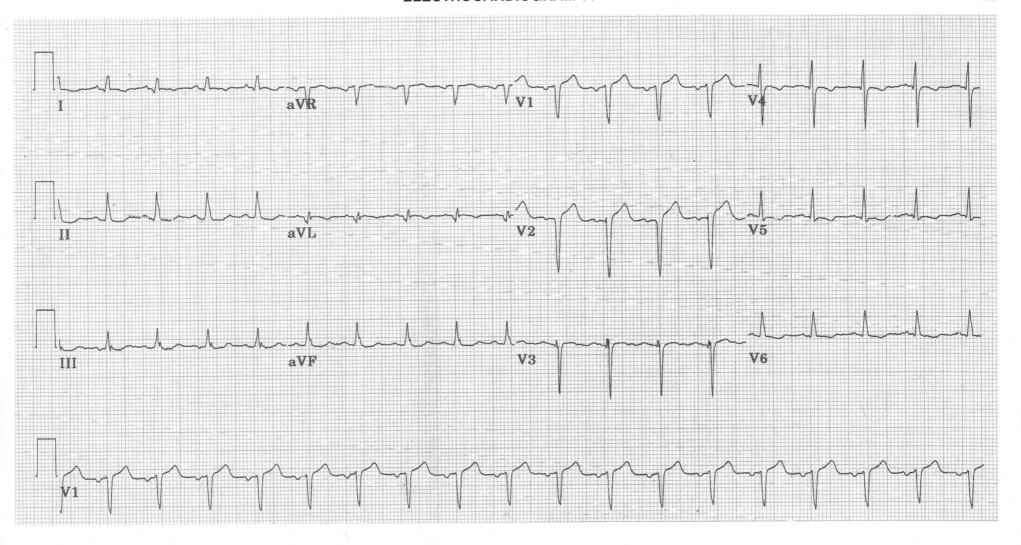

ECG 11 Sixty-six year old gentleman who presented acutely to the hospital with profuse sweating, chest tightness, and dyspnea. A subsequent cardiac catheterization demonstrated multi-vessel coronary artery disease and hypokinesis of the anterior wall. He was referred for successful coronary artery bypass graft surgery.

Interpretation Notes:_____
_____

LEVEL I

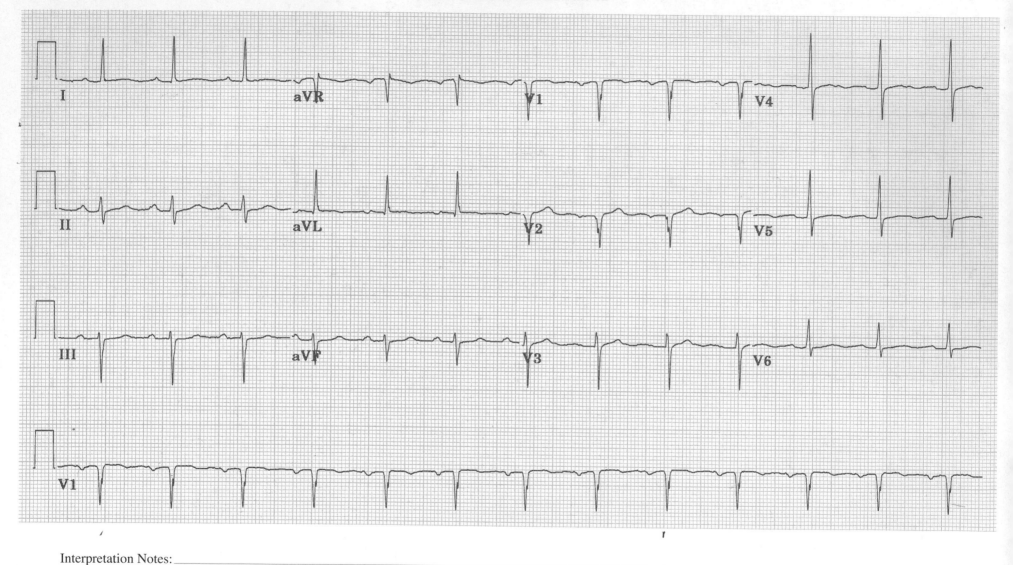

Interpretation Notes: _____

_____

ECG 12 Seventy-six year old gentleman status post two prior coronary artery bypass operations who returns for evaluation of stable angina pectoris and hypertension. This electrocardiogram was obtained as a routine follow-up study.

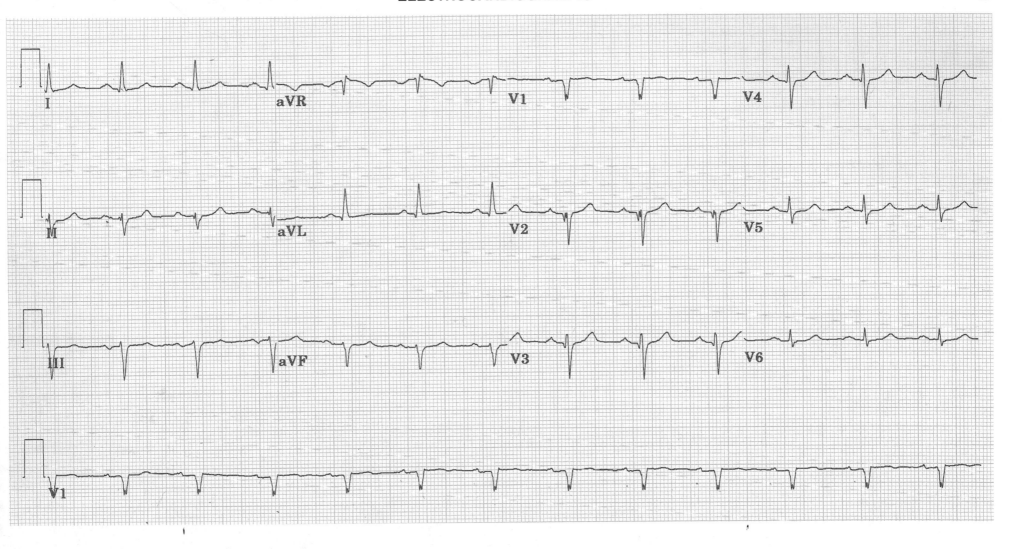

Interpretation Notes: _____
_____
_____

ECG 13 Sixty-two year old gentleman with severe three-vessel coronary artery disease referred for coronary artery bypass graft surgery. A recent cardiac catheterization demonstrated normal left ventricular systolic function without evidence of a prior myocardial infarction. Medications at the time of this electrocardiogram included atenolol, gemfibrozil, and folic acid.

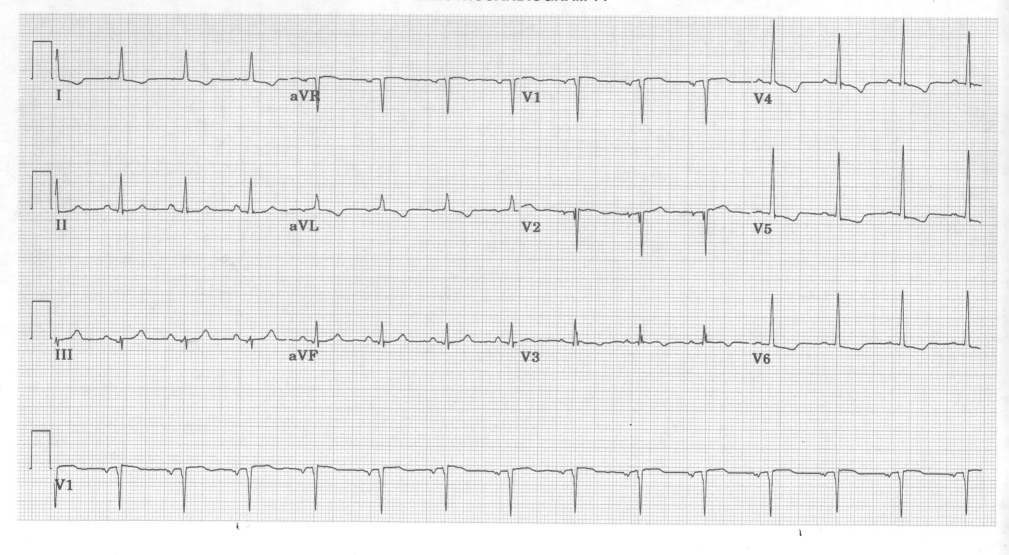

Interpretation Notes: _____

_____

_____

ECG 14 Seventy-two year old woman with advanced emphysema referred for possible lung reduction surgery. An echocardiogram performed three years prior to this electrocardiogram demonstrated normal left ventricular systolic function. By history there was no evidence of a prior myocardial infarction. Medications at the time of this electrocardiogram included theophylline and inhaled bronchodilators.

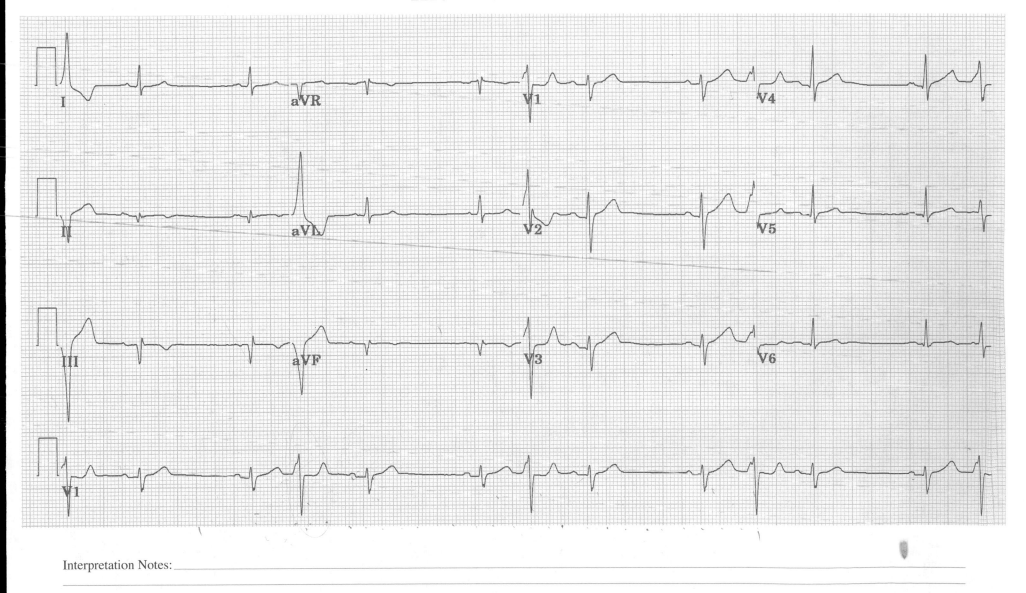

Interpretation Notes: _____

ECG 15 Fifty-two year old gentleman with coronary artery disease who presented to the hospital with an accelerating pattern of angina pectoris. Co-morbid conditions include hyperlipidemia, hypertension, peptic ulcer disease, and chronic anxiety. Medications at the time of this electrocardiogram included aspirin, simvastatin, cholestyramine, a multi-vitamin, metoprolol, and topical nitroglycerin.

ELECTROCARDIOGRAM 16

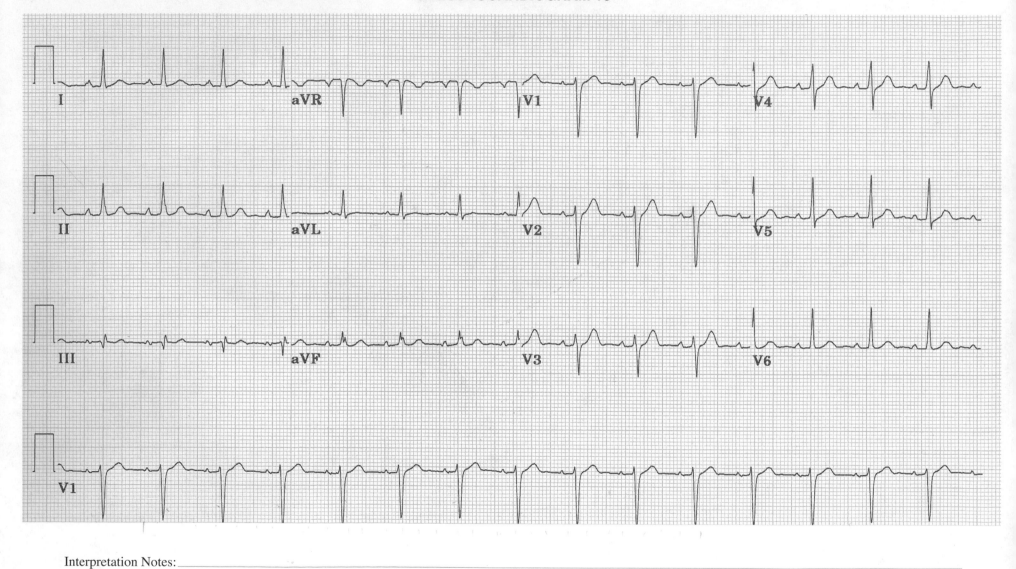

Interpretation Notes: _____

_____

ECG 16 Forty year old gentleman with renal failure secondary to chronic pyelonephritis awaiting renal transplant. His calcium level at the time of this electrocardiogram was greater than 11 mg/dl.

ELECTROCARDIOGRAM 17

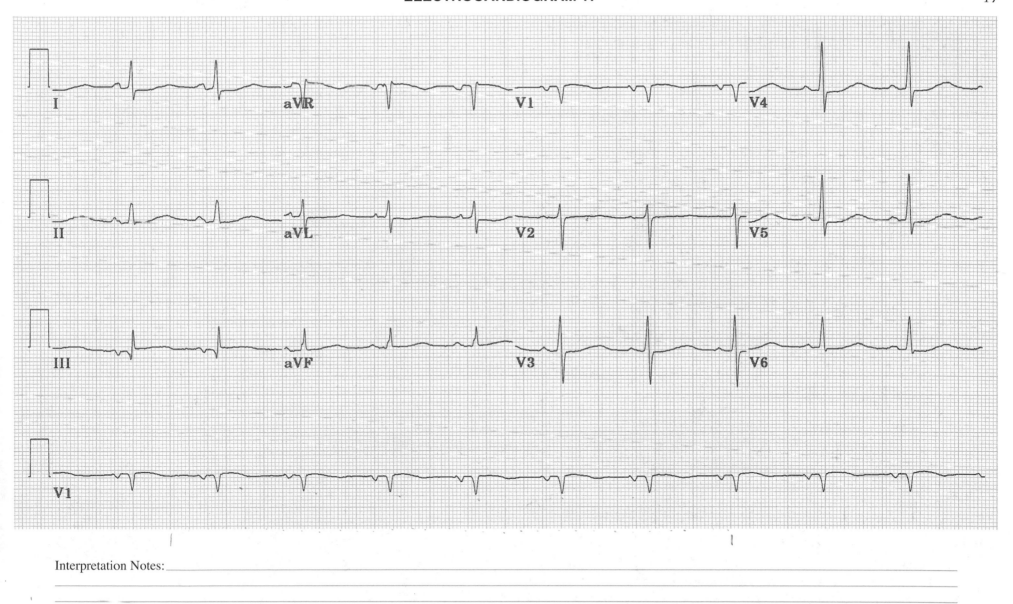

I   aVR   V1   V4

II   aVL   V2   V5

III   aVF   V3   V6

V1

Interpretation Notes: _____

_____

_____

ECG 17 Seventy-two year old gentleman with advanced peripheral vascular disease who is admitted to the hospital for a semi-elective below the knee amputation. His past medical history includes chronic obstructive pulmonary disease, a remote myocardial infarction, and prior pacemaker placement.

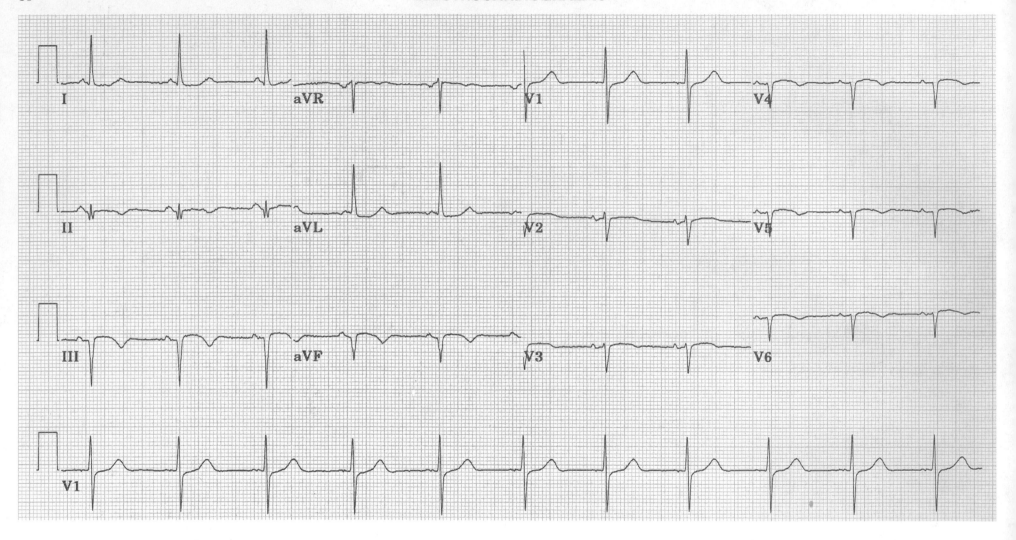

Interpretation Notes: _____

_____

ECG 18 Seventy-nine year old woman with a history of non-insulin requiring diabetes mellitus who was referred to the emergency room from her private physician's office in the setting of acute onset bilateral shoulder discomfort, shortness of breath, and nausea. A cardiac catheterization was performed four days after her hospitalization and demonstrated advanced disease in the right coronary artery which was successfully treated with percutaneous transluminal coronary angioplasty. Medications at the time of this electrocardiogram included aspirin, metoprolol, glyburide, intravenous nitroglycerin, and intravenous heparin.

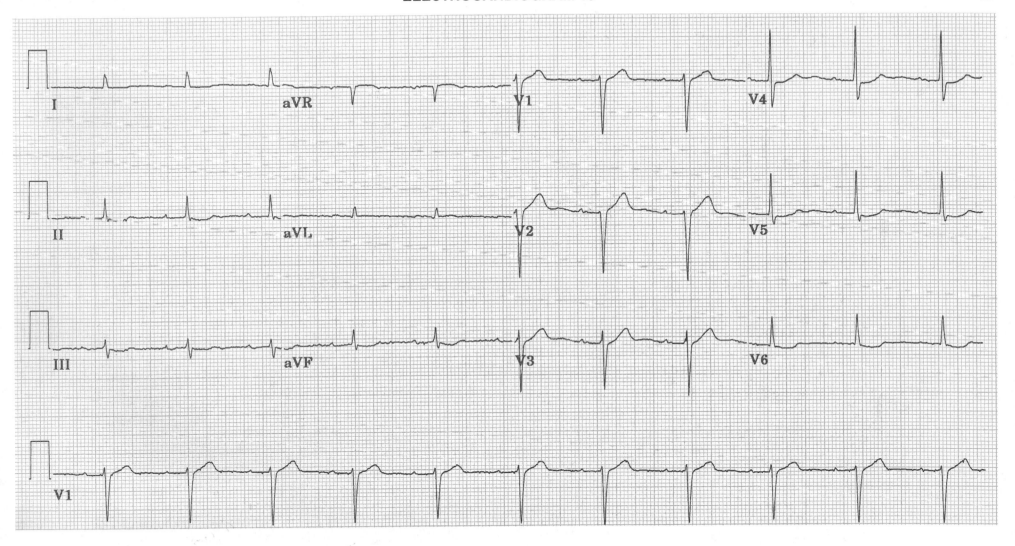

Interpretation Notes: _____

ECG 19 Seventy-two year old gentleman with severe coronary artery disease and severe left ventricular systolic dysfunction who presents for a follow-up cardiac evaluation. Co-morbid conditions include peripheral vascular disease, insulin requiring diabetes mellitus, and hypertension. His medications at the time of this electrocardiogram included captopril, isosorbide mononitrate, furosemide, warfarin, topical nitroglycerin, insulin, and digoxin.

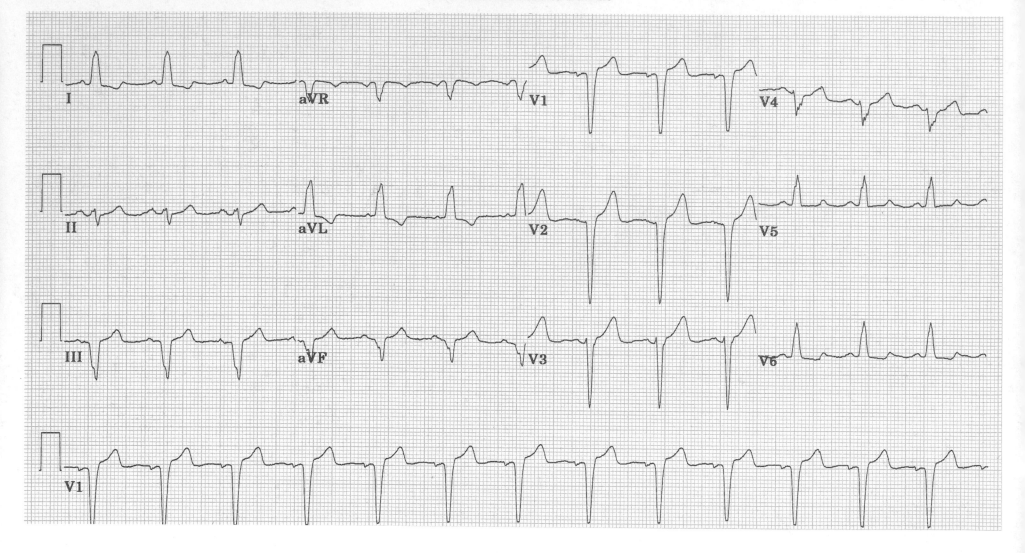

Interpretation Notes: _____

_____

ECG 20 Seventy-nine year old woman with known coronary artery disease and moderately severe left ventricular systolic dysfunction who was re-referred for cardiac evaluation secondary to increasing angina pectoris. Medications at the time of this electrocardiogram included furosemide, metoprolol, premarin, and aspirin.

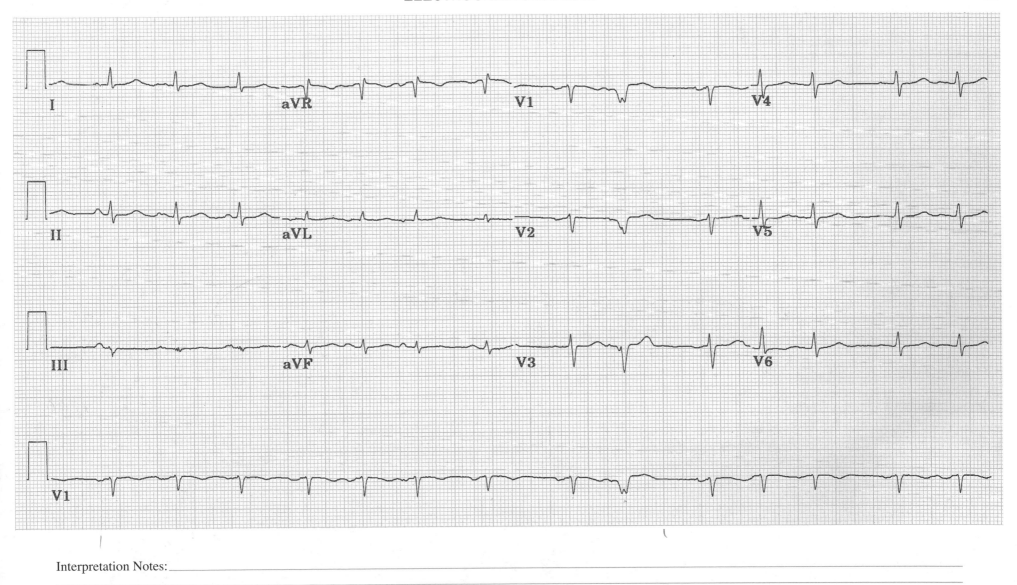

Interpretation Notes: _____

_____

ECG 21 Twenty-five year old woman admitted to the hospital for treatment of chemical dependency and bulimia. She has no known cardiac history. Medications at the time of this electrocardiogram included imipramine and valproic acid.

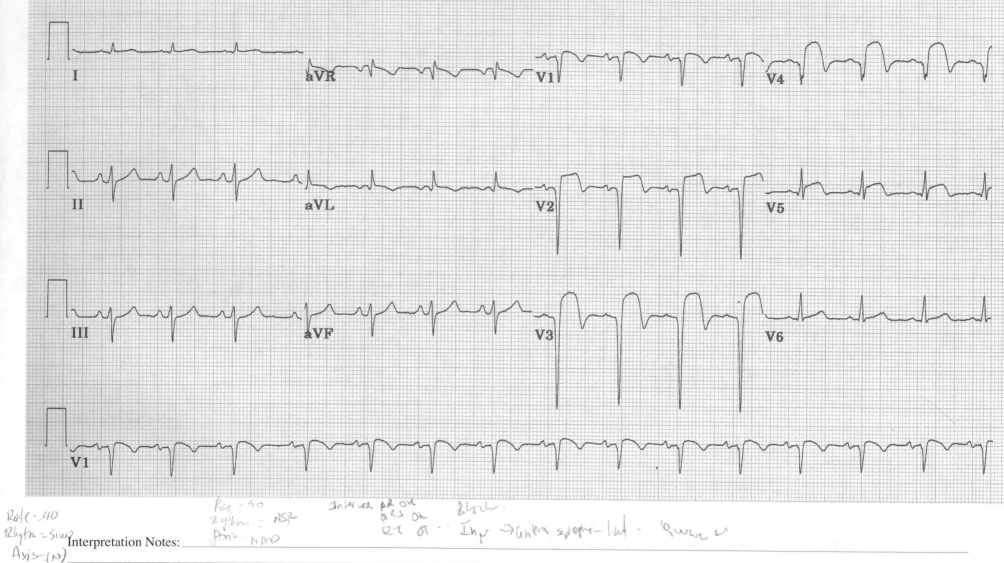

I   aVR   V1   V4

II   aVL   V2   V5

III   aVF   V3   V6

V1

Rate - 90
Rhythm = Sinus
Axis - (N)

Interval
RR OK
QRS OK
Q-J OK

Blocks ∅
Hypertrophy ∅

Rate: 90
Rythm = NSR
Axis: NAD

Interval PR OK
QRS OK
QT OK   Inf → anterolateral → lateral   Q wave in

old in pt.
New = ant. - lat - septal.
INFARCT

Interpretation Notes: _____

_____

ECG 22 Forty-six year old gentleman with a myocardial infarction two years before this electrocardiogram who presented to the emergency room with a six hour history of acute severe substernal chest discomfort. The patient underwent emergent cardiac catheterization and percutaneous transluminal coronary angioplasty of a severe proximal left anterior descending coronary artery stenosis.

ELECTROCARDIOGRAM 23

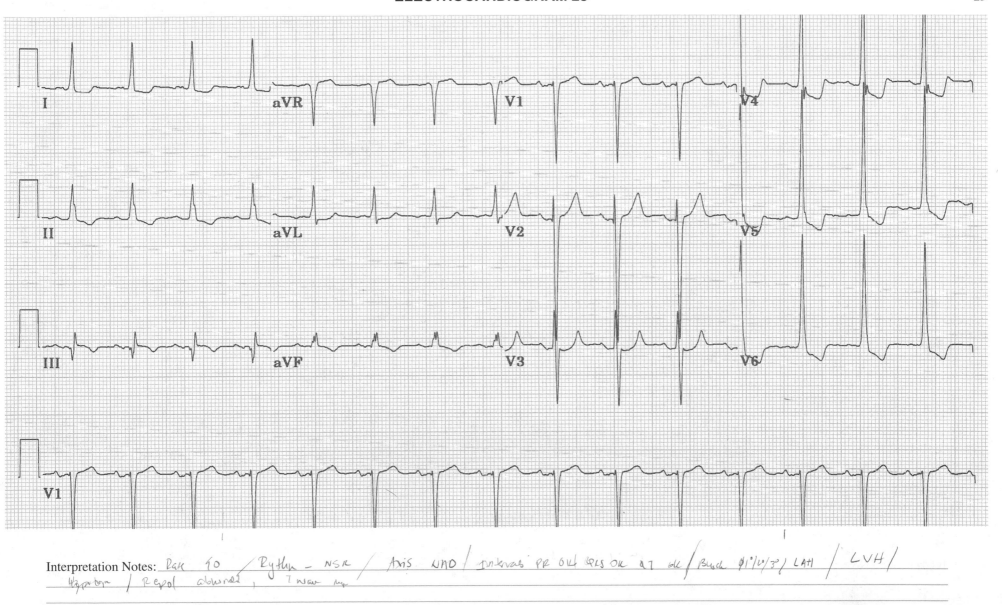

Interpretation Notes: Rate 90 / Rythm - NSR / Axis NAD / Intervals PR OK QRS OK QT ok / Block φ1°/φ°/3° / LAH / LVH / Hyptertp / Repol abnormal, T wave inv

ECG 23 Seventy year old gentleman with a history of paroxysmal atrial arrhythmias who returns for cardiology follow-up. He has coronary artery disease status post a remote inferoposterior myocardial infarction. Co-morbidities include insulin requiring diabetes mellitus and dialysis requiring renal failure. Medications at the time of this electrocardiogram included amiodarone, topical nitroglycerin, and aspirin.

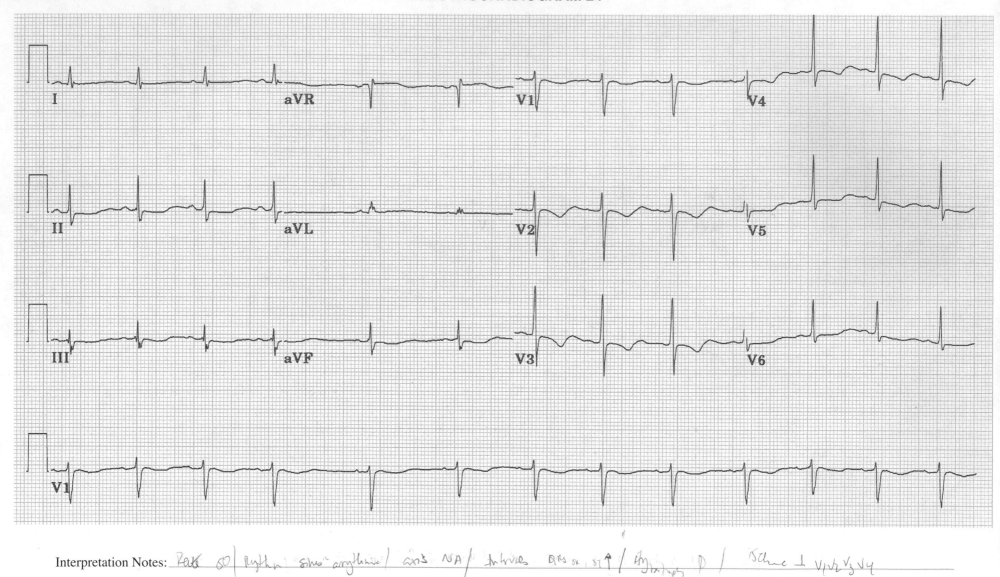

I aVR V1 V4

II aVL V2 V5

III aVF V3 V6

V1

Interpretation Notes: _Rate 80 / Rhythm "sinus" arrythmia / axis NA / intervals QRS ok, ST↑ / hypertrophy Ø / Ischemia ↓ V1 V2 V3 V4_

ECG 24 Twenty-two year old woman hospitalized for inpatient evaluation and treatment of severe depression. Her medications at the time of this electrocardiogram included nortriptyline.

ELECTROCARDIOGRAM 25

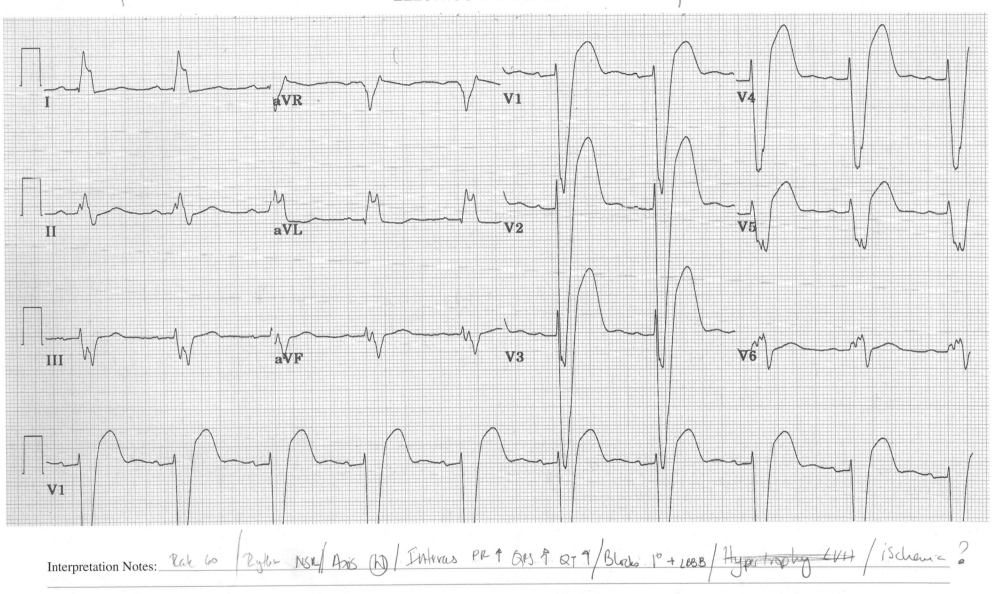

Interpretation Notes: Rate 60 / Rythm NSR / Axis (N) / Intervas PR↑ QRS↑ QT↑ / Blocks 1° + LBBB / Hypertrophy LVH / ischemia ?

ECG 25 Fifty-six year old gentleman with severe left ventricular systolic dysfunction in the setting of normal coronary arteries who is awaiting cardiac transplantation. His medications included thyroxine, furosemide, hydralazine, isosorbide dinitrate, captopril, and amiodarone.

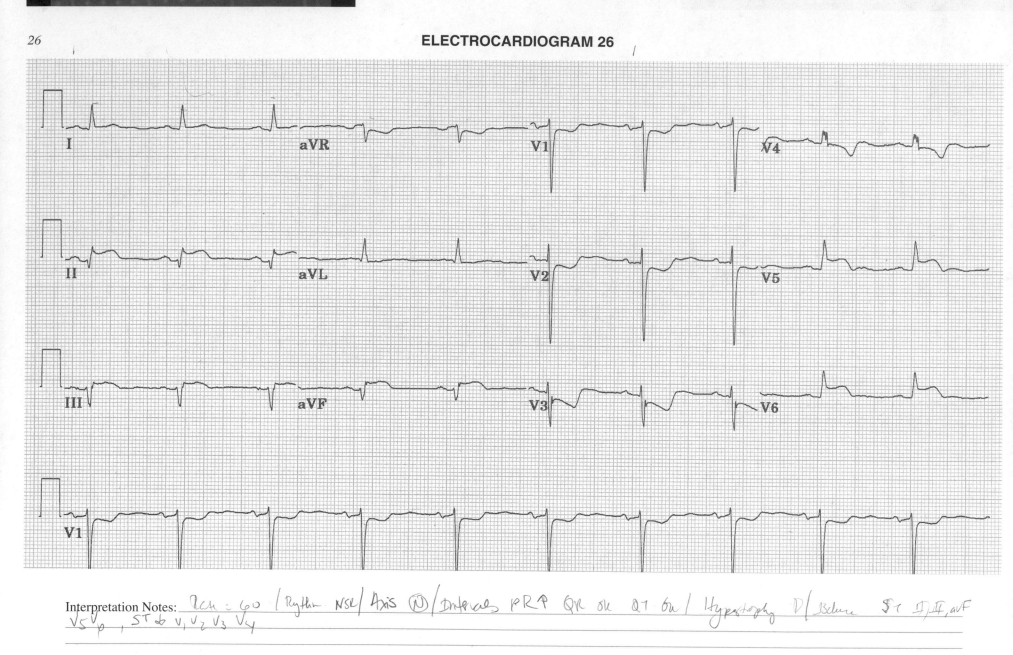

Interpretation Notes: _Rate = 60 / Rhythm NSR / Axis (N) / Intervals PR↑ QRS ok QT ok / Hypertrophy Ø / Ischemia ST↑ I,II,aVF V5 V6 , ST↓ V1 V2 V3 V4_

ECG 26 Sixty-one year old gentleman with coronary artery disease and ischemic left ventricular systolic dysfunction who presents urgently to the hospital with an acute chest discomfort syndrome. His medications included potassium, isosorbide mononitrate, furosemide, glyburide, lisinopril, and warfarin.

ELECTROCARDIOGRAM 27

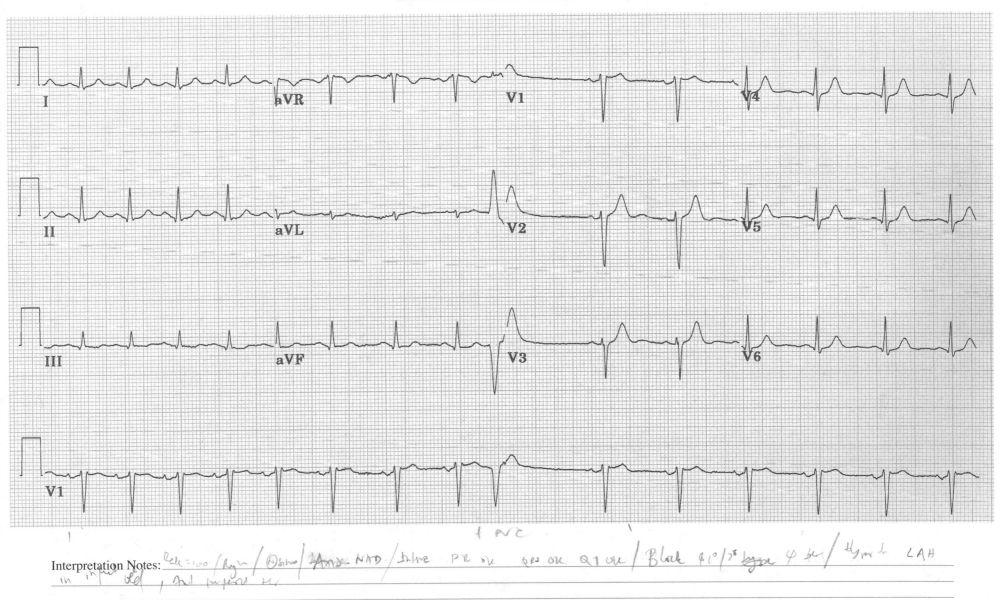

Interpretation Notes: Rate=100/Rgm/Osrw/1An2 NAD./Inline PR ok QRS ok QT ok/Block 8 1°/2° type 4 sec/thyroid LAH in inf old, And infarct M↑

ECG 27 Seventy-eight year old woman with a long history of paroxysmal supraventricular tachycardia seen in routine cardiology follow-up. A recent echocardiogram demonstrated minimal thickening of the aortic valve but otherwise a structurally normal heart. Her medications included propranolol.

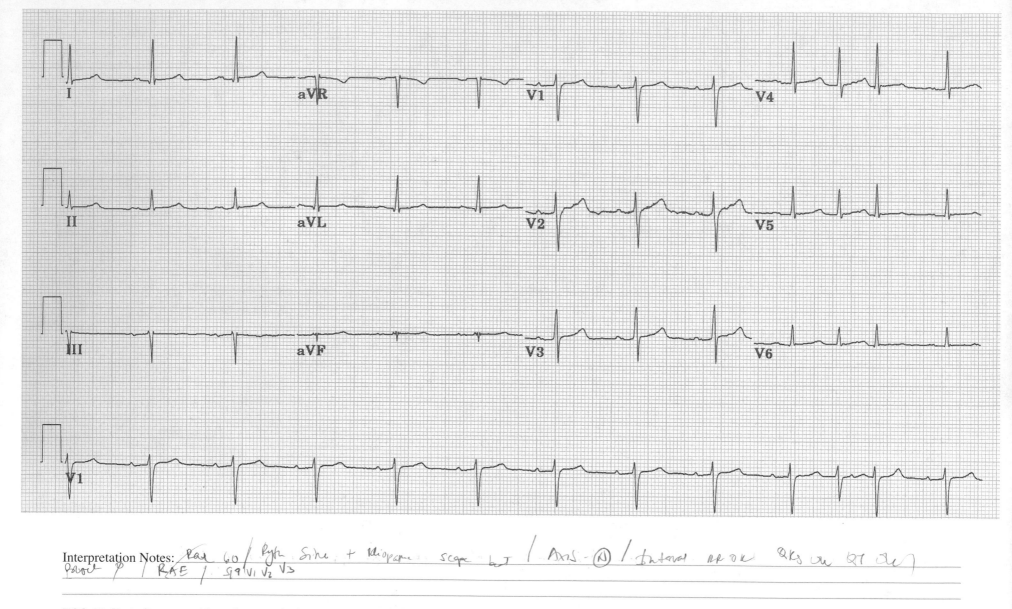

Interpretation Notes: Rate 60 / Rythm Sinus + idiopauic scape bt / Axis -(N) / Interval PR ok QRS ok QT ok)
P-wave p / RAE / Sq V1 V2 V3

ECG 28 Forty-five year old gentleman who is seen in the outpatient infectious disease department following a recent hospitalization for a scrotal infection. His past medical history includes a deep venous thrombosis. His medications included intravenous antibiotics and diphenhydramine.

ELECTROCARDIOGRAM 29

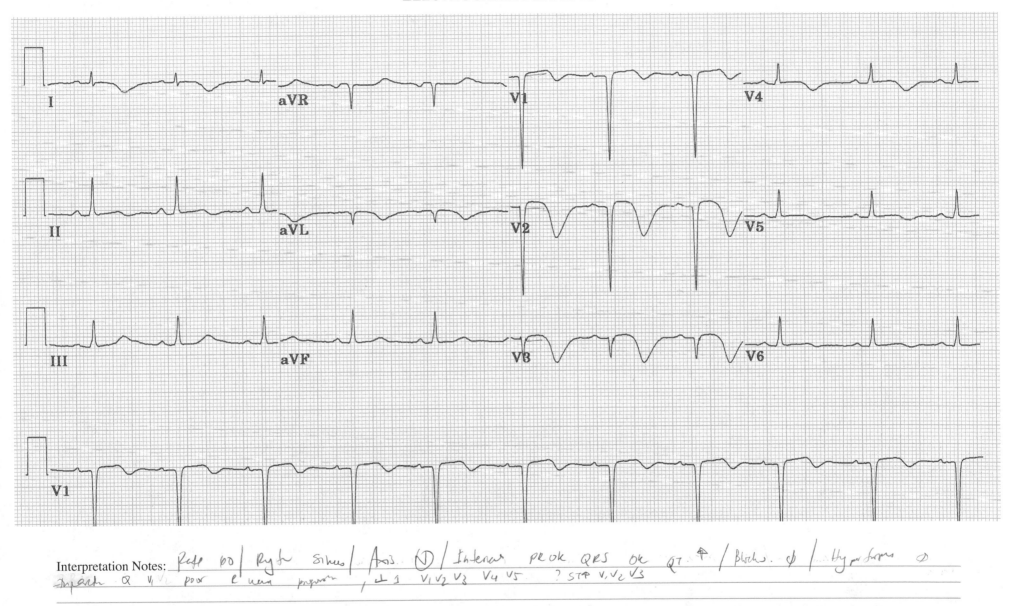

Interpretation Notes: Rate 60 / Rhythm Sinus / Axis (N) / Intervals PR ok QRS ok QT ↑ / Blocks. ∅ / Hypertrophy ∅
Infarct Q V1V2 poor R wave progression / ↓ T V1 V2 V3 V4 V5 ? ST↑ V1 V2 V3

ECG 29 Sixty-six year old woman who presented to a local urgent care facility with acute onset chest, arm, neck, and jaw discomfort in the setting of dyspnea. The patient underwent a cardiac catheterization demonstrating an 80% mid left anterior descending coronary artery stenosis. Left ventricular systolic function was within normal limits. She subsequently underwent percutaneous transluminal coronary angioplasty without complication.

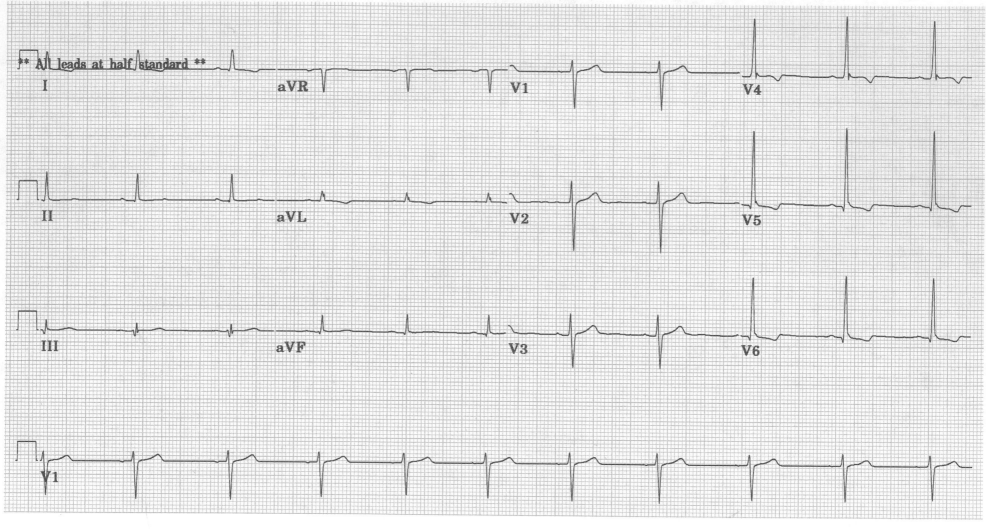

I   ** All leads at half standard **

aVR   **V1**   **V4**

II   **aVL**   **V2**   **V5**

III   **aVF**   **V3**   **V6**

V1

Interpretation Notes: Rate 60/Rythe Sinus / PR ok QRS ok QT ok / Axis Ⓝ / Hypertrophy LVH / Blocks ∅ / Bdwn

1Q III , STb V4 V5 V6

ECG 30 Twenty-nine year old gentleman referred for aortic valve surgery in the setting of severe aortic insufficiency secondary to aortic valve prolapse. He is on no current medications. Transesophageal echocardiography demonstrated a bicuspid aortic valve. The patient subsequently underwent successful aortic valve repair.

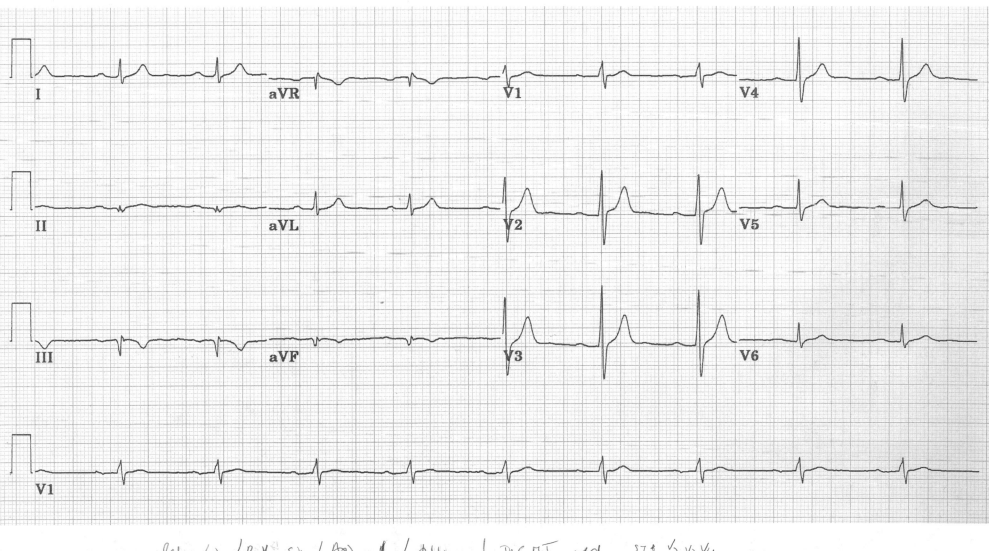

Interpretation Notes: _Rest 60 / Right. sinus / Aos. ll / ϕ Hyp | INF MI _old ST↑ V₂V₃V₄ —_
LAH.

ECG 31 Forty-seven year old gentleman who presented to an outside medical facility with an electrocardiogram consistent with an acute inferior myocardial infarction. He received urgent thrombolytic therapy and was accepted in hospital transfer for cardiac catheterization. Co-morbid conditions included long-term tobacco use and hyper-cholesterolemia. A cardiac catheterization demonstrated severe right coronary artery disease which was treated with percutaneous transluminal coronary angioplasty and a urokinase infusion.

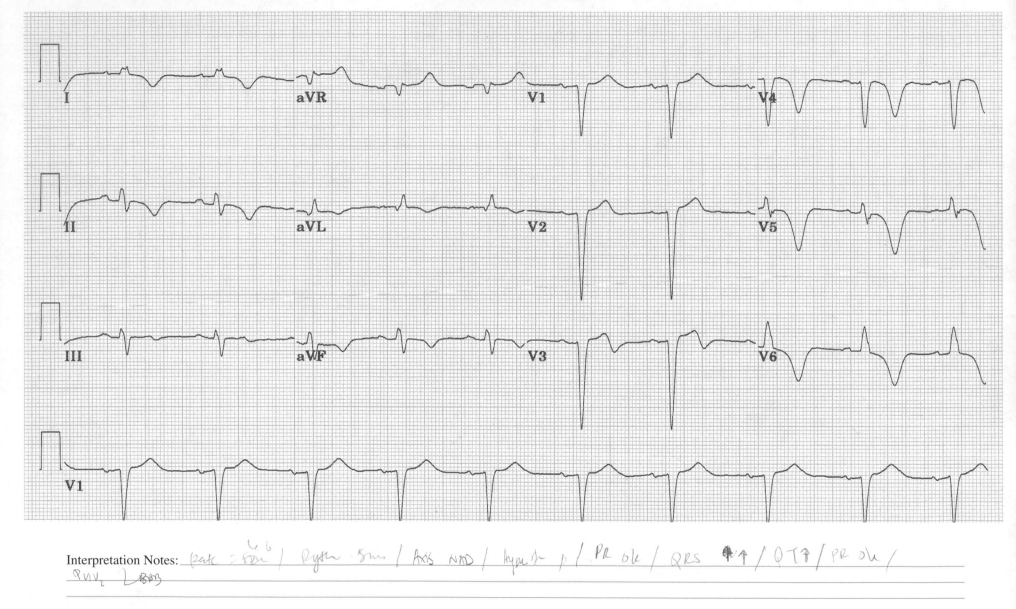

Interpretation Notes: _Rate = 60 / Rythm - Snus / Axis NAD / Ayperte p / PR ole / QRS ↑↑ / QTa / PR ole /_
PVV₂ LBBB

ECG 32 Sixty-six year old woman who was scheduled for an elective stress test at which time the above electrocardiogram was obtained. She was admitted to the hospital to exclude acute myocardial injury. Acute myocardial injury was excluded and subsequent stress testing suggested myocardial ischemia. A cardiac catheterization was performed demonstrating normal left ventricular systolic function and normal coronary arteries.

ELECTROCARDIOGRAM 33

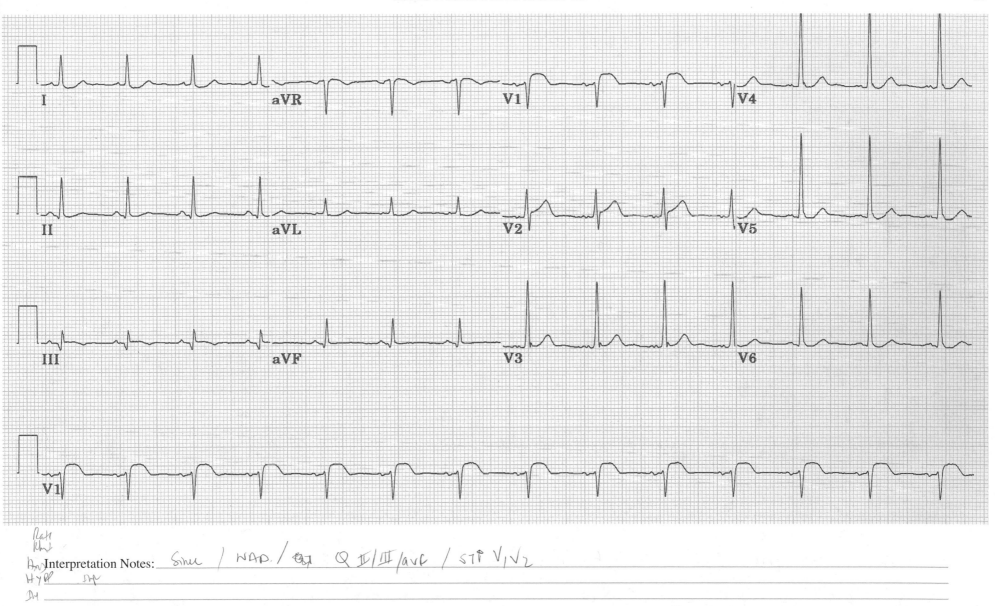

I   aVR   V1   V4

II   aVL   V2   V5

III   aVF   V3   V6

V1

Interpretation Notes: _Sinu / NAD. / &T Q II/III/avF / ST↑ V₁V₂_

ECG 33 Forty-five year old gentleman who presented to an outside emergency room with a one-half hour history of acute chest discomfort radiating to both shoulders and hands. The patient underwent urgent cardiac catheterization which demonstrated a 100% proximal right coronary artery occlusion with superimposed thrombus. The patient underwent successful percutaneous transluminal coronary angioplasty. Cardiac enzymes were positive for acute myocardial injury.

LEVEL I

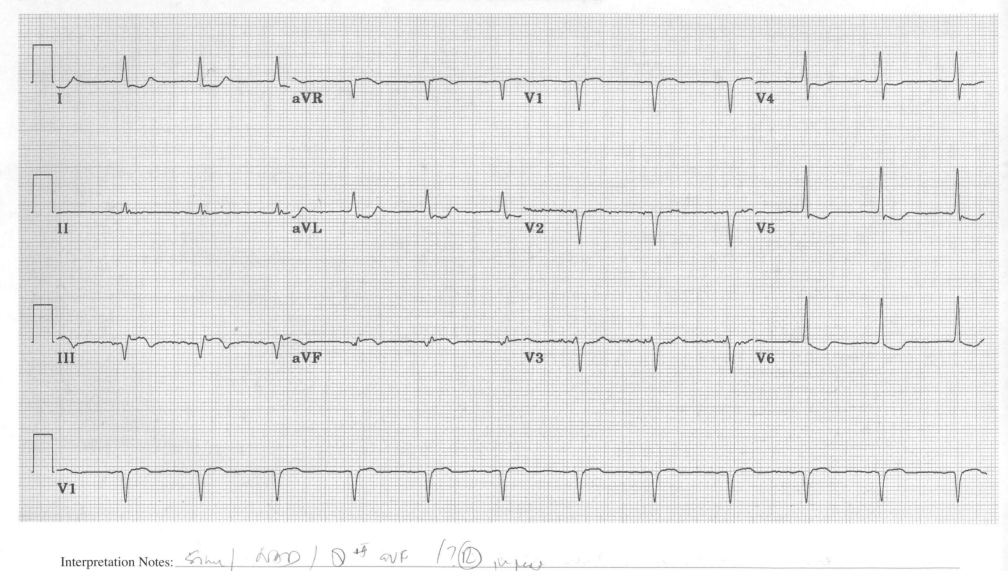

Interpretation Notes: _____

ECG 34 Seventy-two year old woman who presented to the hospital after three hours of severe epigastric pressure with associated vomiting, nausea, and profuse diaphoresis. Serial cardiac enzymes documented acute myocardial injury. Medications at the time of this electrocardiogram included phenytoin, glyburide, ranitidine, lisinopril, intravenous heparin, and intravenous nitroglycerin.

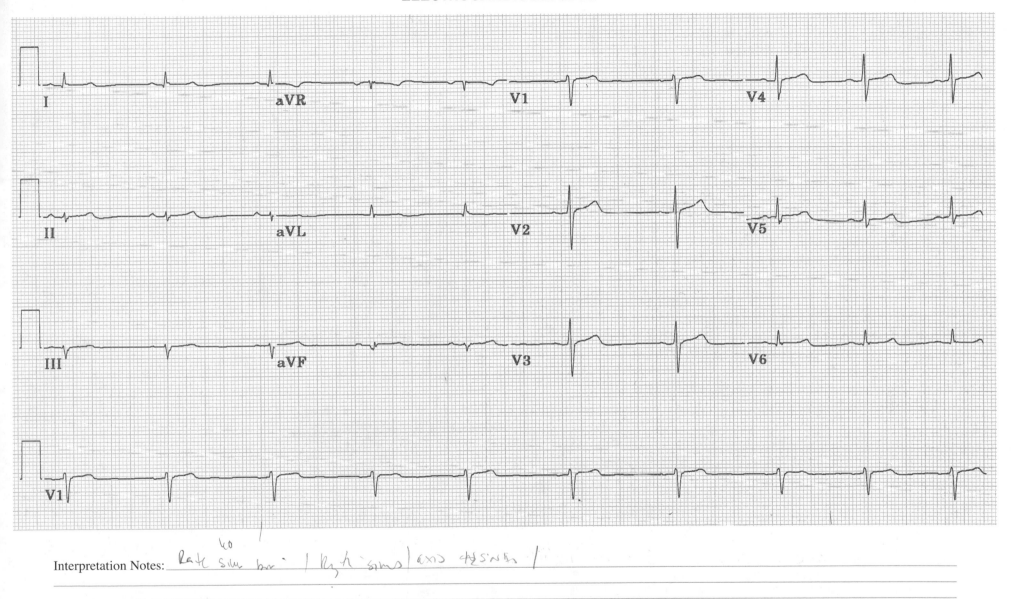

Interpretation Notes: _Rate slow bor: / Rzh sinus/ axis drsinh /_

ECG 35 Thirty-four year old gentleman seen in the Internal Medicine department for a routine physical examination. He has no prior cardiac history and remains in excellent health.

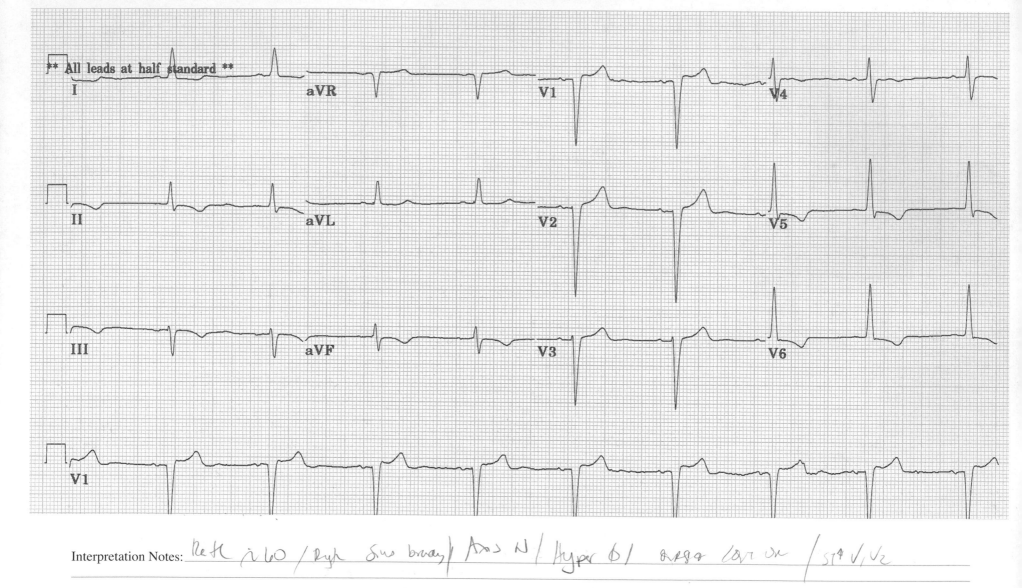

** All leads at half standard **

I   aVR   V1   V4

II   aVL   V2   V5

III   aVF   V3   V6

V1

Interpretation Notes: _Rate 60 / Rythm Sinus brady / Axis N / Hyper Q / QRSa LVH VR / STd V1 V2_

ECG 36 Sixty-one year old gentleman with ischemic heart disease, severe left ventricular systolic dysfunction, and prior coronary artery bypass graft surgery who presents for cardiology clinic follow-up. Co-morbid conditions include severe peripheral vascular disease and hyperlipidemia. His medications included warfarin, lisinopril, digoxin, and furosemide.

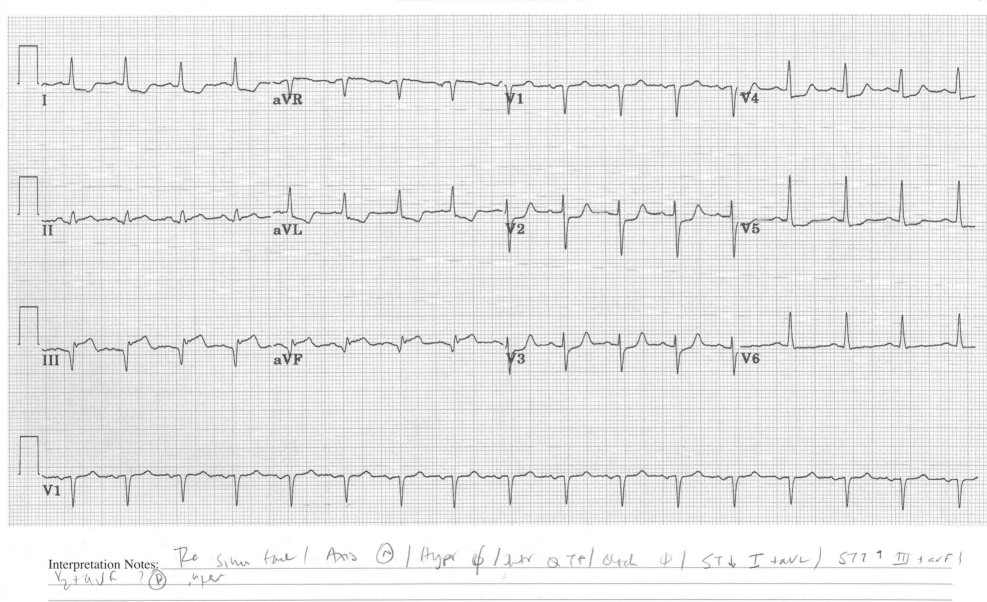

Interpretation Notes: _Re sinu tach / Axis ⓝ / Hyper φ /2nr QT↑/ Blch φ / ST↓ I +aVL / ST↑↑ III +aVF /_
V₂+aVF ? Ⓟ , uper

ECG 37 Seventy-nine year old woman who five days prior to this electrocardiogram experienced acute onset chest discomfort and an electrocardiogram consistent with an acute inferior myocardial infarction. Following her myocardial infarction convalescence, a cardiac catheterization demonstrated severe three-vessel coronary artery disease. This electrocardiogram was obtained prior to anticipated coronary artery bypass graft surgery. Left ventriculography at the time of her cardiac catheterization demonstrated proximal and mid inferior wall akinesis. Her medications included metoprolol, intravenous heparin, intravenous nitroglycerin, and temazepam.

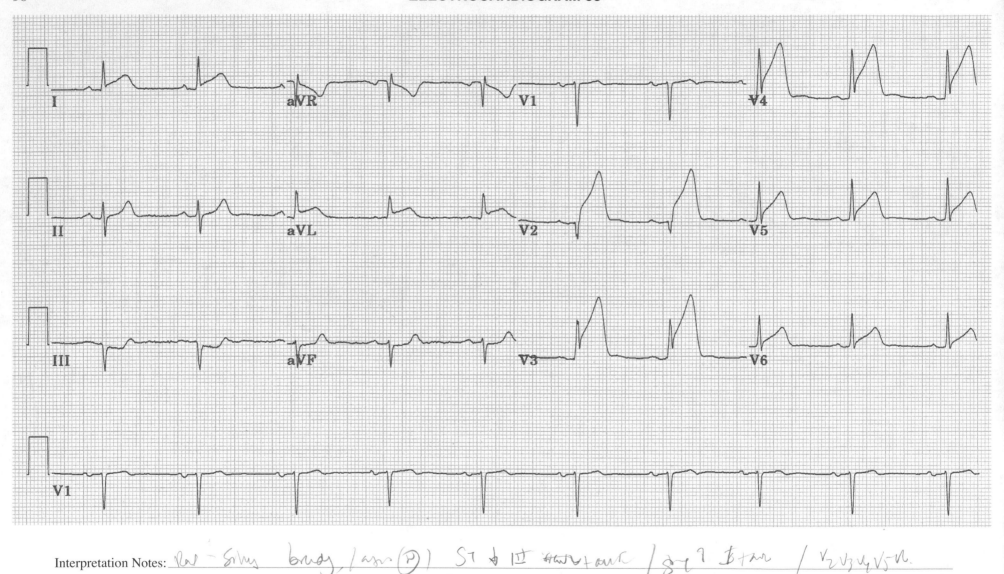

I   aVR   V1   V4

II   aVL   V2   V5

III   aVF   V3   V6

V1

Interpretation Notes: _Rev — sinus brady/arr (P) / ST ↓ II inverior + ant / ST ↑ II + ant / V₂ V₃ V₄ V₅ V₆._

ECG 38 Forty-three year old gentleman admitted in urgent hospital transfer after a one day history of acute chest discomfort. The patient was taken urgently to the cardiac catheterization laboratory where a 90% mid left anterior descending coronary artery stenosis involving a second diagonal branch was present. The patient underwent successful angioplasty and stent deployment.

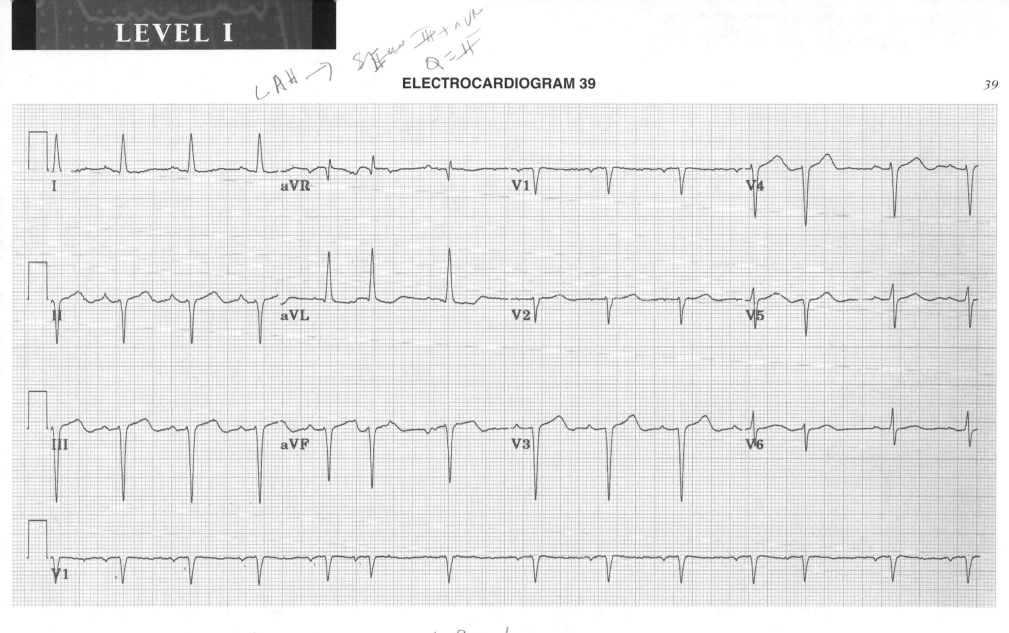

LAH → S↑ III + aVR
Q = II

I   aVR   V1   V4

II   aVL   V2   V5

III   aVF   V3   V6

V1

Interpretation Notes: Regular Sinus   MAT / LAD / RAH / Poor Rwave

ECG 39 Sixty-five year old woman with a history of hypertension and chronic obstructive pulmonary disease who presents to the emergency room with a recent history of generalized weakness and exertional dyspnea. Her medications included inhalers, lisinopril, and furosemide. By history she has not suffered a myocardial infarction.

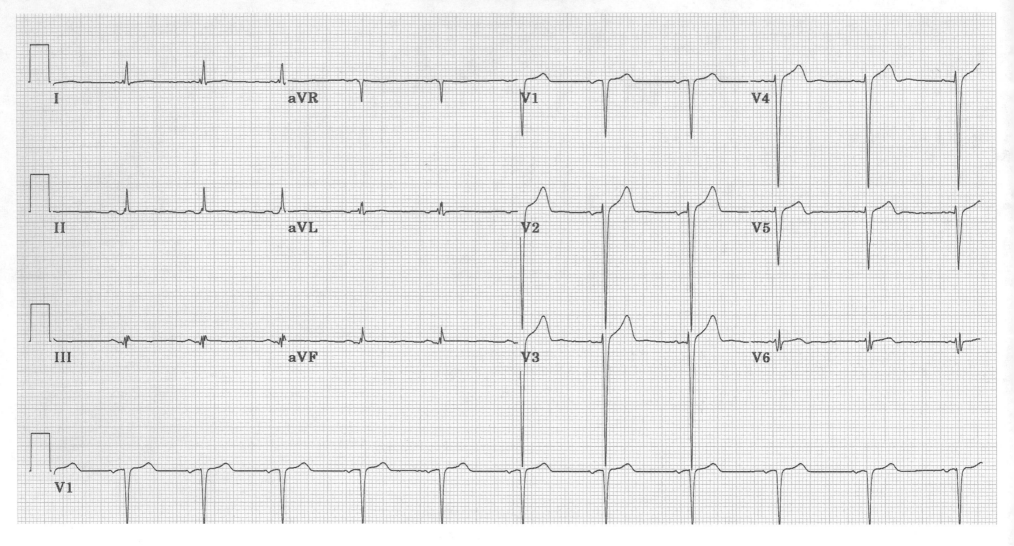

Interpretation Notes: _____

ECG 40 Eighty-one year old woman with a chest discomfort syndrome of ten years duration accepted in transfer from an outside hospital. Further evaluation confirmed the presence of unstable angina and the patient subsequently underwent cardiac catheterization and percutaneous transluminal coronary angioplasty to the left anterior descending coronary artery. Medications at the time of her hospital transfer included triamterene/hydrochlorothiazide, metoprolol, and ibuprofen.

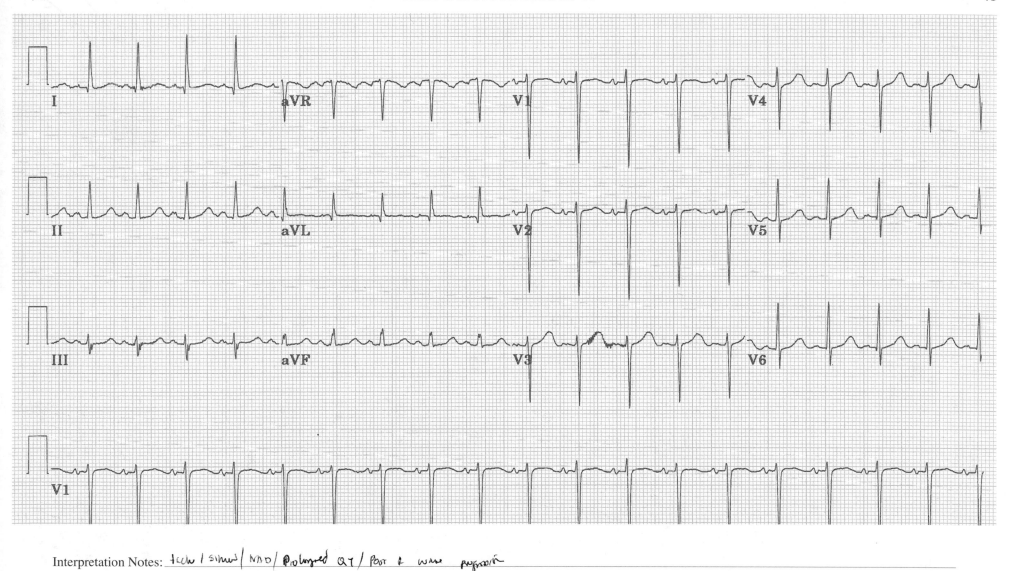

I aVR V1 V4

II aVL V2 V5

III aVF V3 V6

V1

Interpretation Notes: tech / sinus / NAD / Prolonged QT / Poor R wave progression

ECG 41 Forty-eight year old woman with insulin requiring diabetes mellitus and end stage renal disease who presents for an outpatient nephrology follow-up examination. Her medications included prednisone, azathiaprine, furosemide, nifedipine, quinine, metolazone, and warfarin. A serum calcium level was not drawn at the time of this electrocardiogram.

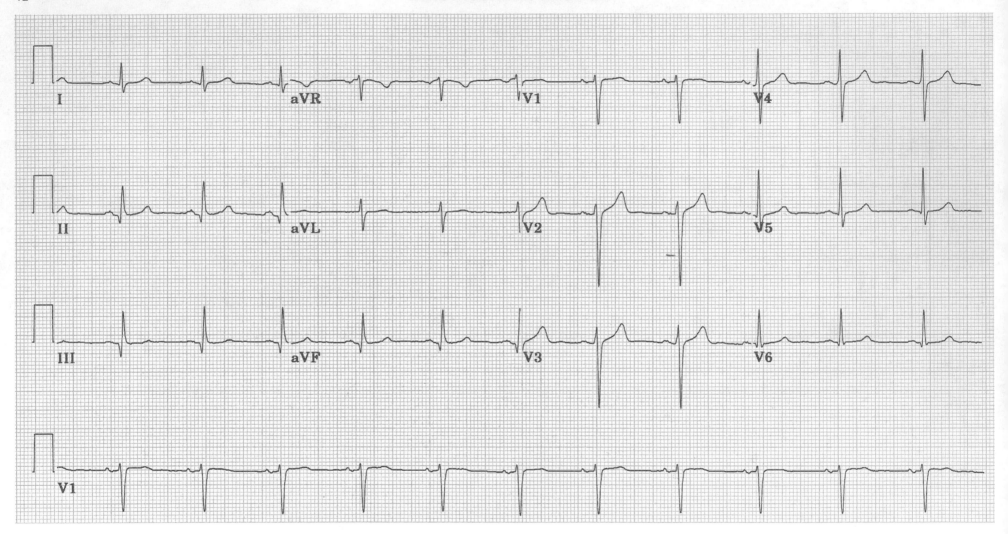

I   aVR   V1   V4

II   aVL   V2   V5

III   aVF   V3   V6

V1

Interpretation Notes: _____

_____

_____

ECG 42 Sixty-five year old gentleman status post an inferior myocardial infarction fourteen years previously. He subsequently underwent coronary artery bypass graft surgery and is currently asymptomatic. The above electrocardiogram was performed as part of his routine follow-up evaluation.

D= wide II

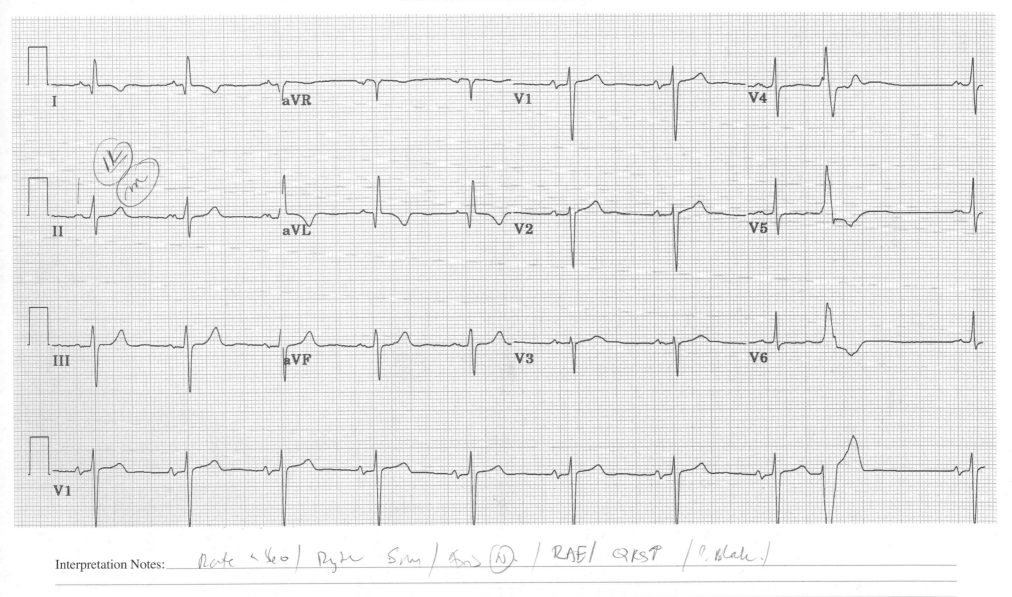

Interpretation Notes: _Rate <60 / Ryth Sm / Axis (N) / RAE / QRST / C. Block /_

ECG 43 Sixty-five year old gentleman referred for coronary artery bypass graft surgery in the setting of pulmonary edema and advanced coronary artery disease. A recent cardiac catheterization demonstrated moderately severe left ventricular systolic dysfunction and anterolateral akinesis. The most advanced coronary artery obstruction was in the diagonal branch of the left anterior descending coronary artery. Medications at the time of this electrocardiogram included atenolol, aspirin, simvastatin, and isosorbide mononitrate. Co-morbidities included hypertension and long-term tobacco use.

44

ELECTROCARDIOGRAM 44

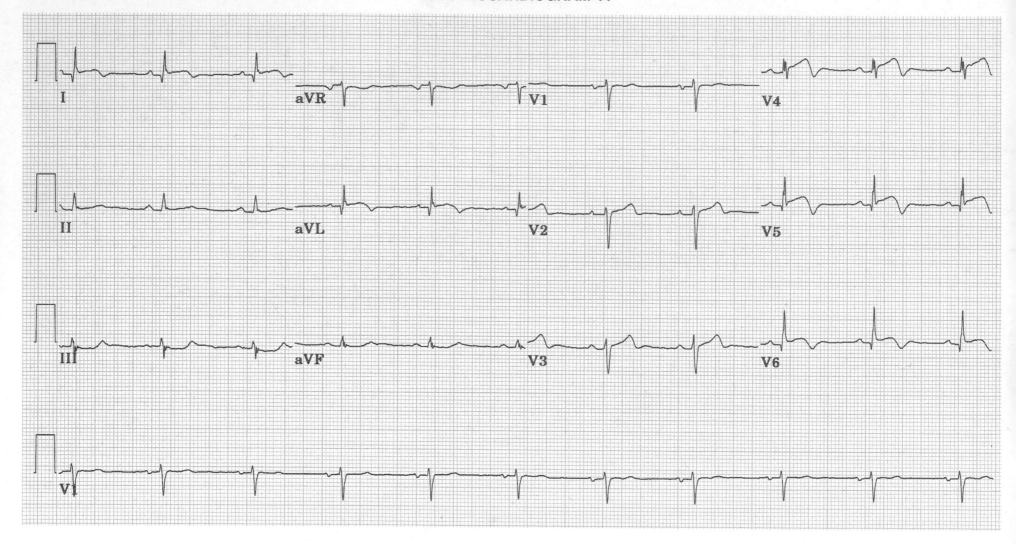

Interpretation Notes: _____

ECG 44 Sixty-six year old gentleman with a several hour history of acute anterior chest discomfort who received urgent intravenous thrombolytic therapy. This electrocardiogram was obtained several hours after thrombolytic administration. The patient subsequently underwent cardiac catheterization which demonstrated moderate diffuse coronary artery disease with the exception of a large second diagonal branch of the left anterior descending coronary artery which was 100% occluded with superimposed thrombus.

LEVEL I

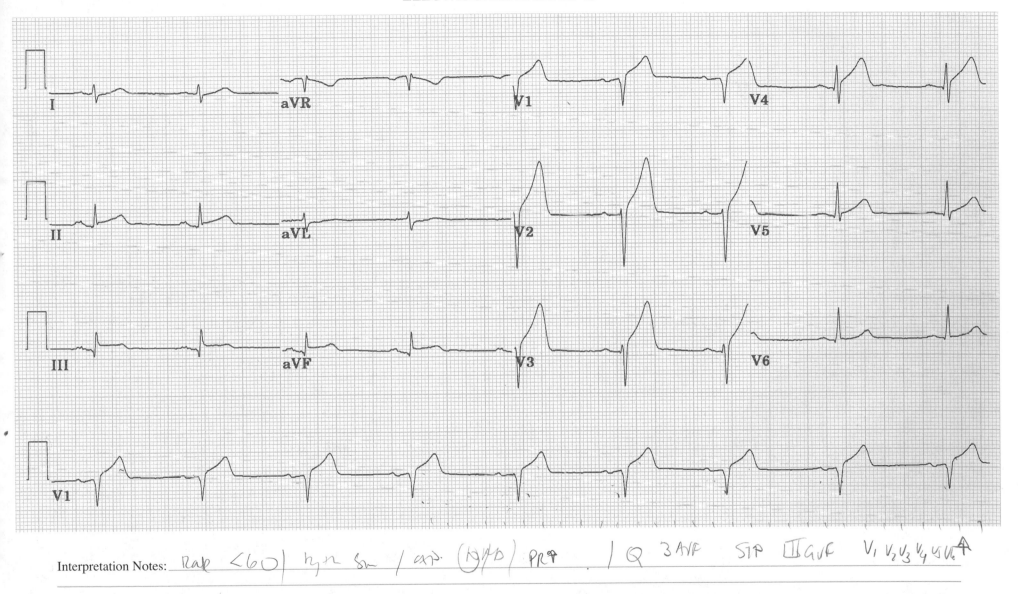

I   aVR   V1   V4
II   aVL   V2   V5
III   aVF   V3   V6
V1

Interpretation Notes: _Rate <60/ hyn sn / ax. (NMD) PR↑ | Q 3 AVF STP II aVF V₁ V₂ V₃ V₄ V₅ V₆ ↑_

ECG 45 Sixty-eight year old gentleman with known coronary artery disease status post coronary artery bypass graft surgery fourteen years prior to this electrocardiogram who is admitted to the hospital with an acute onset chest discomfort syndrome and associated profound shortness of breath. Serial cardiac enzymes documented acute myocardial injury. The patient underwent successful percutaneous transluminal coronary angioplasty and stent placement to the saphenous vein graft subserving the left anterior descending coronary artery.

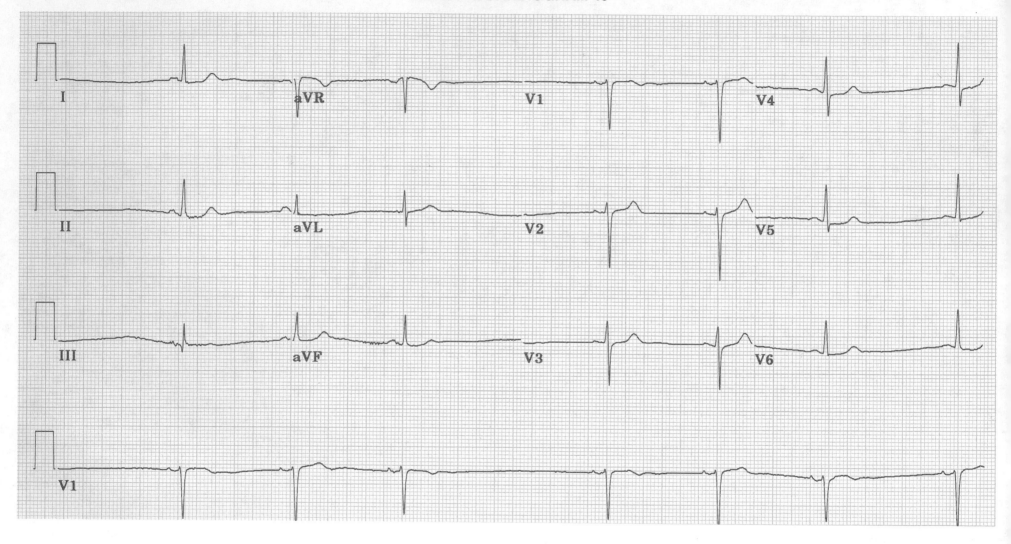

Interpretation Notes: _____

ECG 46 Fifty year old woman with a long-standing history of hypertension and morbid obesity who presented to the hospital with acute left-sided weakness. A computed tomography scan of the brain demonstrated findings consistent with an acute right middle cerebral artery cerebral vascular accident. Medications at the time of this electrocardiogram included aspirin, nifedipine, atenolol, and clonidine.

ELECTROCARDIOGRAM 47

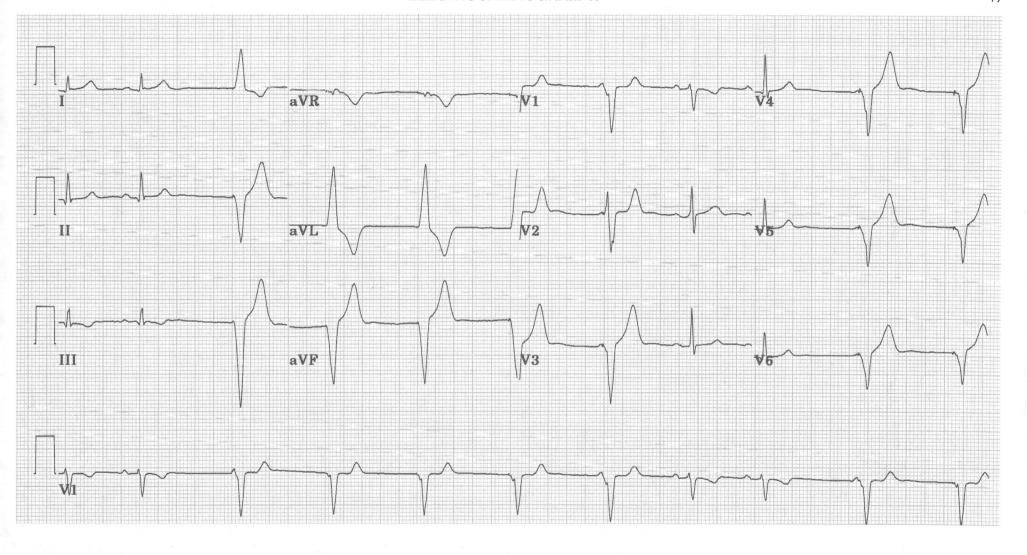

Interpretation Notes: _____

_____

ECG 47 Thirty-seven year old gentleman admitted to the coronary intensive care unit with syncope in the setting of advanced sinus bradycardia. The patient subsequently underwent permanent pacemaker implantation.

LEVEL I

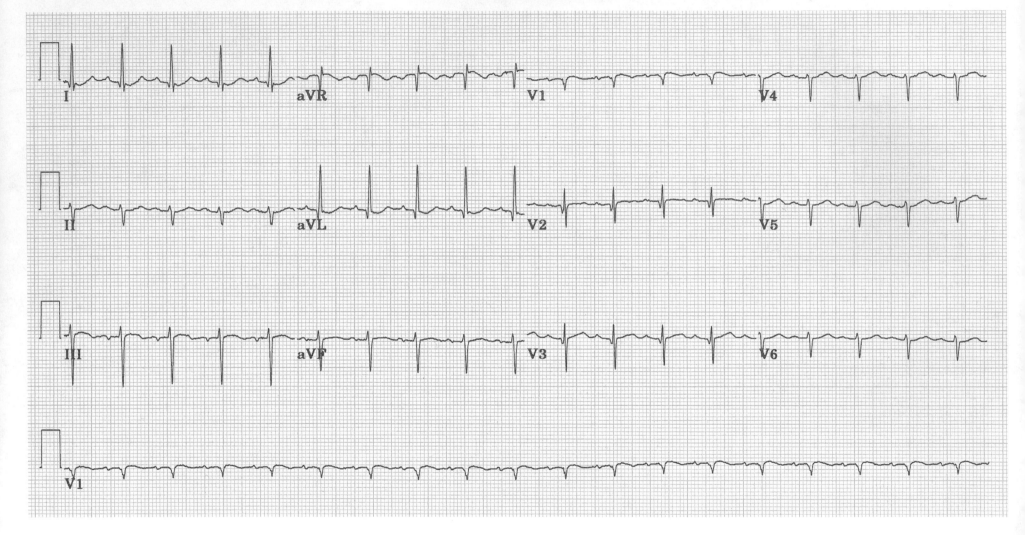

Interpretation Notes: _____

_____

_____

ECG 48 Seventy-four year old gentleman who presents to the Neurology clinic for evaluation of long-standing back discomfort. He has no known cardiac disease and specifically no prior myocardial infarction. Further cardiac evaluation was not pursued. His medications included potassium, ranitidine, a multi-vitamin, and thyroxine.

ELECTROCARDIOGRAM 49

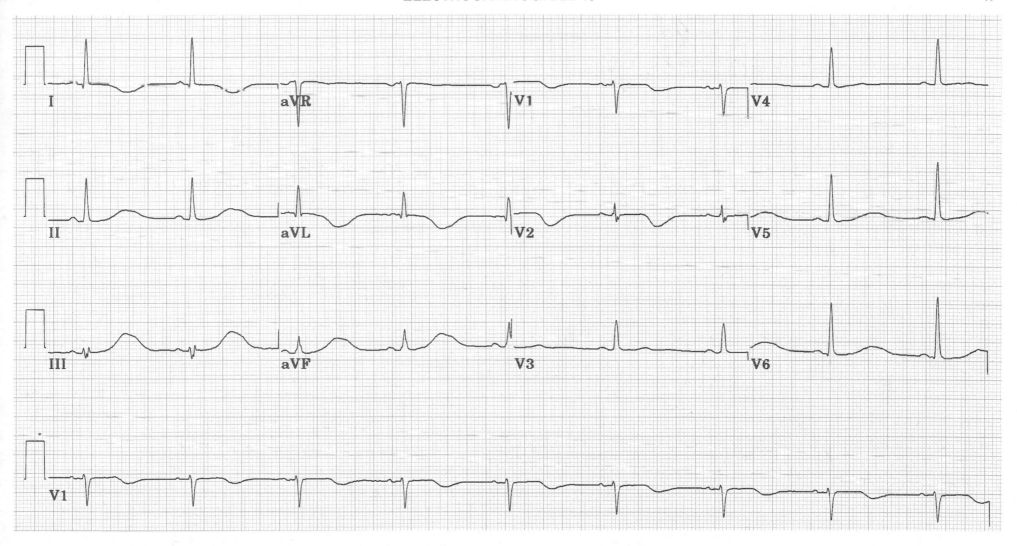

Interpretation Notes: _____

_____

ECG 49 Fifty-nine year old woman who suffered a bradycardic cardiac arrest in the setting of an acute subarachnoid hemorrhage. The patient eventually recovered and was discharged from the hospital. During her hospitalization an echocardiogram demonstrated normal left ventricular function and no evidence of a prior myocardial infarction.

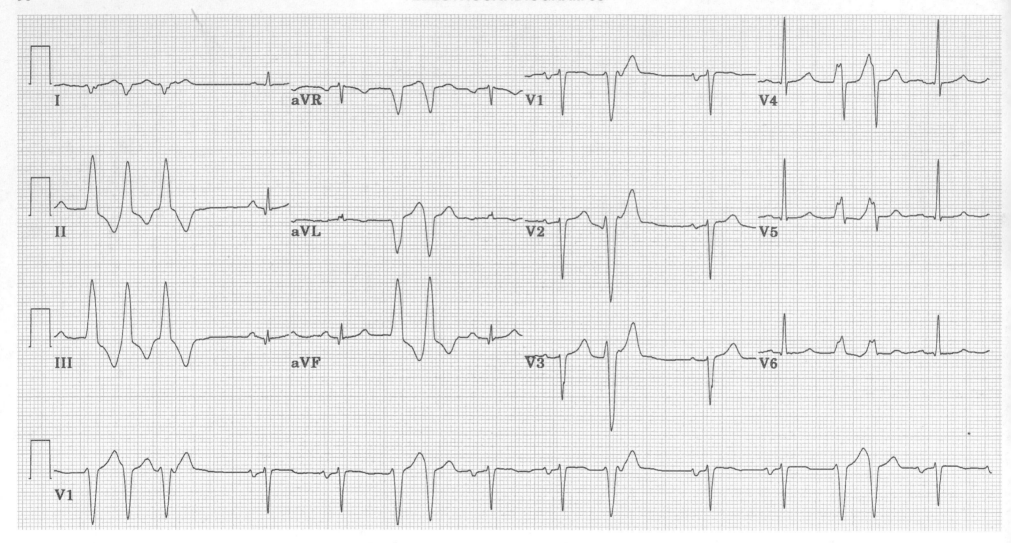

Interpretation Notes: _____
_____
_____

ECG 50 Sixty-five year old gentleman with a non-ischemic dilated cardiomyopathy and moderately severe left ventricular systolic dysfunction who returns for cardiology follow-up in the setting of non-sustained ventricular tachycardia. His medications included mexiletine, aspirin, enalapril, and atenolol. A prior cardiac catheterization demonstrated mild coronary artery disease.

ELECTROCARDIOGRAM 51

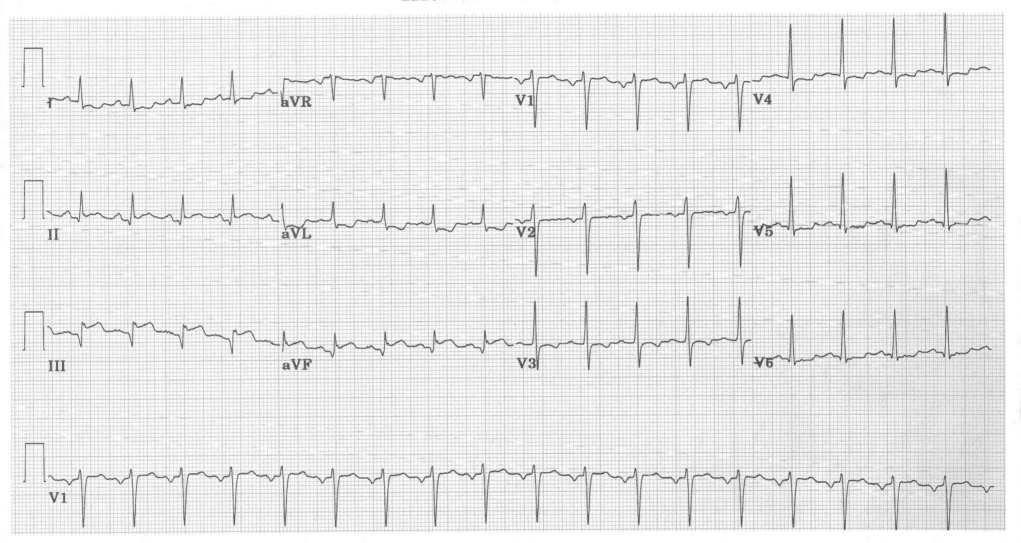

Interpretation Notes: _____

_____

ECG 51 Fifty-four year old gentleman who was urgently transferred from an outside medical center with a two hour history of acute chest discomfort. He received intravenous thrombolytic therapy prior to hospital transfer.

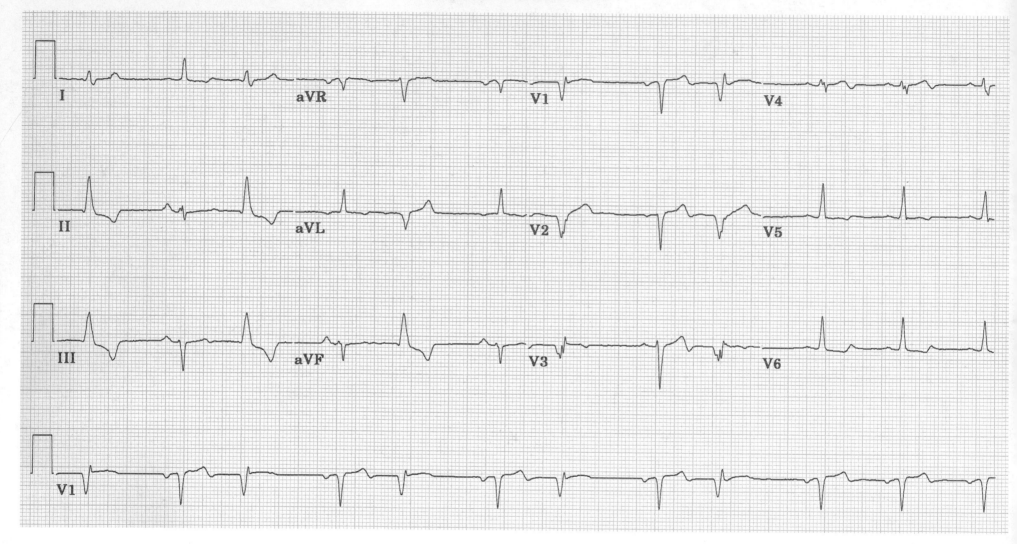

Interpretation Notes: _____

_____

ECG 52 Seventy-eight year old gentleman with a prior anterior myocardial infarction in the setting of a 100% left anterior descending coronary artery occlusion seen in the outpatient department for routine cardiology follow-up. He experienced recent angina pectoris in the setting of urologic surgery. His cardiac medications included amlodipine.

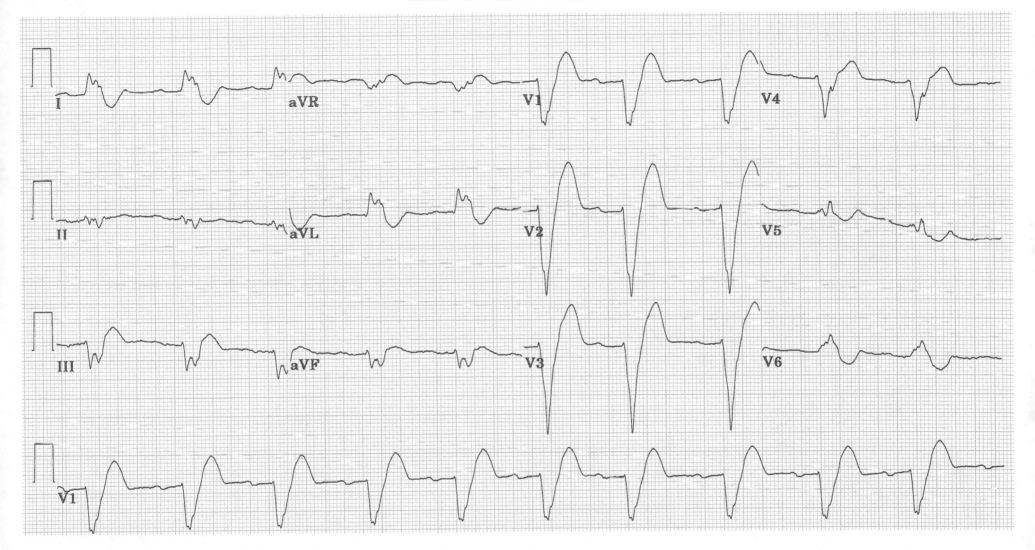

Interpretation Notes:_____

ECG 53 Eighty-one year old gentleman with severe left ventricular systolic dysfunction secondary to ischemic heart disease who returns for outpatient cardiology follow-up. He is status post cardiac defibrillator placement for recurrent ventricular arrhythmias. Medications at the time of this electrocardiogram included ethmozine, mexiletine, isosorbide dinitrate, digoxin, metoprolol, and enalapril.

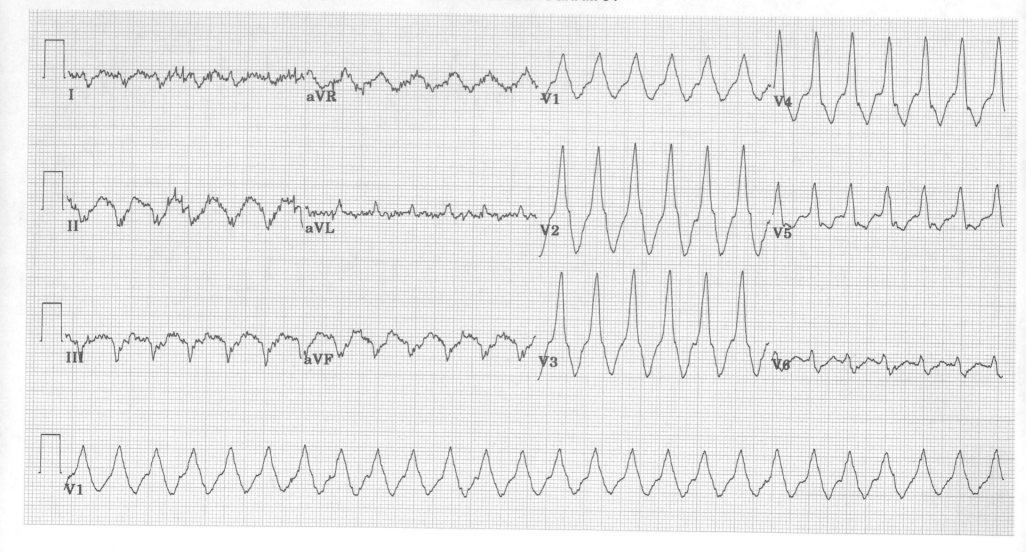

Interpretation Notes:_____

ECG 54 Sixty-five year old gentleman with a nine centimeter thoraco-abdominal aortic aneurysm who is recently status post surgical repair. The patient has minimal coronary artery disease as ascertained by a recent preoperative cardiac catheterization. This electrocardiogram was obtained during hemodialysis. Ventricular tachycardia developed postoperatively and soon thereafter the patient expired.

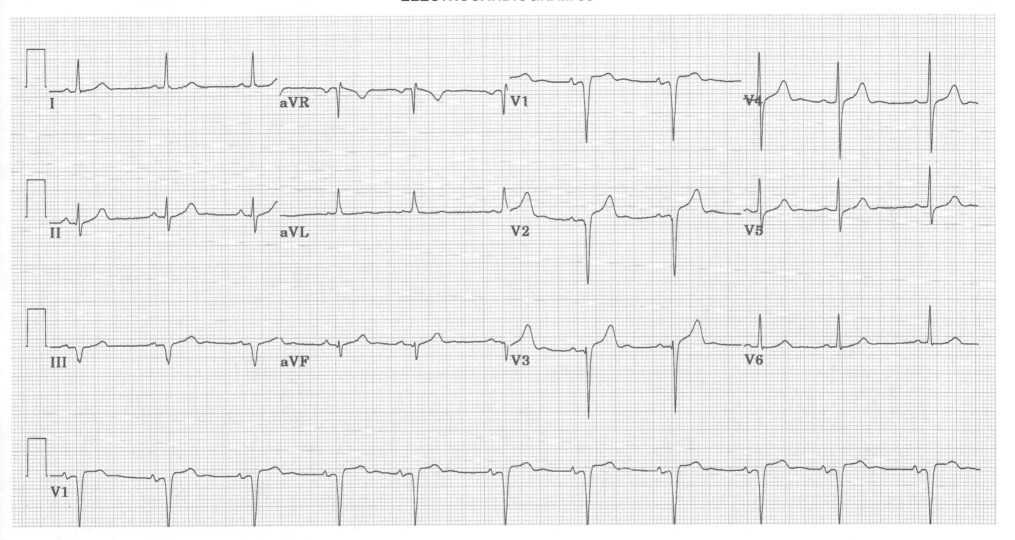

Interpretation Notes: _____

ECG 55 Seventy-nine year old gentleman admitted to the hospital for evaluation of ongoing nasal bleeding. His past medical history includes hypertension and coronary artery disease. A prior catheterization showed "some blockage," however the results are uncertain. Co-morbid conditions include hyperlipidemia and a seizure disorder. His medications at the time of this electrocardiogram included diltiazem, captopril, and carbamazepine.

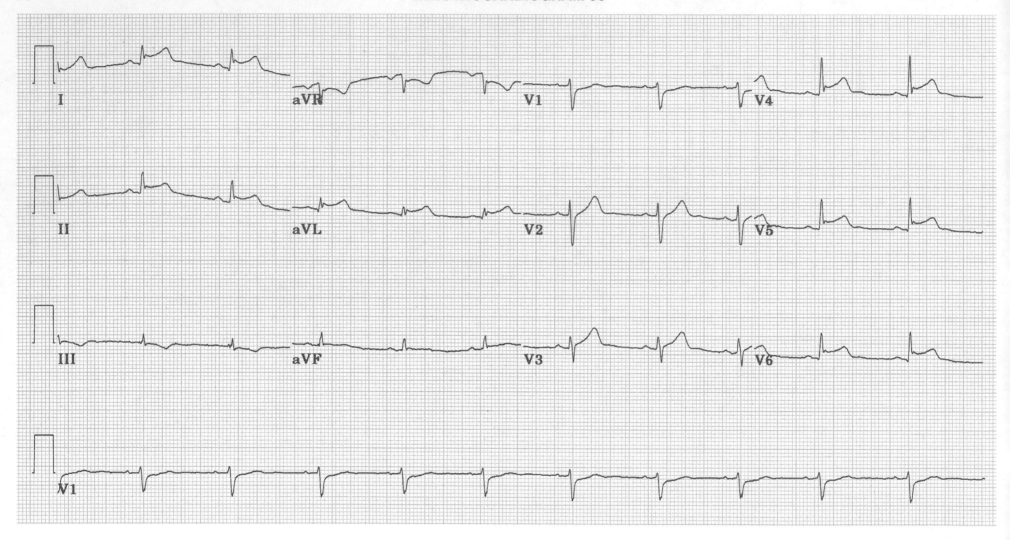

Interpretation Notes: _____

_____

_____

ECG 56 Thirty-five year old gentleman with a history of hyperlipidemia and obesity who presented emergently to the hospital with a several hour history of acute chest heaviness. The discomfort was associated with shortness of breath. A myocardial infarction was subsequently excluded and a cardiac catheterization was normal. The patient was diagnosed with acute pericarditis.

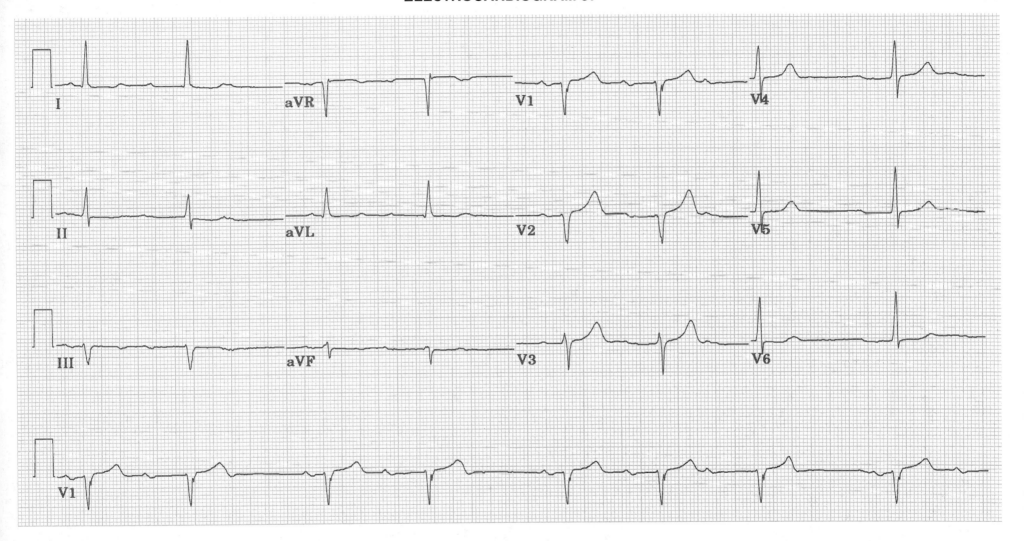

ECG 57 Seventy-seven year old gentleman admitted with a one week history of orthopnea and progressive dyspnea upon exertion. His past medical history includes long-standing non-insulin requiring diabetes mellitus, hypertension, and chronic renal insufficiency. Medications at the time of this electrocardiogram included furosemide, aspirin, topical nitroglycerin, and glucotrol.

Interpretation Notes: _____
_____

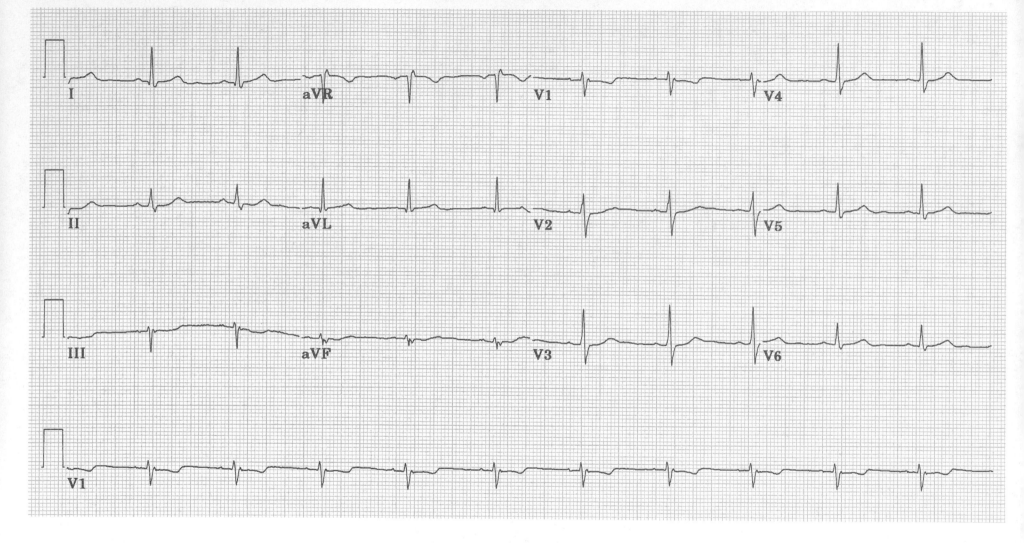

Interpretation Notes: _____
_____
_____

ECG 58 Fifty-eight year old gentleman with a history of adenocarcinoma of the esophagus who returns for cardiology evaluation in the setting of non-sustained ventricular tachycardia and paroxysmal atrial tachycardia. His medications included nadolol.

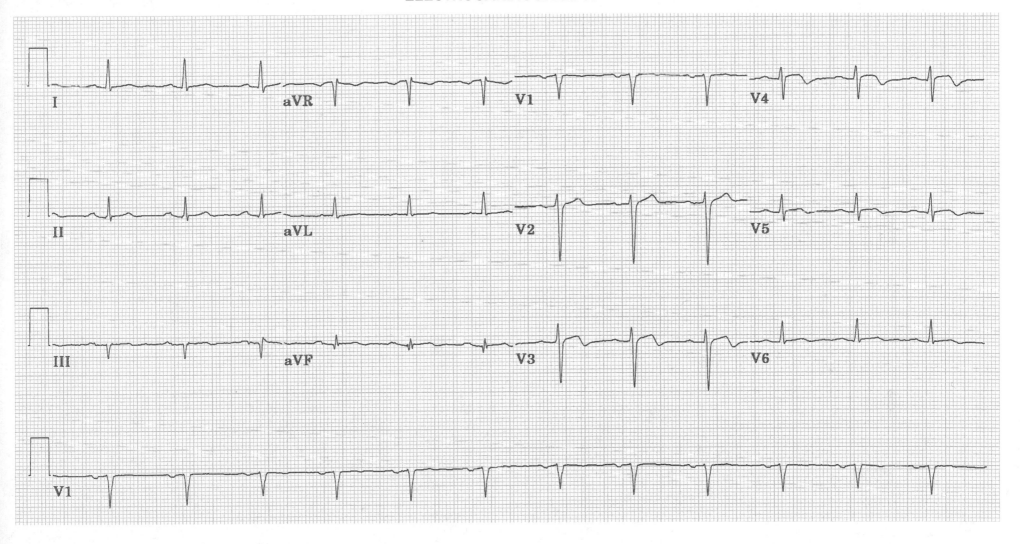

ECG 59 Sixty-eight year old gentleman with a history of coronary artery disease status post coronary artery bypass graft surgery four years prior to this electrocardiogram who presents with a one hour history of acute chest discomfort. The patient was stabilized with intravenous nitroglycerin and intravenous heparin and a near-future cardiac catheterization was planned.

Interpretation Notes:_____
_____

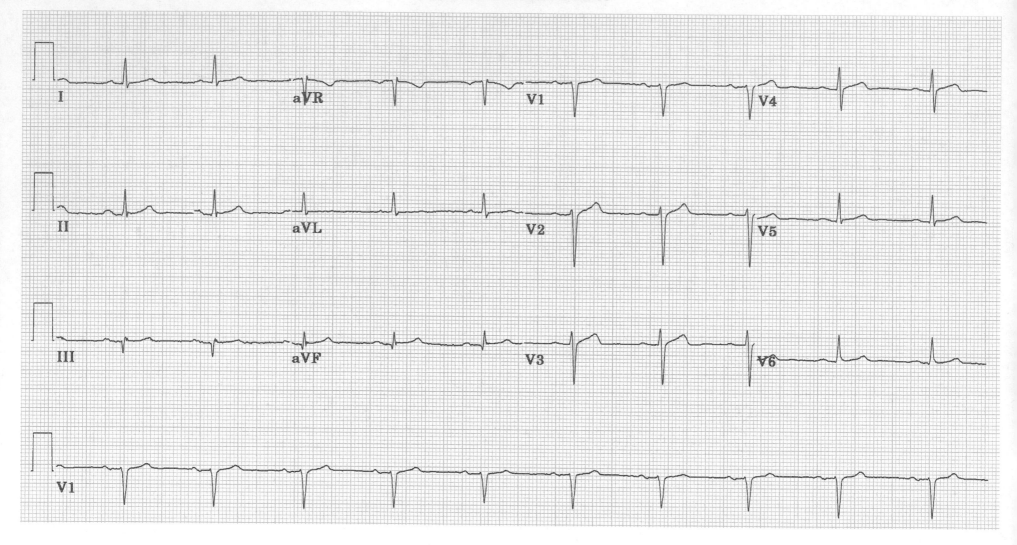

I aVR V1 V4

II aVL V2 V5

III aVF V3 V6

V1

Interpretation Notes: _____

_____

ECG 60 Sixty-eight year old gentleman with a history of coronary artery disease status post coronary artery bypass graft surgery four years prior to this electrocardiogram who presents with a one hour history of acute chest discomfort. The patient was stabilized with intravenous nitroglycerin and intravenous heparin.

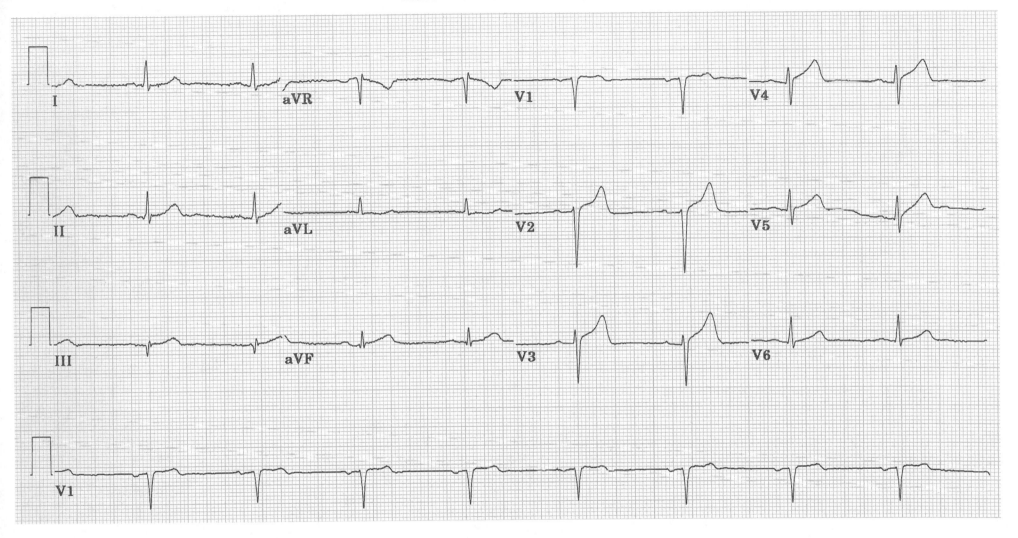

Interpretation Notes: _____

_____

_____

ECG 61 Sixty-eight year old gentleman with a history of coronary artery disease status post coronary artery bypass graft surgery four years prior to this electrocardiogram. The patient underwent an urgent cardiac catheterization demonstrating a subtotal occlusion of the saphenous vein graft supplying the left anterior descending coronary artery. Successful percutaneous transluminal coronary angioplasty with stent placement transpired.

ELECTROCARDIOGRAM 62

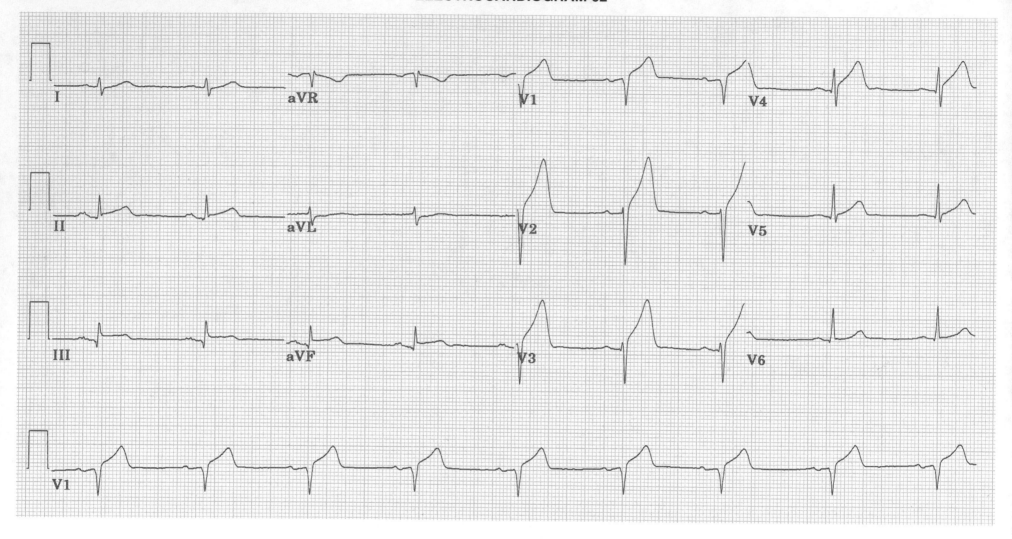

Interpretation Notes: _____

_____

ECG 62 Sixty-eight year old gentleman with a history of coronary artery disease status post coronary artery bypass graft surgery four years prior to this electrocardiogram. The patient underwent an urgent cardiac catheterization demonstrating a subtotal occlusion of the saphenous vein graft supplying the left anterior descending coronary artery. Successful percutaneous transluminal coronary angioplasty with stent placement transpired.

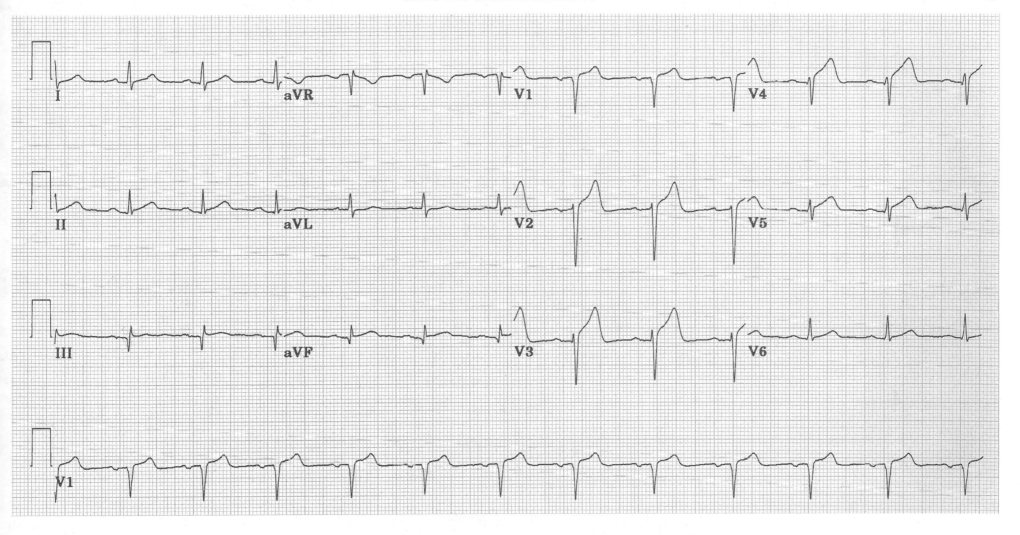

Interpretation Notes: _____

ECG 63 Sixty-eight year old gentleman with a history of coronary artery disease status post coronary artery bypass graft surgery four years prior to this electrocardiogram. The patient underwent an urgent cardiac catheterization demonstrating a subtotal occlusion of the saphenous vein graft supplying the left anterior descending coronary artery. Successful percutaneous transluminal coronary angioplasty with stent placement transpired.

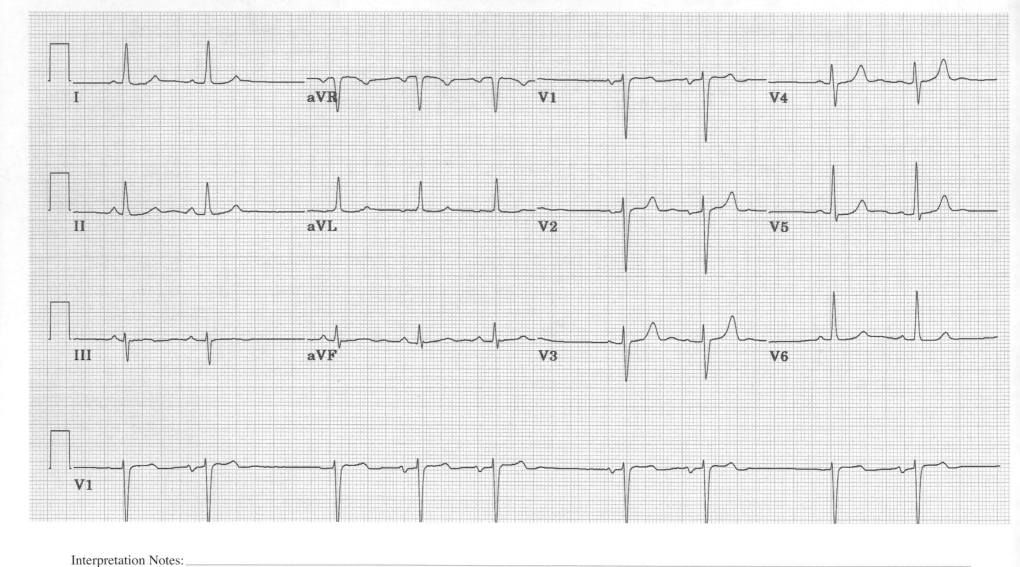

Interpretation Notes: _____

_____

ECG 64 Seventy-eight year old woman with a history of hypertension and insulin requiring diabetes mellitus who is admitted to the hospital with acute onset shortness of breath and a chest X-ray confirming the presence of congestive heart failure. Her past history includes a renal carcinoma resection. Her medications included furosemide, diltiazem, aspirin, metoprolol, isosorbide dinitrate, hydralazine, and insulin.

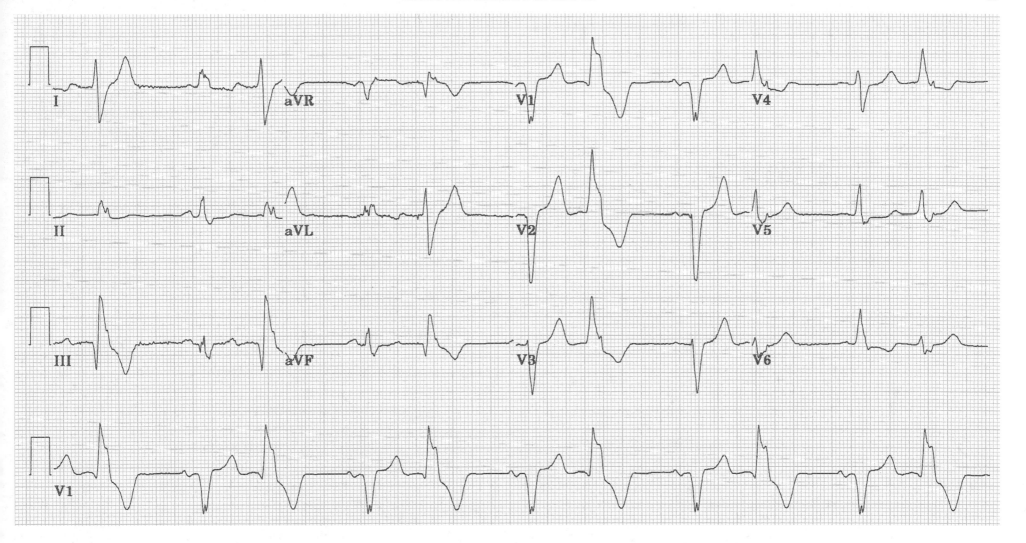

Interpretation Notes: _____

ECG 65 Seventy-six year old gentleman with coronary artery disease who is status post a remote myocardial infarction twenty years prior to this electrocardiogram, location unknown. He returns for a follow-up cardiac evaluation. His interval cardiac history includes coronary artery bypass graft surgery on two separate occasions, the most recent three years prior to this electrocardiogram.

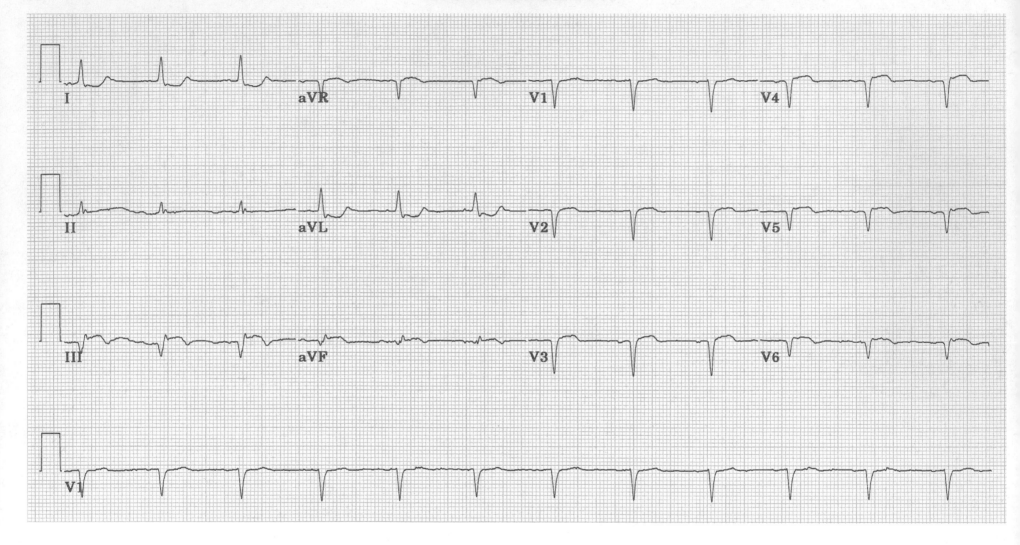

Interpretation Notes: _____

_____

_____

ECG 66 Sixty-four year old gentleman with an acute onset chest discomfort syndrome of two hours duration. Co-morbid conditions include hypertension, hyperlipidemia, and extensive past tobacco use. He has no known prior cardiac history.

ELECTROCARDIOGRAM 67

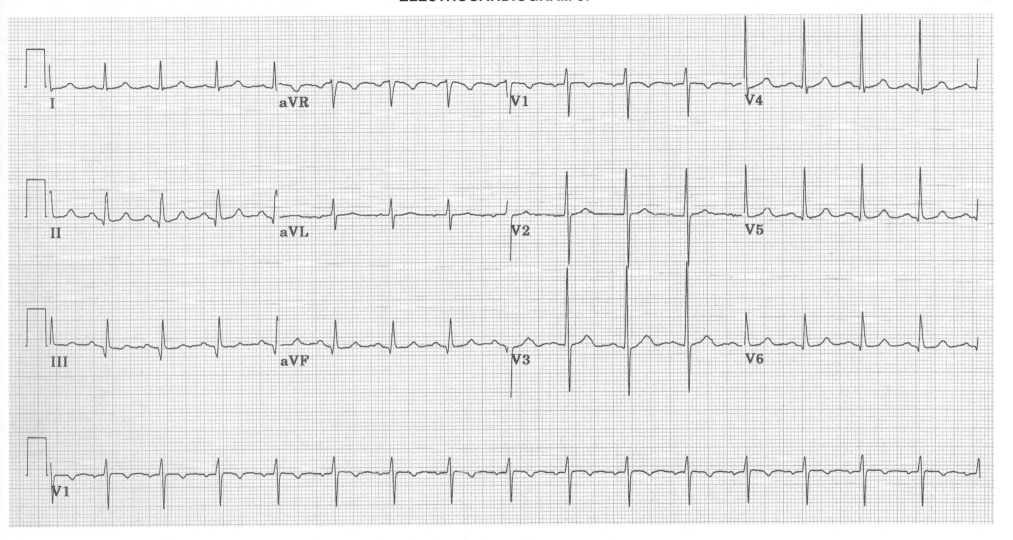

I aVR V1 V4

II aVL V2 V5

III aVF V3 V6

V1

Interpretation Notes: _____

_____

ECG 67 Sixty-eight year old gentleman with obstructive coronary artery disease who is status post a remote inferior myocardial infarction and coronary artery bypass graft surgery ten years prior to this electrocardiogram. He returns for a routine follow-up examination. Co-morbidities include hypercholesterolemia and paroxysmal atrial ar-rhythmias. Medications at the time of this electrocardiogram included aspirin.

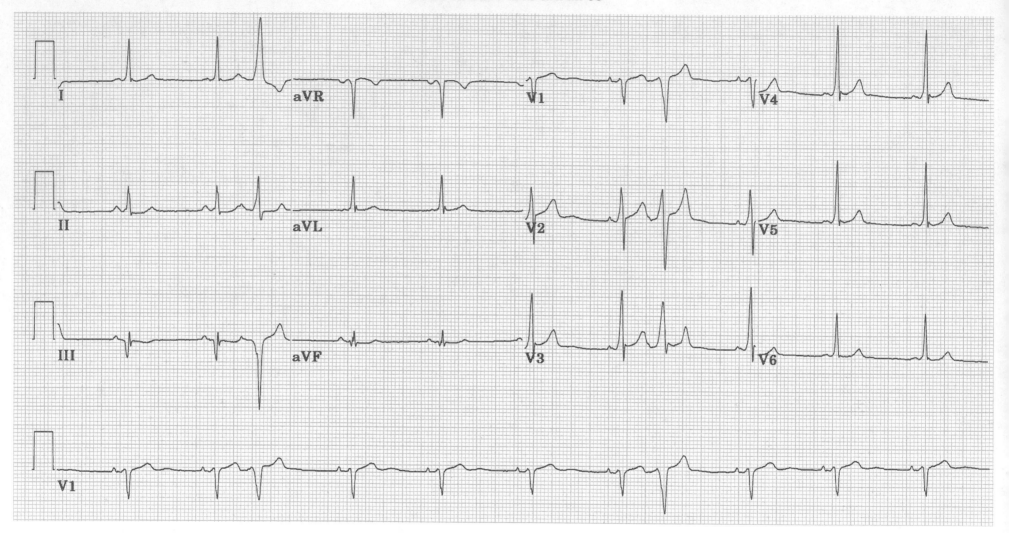

Interpretation Notes: _____

_____

_____

ECG 68 Forty-two year old gentleman who is self-referred for evaluation of heart palpitations. His medications included ibuprofen and ranitidine.

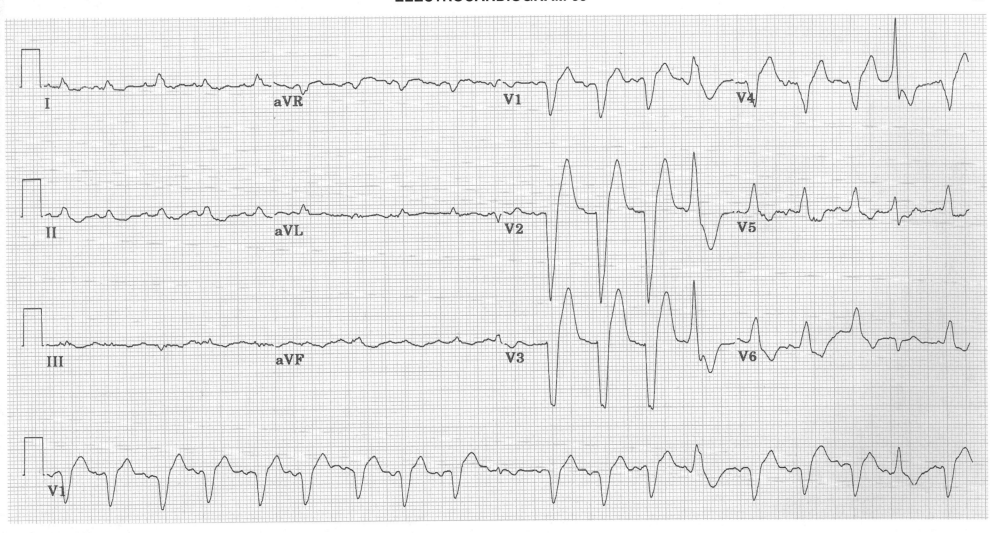

Interpretation Notes:_____

ECG 69 Seventy-one year old gentleman with a two week history of jaundice who presents for further evaluation. The patient's cardiac history includes a remote myocardial infarction and coronary artery bypass graft surgery five years prior to this electrocardiogram. Medications at the time of this electrocardiogram included verapamil and aspirin.

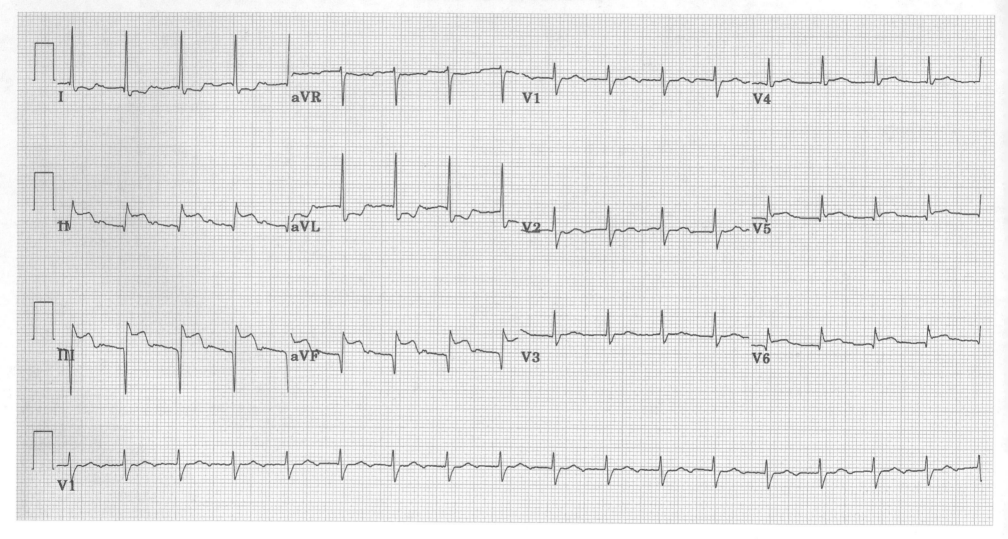

Interpretation Notes: _____

_____

_____

ECG 70 Seventy-four year old woman with acute onset "chest heaviness" who presented to the hospital with the above electrocardiogram. A subsequent cardiac catheterization demonstrated single vessel advanced narrowing of the right coronary artery. This patient underwent successful percutaneous transluminal coronary angioplasty.

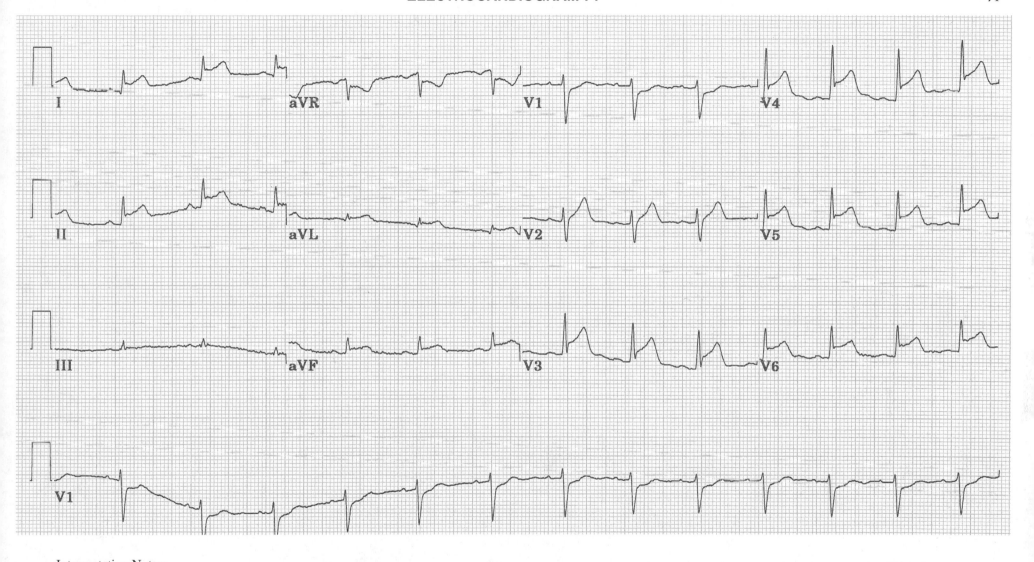

Interpretation Notes: _____

_____

_____

ECG 71 Thirty-five year old gentleman with a history of hyperlipidemia and obesity who presented acutely to the hospital with a several hour history of sudden onset chest heaviness. The discomfort was associated with shortness of breath. A myocardial infarction was excluded and a cardiac catheterization was normal. The patient was diagnosed with acute pericarditis.

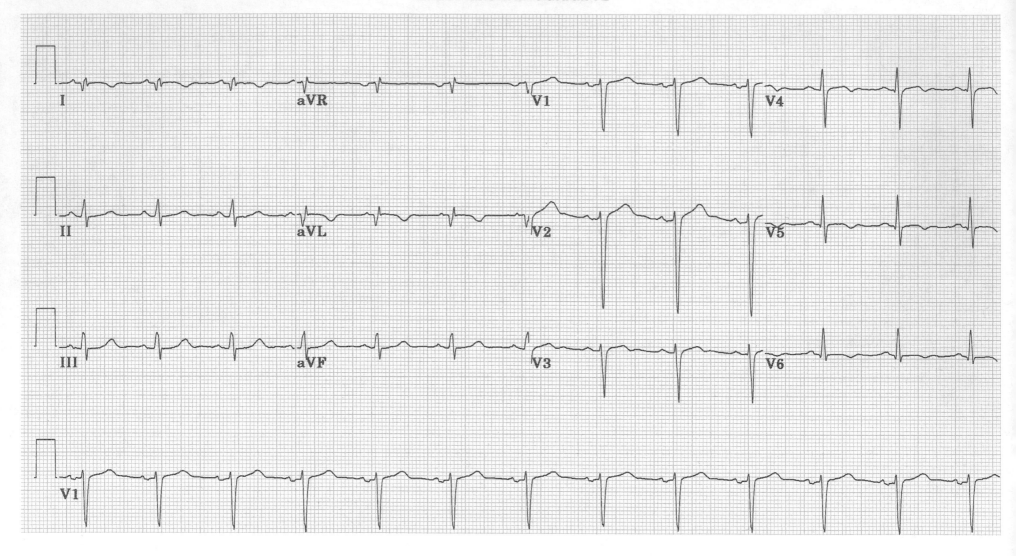

Interpretation Notes:_____

_____

_____

ECG 72 Sixty year old gentleman with coronary artery disease status post coronary artery bypass graft surgery one year prior to this electrocardiogram who was admitted for repair of an abdominal aortic aneurysm. He is not known to have suffered a prior myocardial infarction. Medications included amlodipine and aspirin.

ELECTROCARDIOGRAM 73

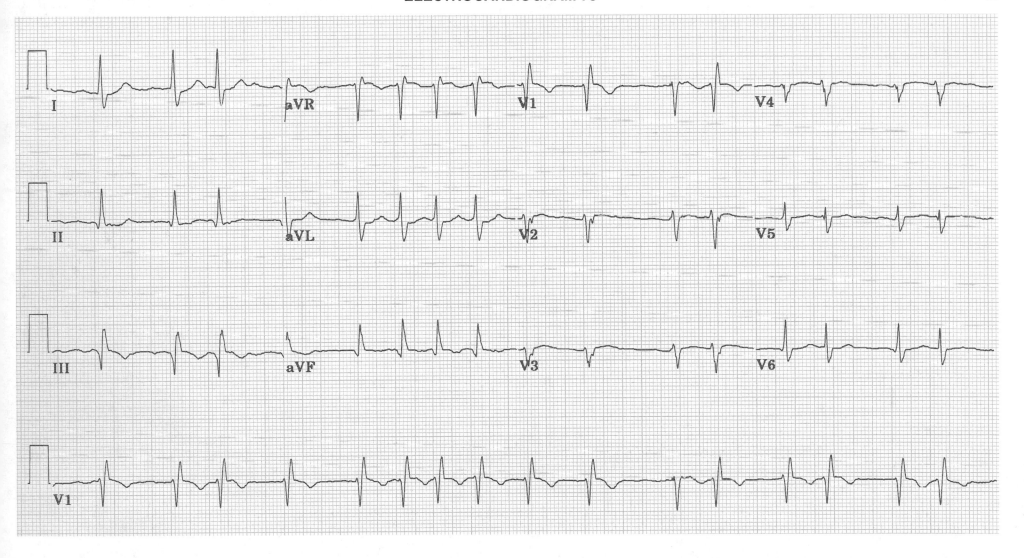

Interpretation Notes: _____

_____

ECG 73 Seventy-two year old woman with recent onset angina pectoris accepted in hospital transfer for planned coronary artery bypass graft surgery. Her medications included glucotrol, thyroxine, omeprazole, lisinopril, and furosemide. Cardiac risk factors include non-insulin requiring diabetes mellitus and hypertension.

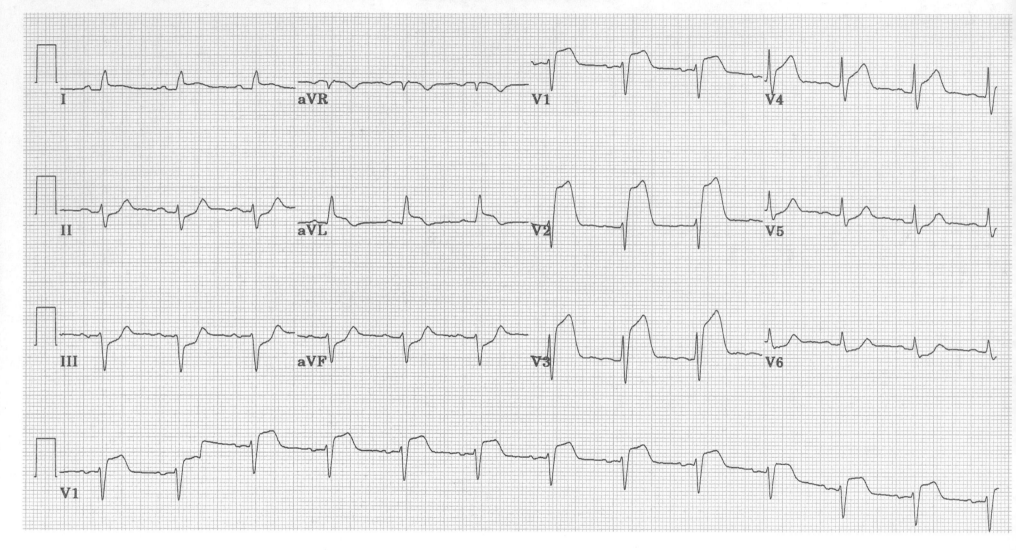

I   aVR   V1   V4

II   aVL   V2   V5

III   aVF   V3   V6

V1

Interpretation Notes: _____

ECG 74 Sixty-four year old gentleman who presented to the emergency room with a two week history of bilateral arm discomfort and numbness. This escalated immediately before presentation and the accompanying electrocardiogram was obtained. An urgent cardiac catheterization demonstrated a 90% proximal left anterior descending coronary artery stenosis, an 80% left circumflex coronary artery stenosis, and an 80% right coronary artery stenosis. Left ventriculography demonstrated antero-apical and infero-apical myocardial infarctions and overall moderate left ventricular systolic dysfunction. The patient was treated medically without further cardiac intervention.

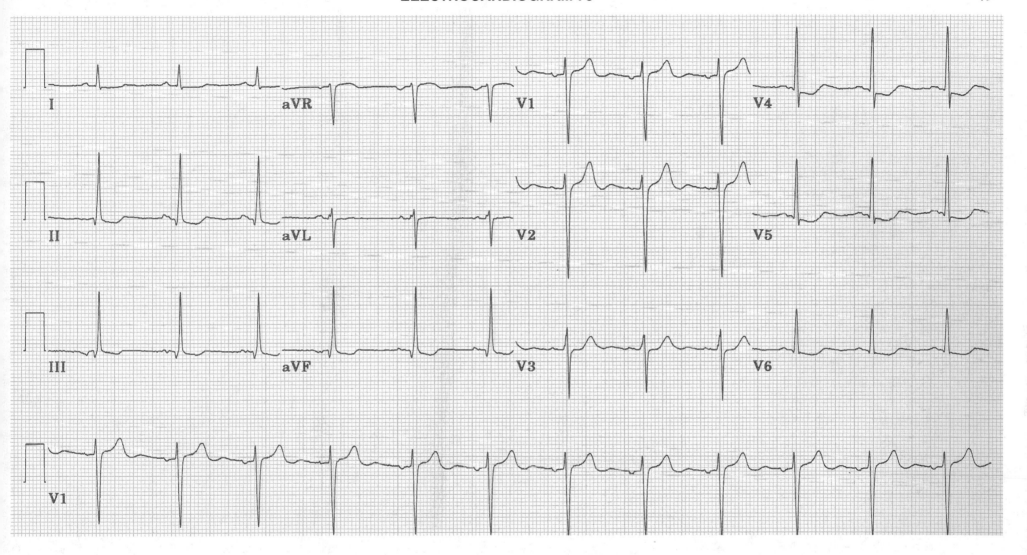

I   aVR   V1   V4

II   aVL   V2   V5

III   aVF   V3   V6

V1

Interpretation Notes: _____

_____

ECG 75 Sixty-two year old gentleman with recent symptoms of accelerating angina pectoris with a subsequent cardiac catheterization demonstrating severe multi-vessel coronary artery disease. This electrocardiogram was obtained prior to anticipated near future coronary artery bypass graft surgery. His cardiac catheterization demonstrated evidence of an age indeterminate inferior myocardial infarction. Medications at the time of this electrocardiogram included metoprolol, furosemide, digoxin, topical nitroglycerin, and captopril.

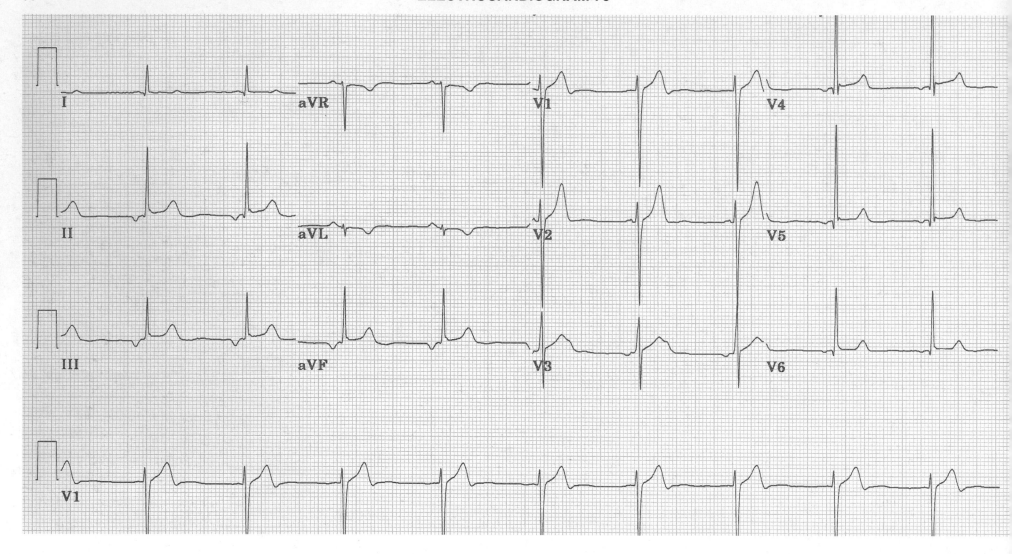

Interpretation Notes: _____

_____

_____

ECG 76 Fifty-five year old gentleman who presents to the emergency room with lightheadedness and a poor appetite. His past medical history is notable for hypertension. His medications included ibuprofen and propranolol.

ELECTROCARDIOGRAM 77

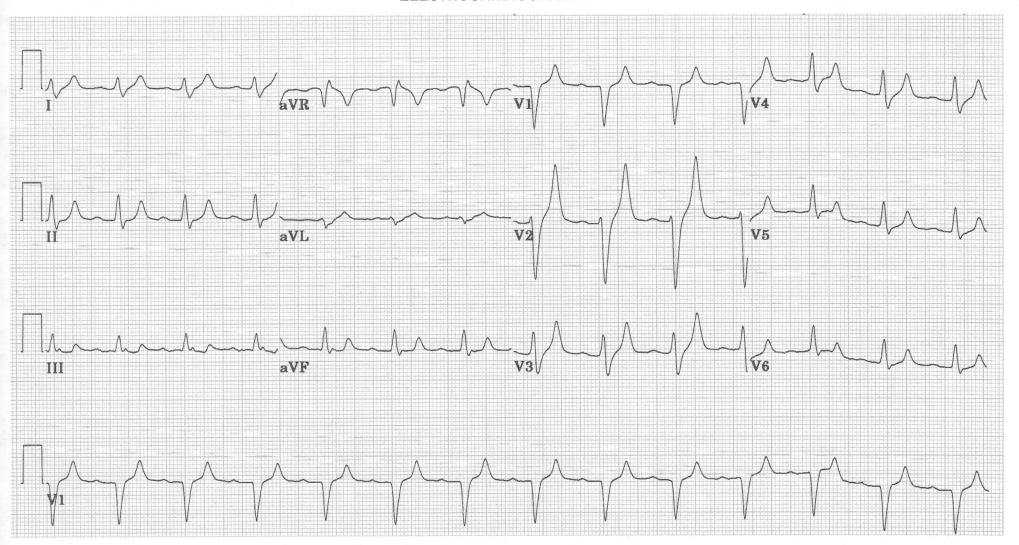

Interpretation Notes: _____

_____

ECG 77 Forty-two year old gentleman with end stage liver disease secondary to chronic hepatitis C infection who presents to the hospital with an altered mental status, acute renal failure, and a serum potassium level of 8.2 meq/L.

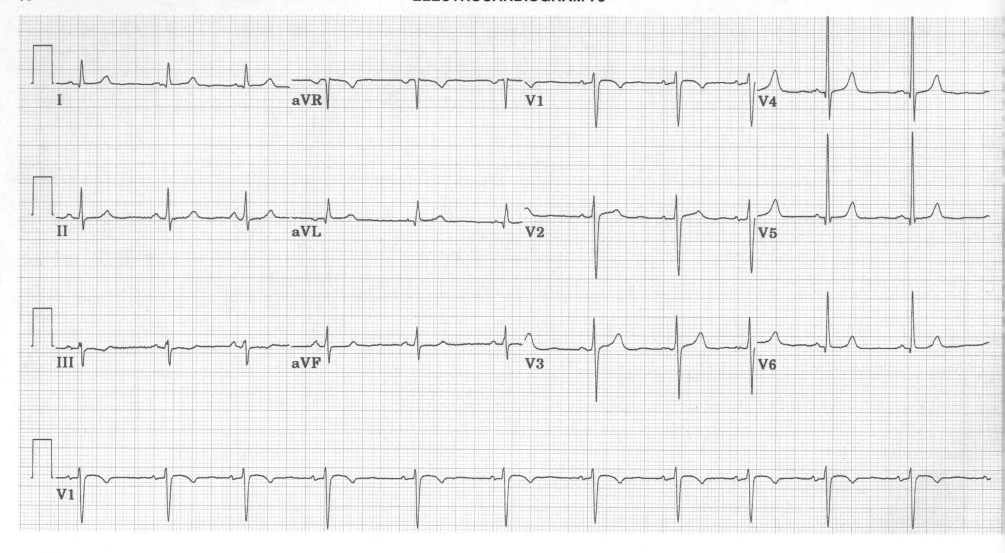

Interpretation Notes: _____

_____

_____

ECG 78 Sixty-one year old woman with long-standing hypertension who presents for a routine physical examination. Her serum potassium level at the time of this electrocardiogram was 4.4 meq/L. Her medications included nonsteroidal anti-inflammatory agents.

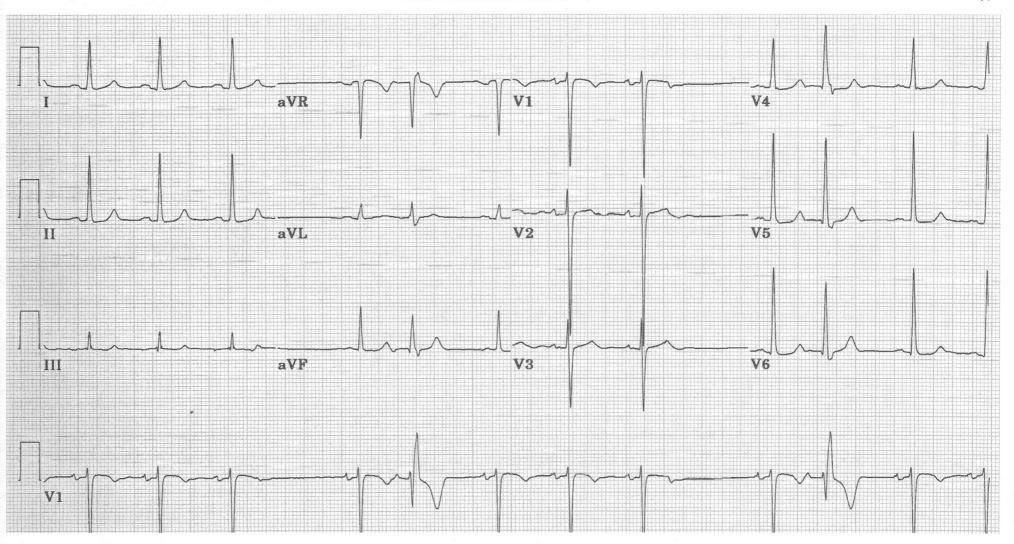

I aVR V1 V4

II aVL V2 V5

III aVF V3 V6

V1

Interpretation Notes: _____

ECG 79 Thirty-five year old woman with a history of mitral valve endocarditis status post St. Jude mitral valve replacement who presents for elective hip replacement. Her medications included warfarin, lisinopril, and meperidine.

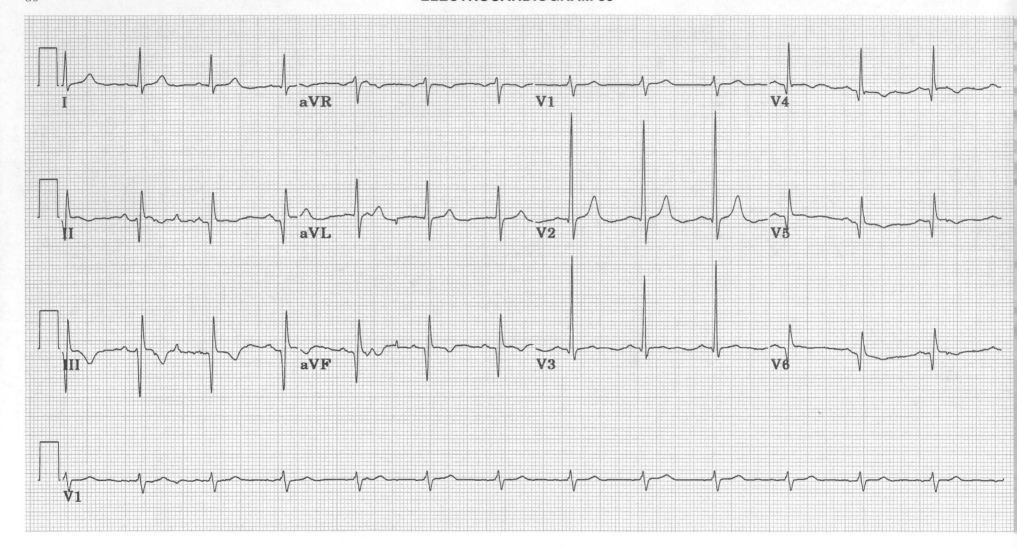

Interpretation Notes: _____

_____

ECG 80 Eighty-seven year old gentleman with a history of gastritis and benign prostatic hypertrophy admitted to the hospital with acute onset abdominal pain. The patient subsequently underwent an exploratory laparotomy for a small bowel obstruction. His past medical history is notable for a myocardial infarction twenty-six years prior to this electrocardiogram.

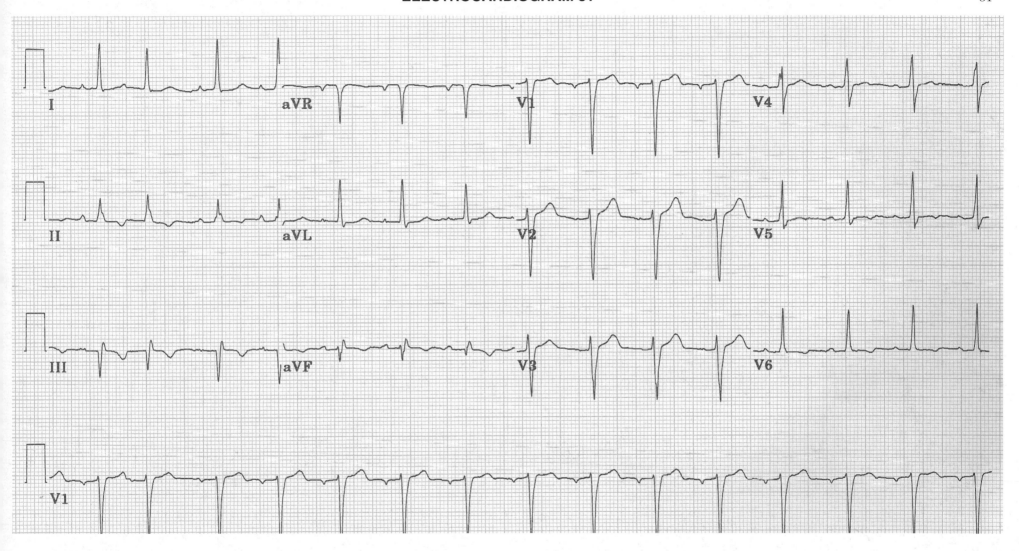

Interpretation Notes: _____

_____

_____

ECG 81 Sixty-one year old gentleman admitted to the hospital for evaluation of recent onset chest discomfort in the setting of coronary artery disease and coronary artery bypass graft surgery five years prior to this electrocardiogram. Medications at the time of this electrocardiogram included aspirin, cimetidine, diltiazem, glipizide, and insulin.

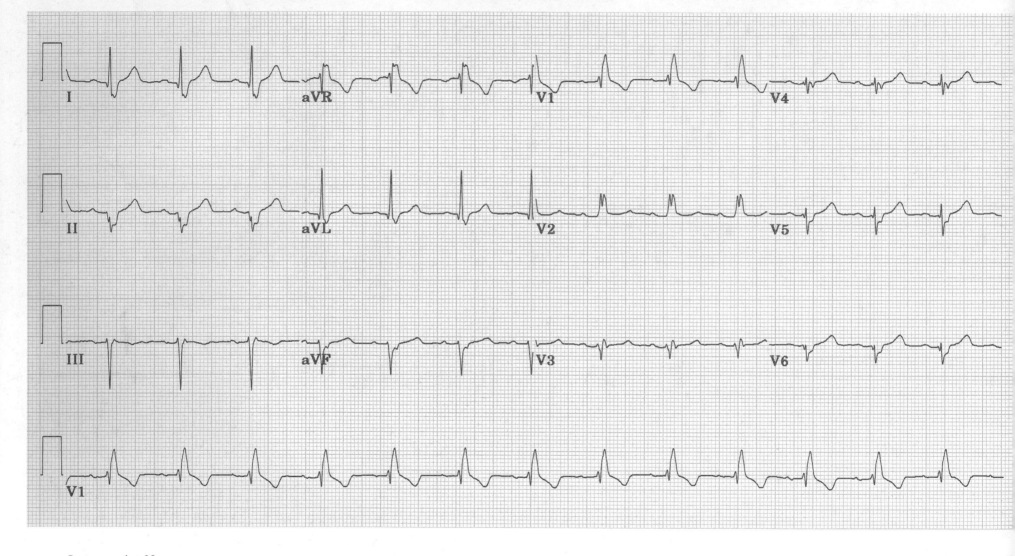

Interpretation Notes: _____

_____

_____

ECG 82 Fifty-five year old woman with a history of hypertension who presents to her primary care physician for a general physical exam and health assessment. Her medications included hydrochlorothiazide. There was no clinical history of a prior myocardial infarction.

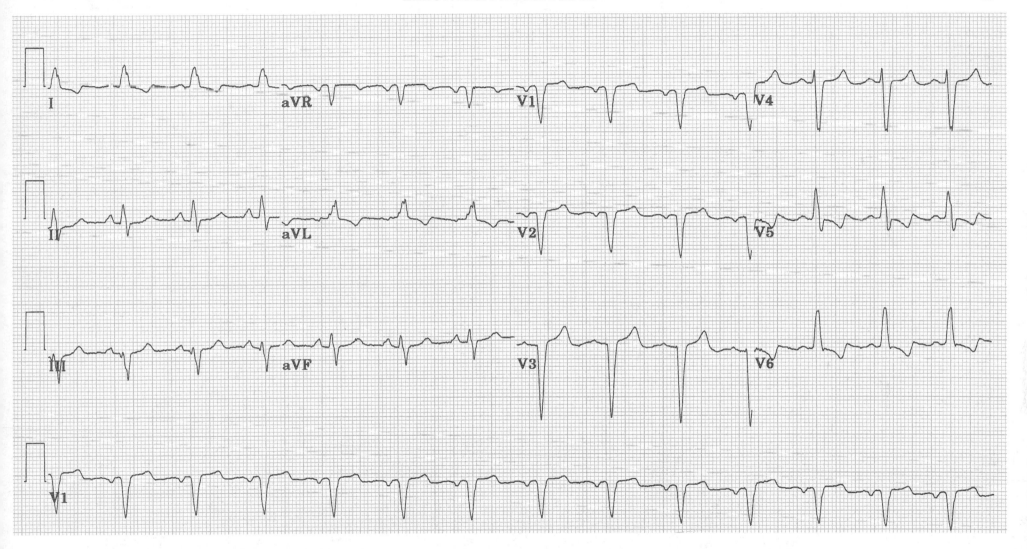

I
aVR
V1
V4

II
aVL
V2
V5

III
aVF
V3
V6

V1

Interpretation Notes: _____

_____

_____

ECG 83 Sixty-nine year old woman accepted in hospital transfer after a recent myocardial infarction for evaluation and treatment of post-infarction angina pectoris. A subsequent cardiac catheterization demonstrated three vessel coronary artery disease. This electrocardiogram was obtained prior to intended coronary artery bypass graft surgery. Medications at the time of this tracing included diltiazem, isosorbide mononitrate, and aspirin.

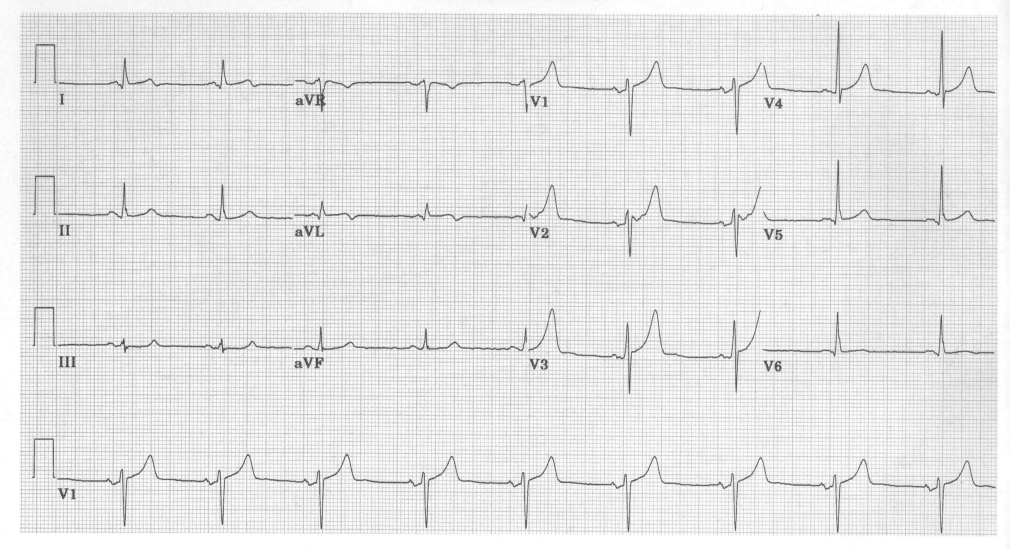

Interpretation Notes: _____

_____

_____

ECG 84 Forty-three year old gentleman who presents acutely to the emergency room with a several hour history of chest discomfort consistent with unstable angina. His medications included atenolol and aspirin. The patient underwent a cardiac catheterization and subsequent percutaneous transluminal coronary angioplasty to his left circumflex coronary artery.

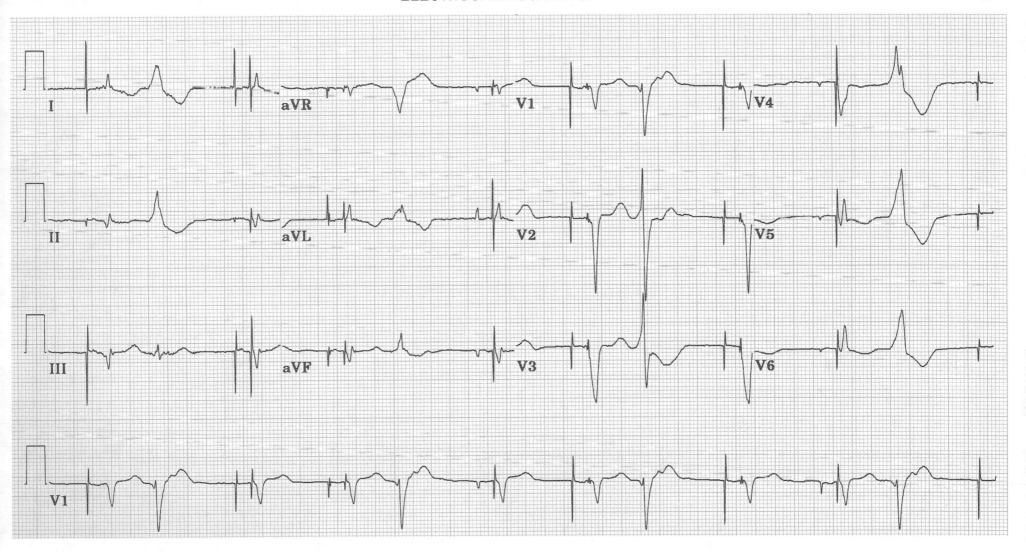

Interpretation Notes: _____

_____

ECG 85 Sixty-four year old gentleman with a history of remote coronary artery bypass graft surgery who presents with recurrent angina pectoris. His past history includes transitional carcinoma of the bladder, non-insulin requiring diabetes mellitus, and peptic ulcer disease. His medications included isosorbide dinitrate, diltiazem, and ferrous sulfate.

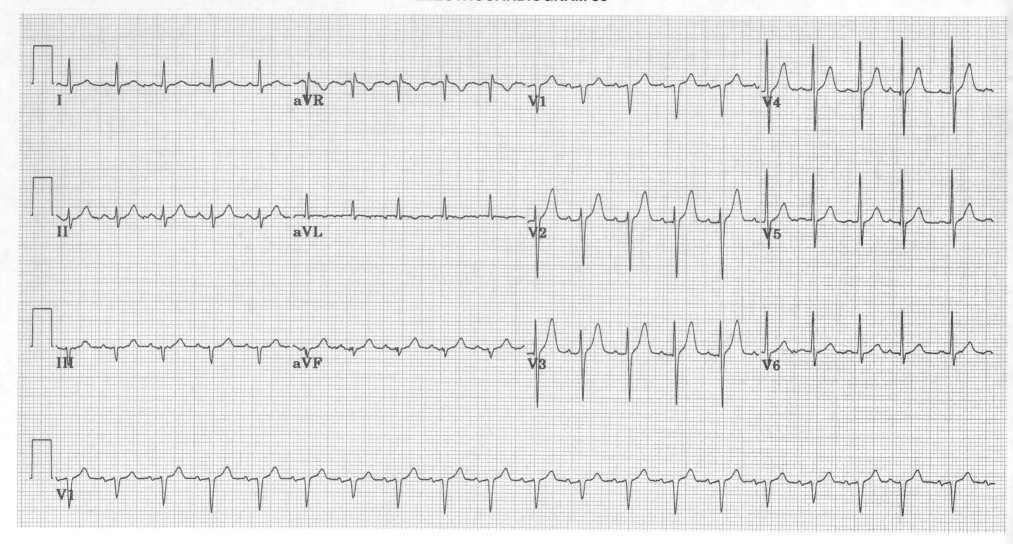

Interpretation Notes: _____

_____

ECG 86 Seventy-two year old gentleman with no known cardiac history who returns for outpatient internal medicine follow-up. This electrocardiogram was obtained as part of his general health evaluation. His medications included aspirin.

LEVEL I

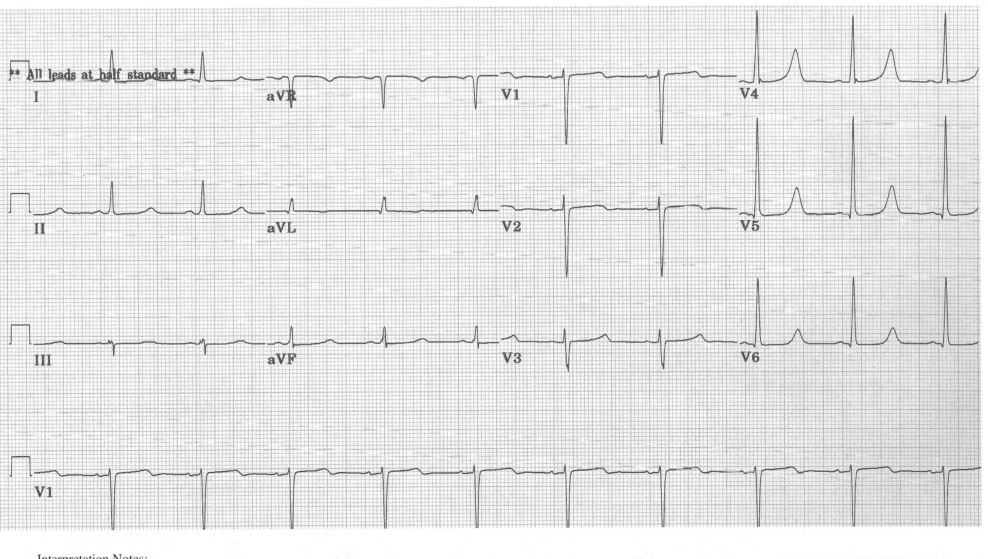

** All leads at half standard **

I aVR V1 V4

II aVL V2 V5

III aVF V3 V6

V1

Interpretation Notes: _____

_____

ECG 87 Forty-seven year old woman with dialysis requiring renal failure secondary to long-standing hypertension who presented to the hospital with recent onset shortness of breath. At the time of this electrocardiogram her serum calcium was 7.2 mg/dl and her serum potassium was 6.4 meq/L.

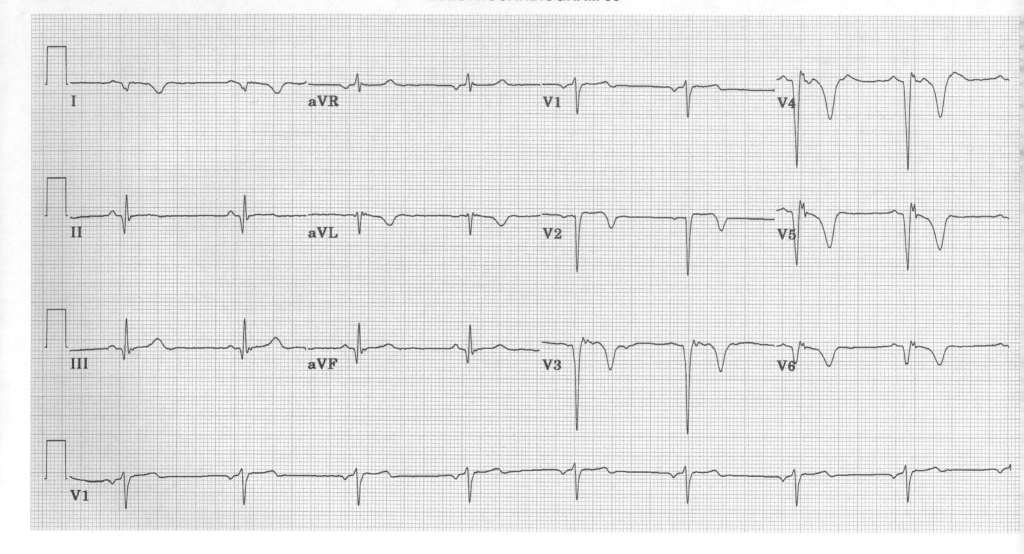

Interpretation Notes: _____

_____

_____

ECG 88 Forty-six year old man with coronary artery disease status post an extensive anterolateral myocardial infarction six years prior to this electrocardiogram who returns for preoperative evaluation prior to implantable cardiac defibrillator generator replacement. His medications included metoprolol, simvastatin, and aspirin.

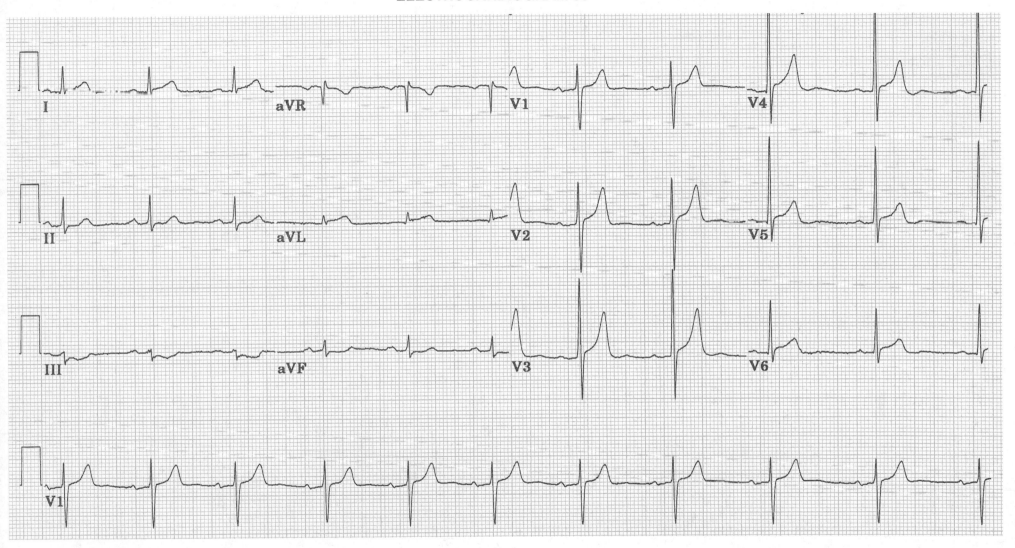

Interpretation Notes: _____

ECG 89 Fifty-eight year old gentleman who presented to the hospital with an acute chest pain syndrome. He underwent a diagnostic cardiac catheterization demonstrating an acute occlusion of the left circumflex coronary artery.

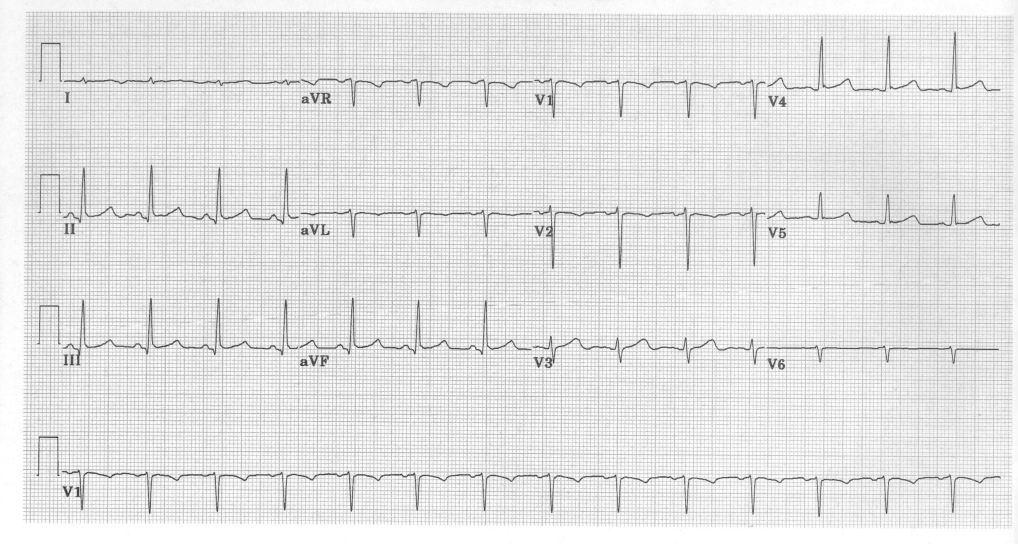

Interpretation Notes: _____

_____

ECG 90 Thirty-three year old woman with severe hypertension and chronic abdominal pain found to have superior mesenteric arterial occlusive disease in the setting of long-standing tobacco use. This patient underwent this electrocardiogram shortly after an abdominal arterial revascularization procedure.

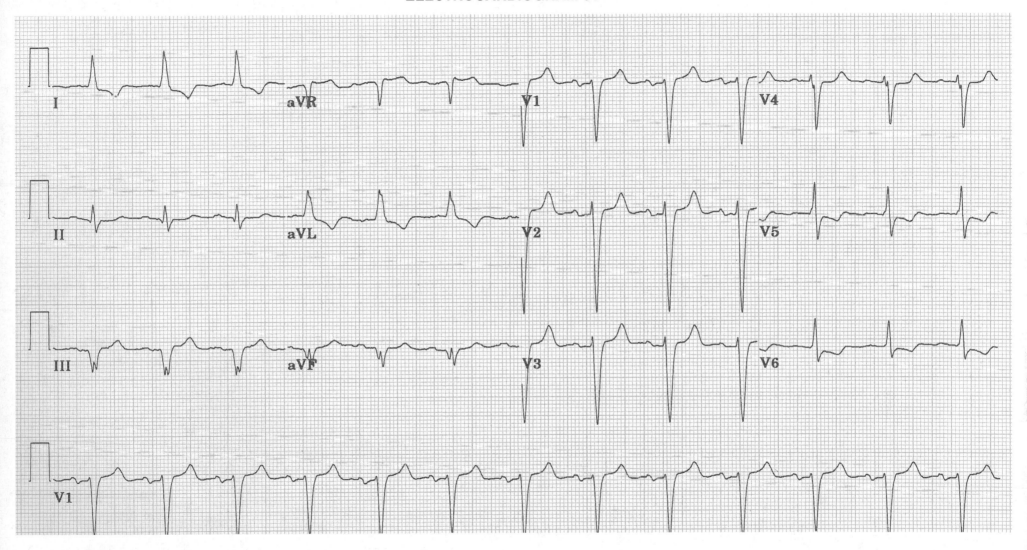

Interpretation Notes: _____

ECG 91 Eighty year old woman with diabetes, hypertension, and advanced peripheral vascular disease who presented acutely to the hospital with a gangrenous right foot. Medications at the time of this electrocardiogram included insulin, topical nitroglycerin, captopril, furosemide, amiodarone, and metolazone.

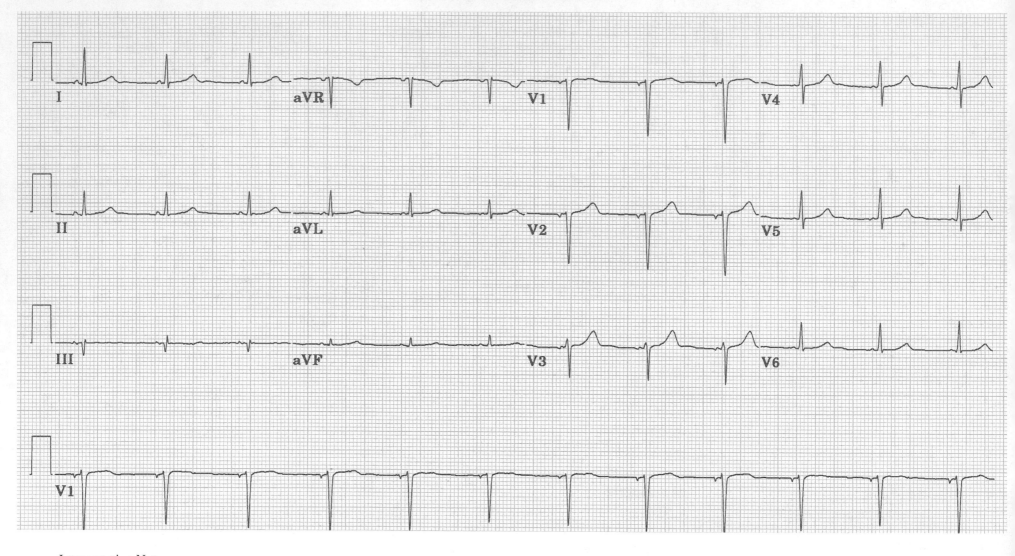

I aVR V1 V4

II aVL V2 V5

III aVF V3 V6

V1

Interpretation Notes: _____

_____

ECG 92 Thirty-four year old woman with a persistent ectopic atrial rhythm felt to represent a supraventricular tachyarrhythmia who is being seen in the outpatient cardiology clinic prior to planned sinus node radiofrequency ablation. Her medications included verapamil.

ELECTROCARDIOGRAM 93

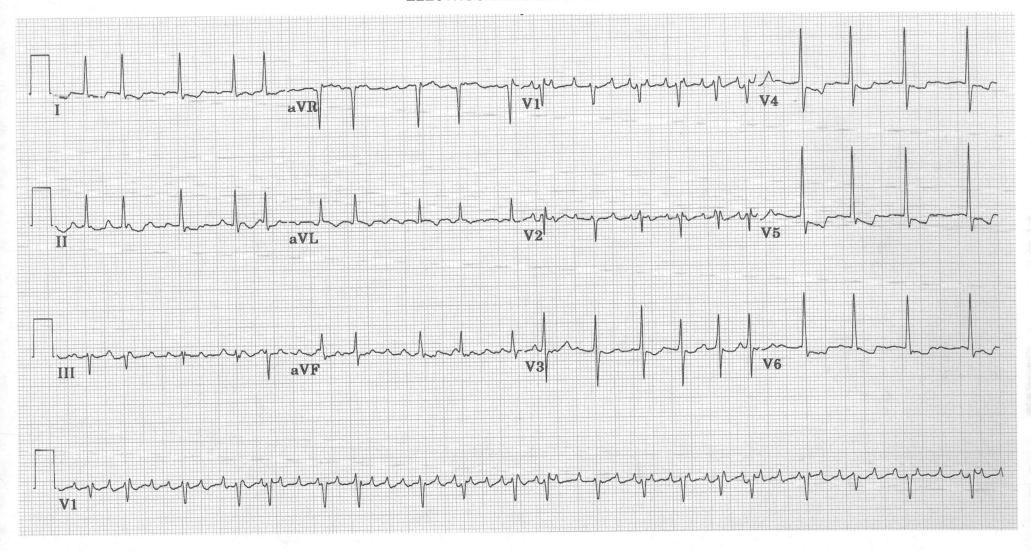

Interpretation Notes: _____

_____

ECG 93 Sixty-six year old woman with drug refractory paroxysmal atrial fibrillation status post permanent pacemaker placement.

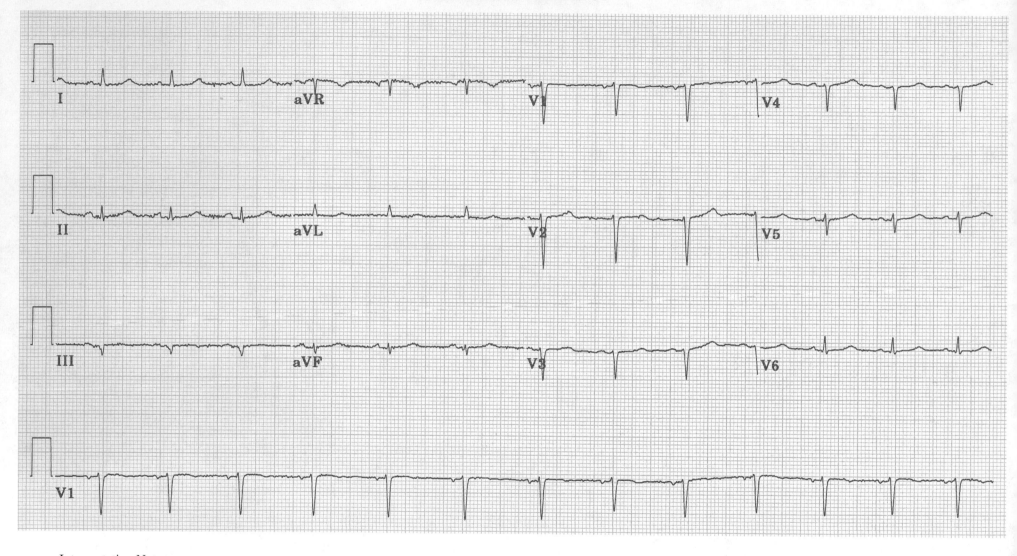

Interpretation Notes: _____

ECG 94 Fifty year old woman with a pattern of accelerating angina admitted for a cardiac catheterization. The patient subsequently underwent coronary artery bypass graft surgery. Co-morbidities include hypertension and hyperlipidemia. Medications at the time of this electrocardiogram included topical nitroglycerin, metoprolol, aspirin, premarin, and amlodipine.

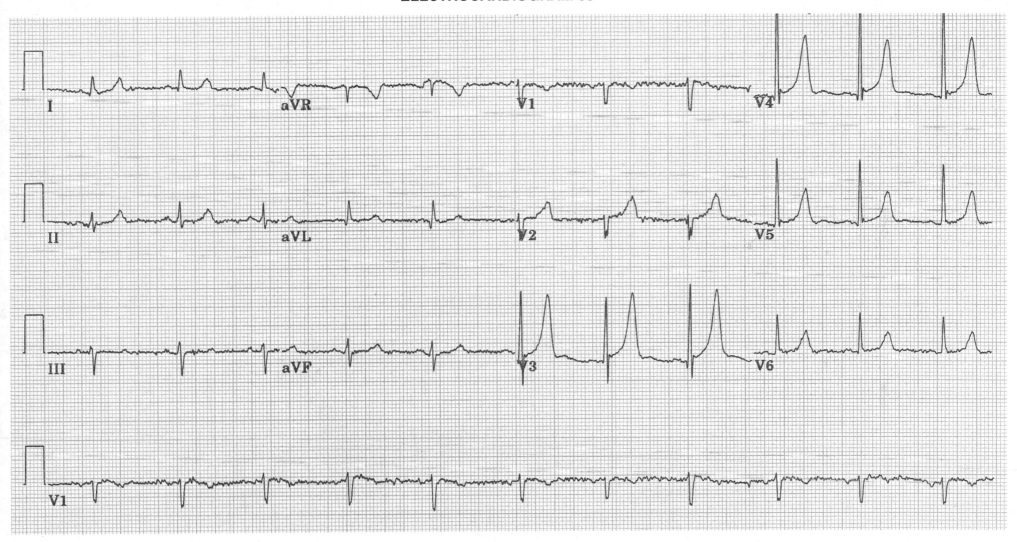

I   aVR   V1   V4

II   aVL   V2   V5

III   aVF   V3   V6

V1

Interpretation Notes: _____

_____

ECG 95 Seventy-three year old gentleman who presented to the emergency room with aphasia and right-sided hemiparesis consistent with an acute stroke. His serum potassium was normal. The patient was on no medications at the time of this electrocardiogram.

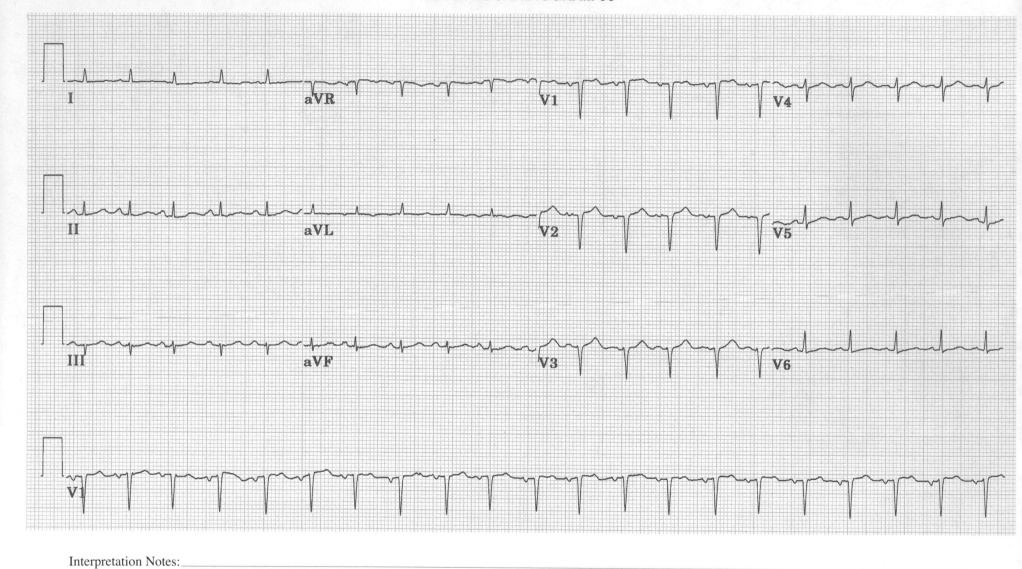

Interpretation Notes: _____

_____

ECG 96 Sixty-nine year old woman admitted to the hospital with acute onset shortness of breath felt to represent an exacerbation of her chronic obstructive pulmonary disease. Co-morbidities include hypertension, insulin requiring diabetes mellitus, and renal insufficiency. Medications at the time of this electrocardiogram included inhalers, insulin, and nifedipine.

ELECTROCARDIOGRAM 97

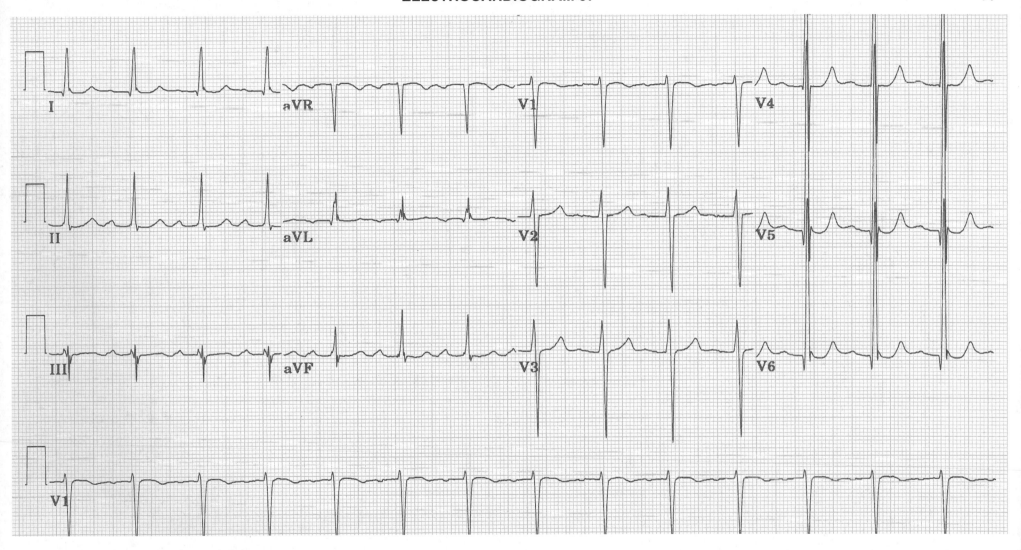

I   aVR   V1   V4

II   aVL   V2   V5

III   aVF   V3   V6

V1

Interpretation Notes: _____

_____

ECG 97 Fifty-one year old gentleman with rheumatic heart disease status post aortic and mitral valve reparative surgery who re-presents with anemia and laboratory studies consistent with hemolysis. A repeat echocardiogram demonstrated severe aortic and mitral insufficiency and the patient was referred for repeat cardiac surgery.

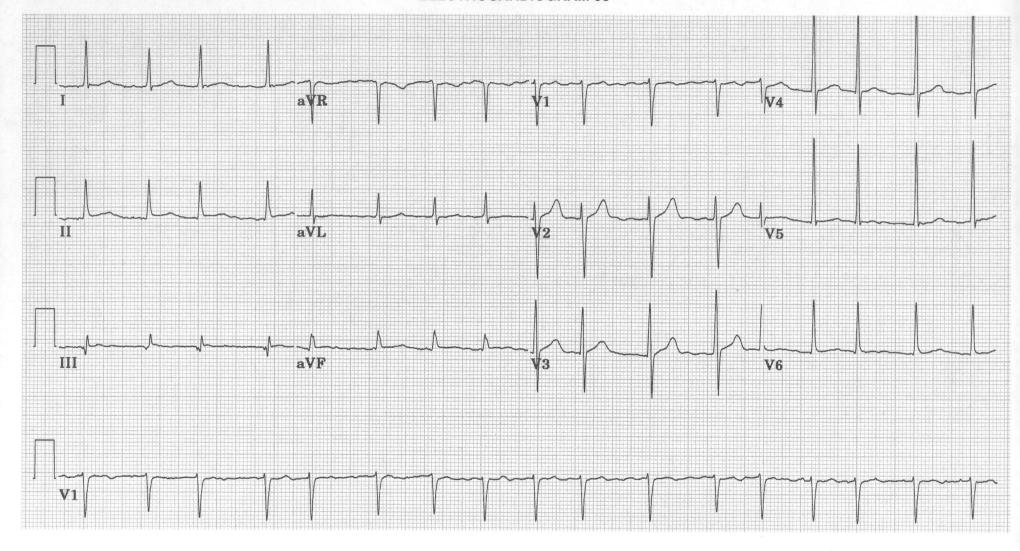

Interpretation Notes: _____

_____

ECG 98 Sixty-five year old gentleman admitted to the hospital for evaluation of acute renal failure in the setting of Wegener's granulomatosis. His past medical history includes paroxysmal atrial fibrillation and hypertension. His medications included prednisone, omeprazole, cyclophosphamide, verapamil, and bumetanide.

ELECTROCARDIOGRAM 99

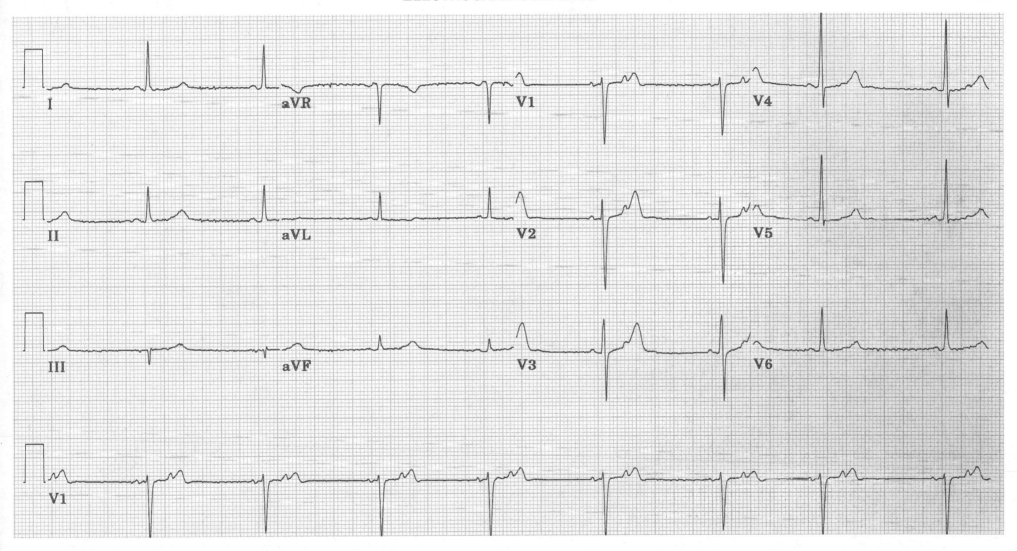

I   aVR   V1   V4

II   aVL   V2   V5

III   aVF   V3   V6

V1

Interpretation Notes: _____

_____

ECG 99 Sixty-five year old gentleman admitted to the hospital for evaluation of acute renal failure in the setting of Wegener's granulomatosis. His past medical history includes paroxysmal atrial fibrillation and hypertension. His medications included prednisone, omeprazole, cyclophosphamide, verapamil, and bumetanide.

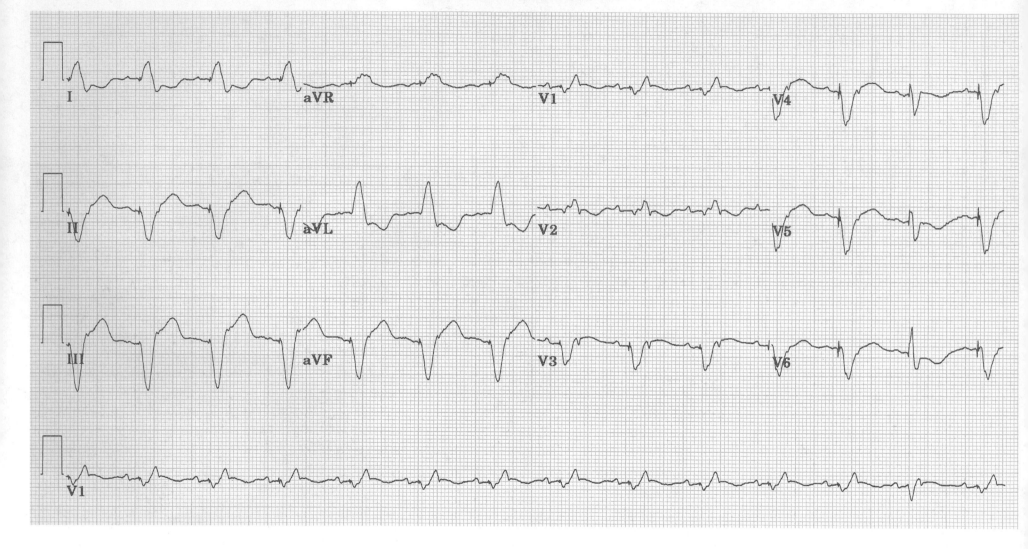

I   aVR   V1   V4

II   aVL   V2   V5

III   aVF   V3   V6

V1

Interpretation Notes: _____

ECG 100 Fifty-nine year old woman with recurrent ventricular tachycardia in the setting of normal coronary arteries documented by cardiac catheterization. Echocardiography demonstrated moderate left ventricular systolic dysfunction and severe right ventricular systolic dysfunction suggesting a non-ischemic cardiomyopathy. Medications at the time of this electrocardiogram included thyroxine, enalapril, and aspirin.

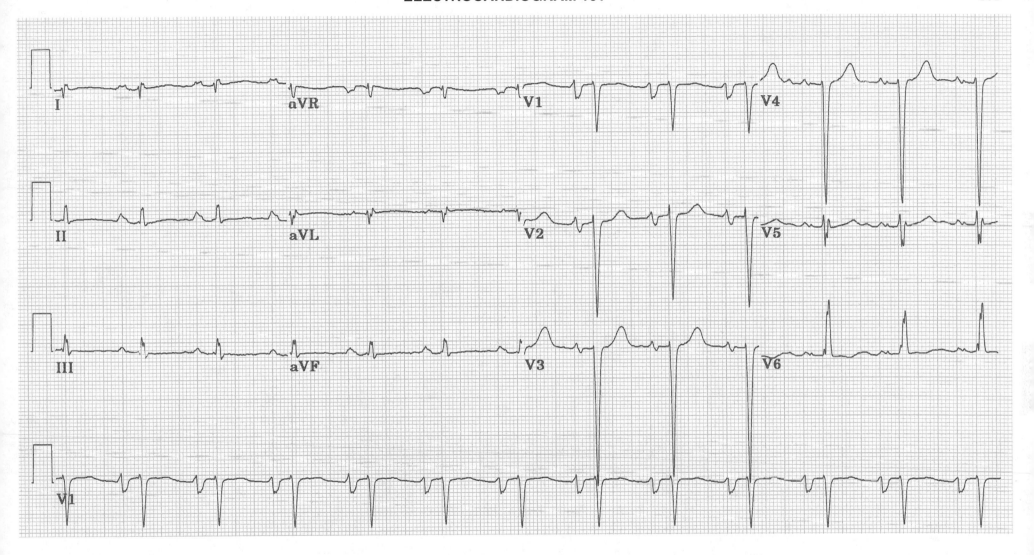

Interpretation Notes: _____

_____

_____

ECG 101 Forty-five year old gentleman with a history of long-term alcohol use who was admitted to the hospital with hemoptysis. An echocardiogram demonstrated severe global left ventricular systolic dysfunction with an estimated left ventricular ejection fraction of 10%. Moderately severe mitral and tricuspid regurgitation were present. Medications at the time of this tracing included furosemide, potassium, digoxin, amiodarone, warfarin, and captopril.

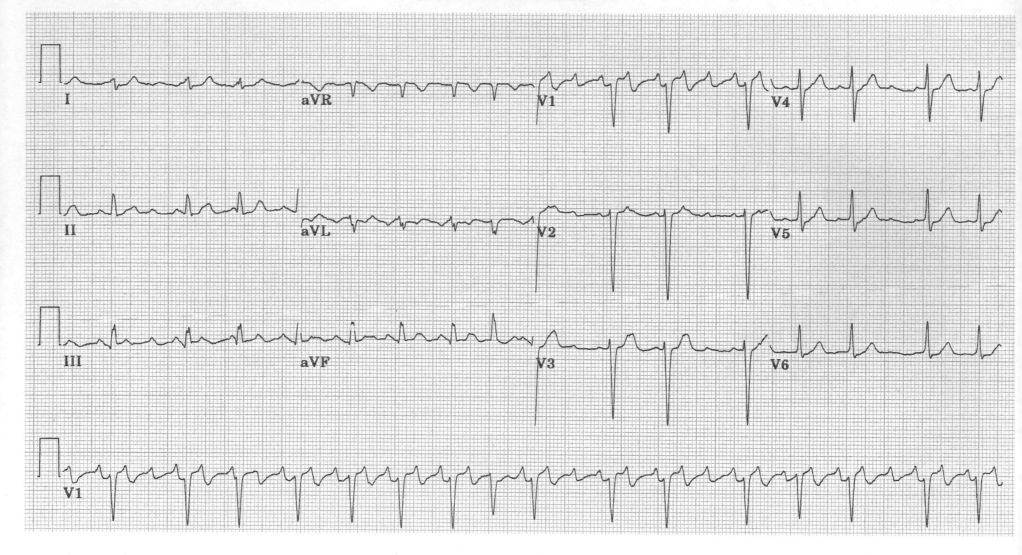

I   aVR   V1   V4

II   aVL   V2   V5

III   aVF   V3   V6

V1

Interpretation Notes: _____

_____

ECG 102 Forty-nine year old woman with a history of rheumatic mitral valvular stenosis who underwent percutaneous mitral valve commissurotomy in the past. She now presents with increasing symptoms of shortness of breath, a resting tachycardia, and moderately severe mitral insufficiency. Medications at the time of this electrocardiogram included verapamil, digoxin, propafenone, and aspirin.

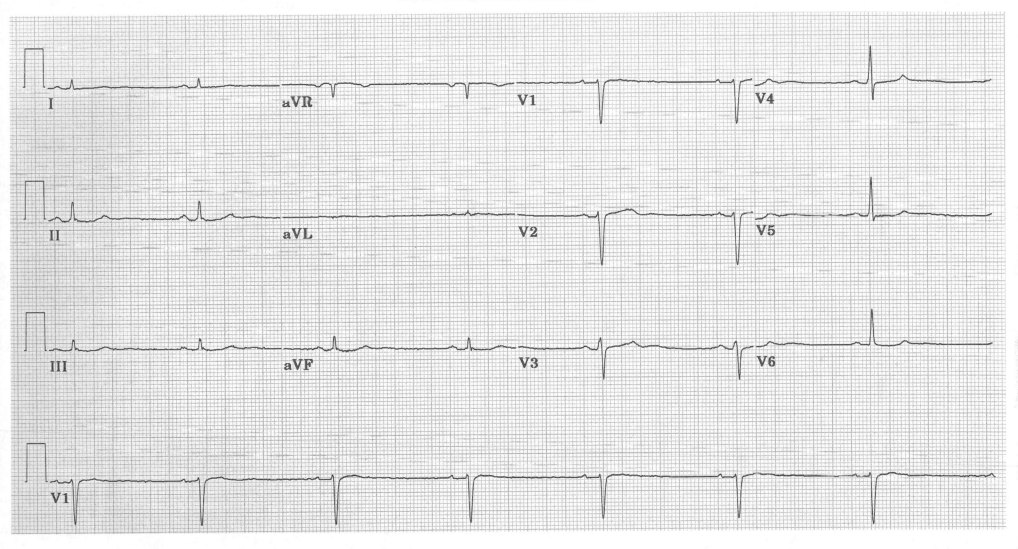

I aVR V1 V4

II aVL V2 V5

III aVF V3 V6

V1

Interpretation Notes: _____

_____

ECG 103 Fifty-six year old gentleman with severe left ventricular systolic dysfunction, mild coronary artery disease, and a suspected non-ischemic cardiomyopathy accepted in transfer from an outside hospital for management of both recurrent atrial and ventricular dysrhythmias. His medications at the time of this electrocardiogram included furosemide, captopril, potassium, digoxin, and lidocaine.

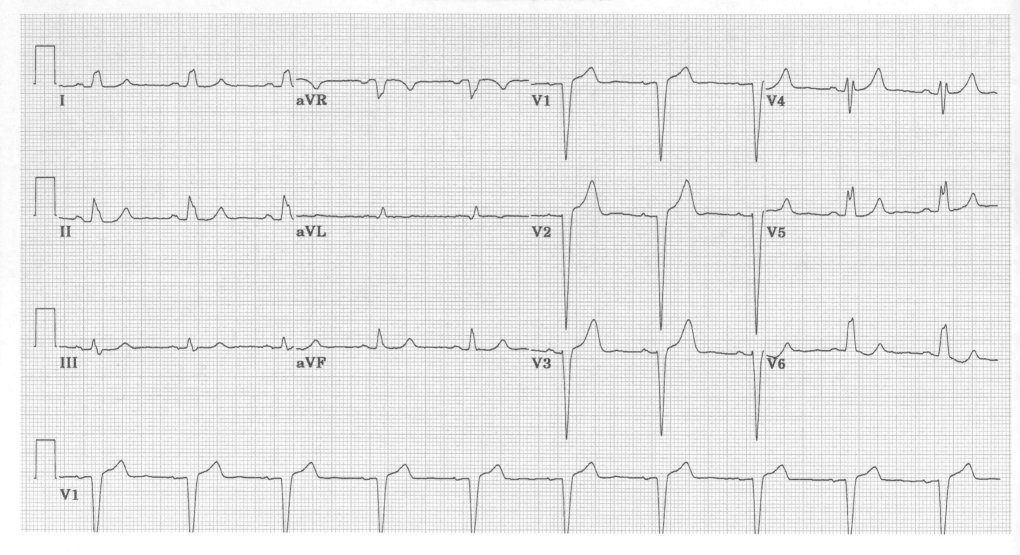

Interpretation Notes: _____

_____

ECG 104 Fifty-three year old woman who is being evaluated in the breast clinic for a recently performed abnormal mammogram. She has no known cardiac conditions and is on no current medications.

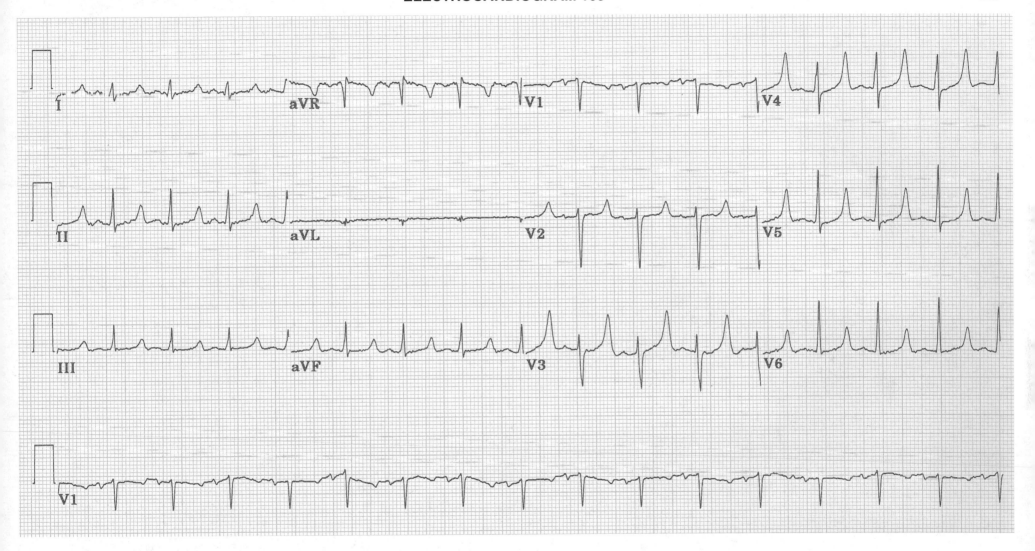

I aVR V1 V4

II aVL V2 V5

III aVF V3 V6

V1

Interpretation Notes: _____

ECG 105 Nineteen year old gentleman with dialysis requiring end stage renal disease of unknown etiology who presented to the hospital with symptoms of shortness of breath and chest x-ray confirmation of pulmonary edema. His serum potassium at the time of admission was 6.8 meq/L. His serum calcium was 6.0 mg/dl.

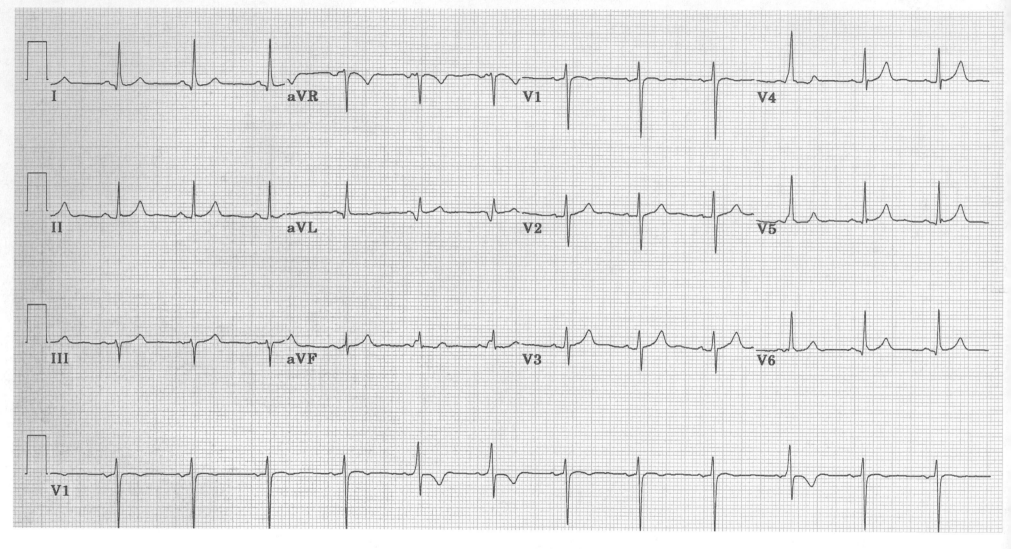

Interpretation Notes: _____

_____

ECG 106 Thirty-three year old woman seen in the outpatient clinic after a recent hospitalization for an asthma exacerbation. She also has a history of palpitations but no prior diagnosis of the Wolff-Parkinson-White syndrome. Medications at the time of this electrocardiogram included amitriptyline, ranitidine, aspirin, and inhalers.

ELECTROCARDIOGRAM 107

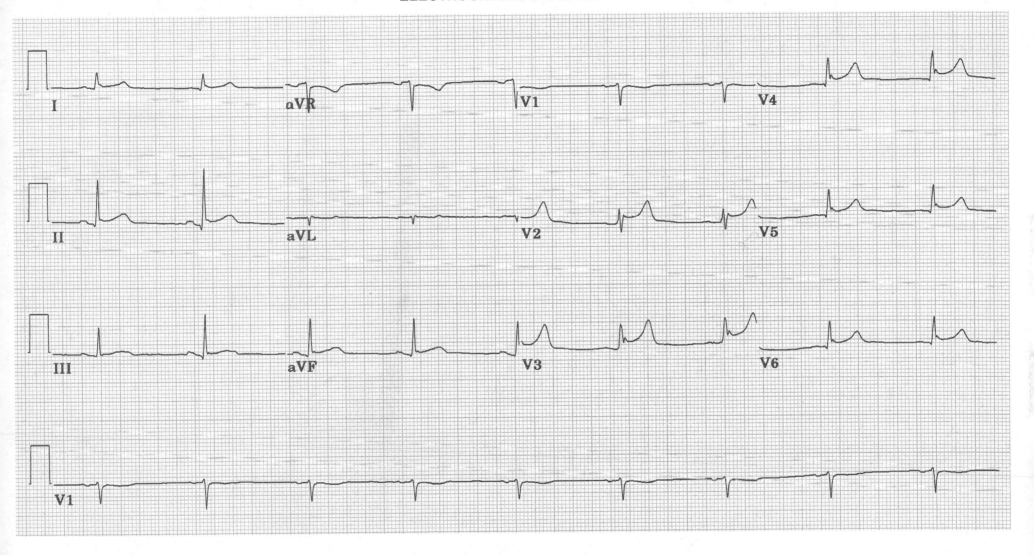

Interpretation Notes:_____

ECG 107 Seventy-one year old gentleman status post coronary artery bypass graft surgery. This electrocardiogram was obtained on the first postoperative day.

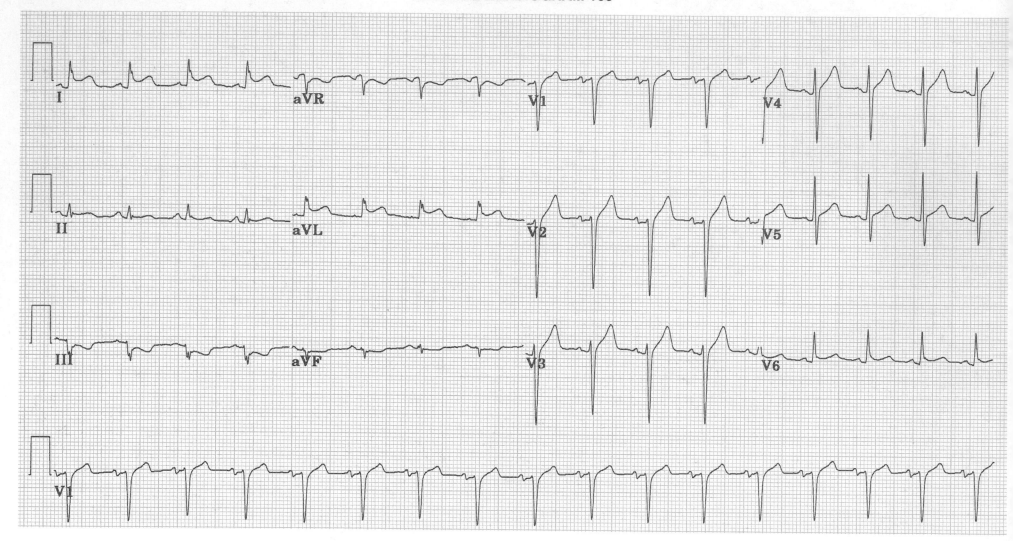

Interpretation Notes: _____

_____

_____

ECG 108 Fifty-nine year old gentleman with coronary artery disease. He is status post recent coronary artery bypass graft surgery.

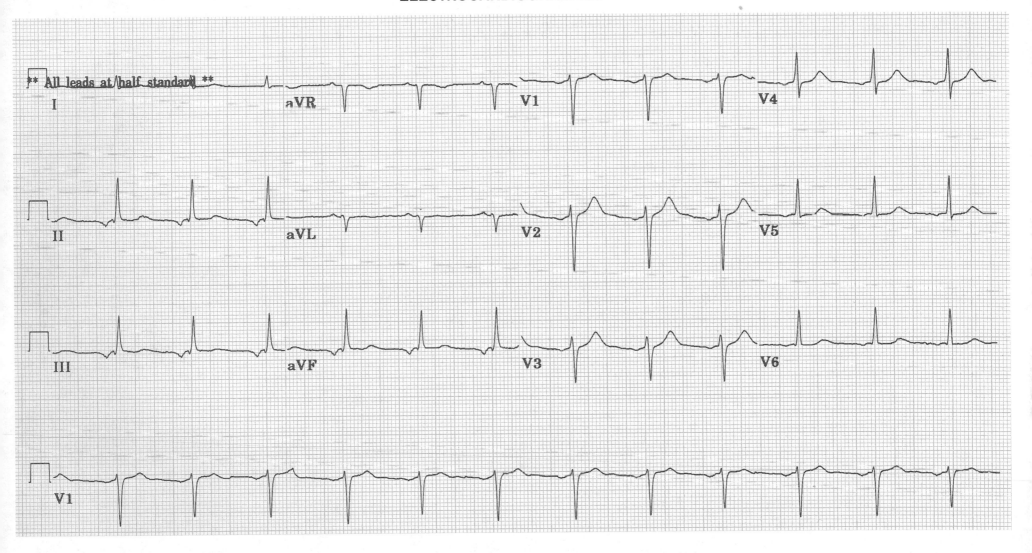

** All leads at half standard **

I aVR V1 V4

II aVL V2 V5

III aVF V3 V6

V1

Interpretation Notes: _____

ECG 109 Seventy-three year old gentleman admitted acutely to the hospital with profound shortness of breath and a blood pressure of 215/130. The patient was intubated. His past medical history includes an abdominal aortic aneurysm, hypertension, and chronic obstructive pulmonary disease. Medications at the time of this electrocardiogram included minoxidil, isosorbide mononitrate, furosemide, and inhalers.

LEVEL I

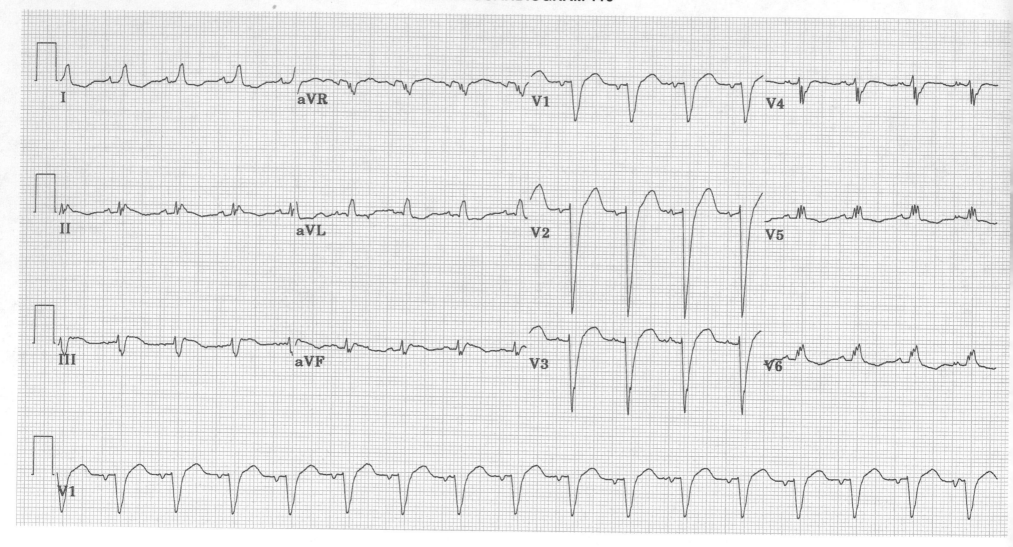

Interpretation Notes: _____

_____

ECG 110 Fifty-two year old gentleman with advanced ischemic heart disease and severe left ventricular systolic dysfunction who is recently postoperative coronary artery bypass graft surgery.

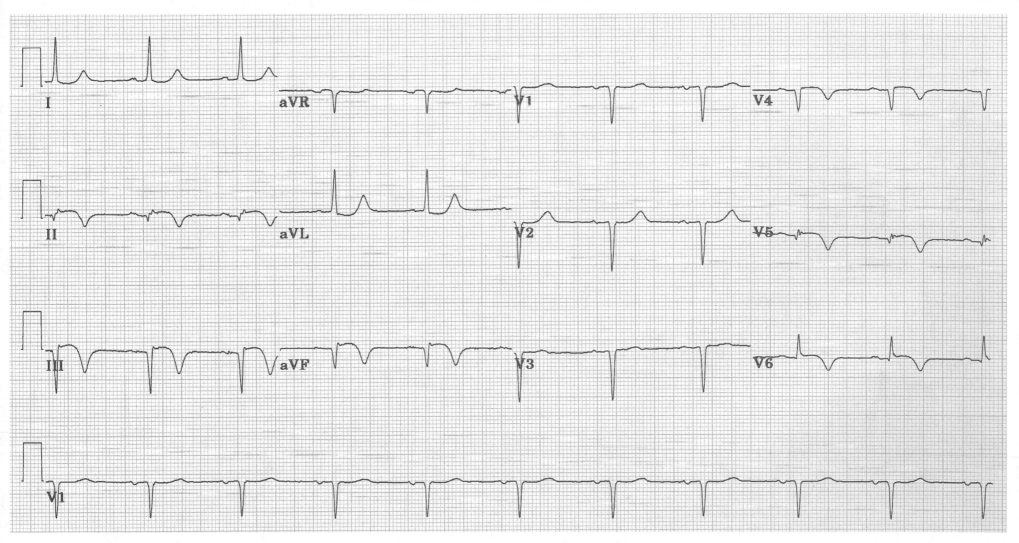

Interpretation Notes: _____

_____

_____

ECG 111 Seventy-seven year old woman who was accepted in hospital transfer after suffering an acute inferior myocardial infarction ten days prior to this electrocardiogram. Co-morbidities include hypertension and a prior cerebral aneurysm repair. Her medications included nifedipine, triamterene/hydrochlorothiazide, and aspirin.

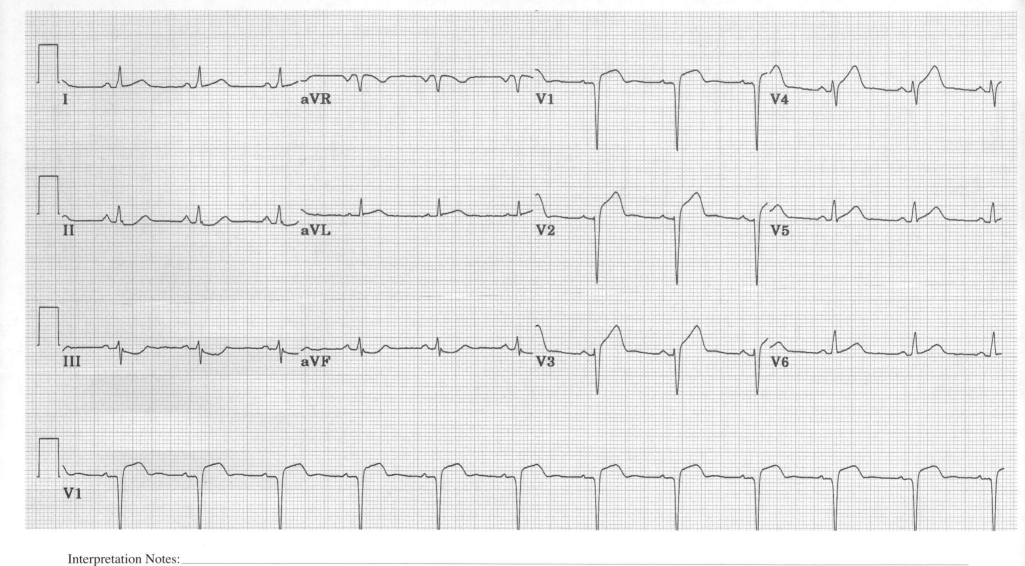

Interpretation Notes: _____

ECG 112 Fifty-one year old gentleman with multiple cardiac risk factors who is accepted in urgent hospital transfer. A cardiac catheterization demonstrated a 100% proximal left anterior descending coronary artery obstruction and moderate left ventricular systolic dysfunction. The patient suffered recurrent myocardial ischemia and was subsequently referred for successful coronary artery bypass graft surgery.

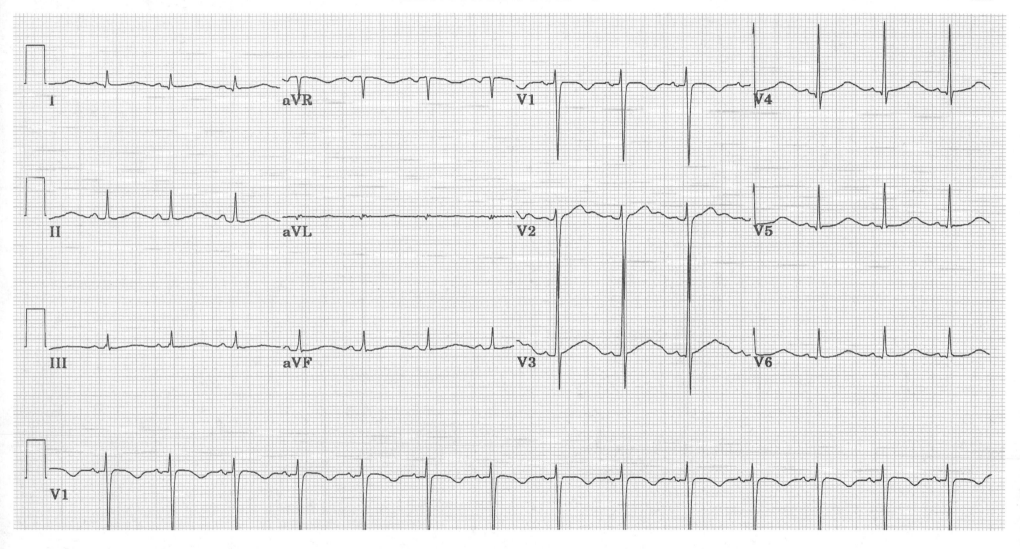

Interpretation Notes:_____

ECG 113 Twenty-eight year old gentleman status post orthotopic liver transplantation secondary to chronic hepatitis B infection contracted ten years prior to this electro-cardiogram who re-presents to the hospital with epigastric pain, nausea, and hematemesis. His medications at the time of this electrocardiogram included cyclosporine, prednisone, and omeprazole. His admission serum chemistries were notable for a serum potassium level of 2.3 meq/L.

LEVEL I

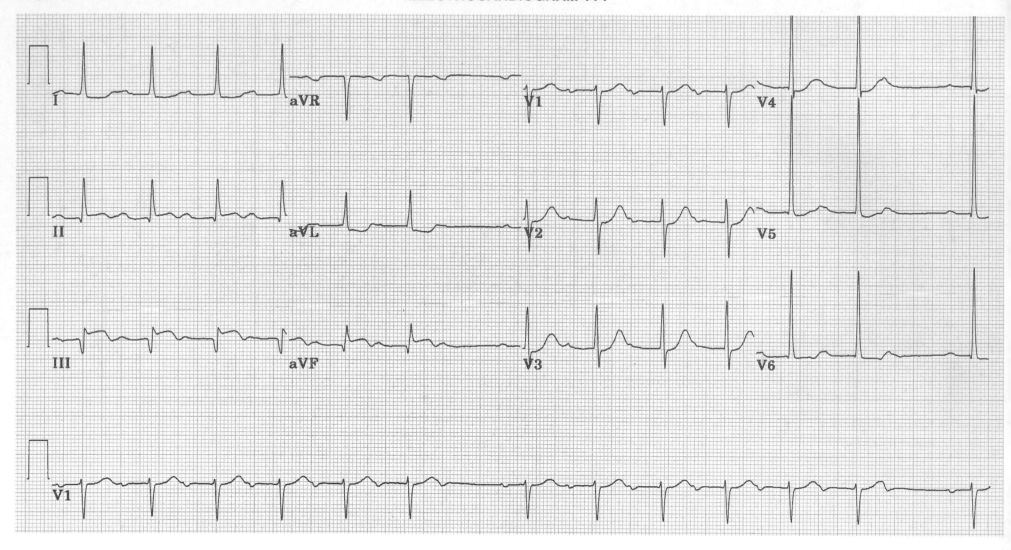

Interpretation Notes:_____

_____

_____

ECG 114 Seventy-four year old gentleman who presents to the hospital with sudden onset anterior chest discomfort and the accompanying electrocardiogram. An urgent cardiac catheterization was followed by a percutaneous transluminal coronary angioplasty to the right coronary artery as acute thrombus was present. Medications at the time of this electrocardiogram included intravenous heparin, intravenous nitroglycerin, aspirin, and metoprolol.

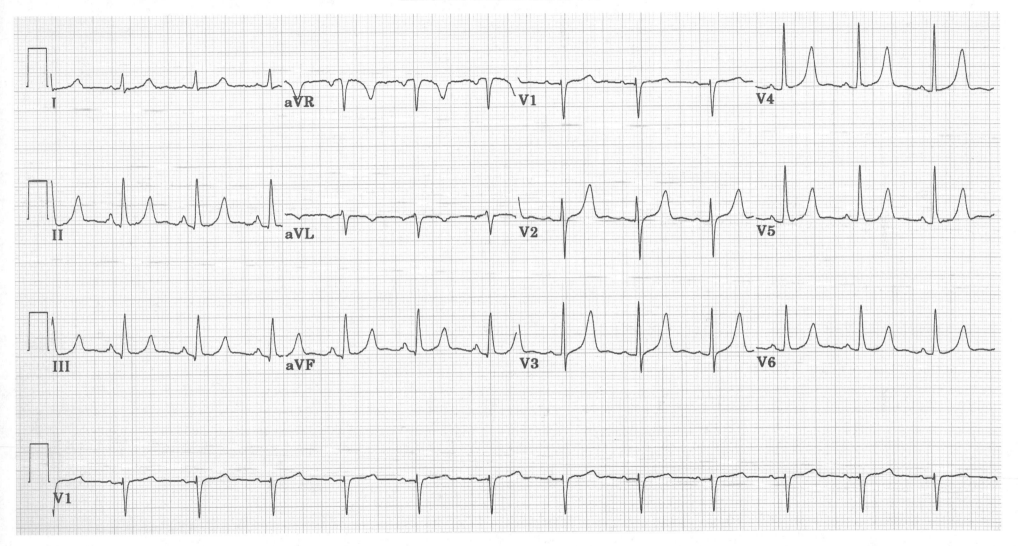

Interpretation Notes: _____

_____

ECG 115 Sixty-seven year old woman on hemodialysis secondary to long-standing hypertension who is urgently admitted to the hospital with sudden onset sharp abdominal pain. Her medications included atenolol, famotidine, timolol eye drops, and hydralazine. Her serum potassium at the time of this electrocardiogram was 4.4 meq/L.

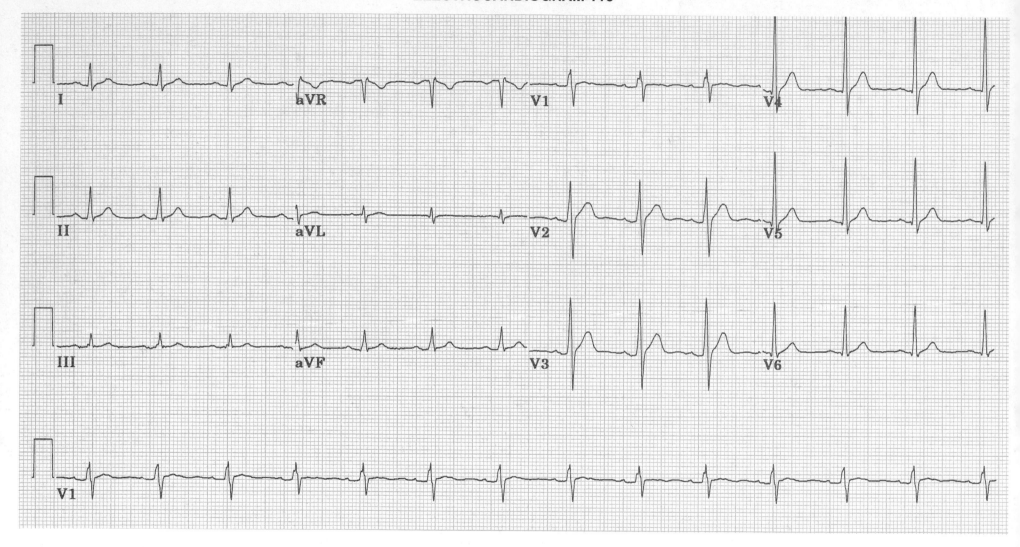

Interpretation Notes: _____

_____

ECG 116 Fifty year old gentleman with recently diagnosed multiple myeloma and a serum calcium level of 13.1 mg/dl.

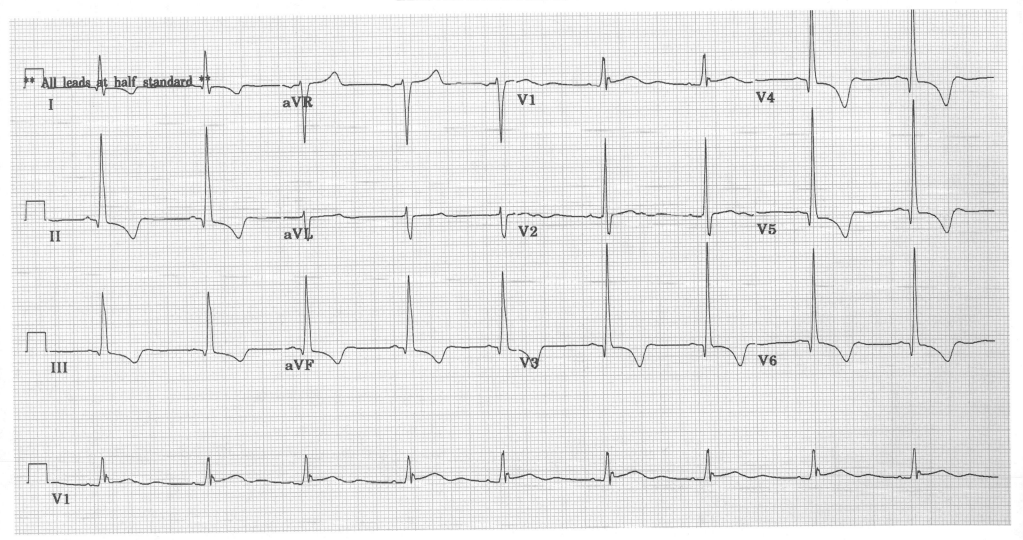

** All leads at half standard **

I aVR V1 V4

II aVL V2 V5

III aVF V3 V6

V1

Interpretation Notes: _____

ECG 117 Seventy-four year old gentleman with hypertrophic obstructive cardiomyopathy who is being seen in follow-up in the psychiatry department for chronic depression. His cardiac medications included verapamil and atenolol.

ELECTROCARDIOGRAM 118

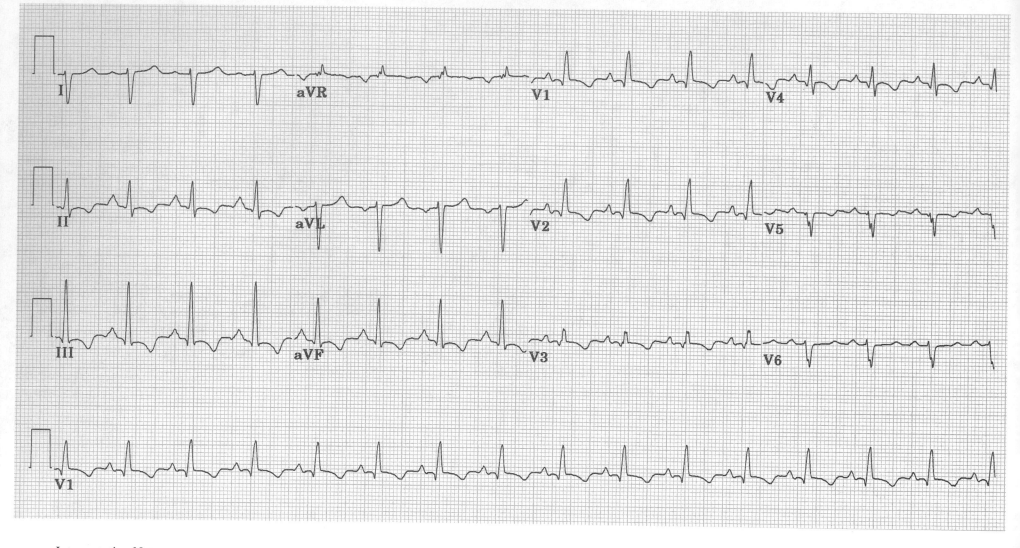

Interpretation Notes: _____

_____

_____

ECG 118 Forty year old woman with primary pulmonary hypertension and severe right ventricular systolic dysfunction admitted for further evaluation and treatment of worsening right-sided congestive heart failure. Her medications included warfarin, nifedipine, furosemide, potassium, and inhaled bronchodilators.

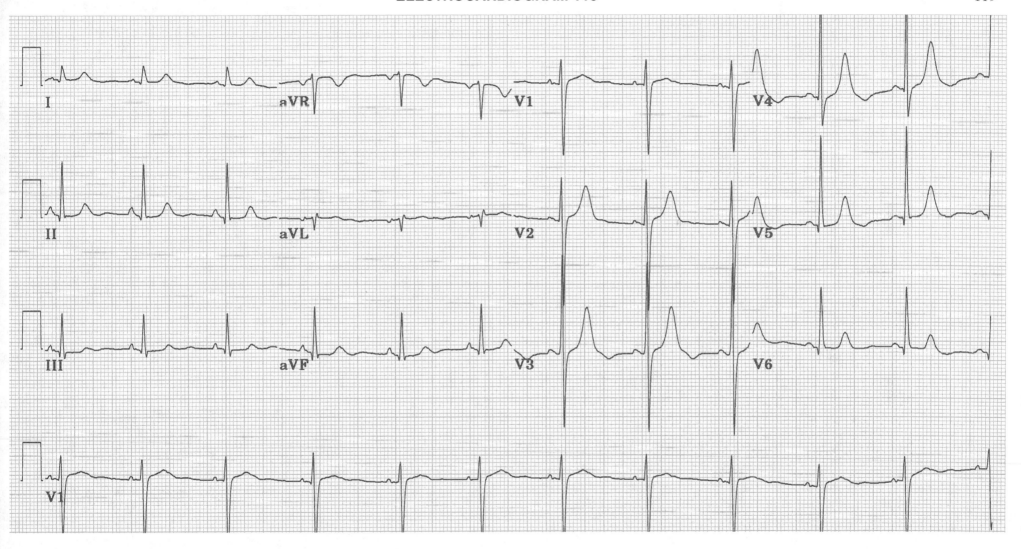

ECG 119 Fifty-three year old woman who was seen in the emergency room with an acute upper GI distress syndrome. She has a long-standing history of tobacco use. Her medications included ranitidine. A serum potassium level was not checked at the time of this electrocardiogram.

Interpretation Notes:_____
_____
_____

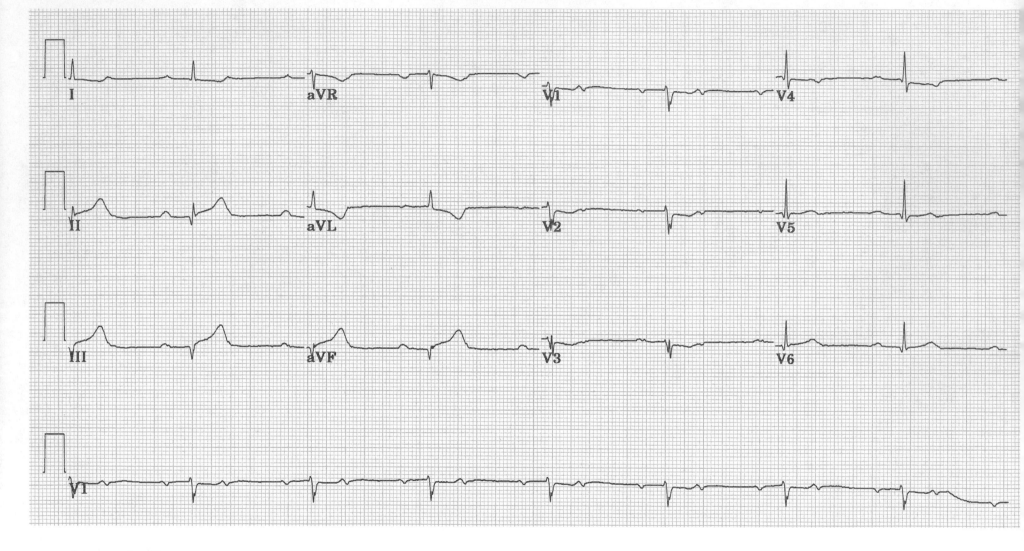

Interpretation Notes: _____

_____

_____

ECG 120 Sixty-four year old gentleman who presented to an outside emergency room with an acute onset chest discomfort syndrome accepted in urgent hospital transfer for cardiac catheterization. The patient received immediate thrombolytic therapy. A cardiac catheterization demonstrated a 100% distal occlusion of a saphenous vein graft to the right coronary artery which was successfully angioplastied.

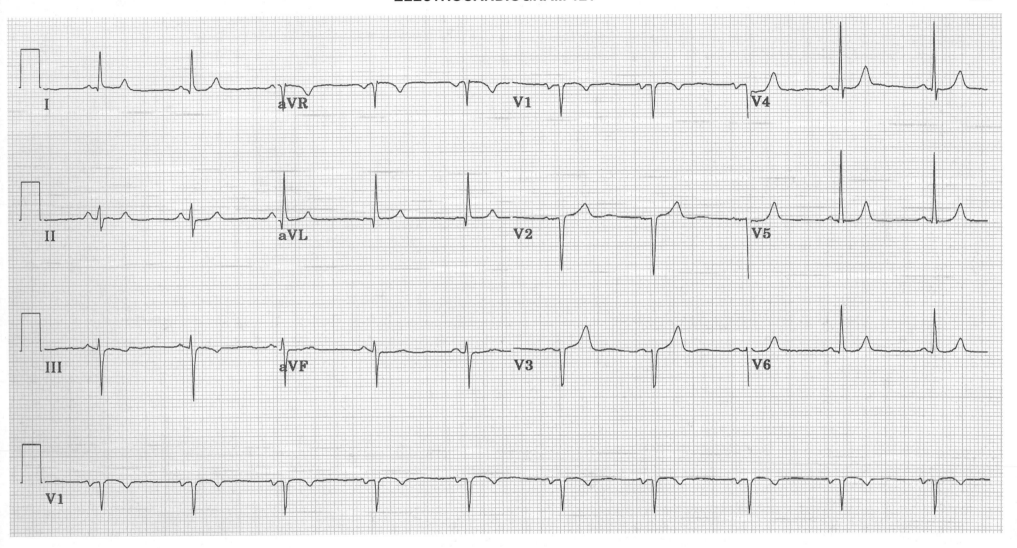

Interpretation Notes: _____

_____

ECG 121 Sixty-seven year old woman with a history of essential thrombocytosis, hypertension, and glaucoma seen in routine follow-up. She had no active cardiac symptoms and a potassium level was normal at the time of this electrocardiogram.

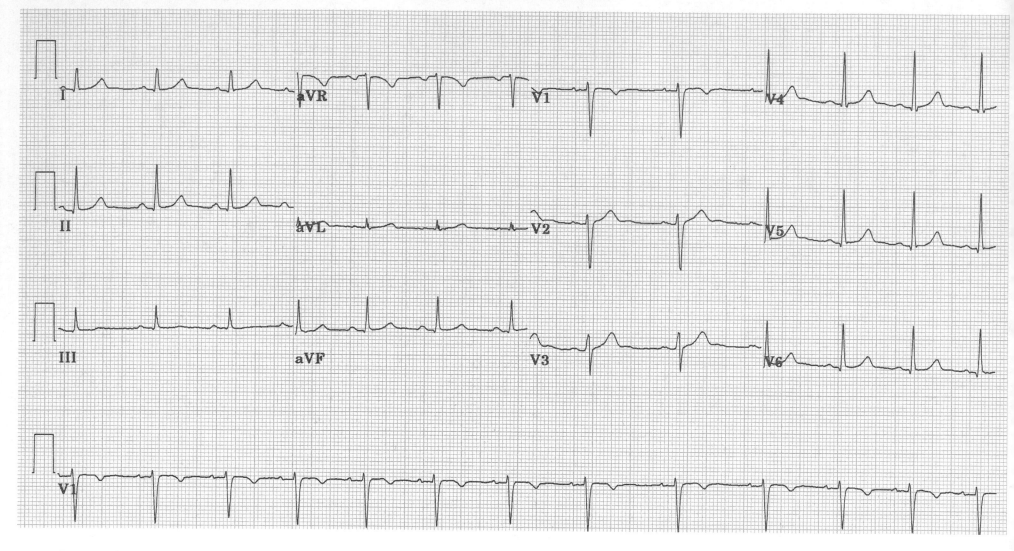

Interpretation Notes:_____

ECG 122 Twenty-two year old woman who presents for evaluation of headaches. Her past medical history includes asthma. Her medications included inhalers for her asthma.

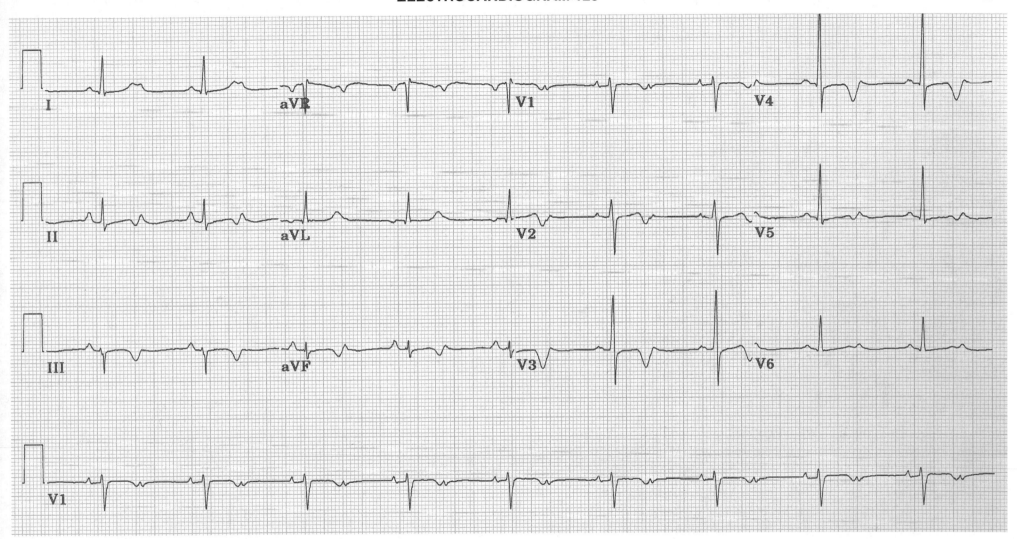

I aVR V1 V4

II aVL V2 V5

III aVF V3 V6

V1

Interpretation Notes: _____

ECG 123 Sixty-three year old gentleman with non-insulin requiring diabetes mellitus referred to the cardiac arrhythmia clinic for consideration of permanent pacemaker placement. He recently was diagnosed with endocarditis related to a prior pacemaker which necessitated lead extraction. His medications included vancomycin and ceftazidime.

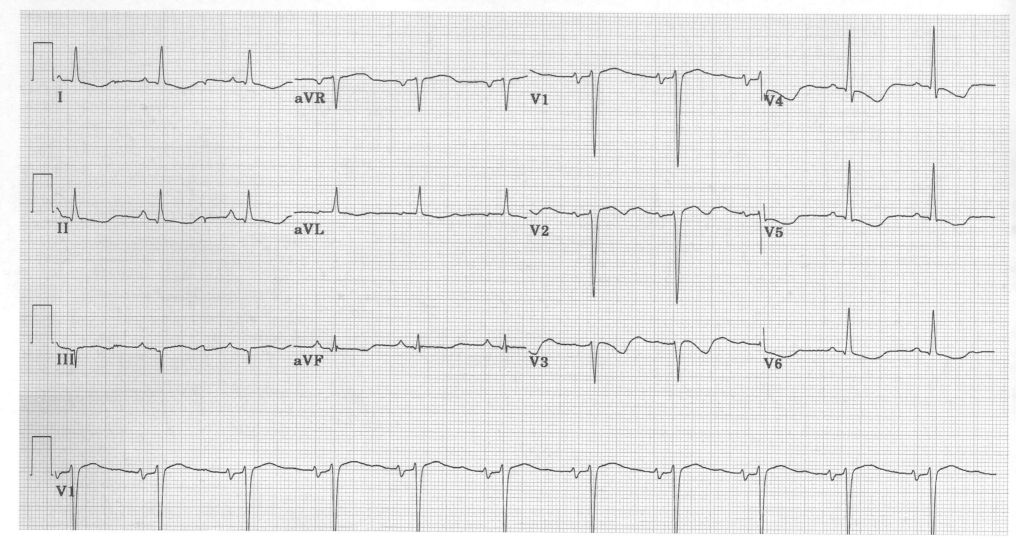

Interpretation Notes: _____

_____

ECG 124 Sixty-seven year old woman admitted with mental status changes and a confirmed subarachnoid hemorrhage. Co-morbid conditions include liver cirrhosis, hypertension, and paroxysmal atrial fibrillation. Medications at the time of this electrocardiogram included isosorbide mononitrate, spironolactone, and disopyramide.

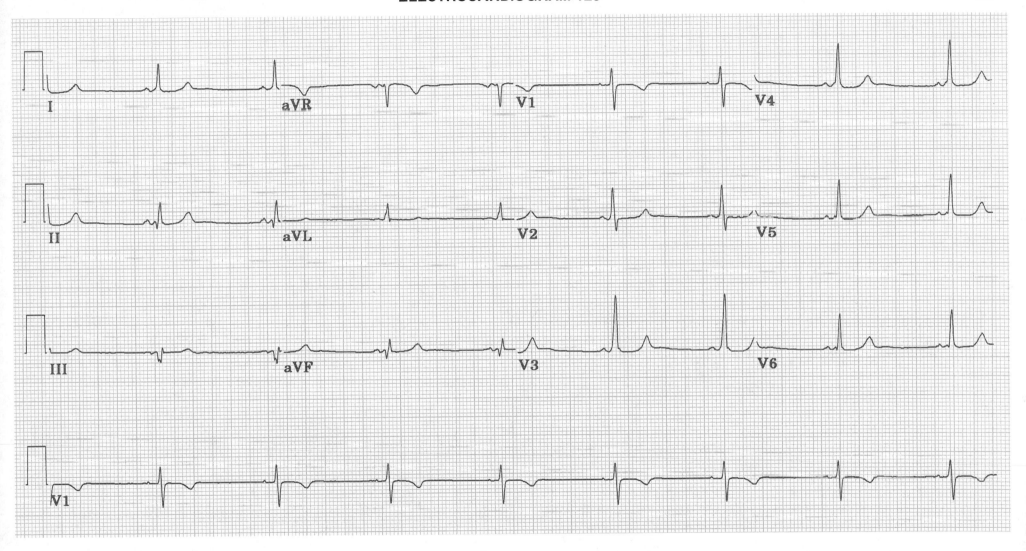

I   aVR   V1   V4

II   aVL   V2   V5

III   aVF   V3   V6

V1

Interpretation Notes: _____

ECG 125 Forty-five year old gentleman with a recent history of documented atrial fibrillation in the setting of the Wolff-Parkinson-White syndrome. He underwent successful radiofrequency ablation of a left posterolateral accessory pathway shortly after this electrocardiogram was obtained.

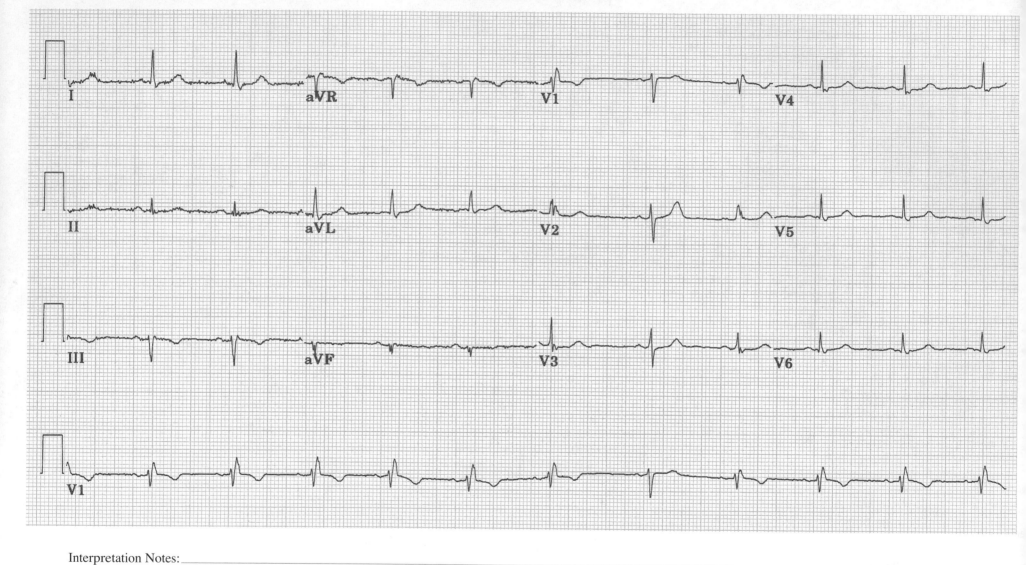

I   aVR   V1   V4

II   aVL   V2   V5

III   aVF   V3   V6

V1

Interpretation Notes: _____

_____

ECG 126 Seventy-five year old woman without a prior cardiac history who is being evaluated preoperatively for a right hip replacement.

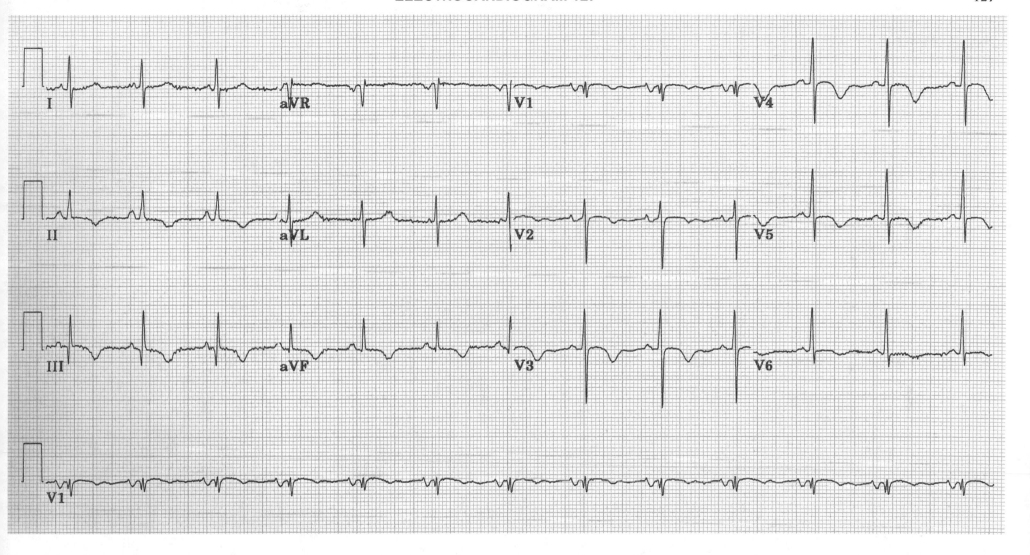

I aVR V1 V4

II aVL V2 V5

III aVF V3 V6

V1

Interpretation Notes: _____

_____

ECG 127 Eighty-two year old woman who presents to the hospital with acute onset severe shortness of breath. Her past medical history includes hypertension and gout. Her admission blood gas demonstrated advanced hypoxemia and a V/Q scan was interpreted as high probability for a pulmonary embolism.

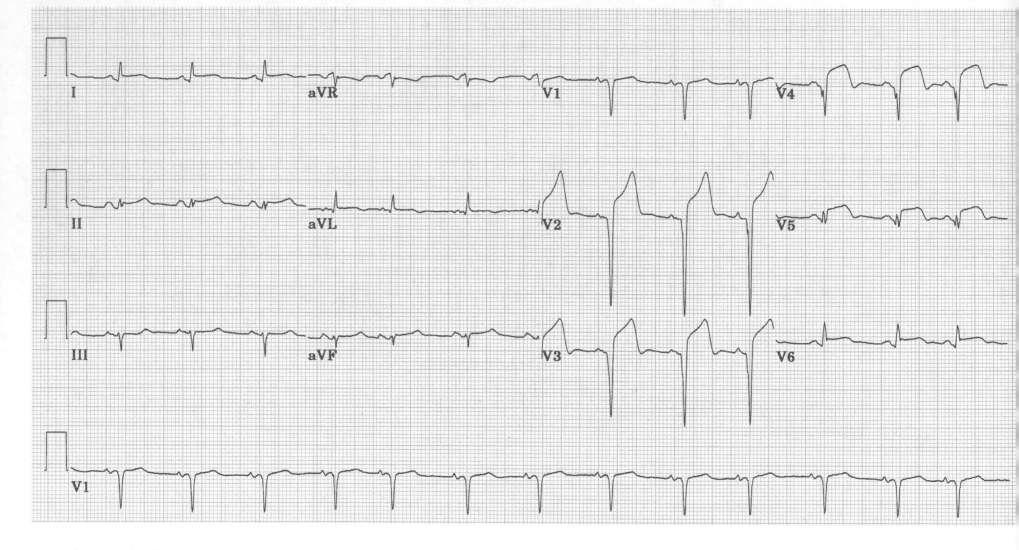

I aVR V1 V4

II aVL V2 V5

III aVF V3 V6

V1

Interpretation Notes: _____

ECG 128 Seventy-three year old gentleman who presented to the emergency room with severe constant chest discomfort and an electrocardiogram consistent with an extensive acute myocardial infarction. The patient developed cardiogenic shock and was taken to the cardiac catheterization laboratory where an urgent angioplasty of a 100% proximal left anterior descending occlusion was performed. The patient developed pneumonia, hypotension, and subsequently expired.

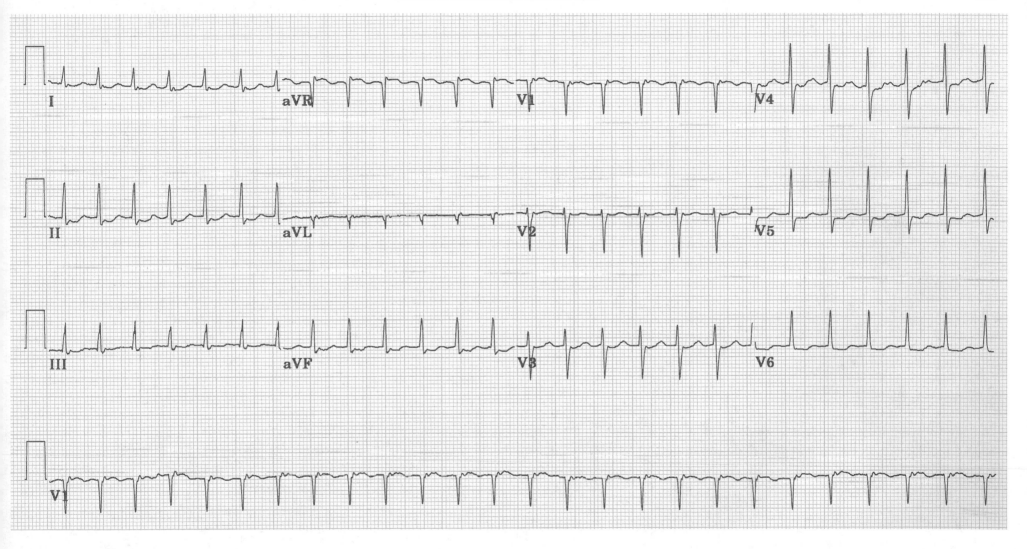

I aVR V1 V4

II aVL V2 V5

III aVF V3 V6

V1

Interpretation Notes: _____

ECG 129 Forty-four year old woman with a several hour history of "rapid heart beating" and mild shortness of breath. Her past medical history includes hypertension. Her medications included lisinopril. The patient received intravenous adenosine which promptly converted this dysrhythmia to normal sinus rhythm.

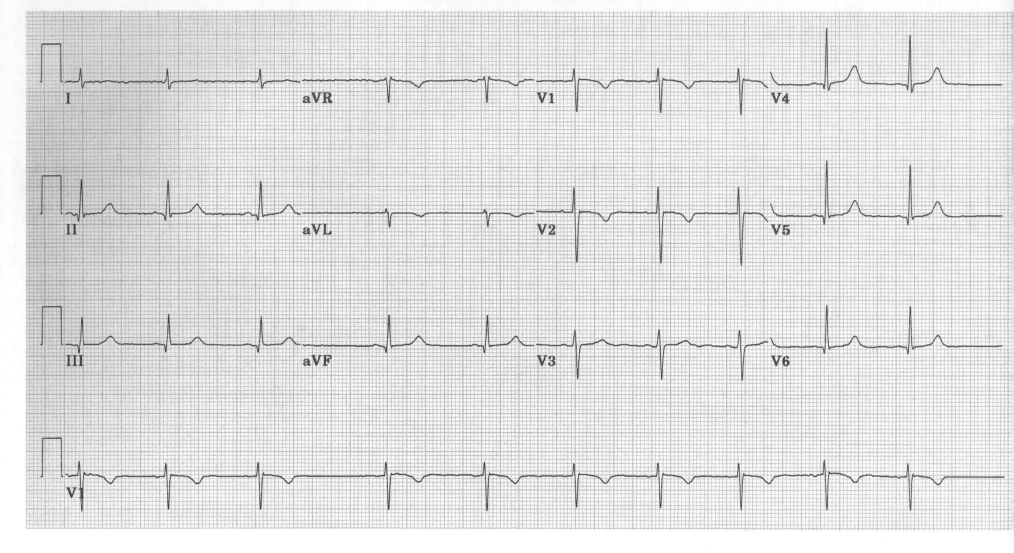

Interpretation Notes: _____

_____

ECG 130 Thirty-four year old woman who presents to the hospital with acute onset epigastric pain, diarrhea, and dizziness. Her past medical history includes migraine headaches and nephrolithiasis.

ELECTROCARDIOGRAM 131

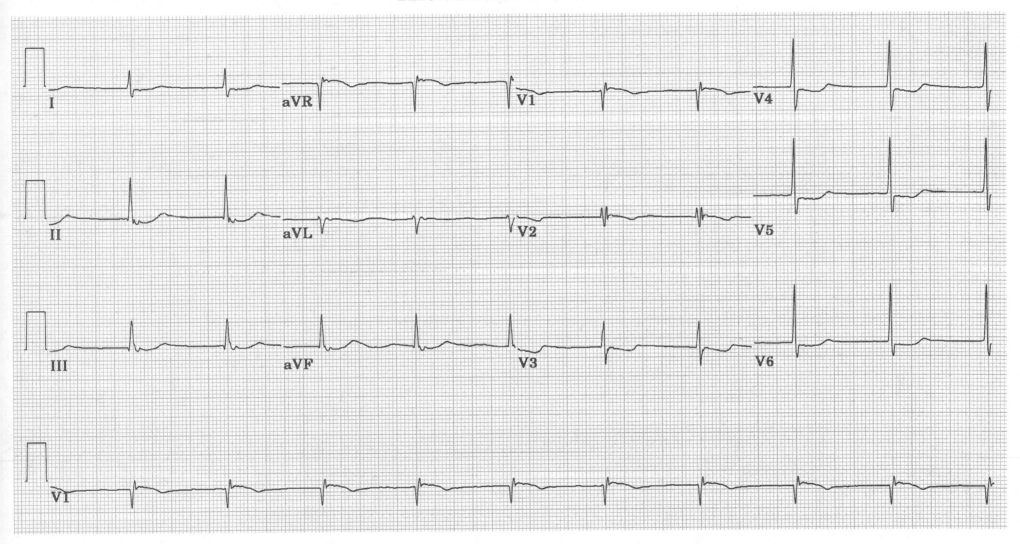

Interpretation Notes: _____

ECG 131 Seventy-two year old woman recently status post aortic valve replacement, pericardial patch closure of an atrial septal defect and ascending aorta replacement with a synthetic graft for an ascending aortic aneurysm. Her medications included digoxin, warfarin, metoprolol, and amlodipine.

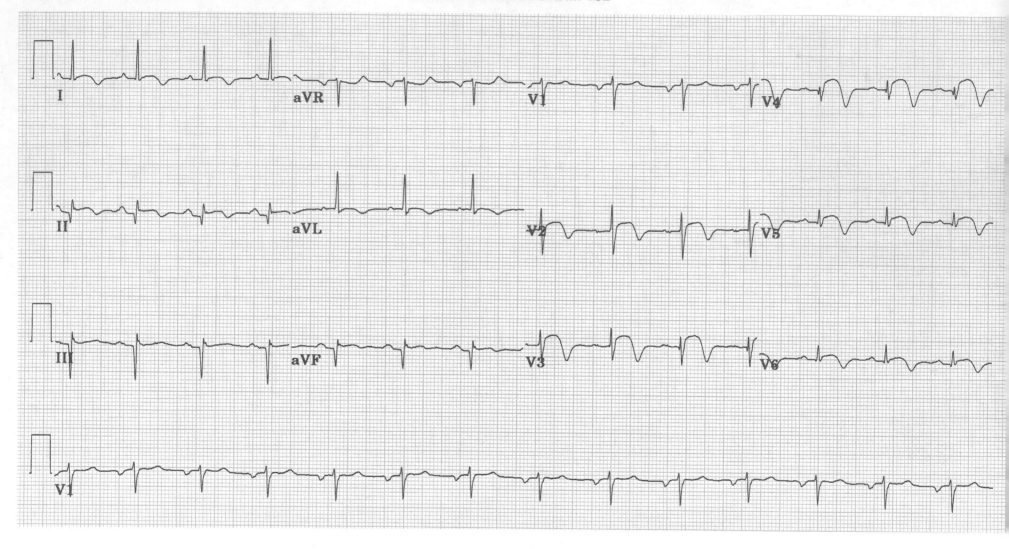

I   aVR   V1   V4

II   aVL   V2   V5

III   aVF   V3   V6

V1

Interpretation Notes: _____

_____

ECG 132 Seventy year old gentleman who presented to the emergency room with a two day history of chest pressure, nausea, and vomiting. Serial serum cardiac enzyme analysis demonstrated evidence of acute myocardial injury. A cardiac catheterization demonstrated a 100% stenosis of the left anterior descending coronary artery and a 50% stenosis of the right coronary artery.

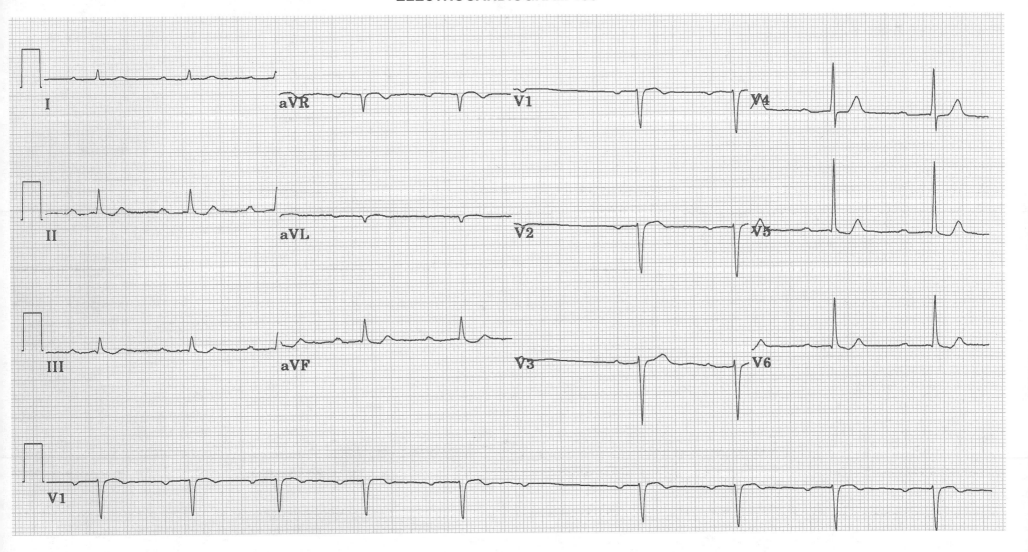

Interpretation Notes:

ECG 133 Fifty-seven year old woman hospitalized with advanced congestive heart failure requiring intubation in the setting of severe aortic and mitral insufficiency. She underwent successful St. Jude mitral and aortic valve replacements. Medications at the time of this electrocardiogram included furosemide, enalapril, topical nitroglycerin, potassium, and digoxin.

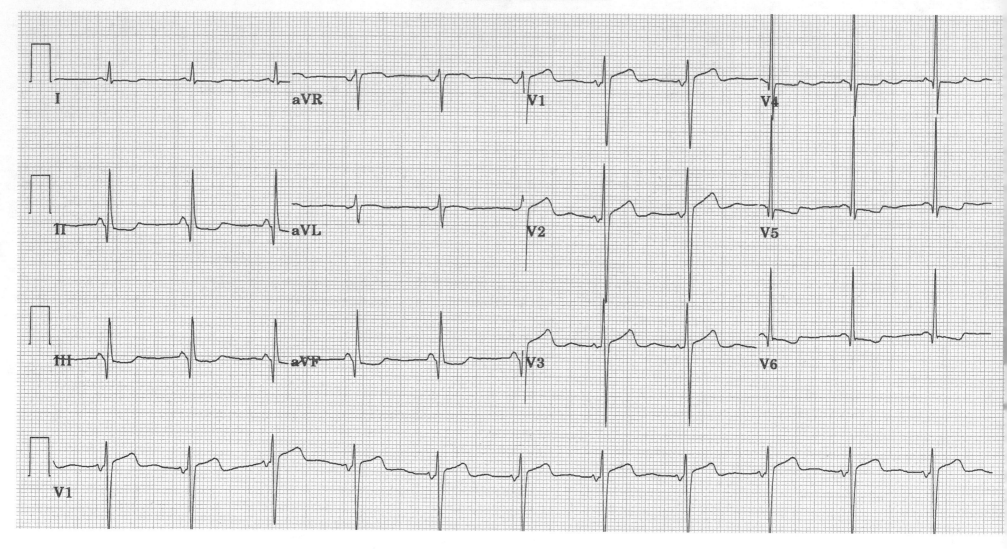

I aVR V1 V4

II aVL V2 V5

III aVF V3 V6

V1

Interpretation Notes: _____

ECG 134 Sixty-one year old gentleman with insulin requiring diabetes mellitus who presented to the hospital with a 24 hour history of fatigue, chills, and weakness. A subsequent evaluation included positive blood cultures for a gram negative organism.

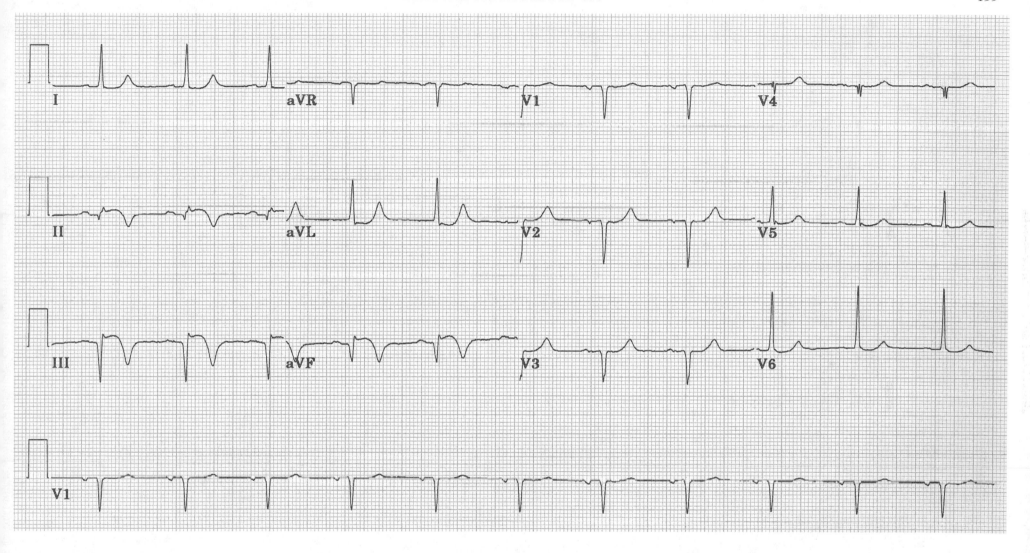

I aVR V1 V4

II aVL V2 V5

III aVF V3 V6

V1

Interpretation Notes: _____

_____

ECG 135 Seventy-seven year old woman who was accepted in hospital transfer after suffering an acute inferior myocardial infarction ten days prior to this electrocardiogram. Co-morbidities include hypertension and a prior cerebral aneurysm repair. Her medications included nifedipine, triamterene/hydrochlorothiazide, and aspirin.

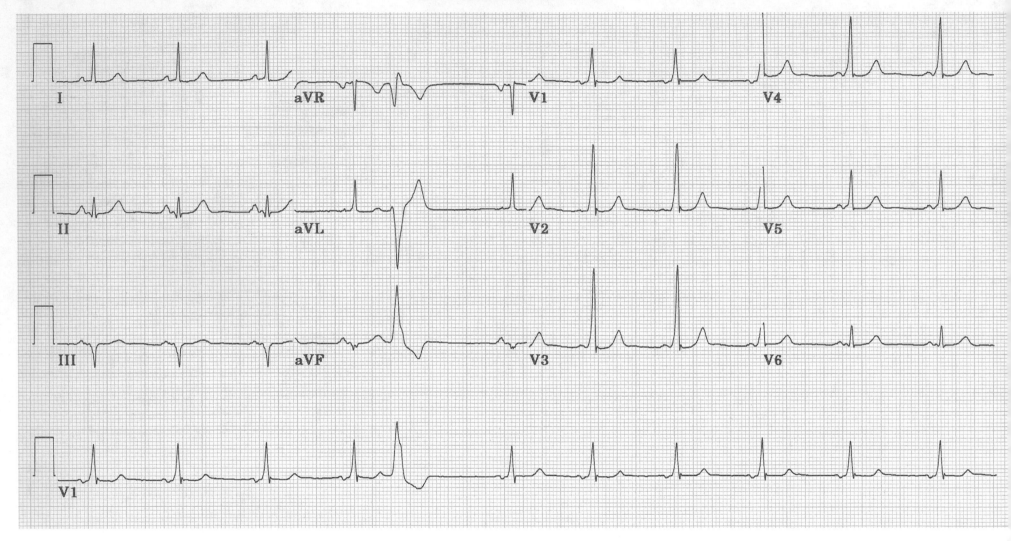

I

aVR

V1

V4

II

aVL

V2

V5

III

aVF

V3

V6

V1

Interpretation Notes:_____

ECG 136 Fifty-eight year old woman who is being evaluated preoperatively prior to a bilateral mastectomy for cancer of the breast. Her cardiac history includes a normal cardiac catheterization prompted by a chest discomfort syndrome two years before this electrocardiogram. There is no clinical history of palpitations, pre-syncope, or a prior myocardial infarction.

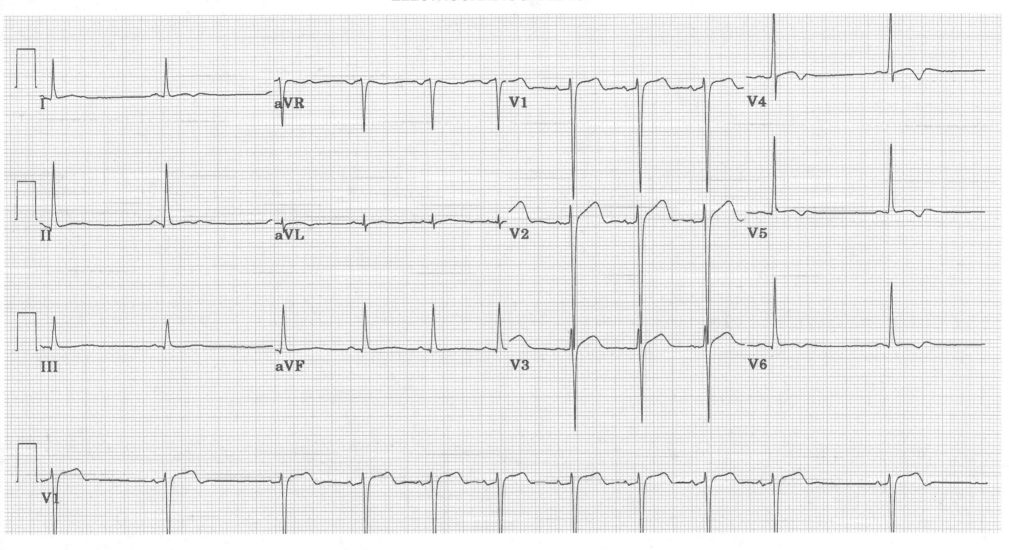

Interpretation Notes:_____

_____

ECG 137 Thirty-two year old gentleman with a history of hepatitis and alcohol use who presents for further evaluation of dyspnea. Medications at the time of this electrocardiogram included enalapril, furosemide, and a multi-vitamin.

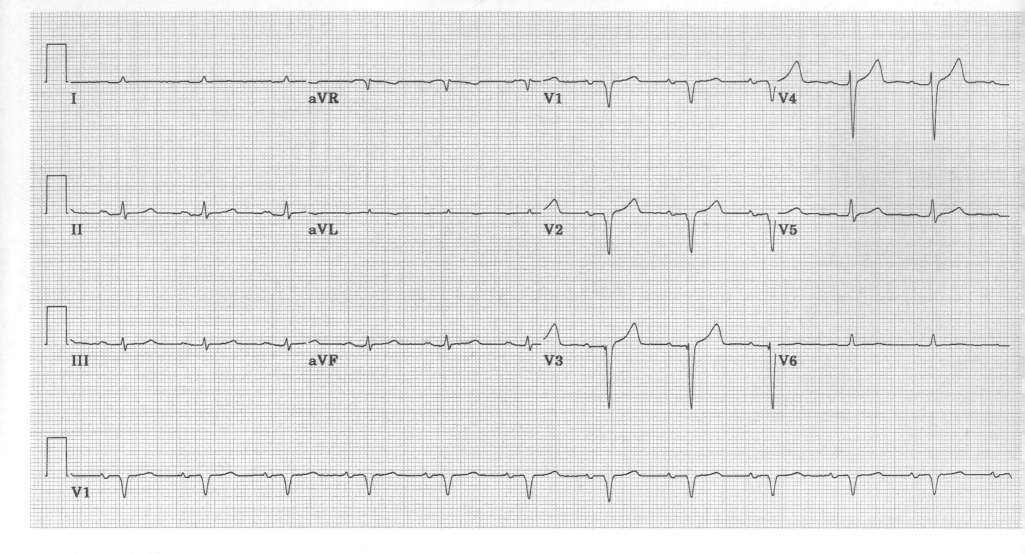

Interpretation Notes: _____

_____

_____

ECG 138 Fifty-one year old gentleman with dialysis requiring renal failure and a recent positive stress echocardiogram referred for a cardiac catheterization. The cardiac catheterization demonstrated multi-vessel coronary artery obstructive disease. No left ventriculogram was performed secondary to the patient's history of renal failure.

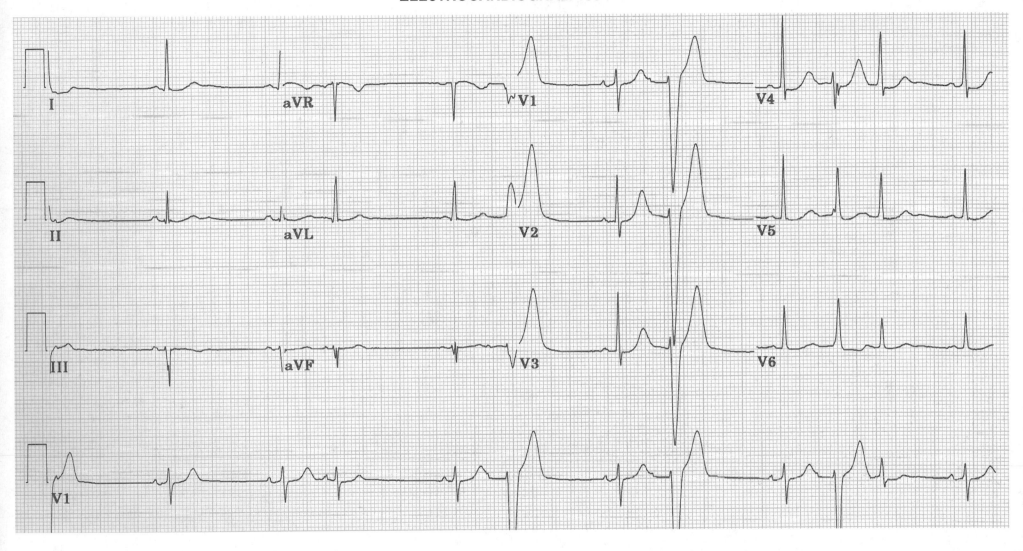

Interpretation Notes: _____

_____

ECG 139 Fifty-six year old gentleman with rheumatoid arthritis who is seen in the outpatient department for a follow-up evaluation. He has no cardiac history and is on no cardiac medications.

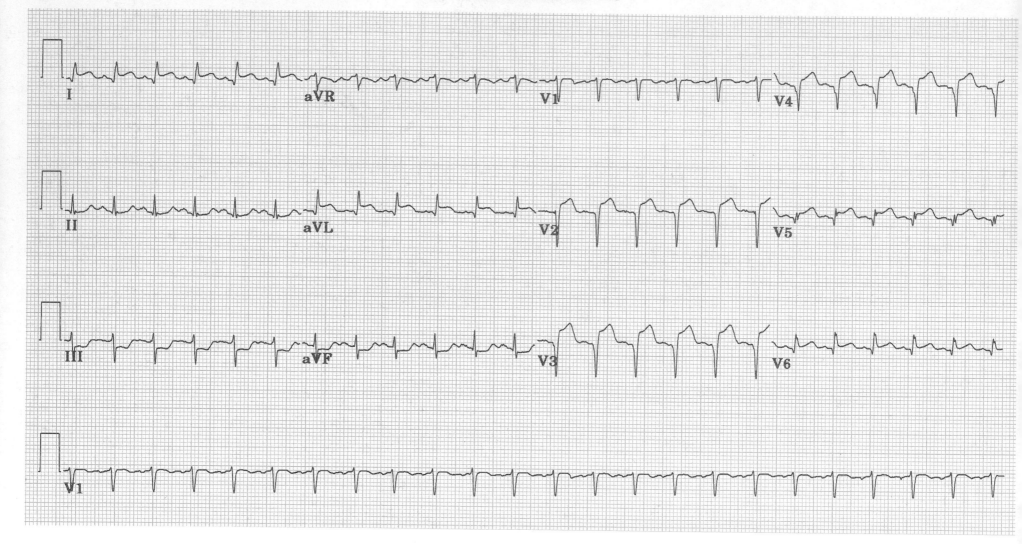

I   aVR   V1   V4

II   aVL   V2   V5

III   aVF   V3   V6

V1

Interpretation Notes: _____

_____

ECG 140 Sixty-six year old woman who underwent persantine thallium stress testing demonstrating a large area of myocardial ischemia. The patient subsequently underwent an angioplasty to her left anterior descending coronary artery complicated by acute closure and infarction. This electrocardiogram was obtained at the time of the percutaneous transluminal coronary angioplasty.

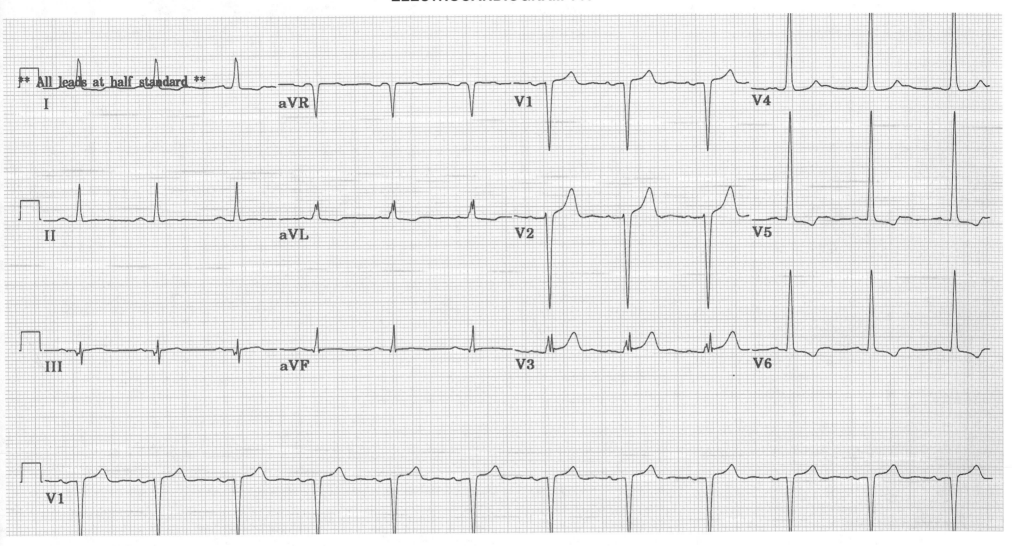

** All leads at half standard **

I · aVR · V1 · V4
II · aVL · V2 · V5
III · aVF · V3 · V6
V1

Interpretation Notes: _____

_____

ECG 141 Twenty-six year old gentleman with severe rheumatic aortic insufficiency seen in preoperative cardiac evaluation prior to anticipated aortic valve replacement. A recent echocardiogram demonstrated severe aortic insufficiency, a dilated left ventricle with mildly reduced left ventricular systolic function, and left ventricular hypertrophy.

LEVEL I

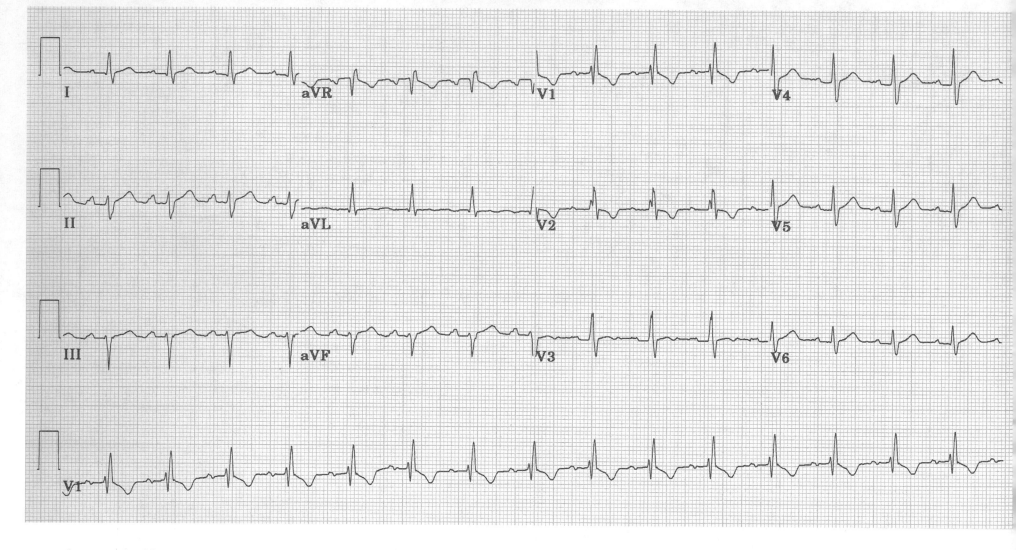

I   aVR   V1   V4

II   aVL   V2   V5

III   aVF   V3   V6

V1

Interpretation Notes: _____

ECG 142 Seventeen year old gentleman with an ostium primum atrial septal defect and cleft mitral valve who underwent this electrocardiogram prior to cardiac surgical repair.

ELECTROCARDIOGRAM 143

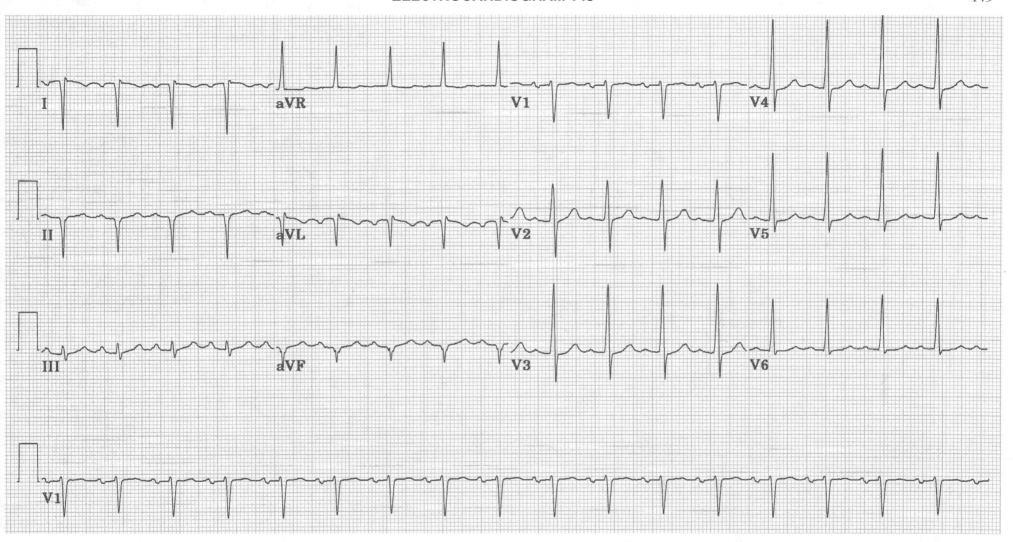

Interpretation Notes: _____

_____

_____

ECG 143 Forty-four year old gentleman with severe peripheral vascular disease admitted for lower extremity revascularization surgery. He has known coronary artery disease and is status post a myocardial infarction in the remote past, location unknown. His medications included insulin, carbamazepine, amitryptiline, and warfarin.

LEVEL I

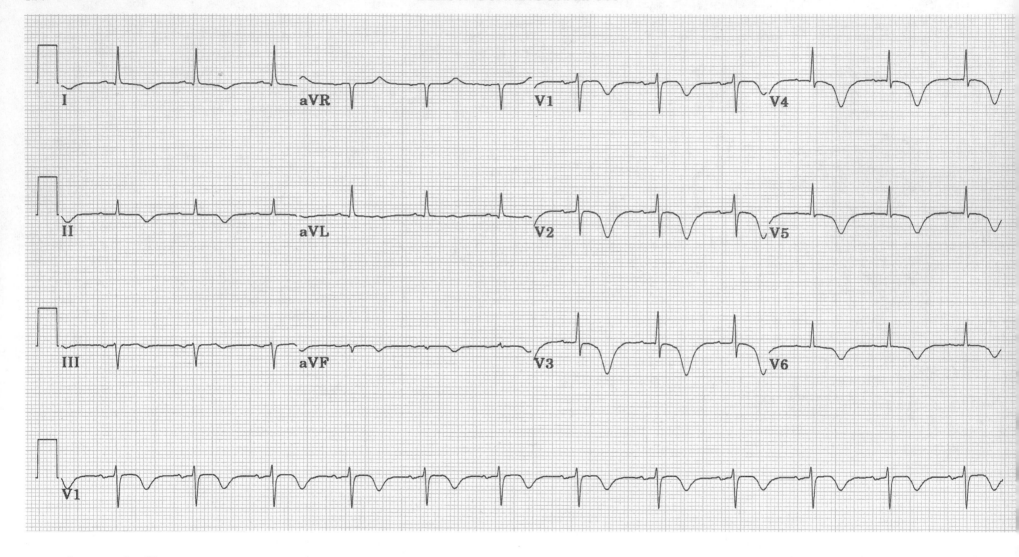

Interpretation Notes: _____

_____

_____

ECG 144 Seventy-two year old woman with a history of insulin requiring diabetes mellitus who is accepted in hospital transfer with the suspected diagnosis of status epilepticus. The patient was diagnosed with a metabolic encephalopathy. Her neurological status failed to improve and she subsequently expired.

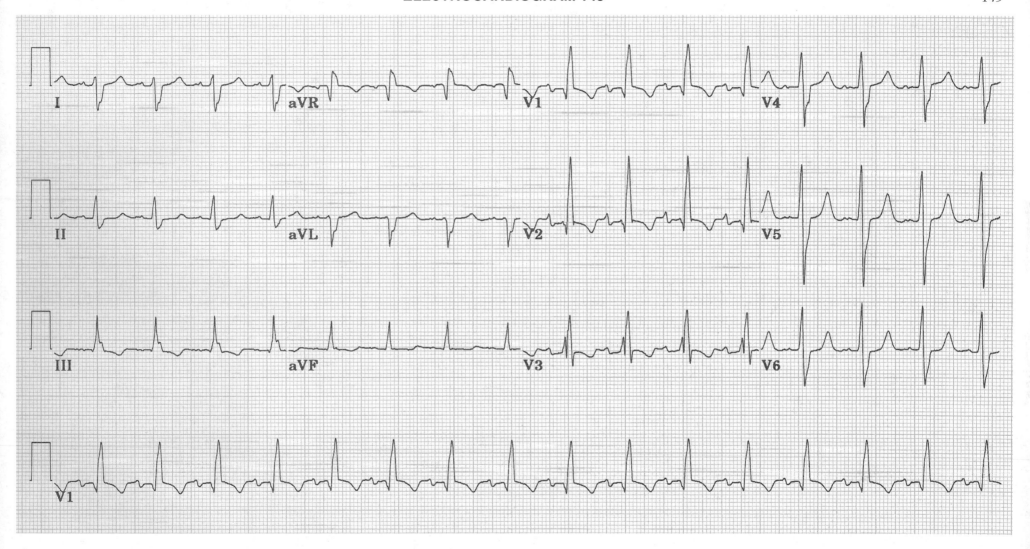

I   aVR   V1   V4

II   aVL   V2   V5

III   aVF   V3   V6

V1

Interpretation Notes: _____

_____

ECG 145 Sixty-six year old woman with coronary artery disease who is recently status post coronary artery bypass graft surgery. Her co-morbidities include non-insulin requiring diabetes mellitus, hypertension, hypothyroidism, and moderate restrictive lung disease. Her medications at the time of this electrocardiogram included aspirin, hydralazine, omeprazole, thyroxine, metoprolol, and prednisone.

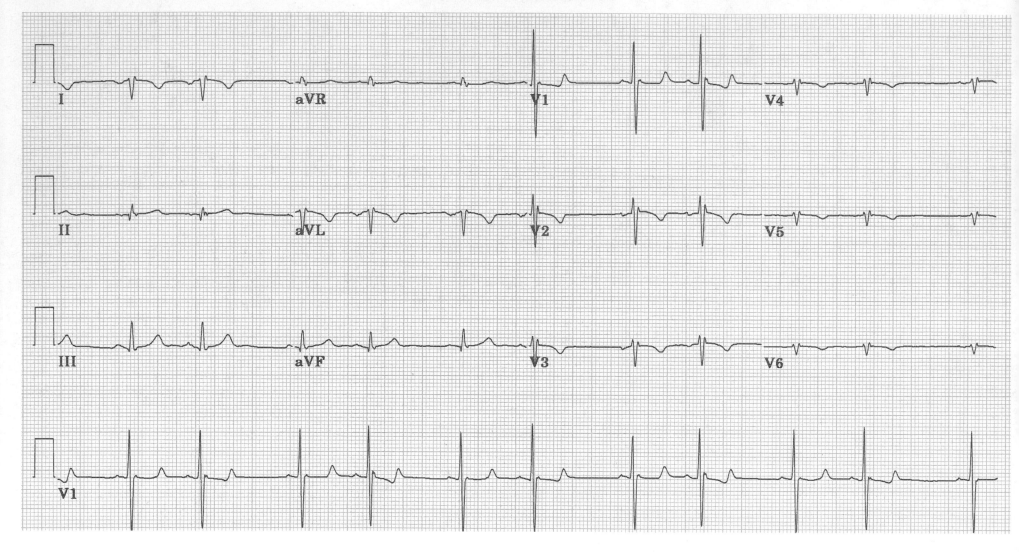

Interpretation Notes: _____

_____

ECG 146 Twenty-two year old woman who presents for evaluation of dysplastic nevi. She has known dextrocardia and is on no current medications.

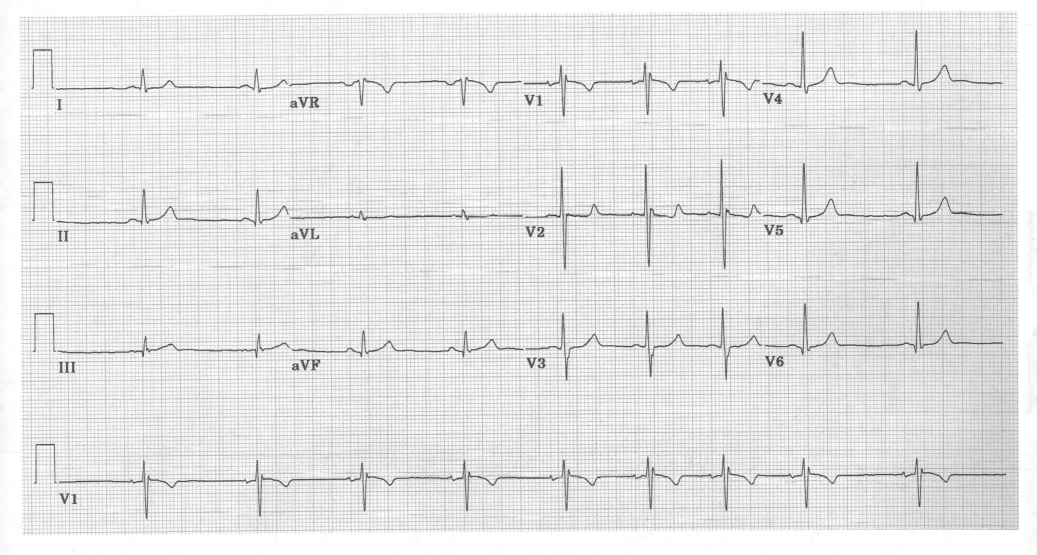

I aVR V1 V4

II aVL V2 V5

III aVF V3 V6

V1

Interpretation Notes: _____

_____

ECG 147 Twenty-two year old woman who presents for evaluation of dysplastic nevi. She has known dextrocardia and is on no current medications.

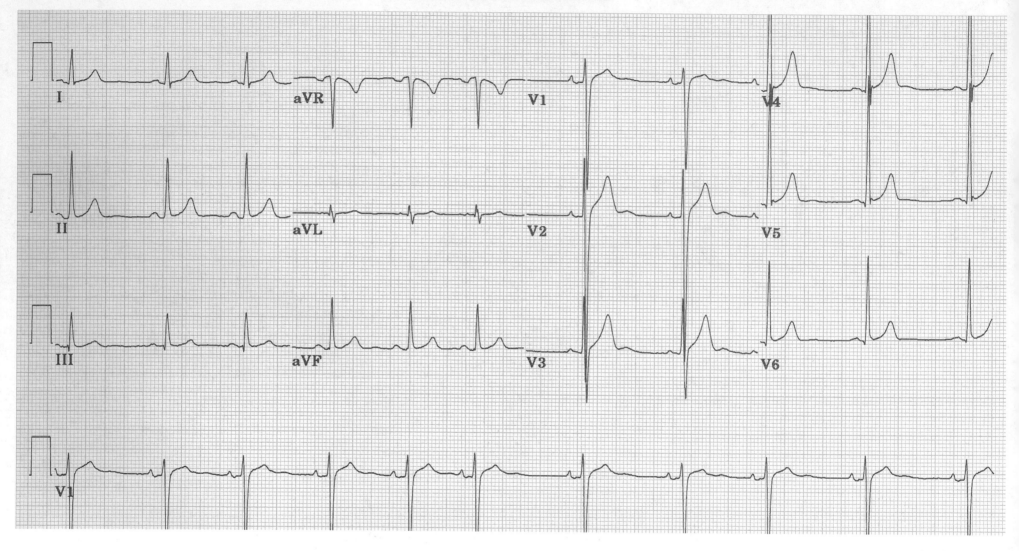

Interpretation Notes: _____

_____

ECG 148 Nineteen year old gentleman with a history of a seizure disorder admitted for evaluation after an intentional carbamazepine overdose.

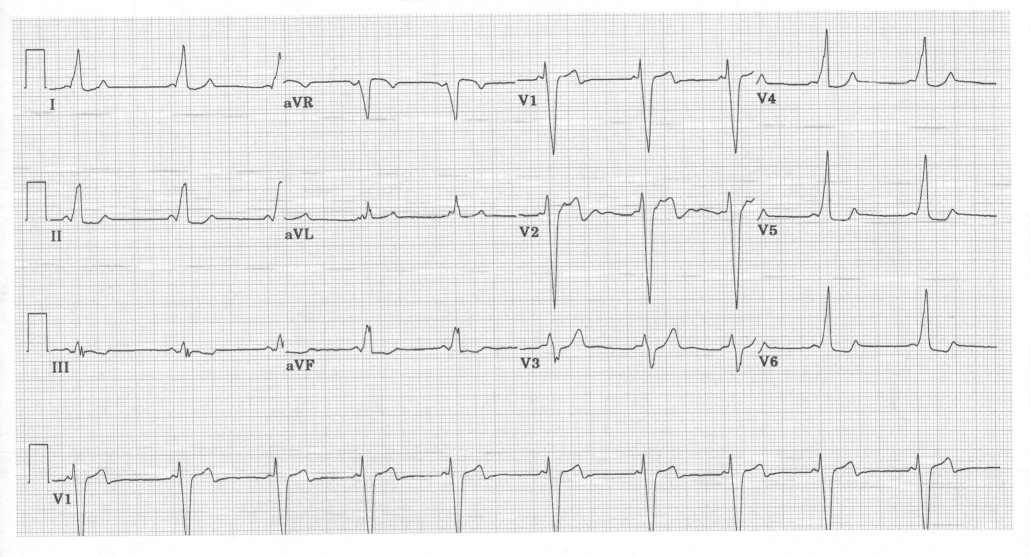

Interpretation Notes:

ECG 149 Twenty-two year old gentleman seen prior to a planned radiofrequency ablation of a right anterior para-septal accessory pathway. He is on no current medications. The patient suffers from frequent palpitations but no pre-syncope.

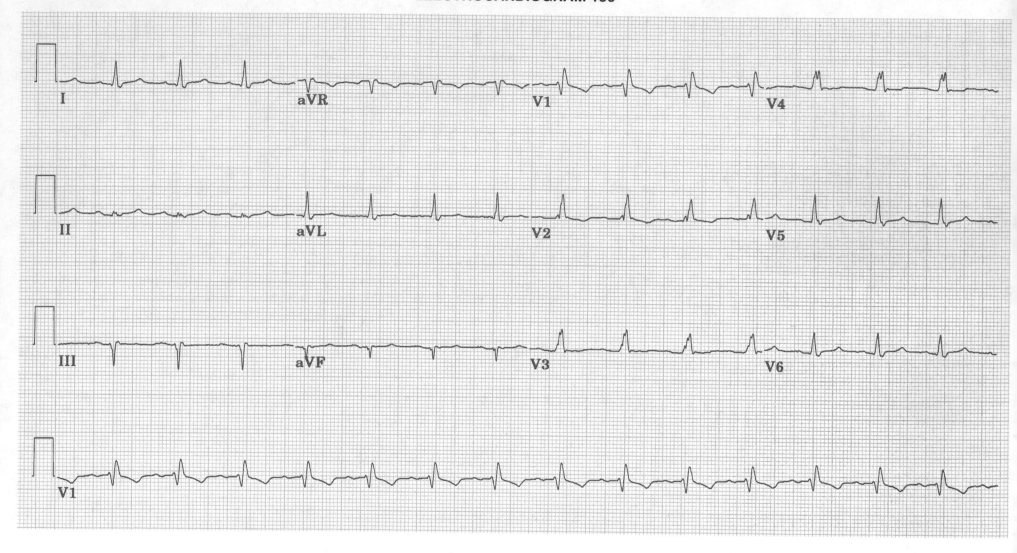

Interpretation Notes: _____

_____

ECG 150 Sixty-eight year old gentleman with recent onset angina pectoris whose cardiac catheterization demonstrated severe coronary artery obstructive disease. This electrocardiogram was obtained shortly after coronary artery bypass graft surgery.

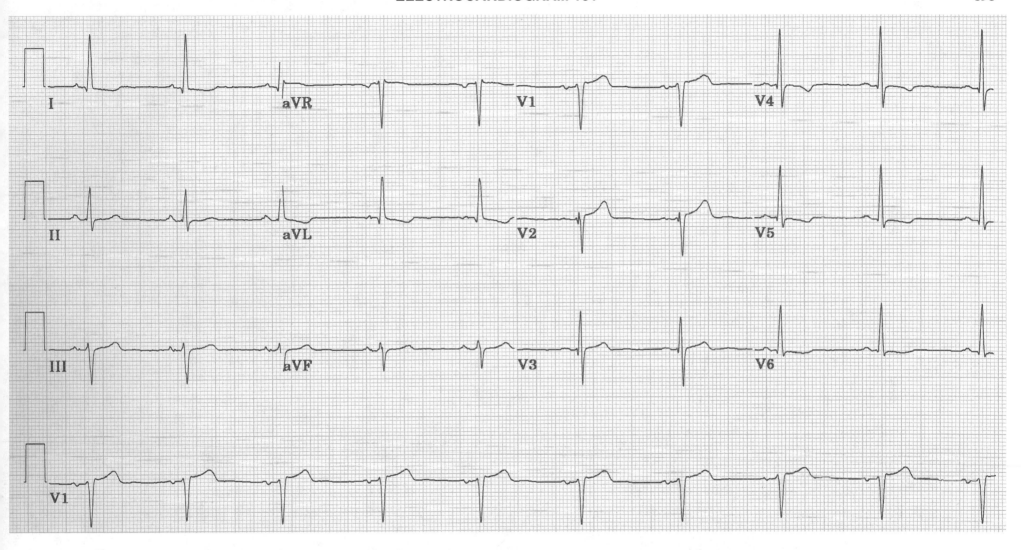

I aVR V1 V4

II aVL V2 V5

III aVF V3 V6

V1

Interpretation Notes: _____

_____

ECG 151 Eighty year old gentleman with severe aortic stenosis who is awaiting aortic valve surgery. A recent echocardiogram demonstrated normal left ventricular systolic function without evidence of a prior myocardial infarction. His medications at the time of this electrocardiogram included fosinopril, aspirin, and a multi-vitamin.

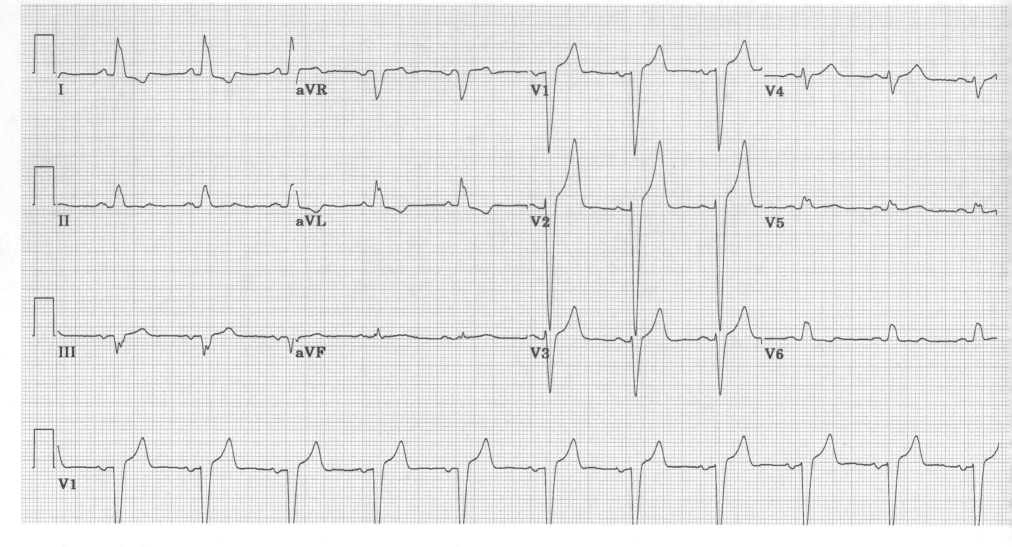

Interpretation Notes: _____

_____

ECG 152 Seventy year old gentleman status post remote coronary artery bypass graft surgery and a prior myocardial infarction, location unknown, who is now being seen preoperatively prior to anticipated knee replacement surgery. The patient is currently asymptomatic. His cardiac medications included metoprolol and aspirin.

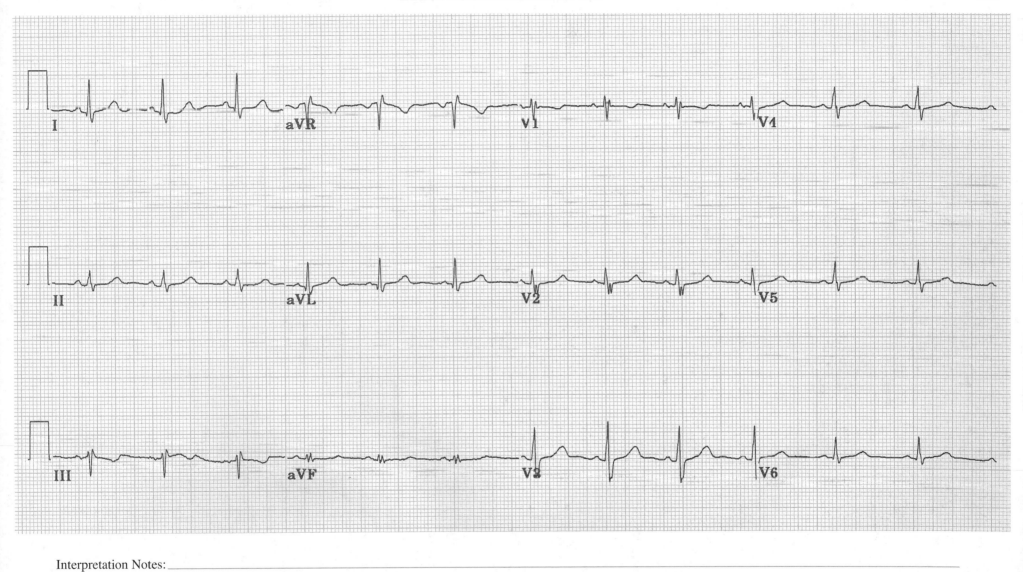

Interpretation Notes: _____

_____

ECG 153 Twenty-seven year old woman two days status post corrective cardiac surgical repair for an ostium secundum atrial septal defect.

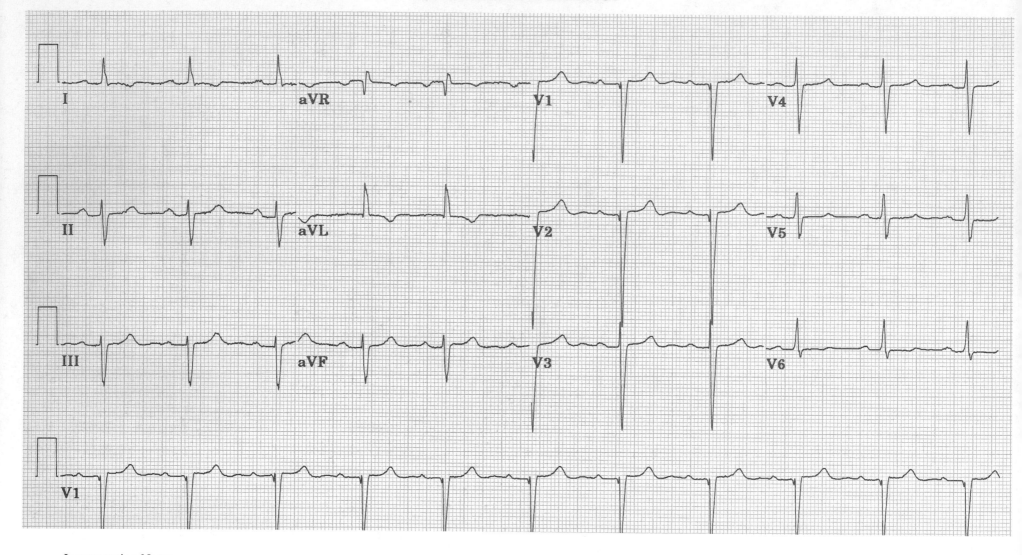

Interpretation Notes: _____

_____

ECG 154 Forty-seven year old woman with a history of sarcoidosis, asthma, and corrected transposition of the great vessels who returns for pulmonary medicine follow-up. Her medications included premarin and a steroid eye drop preparation.

ELECTROCARDIOGRAM 155

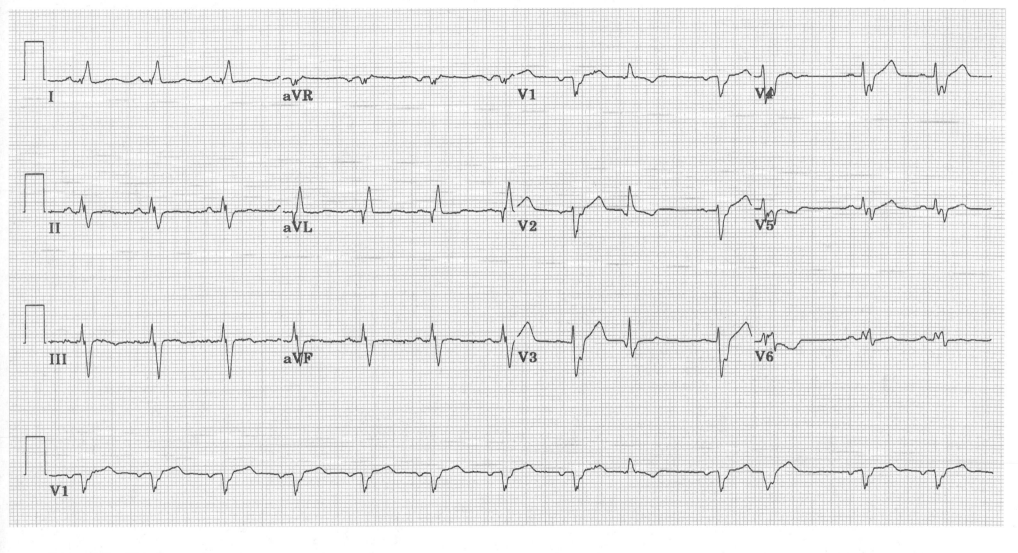

Interpretation Notes:_____

_____

ECG 155 Fifty-five year old gentleman recently admitted to the hospital after an acute lateral myocardial infarction. He has a history of a remote anterior myocardial infarction and severe left ventricular systolic dysfunction. This electrocardiogram was obtained as part of the patient's evaluation for possible coronary artery bypass graft surgery. Medications at the time of this electrocardiogram included lisinopril, metoprolol, furosemide, and aspirin.

LEVEL I

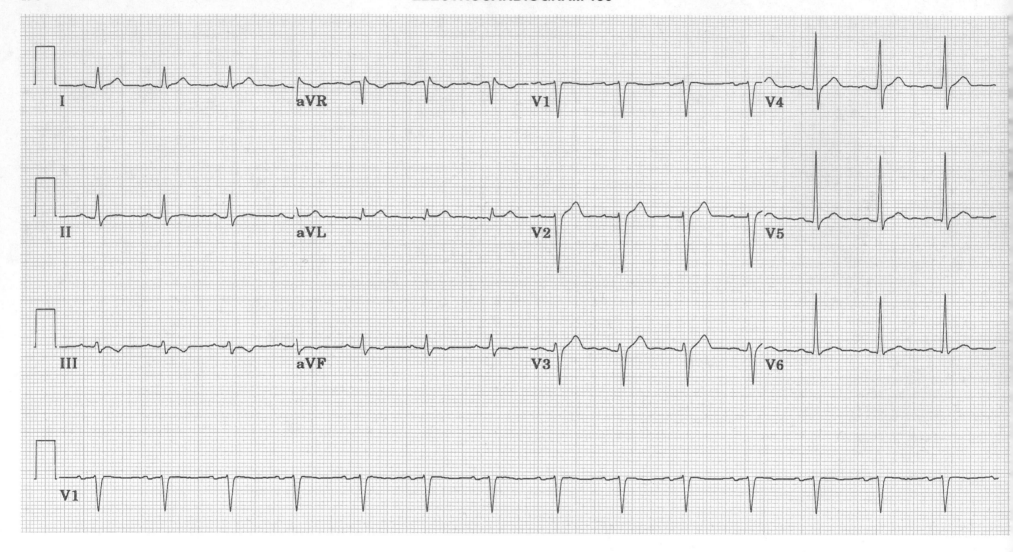

I aVR V1 V4

II aVL V2 V5

III aVF V3 V6

V1

Interpretation Notes: _____

_____

_____

ECG 156 Forty-three year old gentleman with a six day history of abrupt onset fever, and chills, pruritic rash, and headache. The patient was seen in the emergency room and subsequently admitted to the hospital. This tracing represented his admission electrocardiogram. His admission serum calcium level was not elevated at 8.9 mg/dl. His serum protein, and albumin were both within normal limits.

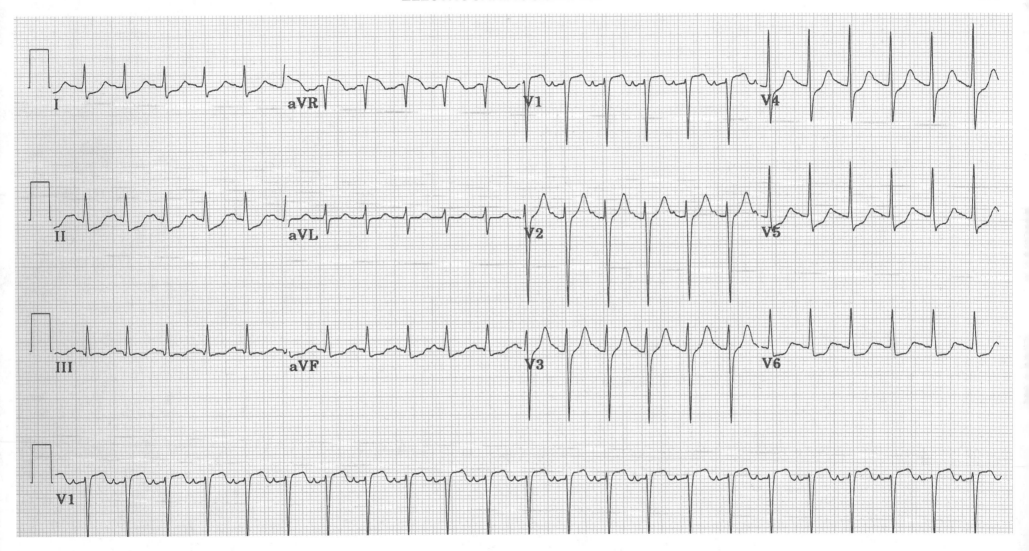

Interpretation Notes: _____

ECG 157 Forty-three year old woman with a history of sarcoidosis and bronchiolitis obliterans who is admitted to the hospital with a two day history of shortness of breath. Her past medical history includes hypertension and hepatitis C. Medications at the time of this electrocardiogram included prednisone, nebulized inhalers, hydrochlorothiazide, furosemide, and potassium.

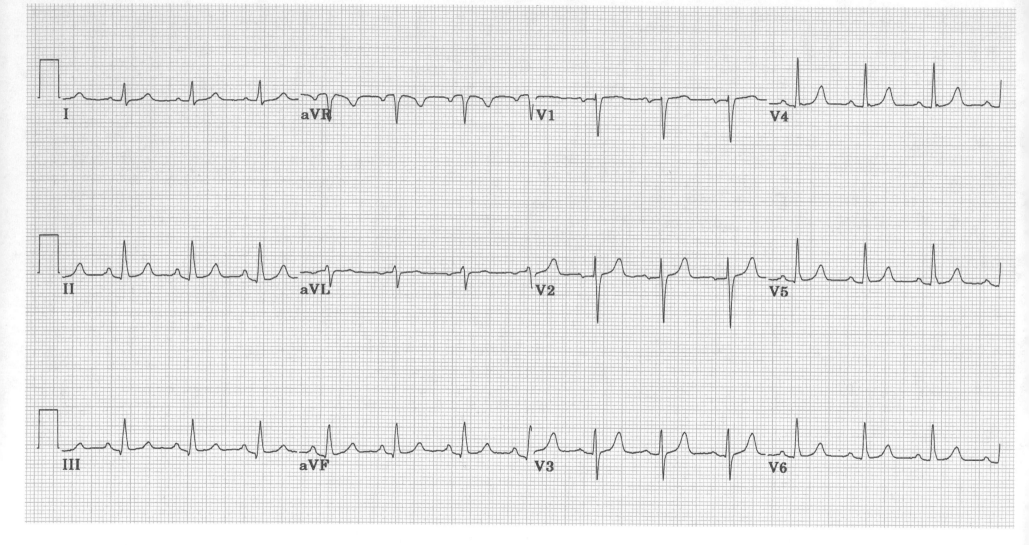

Interpretation Notes:_____

_____

_____

ECG 158 Sixty-seven year old woman with dialysis requiring renal failure being seen in the outpatient nephrology clinic.

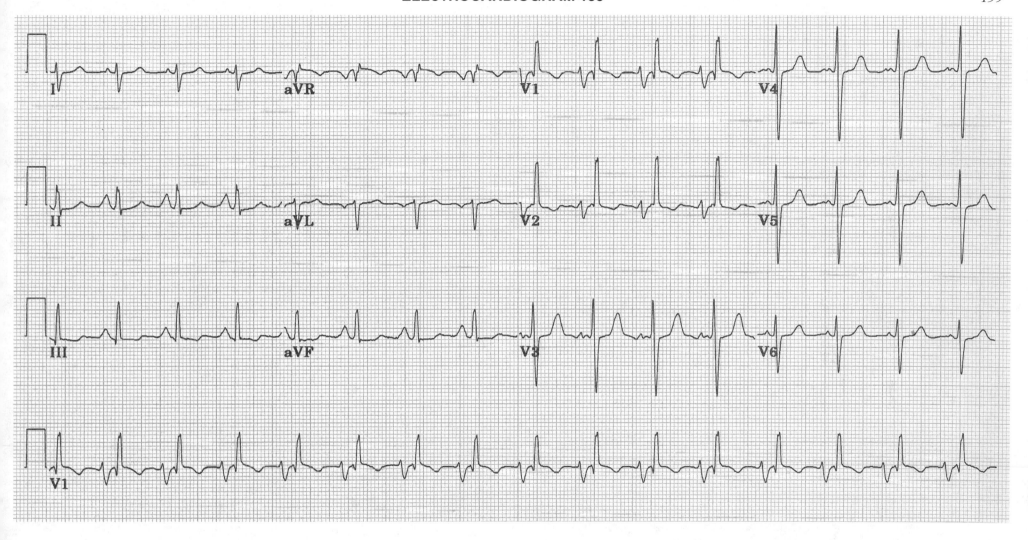

Interpretation Notes: _____

_____

_____

ECG 159 Forty-eight year old gentleman with severe mitral stenosis referred for mitral valve reparative surgery. He is on no current medications. A recent echocardiogram confirmed the presence of severe mitral stenosis, a dilated right ventricle with moderately severe systolic dysfunction, moderately severe tricuspid insufficiency, and severe pulmonary hypertension.

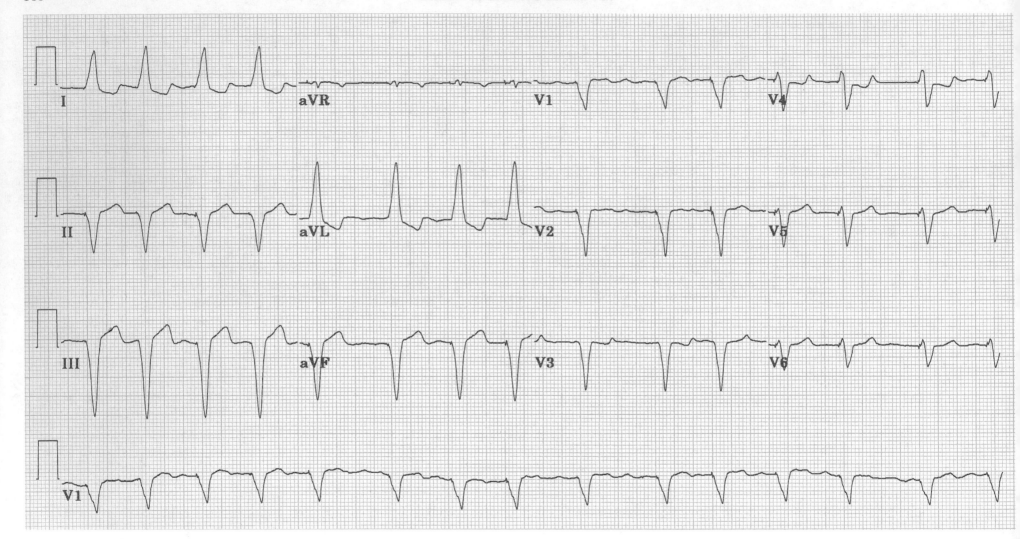

Interpretation Notes: _____

ECG 160 Seventy-four year old woman with a history of severe coronary artery obstructive disease status post coronary artery stenting and remote mechanical aortic valve replacement who is admitted to the hospital with signs and symptoms of congestive heart failure. Her past history includes rheumatic mitral and aortic valvular heart disease. Her medications included diltiazem, furosemide, potassium, atenolol, and aspirin.

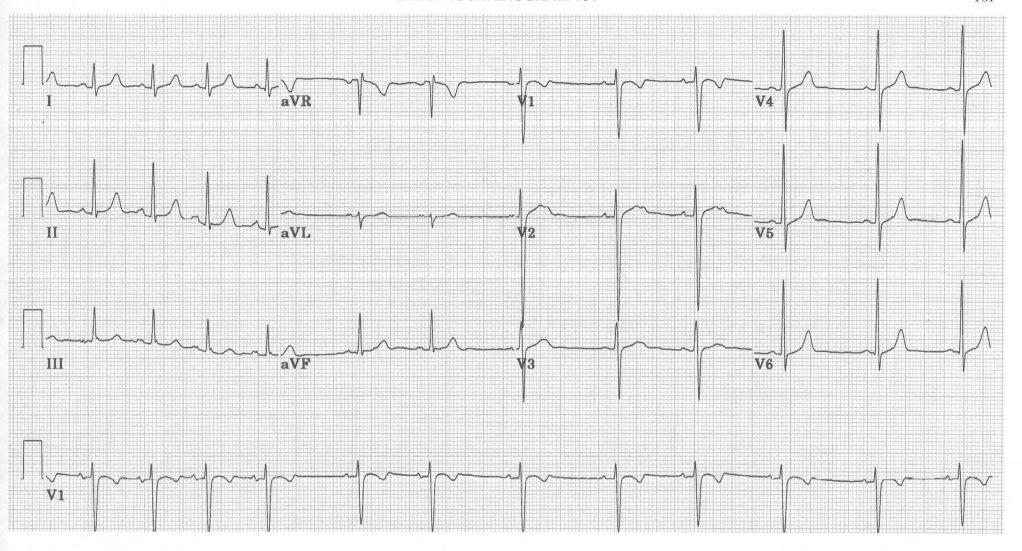

ECG 161 Sixteen year old gentleman admitted acutely to the hospital for further evaluation of suicidal ideation and depression. He has no known cardiac history.

Interpretation Notes: _____
_____
_____

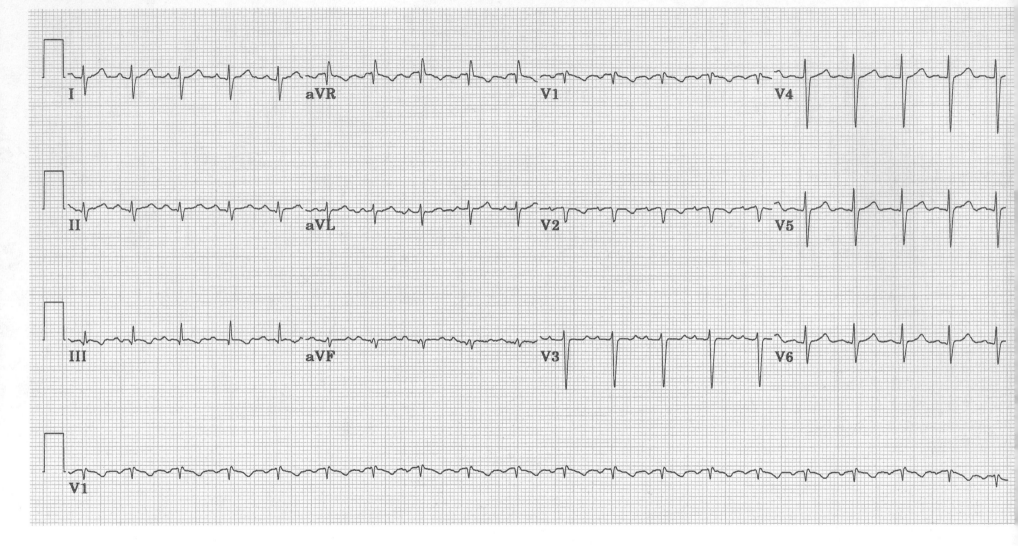

Interpretation Notes: _____

ECG 162 Sixty year old gentleman with respiratory failure secondary to chronic obstructive pulmonary disease admitted to the intensive care unit for mechanical ventilation and further therapy. Co-morbid conditions include congestive heart failure, non-insulin requiring diabetes mellitus, and hypertension. His medications included furosemide, potassium, lisinopril, and inhalers.

ELECTROCARDIOGRAM 163

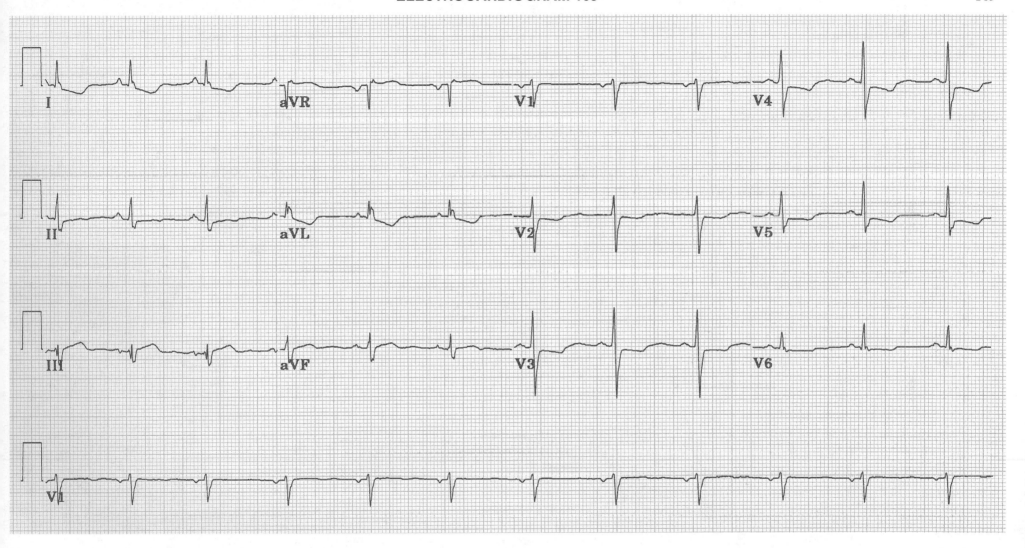

Interpretation Notes: _____

_____

ECG 163 Seventy-seven year old woman admitted to the hospital with an acute inferior myocardial infarction who is now referred for coronary artery bypass graft surgery. An echocardiogram confirmed inferoposterior akinesis. Her medications included aspirin, intravenous heparin, intravenous nitroglycerin, and metoprolol.

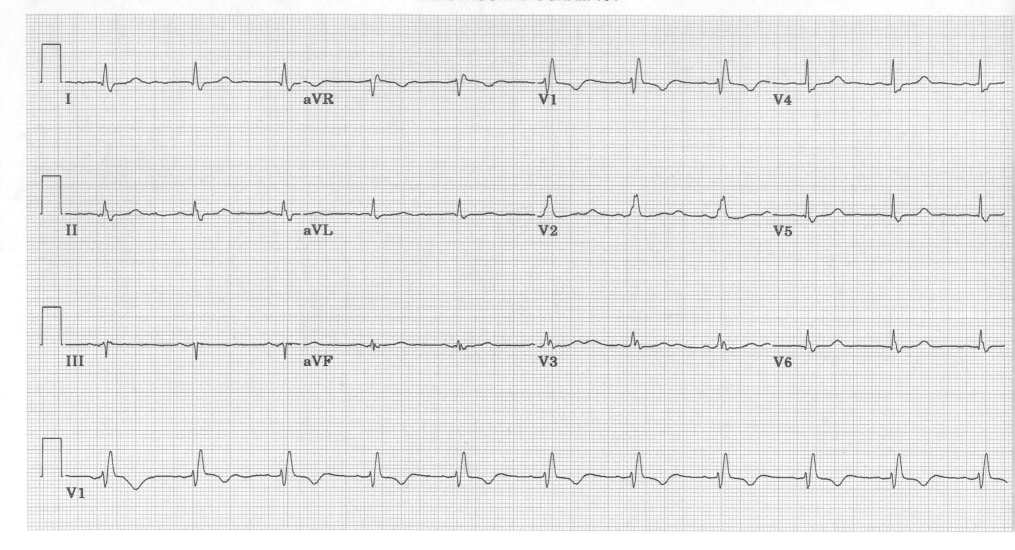

Interpretation Notes: _____

_____

_____

ECG 164 Eighty-eight year old gentleman with a history of long-standing hypertension and multi-vessel coronary artery obstructive disease who is recently status post coronary artery bypass graft surgery.

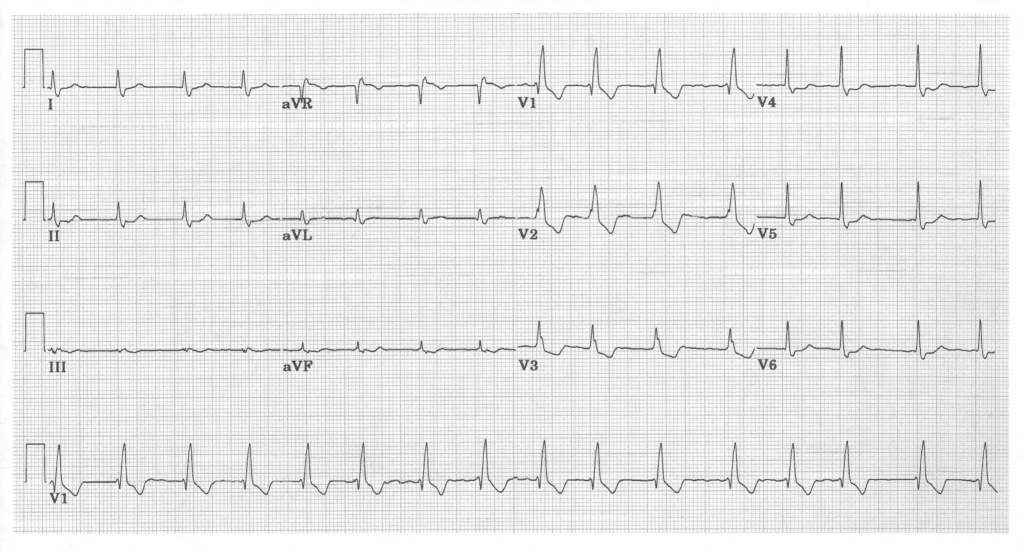

Interpretation Notes: _____

ECG 165 Sixty-three year old gentleman with a history of esophageal carcinoma who is recently status post esophagogastrectomy. He has a history of chronic atrial fibrillation. His medications at the time of this electrocardiogram included diltiazem, furosemide, digoxin, warfarin, and potassium.

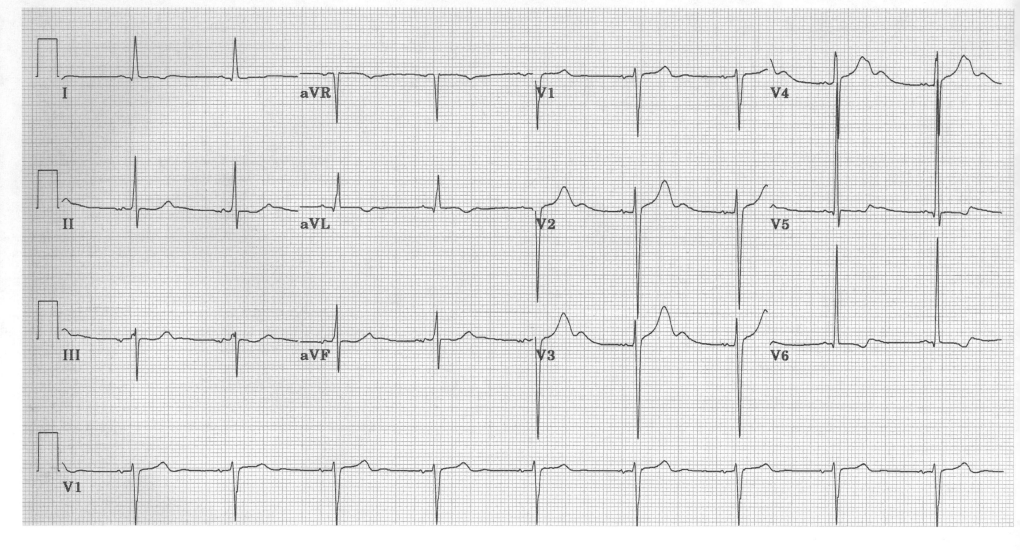

Interpretation Notes: _____

ECG 166 Fifty year old woman status post remote surgical correction of an aortic coarctation, long-standing hypertension, and hypertensive heart disease referred for further evaluation of recurrent atrial dysrhythmias and congestive heart failure. Her medications included captopril, disopyramide, and aspirin.

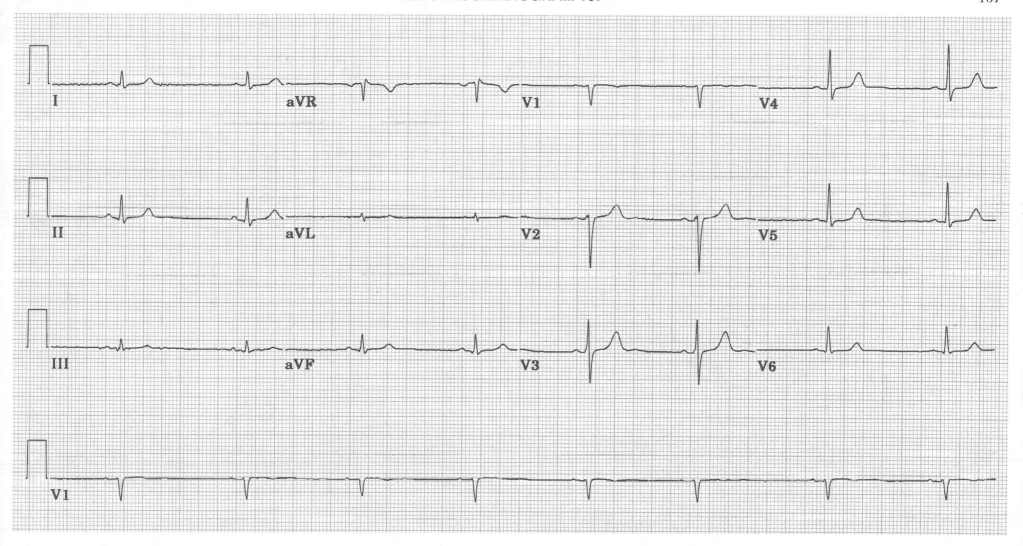

Interpretation Notes: _____

_____

_____

ECG 167 Forty-six year old woman referred for evaluation of suspected long-standing pulmonic stenosis. She is on no medications. A recent echocardiogram demonstrated mild pulmonic stenosis and otherwise was normal.

LEVEL I

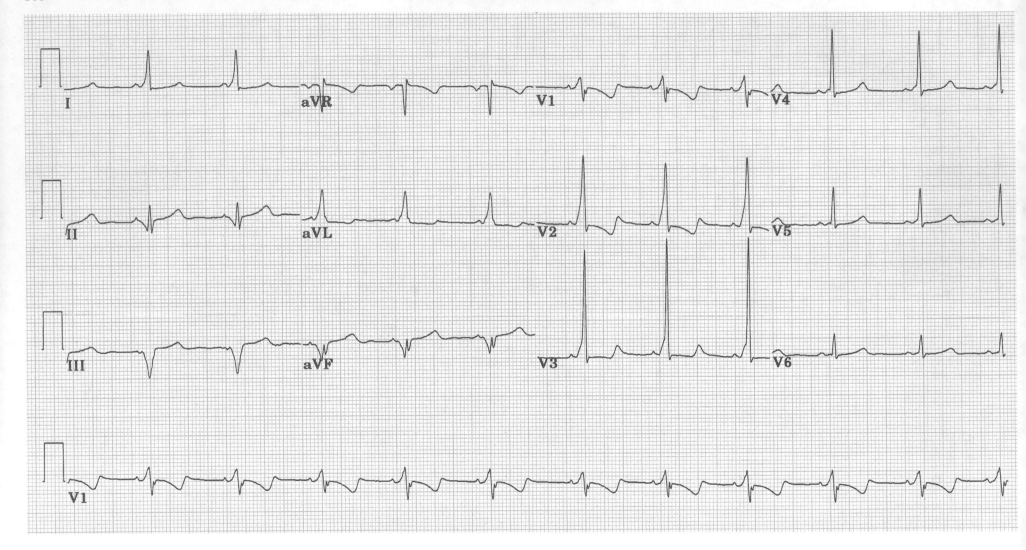

Interpretation Notes:_____

ECG 168 Thirty-seven year old woman with Wolff-Parkinson-White syndrome who returns for a repeat evaluation in the setting of medication-induced fatigue and persistent palpitations. Her medications included propranolol. The patient subsequently underwent successful radiofrequency ablation of a right ventricular posteroseptal accessory pathway.

ELECTROCARDIOGRAM 169

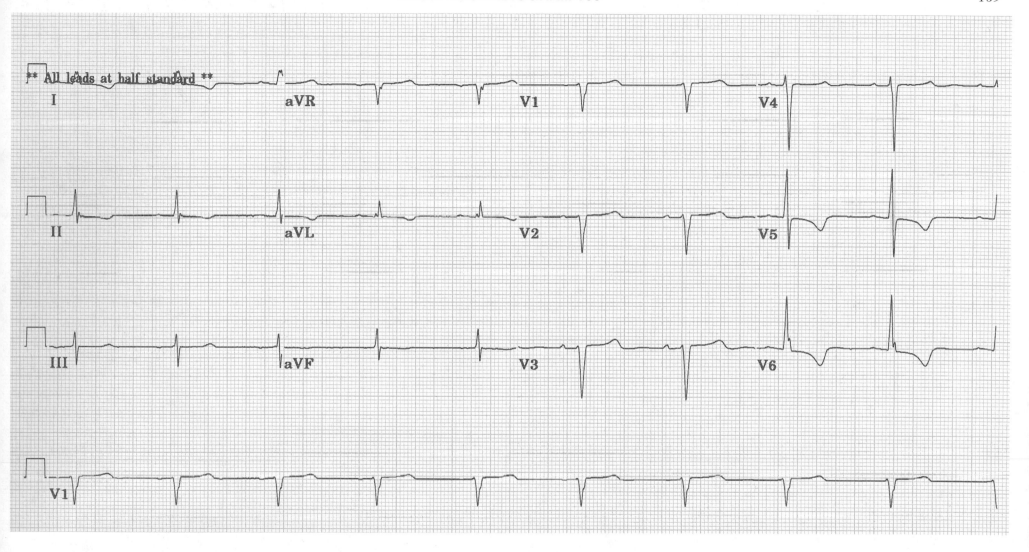

** All leads at half standard **

I	aVR	V1	V4
II	aVL	V2	V5
III	aVF	V3	V6

V1

Interpretation Notes: _____

_____

ECG 169 Forty-five year old woman with valvular heart disease who is recently status post mitral valve reparative surgery for mitral insufficiency and a septal myectomy for hypertrophic obstructive cardiomyopathy. Her medications included metoprolol, furosemide, warfarin, and atorvastatin.

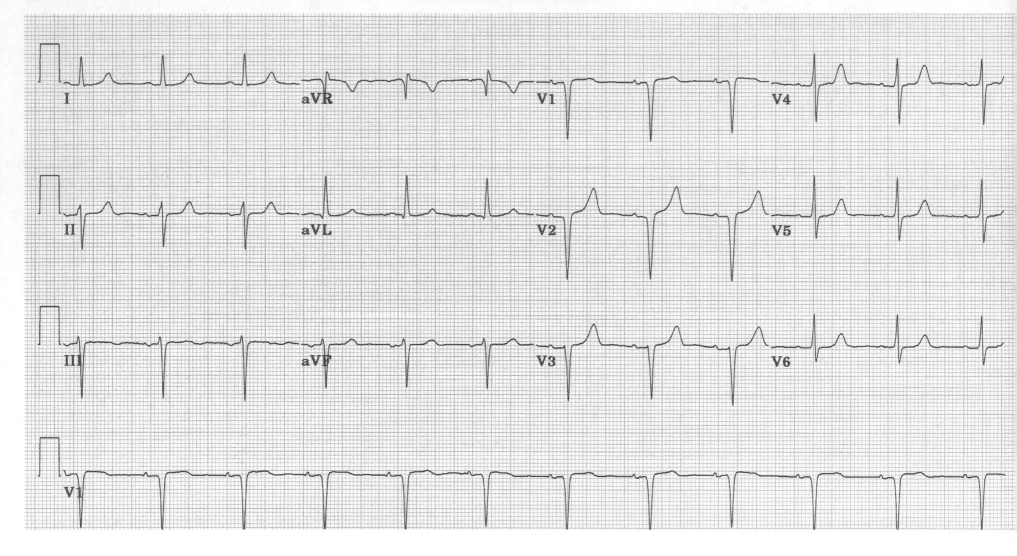

Interpretation Notes: _____

_____

_____

ECG 170 Eighty year old woman admitted to the hospital with a severe upper respiratory tract infection. She is on no current medications and has no prior cardiac history.

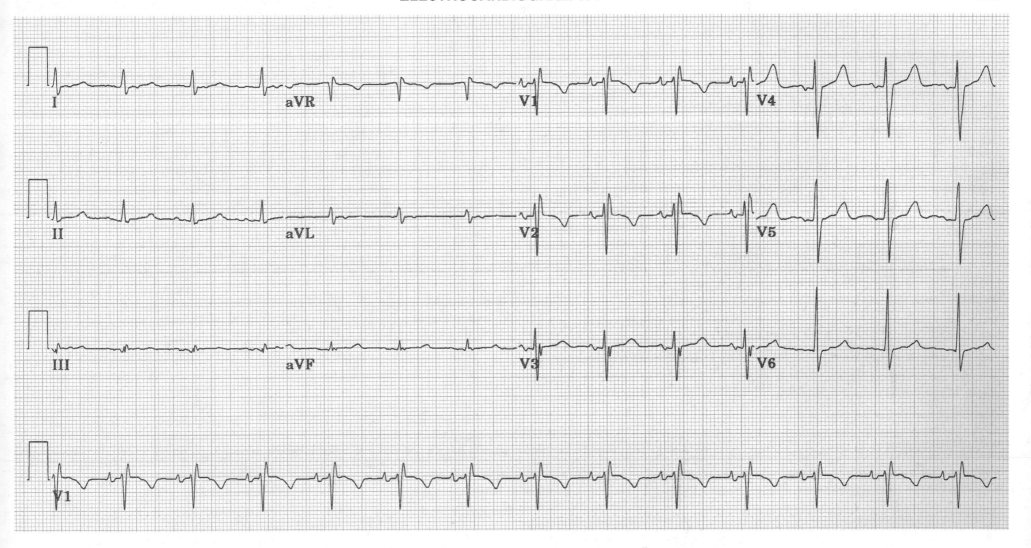

ECG 171 Fifty-nine year old gentleman status post cardiac transplantation three years prior to this electrocardiogram secondary to severe ischemic left ventricular systolic dysfunction who is now seen in the cardiology outpatient clinic. He overall feels well without symptoms of congestive heart failure. His medications include prednisone, aza-thioprine, labetalol, diltiazem, minoxidil, glyburide, and famotidine.

LEVEL I

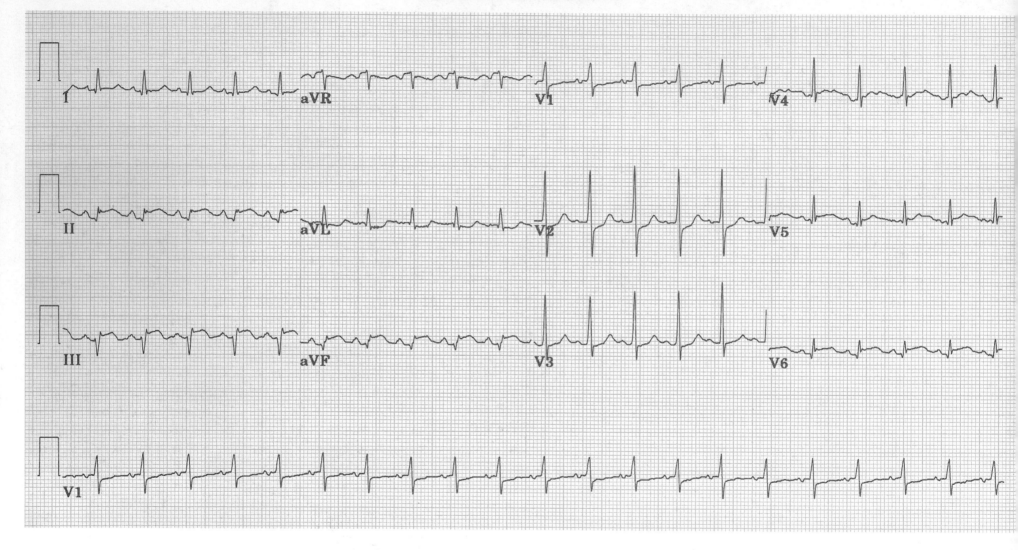

Interpretation Notes: _____

_____

ECG 172 Seventy-one year old woman status post a myocardial infarction twenty-five years prior to this electrocardiogram who presents with acute onset chest discomfort. Co-morbidities include tobacco use, primary hyperthyroidism, and long-standing hypertension. Serial cardiac enzyme analysis confirmed acute myocardial injury.

LEVEL I

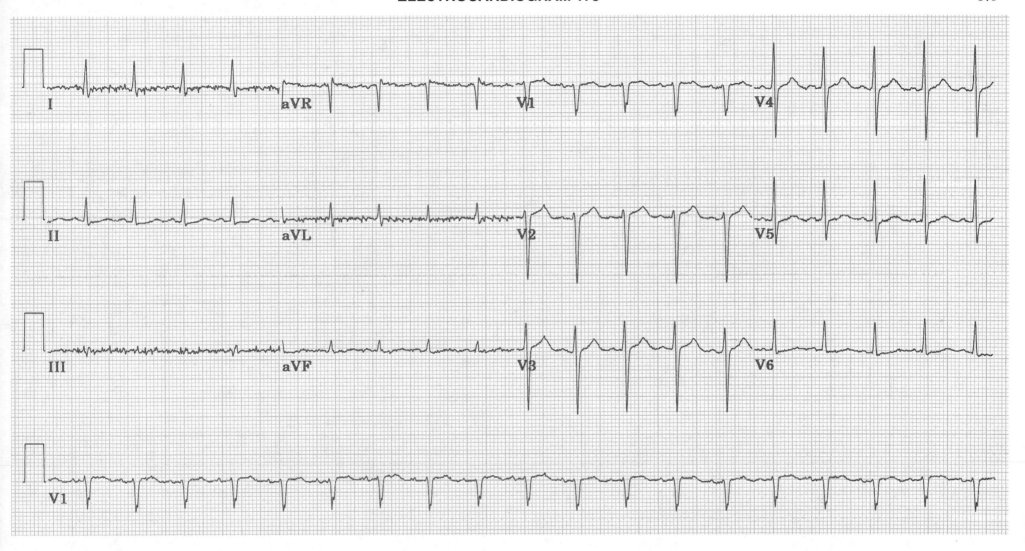

I   aVR   V1   V4

II   aVL   V2   V5

III   aVF   V3   V6

V1   V1

Interpretation Notes: _____

_____

_____

ECG 173 Twenty-five year old woman with insulin requiring diabetes of long-standing duration who presents to the hospital with signs and symptoms of sinusitis. She has renal failure and is dialysis dependent. Medications at the time of this electrocardiogram included furosemide, diltiazem, insulin, and clonidine.

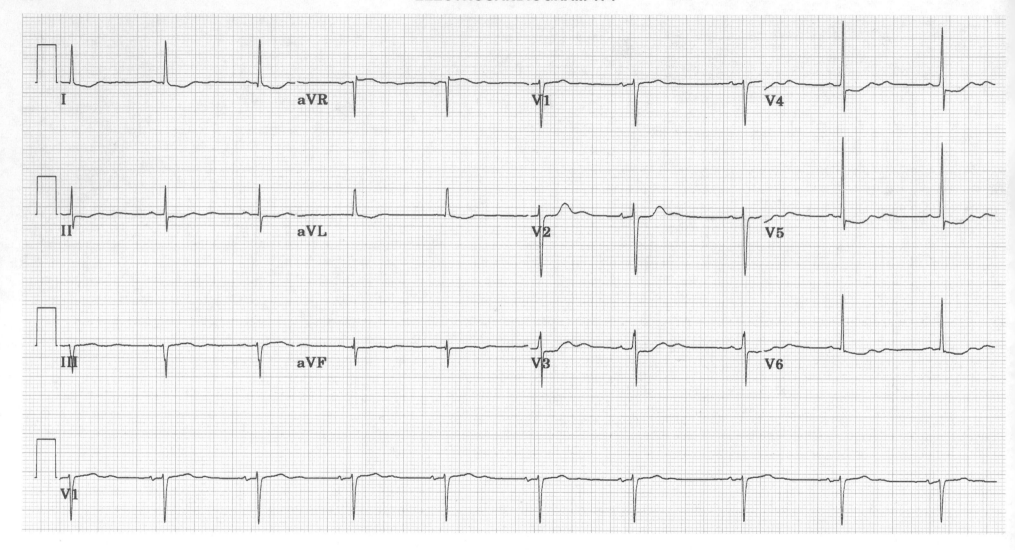

ECG 174 Seventy-five year old woman with long-standing hypertension who is referred for a cardiac evaluation. Her medications included amlodipine and digoxin. Her serum electrolytes were all within normal limits.

Interpretation Notes: _____

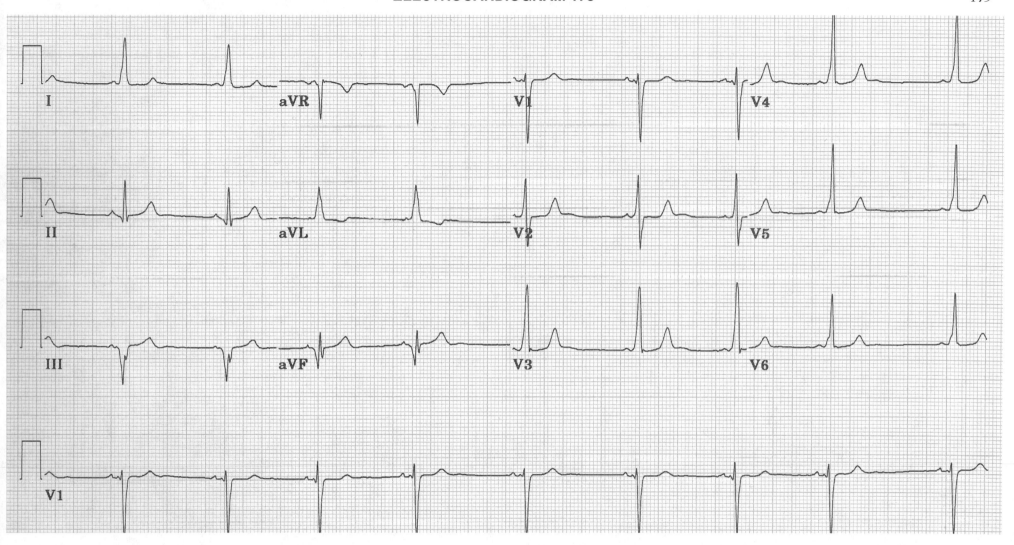

I   aVR   V1   V4

II   aVL   V2   V5

III   aVF   V3   V6

V1

Interpretation Notes: _____

_____

ECG 175 Twenty-two year old woman with symptomatic palpitations who underwent a successful radiofrequency catheter ablation of a right posteroseptal accessory pathway. This electrocardiogram was obtained prior to her radiofrequency ablation.

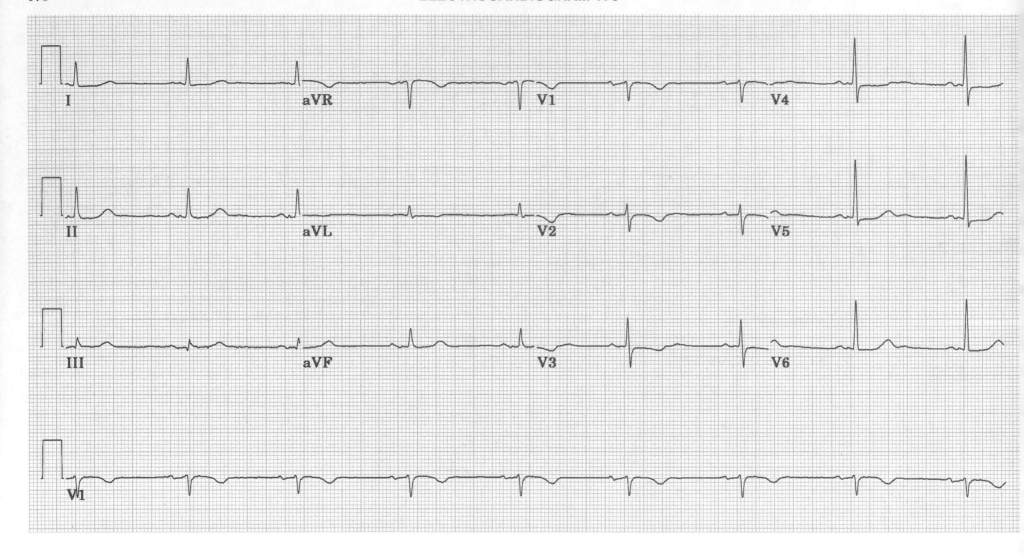

Interpretation Notes:_____

ECG 176 Seventy-four year old woman who is being seen in the breast clinic. Her past medical history includes hypertension, atrial fibrillation, and mitral valve prolapse. Her medications included propafenone, triamterene/hydrochlorothiazide, and atenolol. Her serum electrolytes were normal at the time of this electrocardiogram.

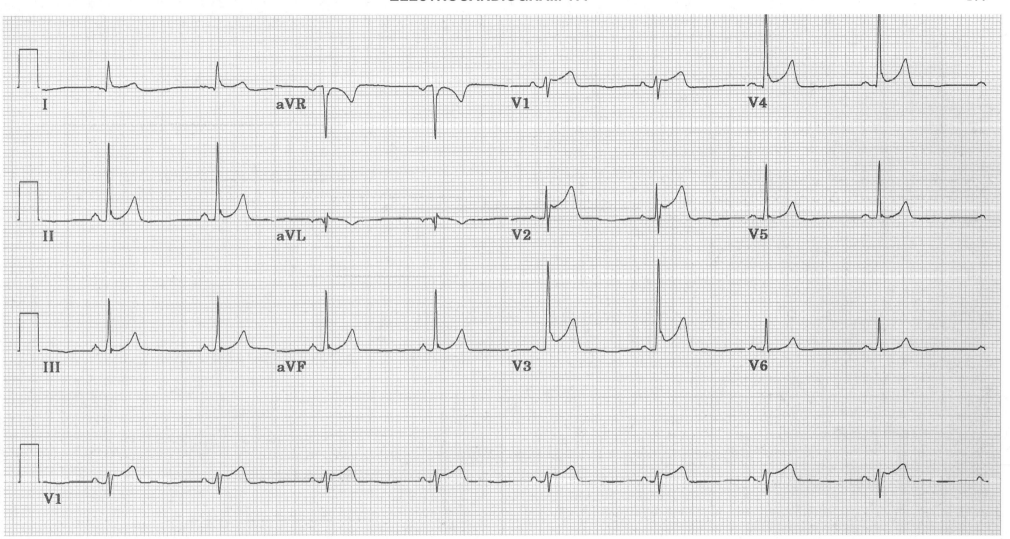

I aVR V1 V4
II aVL V2 V5
III aVF V3 V6
V1

Interpretation Notes:_____

_____

ECG 177 Thirty-eight year old gentleman with acute onset chest discomfort felt non-cardiac and most likely musculoskeletal in origin. He has no known prior health problems.

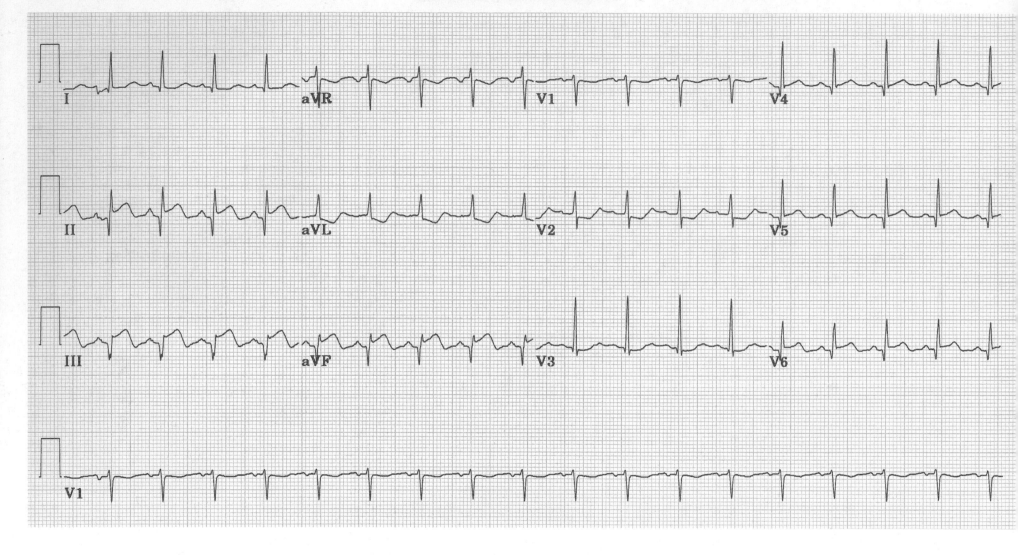

Interpretation Notes: _____

_____

ECG 178 Seventy-one year old woman with acute onset chest discomfort of two hours duration who presented to the emergency room. The above electrocardiogram was obtained. An urgent cardiac catheterization demonstrated a 90% proximal right coronary artery obstruction with thrombus. Successful acute percutaneous transluminal coronary angioplasty was performed without complication.

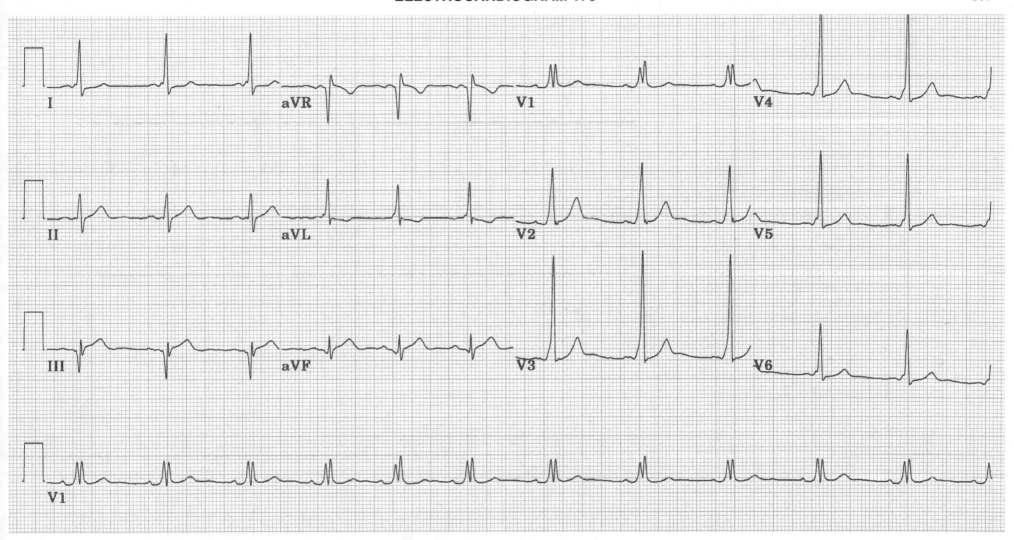

I   aVR   V1   V4

II   aVL   V2   V5

III   aVF   V3   V6

V1

Interpretation Notes: _____

_____

_____

ECG 179 Twenty-nine year old gentleman who presented to an outside hospital with a wide complex tachycardia in the setting of perceived intermittent palpitations of one year duration. The patient was placed on intravenous procainamide and he converted to normal sinus rhythm. His resting electrocardiogram demonstrated the Wolff-Parkinson-White syndrome. He underwent successful radiofrequency ablation of his left posterior ventricular accessory pathway.

LEVEL I

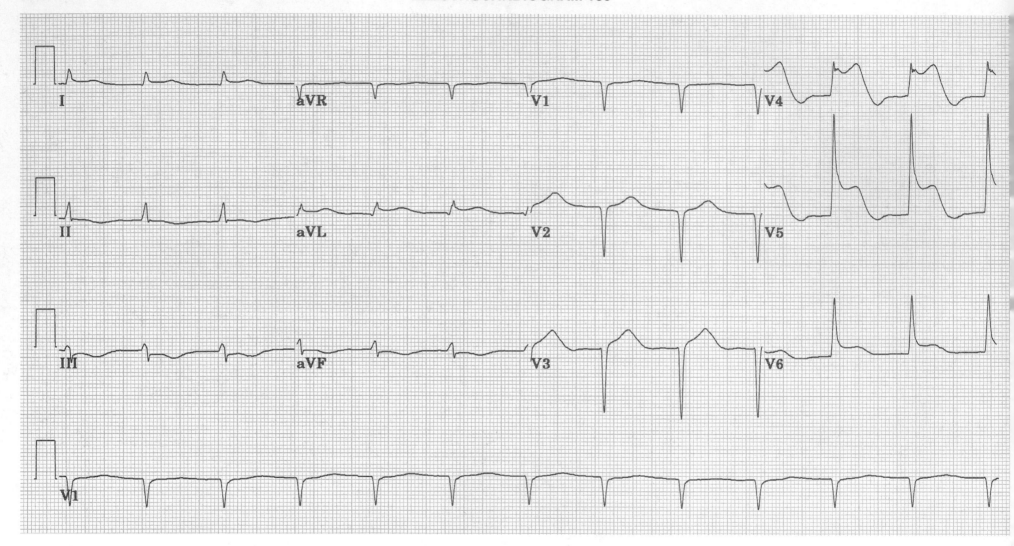

Interpretation Notes: _____

_____

_____

ECG 180 Seventy-four year old woman with coronary artery disease who presents to the hospital with a one hour history of acute chest discomfort consistent with myocardial injury.

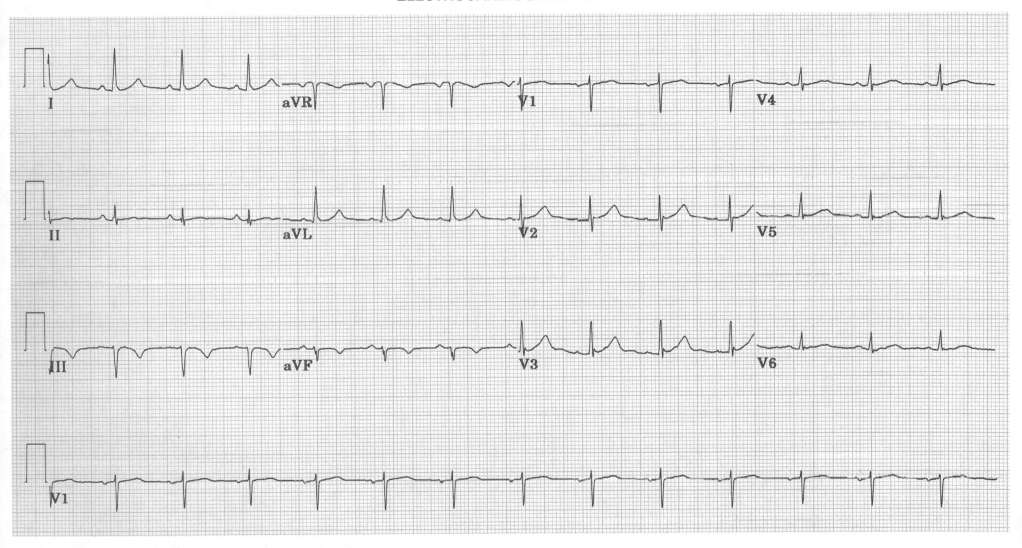

Interpretation Notes: _____

_____

ECG 181 Fifty year old gentleman who presented to the emergency room two hours after severe chest discomfort onset. The accompanying electrocardiogram was obtained and a cardiac catheterization transpired shortly thereafter demonstrating a subtotal mid right coronary artery stenosis with superimposed thrombus. A successful stent was placed to the mid right coronary artery.

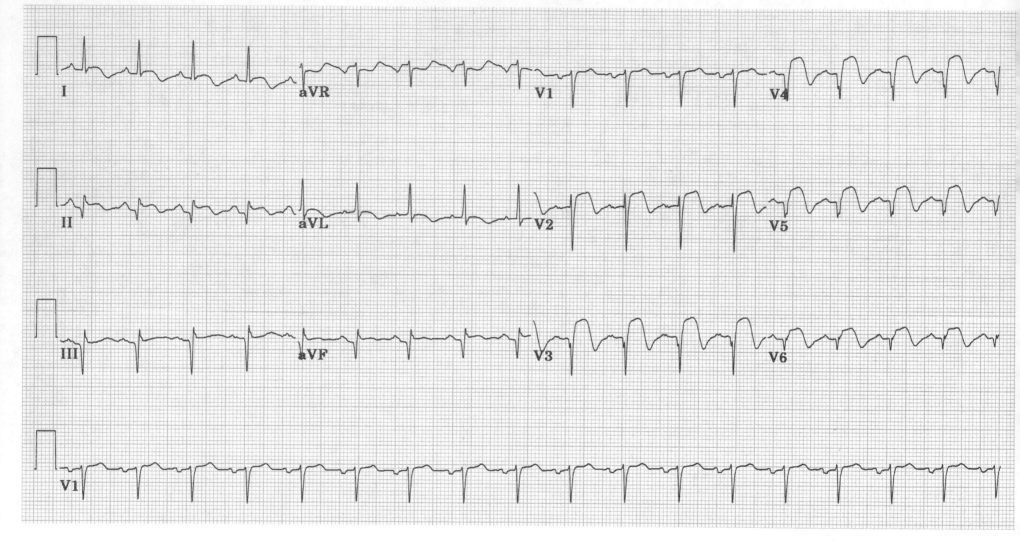

Interpretation Notes: _____

ECG 182 Seventy year old gentleman with a two day history of intermittent chest discomfort, nausea, and vomiting who presented acutely to the hospital emergency room. A subsequent urgent cardiac catheterization demonstrated a 100% left anterior descending coronary artery occlusion with apical left ventricular aneurysm formation.

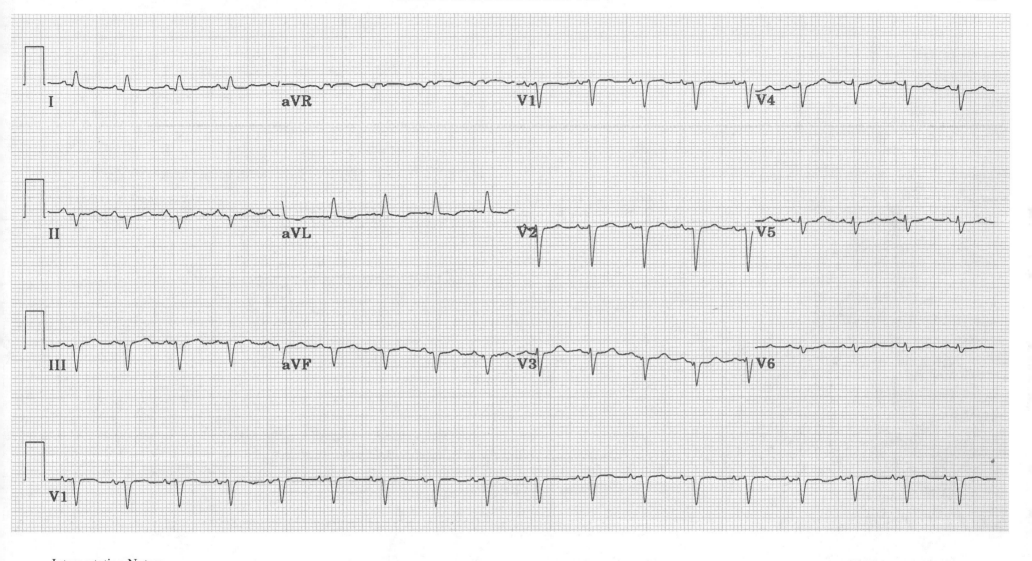

Interpretation Notes: _____

_____

ECG 183 Seventy-four year old woman with a prior surgical resection of squamous cell esophageal cancer who re-presents to the hospital with increasing shortness of breath and orthopnea. An echocardiogram demonstrated a large pericardial effusion and normal left ventricular wall motion. The patient is not known to have a history of a prior myocardial infarction and no prior cardiac evaluation has been undertaken.

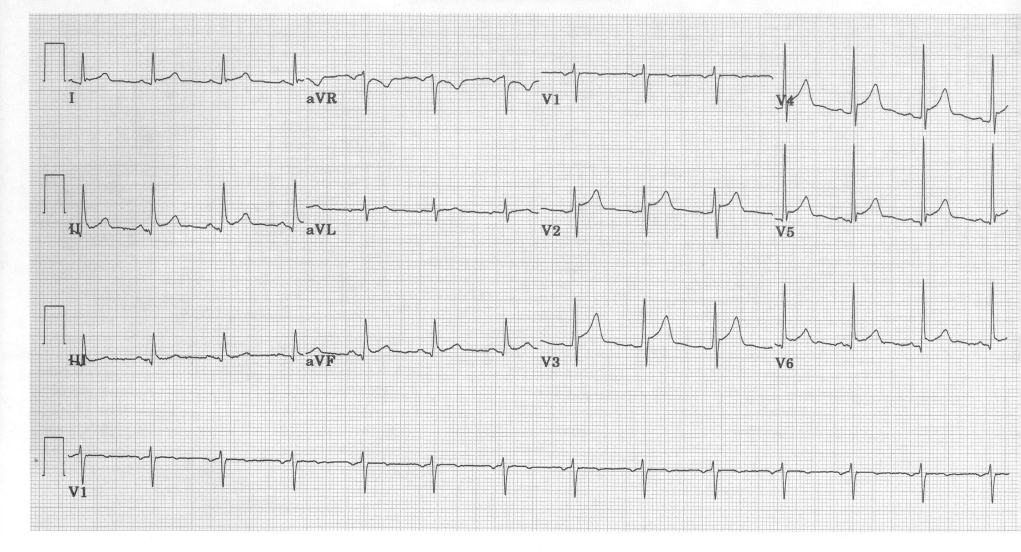

Interpretation Notes: _____

ECG 184 Sixty-four year old gentleman recently status post coronary artery bypass graft surgery.

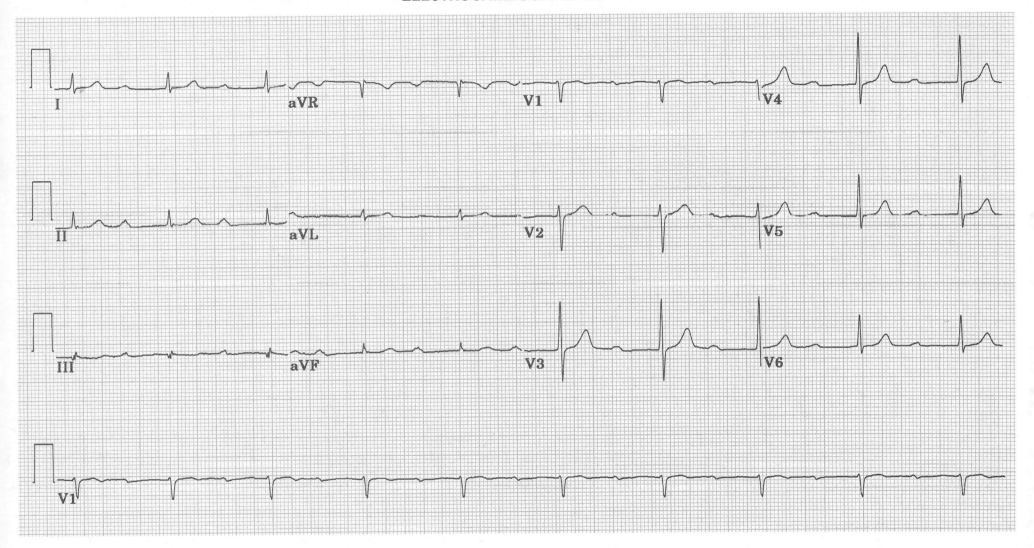

I aVR V1 V4

II aVL V2 V5

III aVF V3 V6

V1

Interpretation Notes: _____

ECG 185 Sixty-seven year old gentleman with a history of coronary artery disease and stable angina pectoris who returns for cardiology follow-up. His medications included diltiazem, gemfibrozil, and aspirin. A recent stress echocardiogram was negative for inducible myocardial ischemia.

LEVEL I

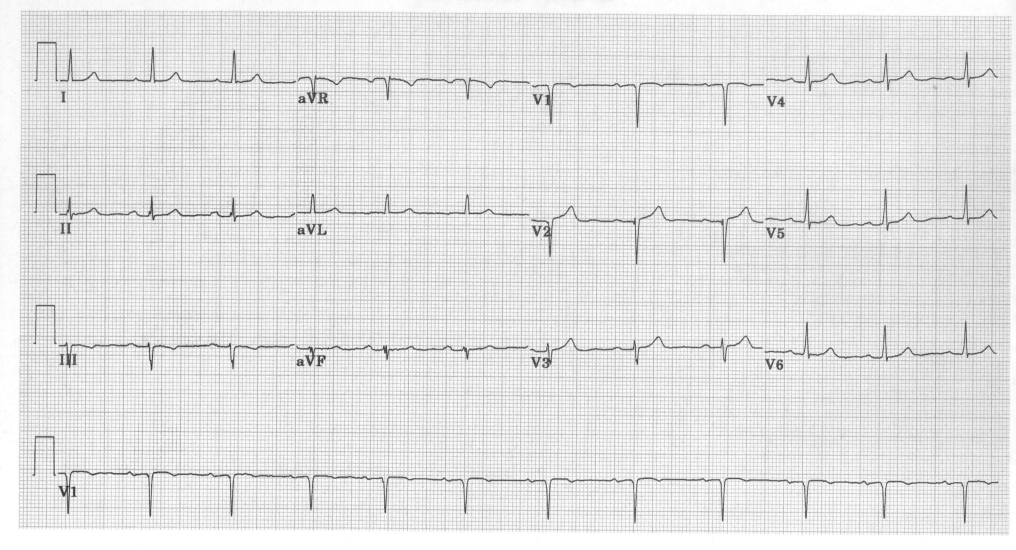

Interpretation Notes: _____

_____

_____

ECG 186 Seventy-seven year old woman who presented to the hospital with a four day history of intermittent chest burning with radiation to the back. Subsequent serum cardiac enzyme analysis and echocardiography confirmed a recent septal myocardial infarction.

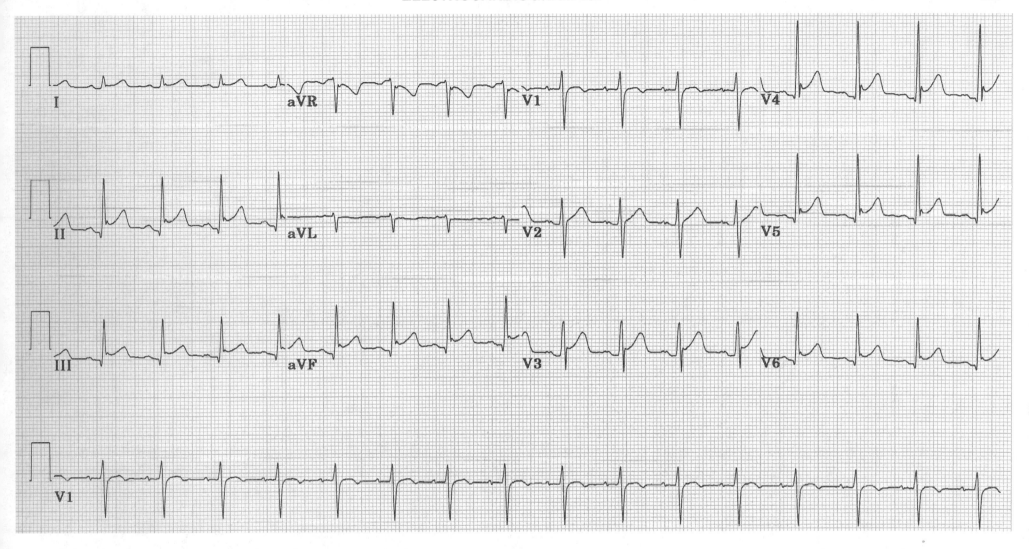

Interpretation Notes:_____

ECG 187 Thirty-nine year old gentleman admitted with a two day history of chest discomfort, worse with inspiration and a supine position, relieved with leaning forward. The patient was treated with oral nonsteroidal anti-inflammatory agents with symptomatic improvement. A myocardial infarction was excluded by serial cardiac enzyme analysis.

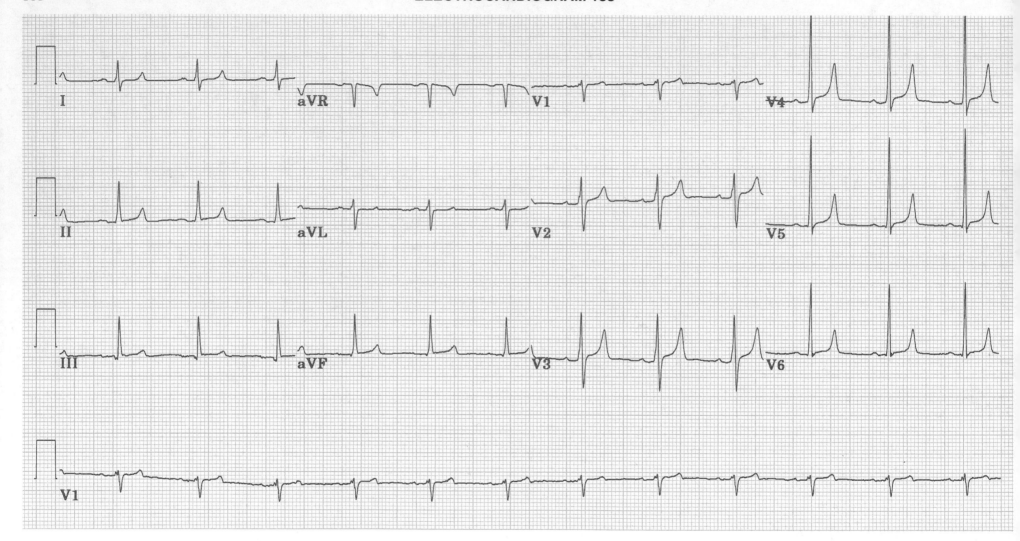

Interpretation Notes: _____

_____

ECG 188 Twenty-eight year old gentleman with dialysis requiring renal failure awaiting kidney transplantation. He has a past history of advanced hypertension. His serum potassium level at the time of this electrocardiogram was 6.3 meq/L.

ELECTROCARDIOGRAM 189

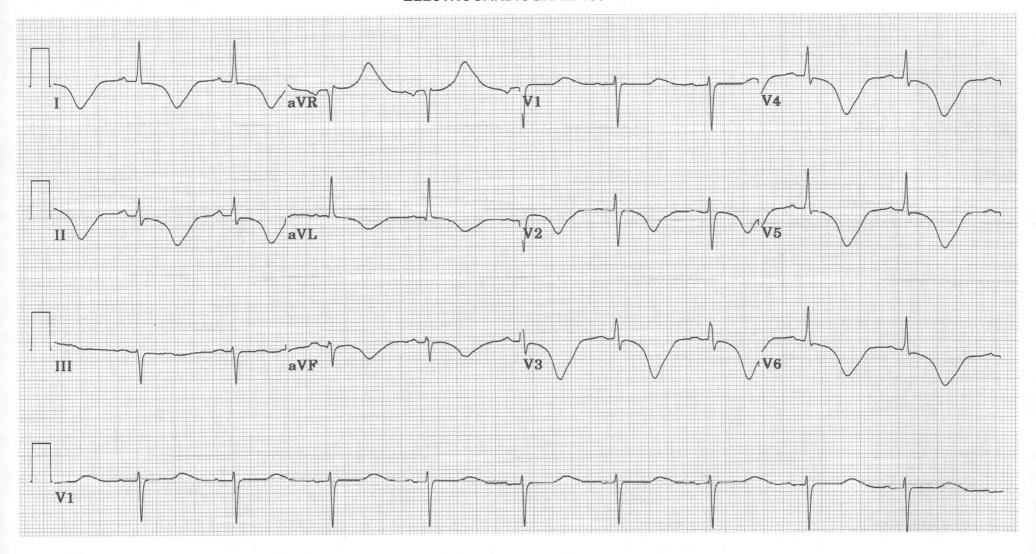

Interpretation Notes: _____

ECG 189 Fifty-nine year old woman who presented with a chest discomfort syndrome and the above electrocardiogram. She subsequently underwent cardiac catheterization demonstrating normal coronary arteries and global mild left ventricular systolic dysfunction. Neurology was consulted for the possibility of a subarachnoid hemorrhage and this was excluded. Her past medical history includes hypertension.

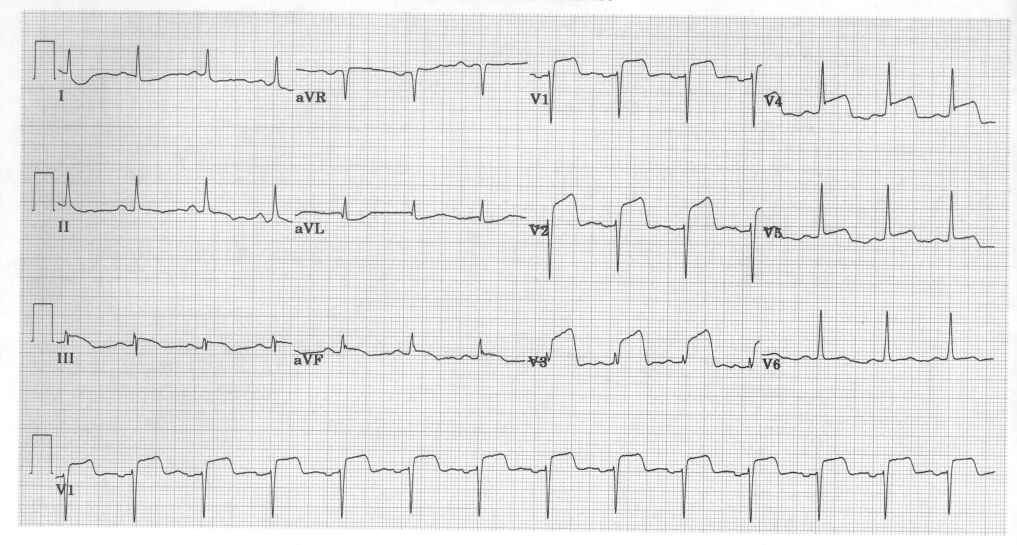

Interpretation Notes: _____

_____

ECG 190 Fifty year old gentleman with a history of a prior anterior myocardial infarction and percutaneous transluminal coronary angioplasty to his left anterior descending coronary artery who re-presents with an acute chest discomfort syndrome and the accompanying electrocardiogram. Co-morbid conditions include diabetes mellitus, hypertension and chronic renal insufficiency. His medications included furosemide, metoprolol, topical nitroglycerin, hydralazine, insulin, and aspirin.

ELECTROCARDIOGRAM 191

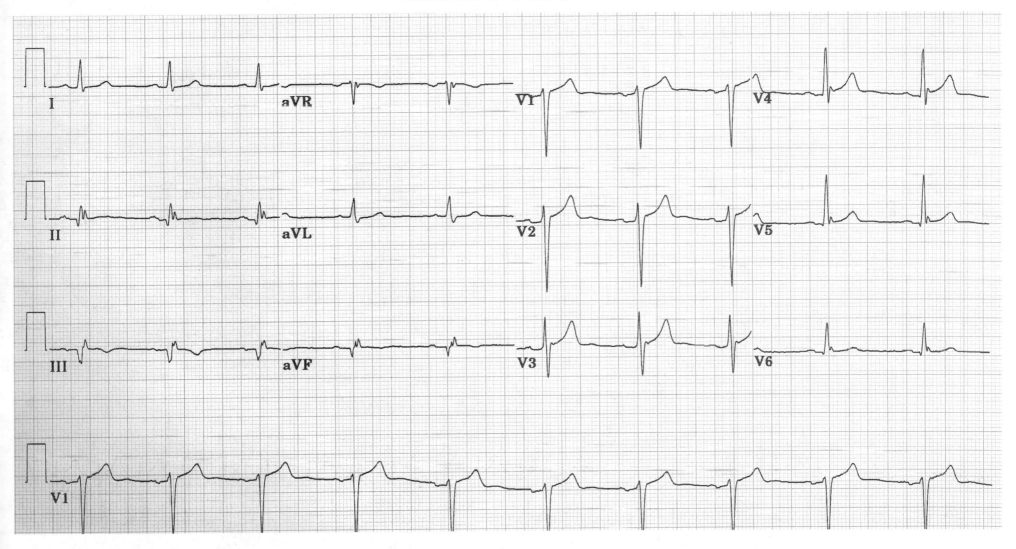

I aVR V1 V4

II aVL V2 V5

III aVF V3 V6

V1

Interpretation Notes: _____

ECG 191 Forty-seven year old gentleman with coronary artery disease status post an inferior myocardial infarction two years prior to this electrocardiogram. He subsequently underwent four-vessel coronary artery bypass graft surgery. He is now admitted to the hospital for evaluation of recent onset non-sustained ventricular tachycardia.

ELECTROCARDIOGRAM 192

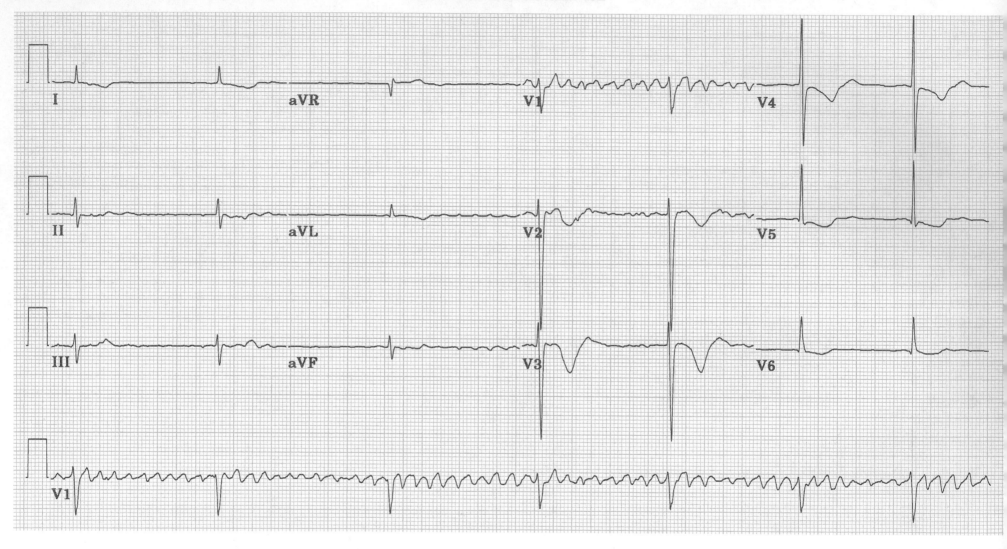

I aVR V1 V4

II aVL V2 V5

III aVF V3 V6

V1

Interpretation Notes: _____

_____

_____

ECG 192 Fifty-nine year old woman with a history of hypertension and atrial dysrhythmias who is admitted acutely to the hospital for evaluation of a cerebrovascular accident.

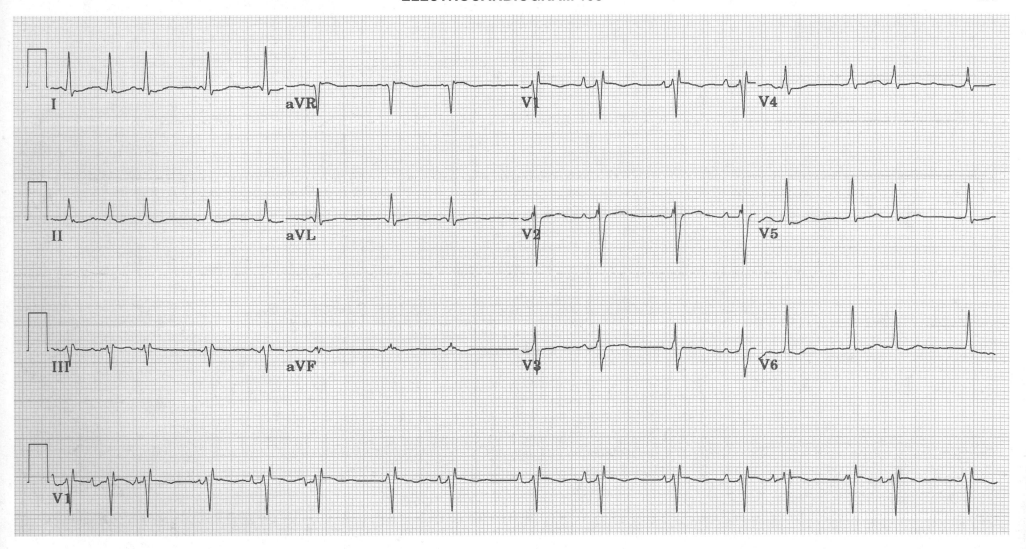

Interpretation Notes: _____

_____

_____

ECG 193 Sixty-seven year old gentleman with non-Hodgkin's lymphoma who presents for follow-up evaluation and chemotherapy administration. His past medical history includes hypertension.

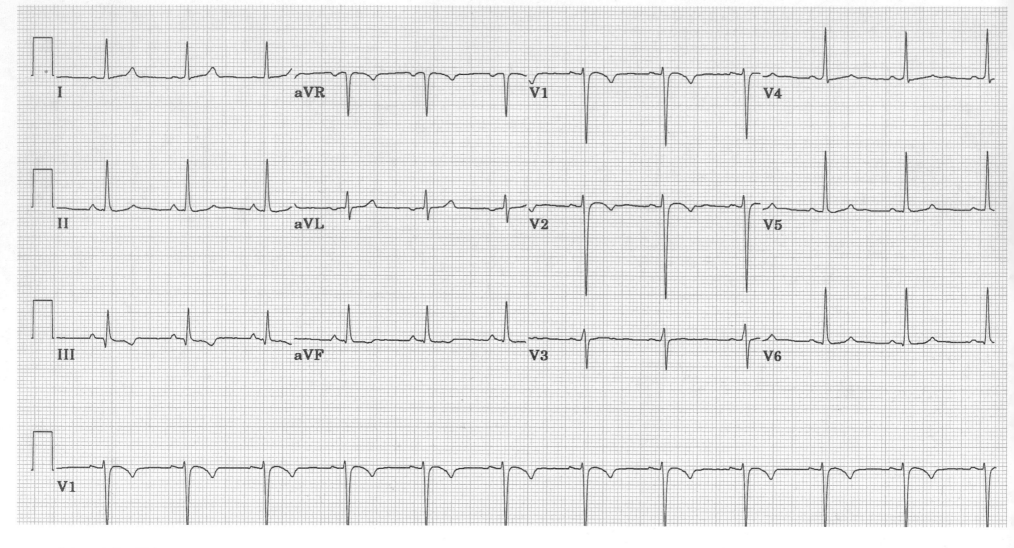

Interpretation Notes: _____

_____

_____

ECG 194 Twenty-two year old woman admitted to the hospital for evaluation and treatment of schizophrenia. She is on no current medications.

ELECTROCARDIOGRAM 195

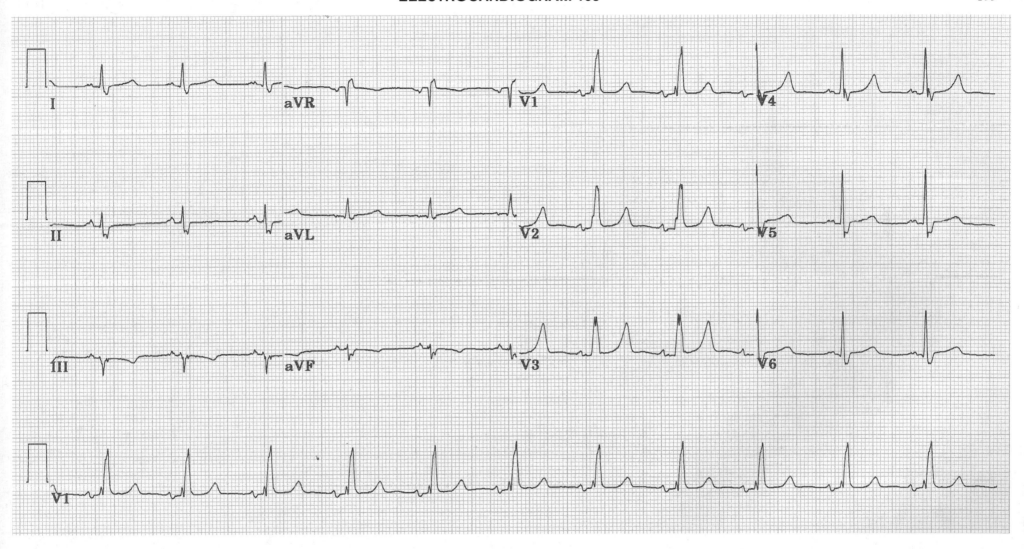

I   aVR   V1   V4

II   aVL   V2   V5

III   aVF   V3   V6

V1

Interpretation Notes: _____

ECG 195 Sixty-five year old gentleman with advanced peripheral vascular disease scheduled for a cardiac catheterization prior to a lower extremity arterial revascularization procedure. This electrocardiogram was obtained at the time of his cardiac catheterization. The cardiac catheterization demonstrated an 80% to 90% proximal stenosis of a large ramus intermedius coronary artery. Otherwise the coronary arteries were without significant obstructive lesions.

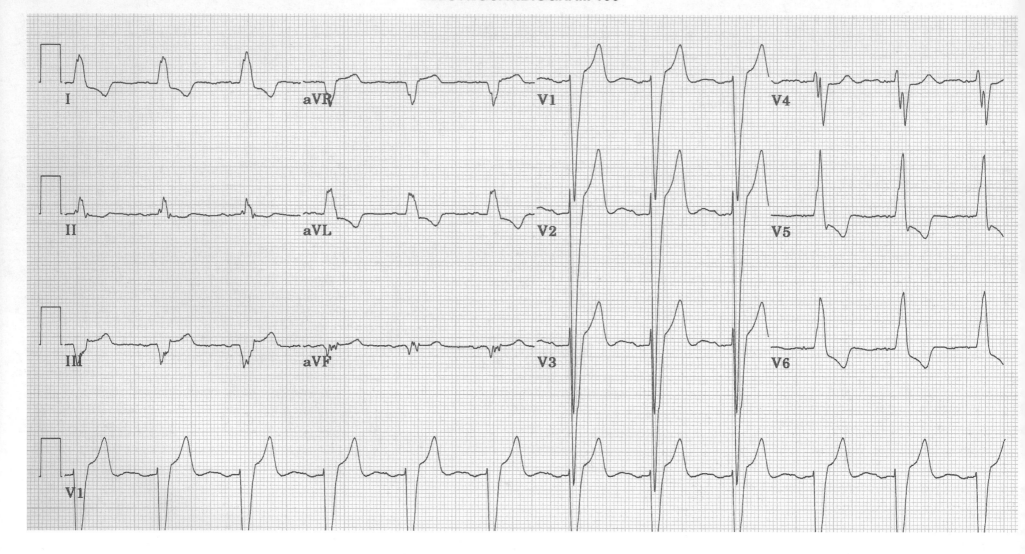

Interpretation Notes: _____

_____

ECG 196 Seventy-four year old gentleman who presents to the outpatient clinic with accelerating angina pectoris over the past two months. His past medical history includes coronary artery disease, hypertension, and hyperlipidemia. His medications included topical nitroglycerin, amlodipine, metoprolol, digoxin, and aspirin. A repeat cardiac catheterization demonstrated compromised blood flow to the left circumflex coronary artery territory.

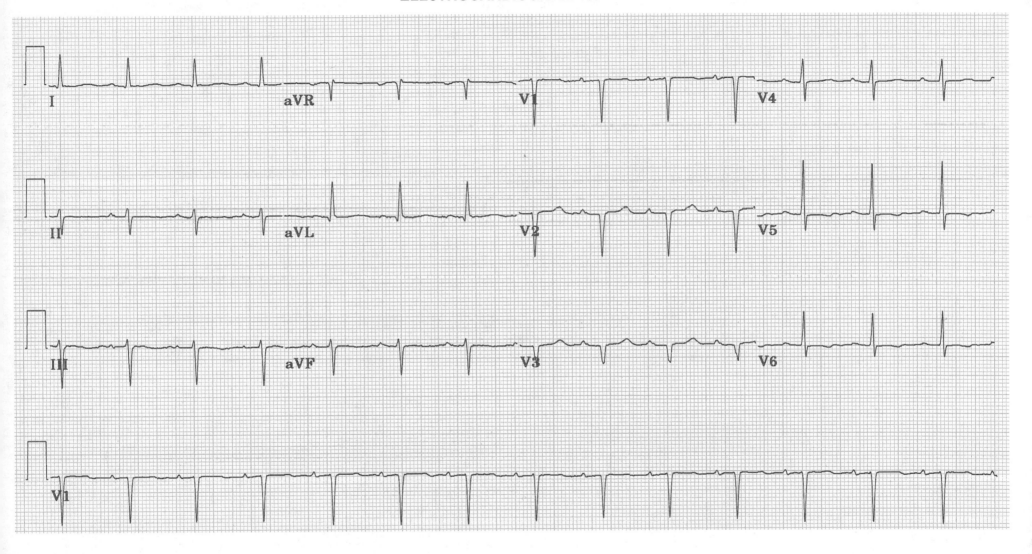

Interpretation Notes:_____

ECG 197 Seventy year old gentleman undergoing preoperative evaluation prior to planned bilateral total knee replacement. He has no known cardiac disease. Co-morbid conditions include severe debilitating rheumatoid arthritis requiring chronic steroid therapy, glucose intolerance, and restrictive lung disease. Medications at the time of this electrocardiogram included prednisone and thyroxine.

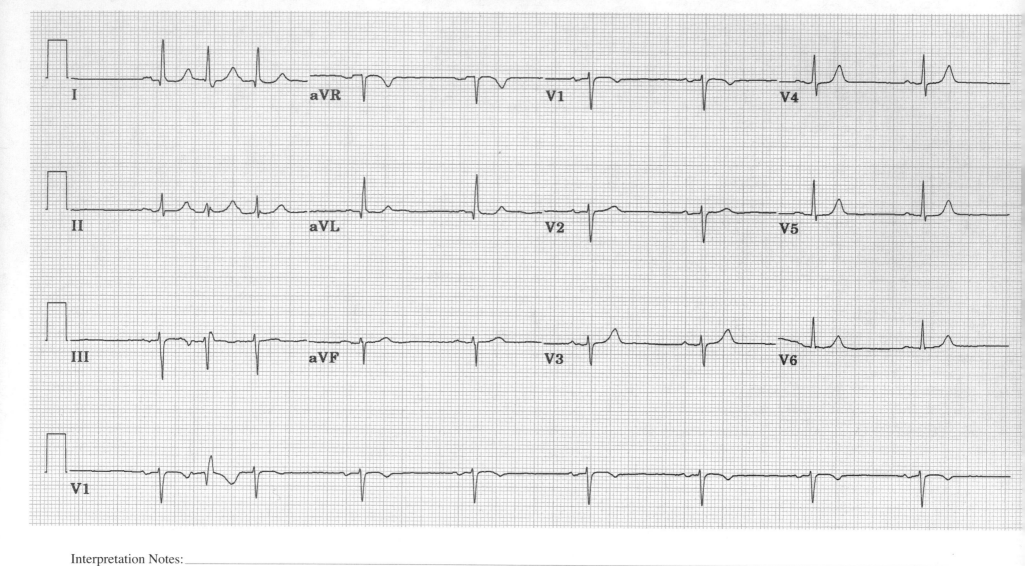

I aVR V1 V4

II aVL V2 V5

III aVF V3 V6

V1

Interpretation Notes: _____

_____

ECG 198 Seventy-six year old woman with a history of hypertension who received a preoperative electrocardiogram prior to subsequent gynecologic surgery. She has no known prior cardiac history.

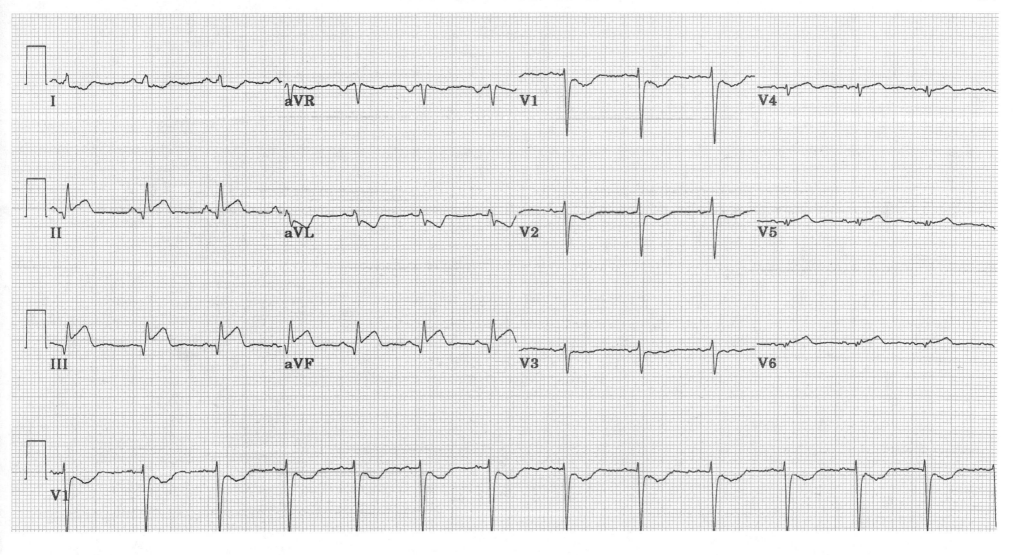

I aVR V1 V4

II aVL V2 V5

III aVF V3 V6

V1

Interpretation Notes:_____

ECG 199 Sixty-seven year old woman with severe left ventricular systolic dysfunction secondary to ischemic heart disease who re-presents to the hospital with an acute chest discomfort syndrome, persistent vomiting, and blurred vision. The patient has severe chronic congestive heart failure and is currently on home dobutamine. She is status post remote coronary artery bypass graft surgery and ventricular aneurysmectomy.

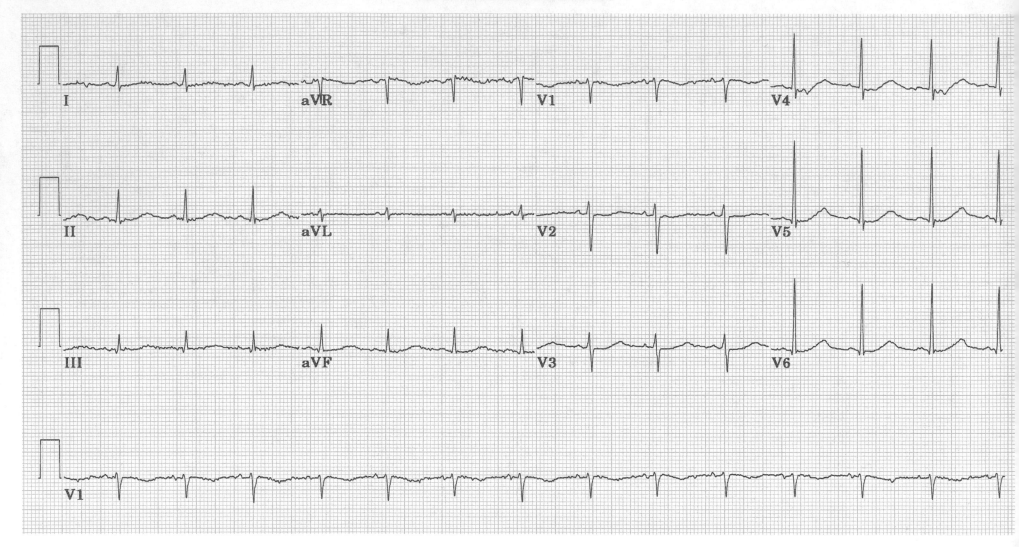

Interpretation Notes: _____

_____

_____

ECG 200 Fifty-one year old woman with metastatic breast carcinoma admitted for a bone marrow transplantation. Her potassium level at the time of this tracing was 3.1 meq/L.

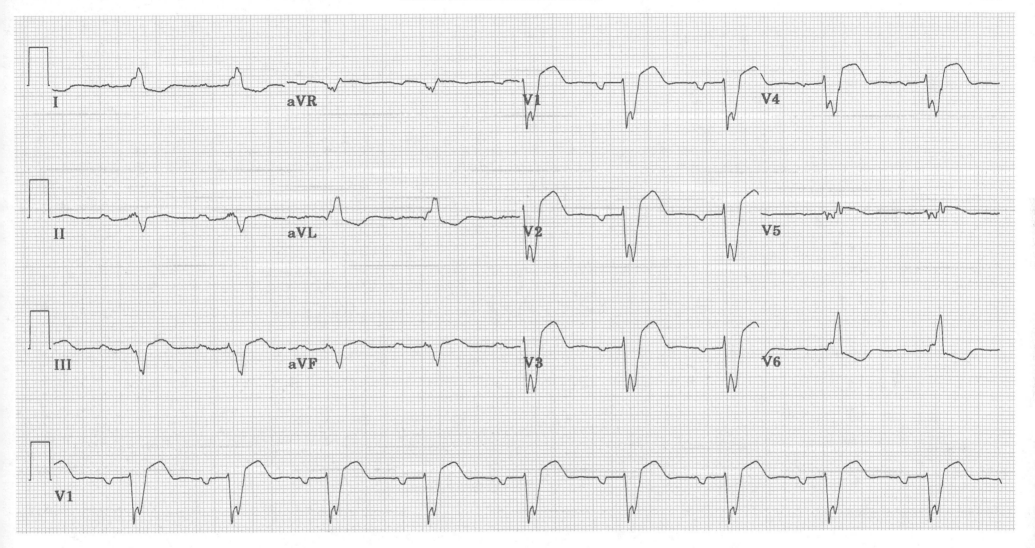

I   aVR   V1   V4

II   aVL   V2   V5

III   aVF   V3   V6

V1

Interpretation Notes: _____

_____

ECG 201 Sixty-six year old gentleman with advanced coronary artery disease and prior coronary artery bypass graft surgery. He has severe left ventricular systolic dysfunction. He now returns for a follow-up cardiac evaluation. He currently complains of fatigue but otherwise feels well. Medications at the time of this electrocardiogram included digoxin, furosemide, isosorbide mononitrate, and amiodarone.

ELECTROCARDIOGRAM 202

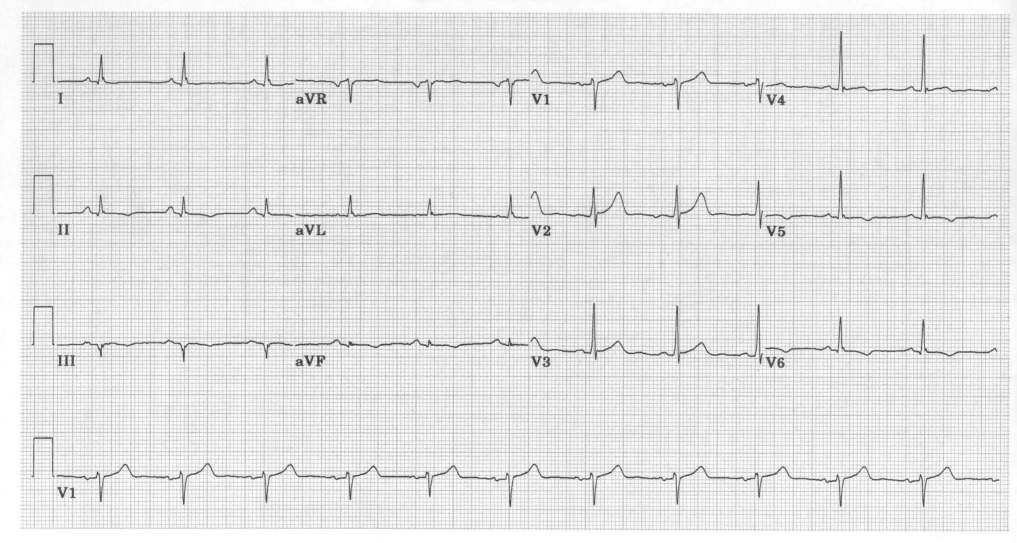

Interpretation Notes: _____

_____

_____

ECG 202 Fifty-six year old gentleman status post a remote inferior myocardial infarction and subsequent percutaneous transluminal coronary angioplasty of a dominant right coronary artery who returns for follow-up cardiac evaluation. At the time of this electrocardiogram the patient felt well without recurrent angina pectoris. His medications included propranolol and aspirin.

ELECTROCARDIOGRAM 203

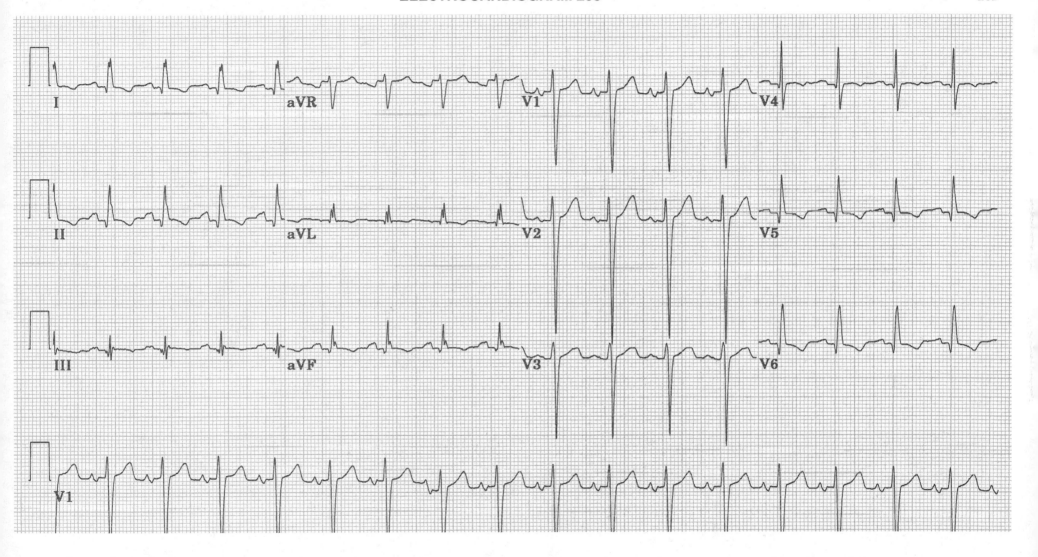

I aVR V1 V4

II aVL V2 V5

III aVF V3 V6

V1

Interpretation Notes: _____

ECG 203 Twenty-one year old gentleman status post mitral and aortic St. Jude valve replacements secondary to rheumatic valvular heart disease who returns for outpatient cardiology reassessment. His medications included warfarin, digoxin, and verapamil. There was no prior myocardial infarction history.

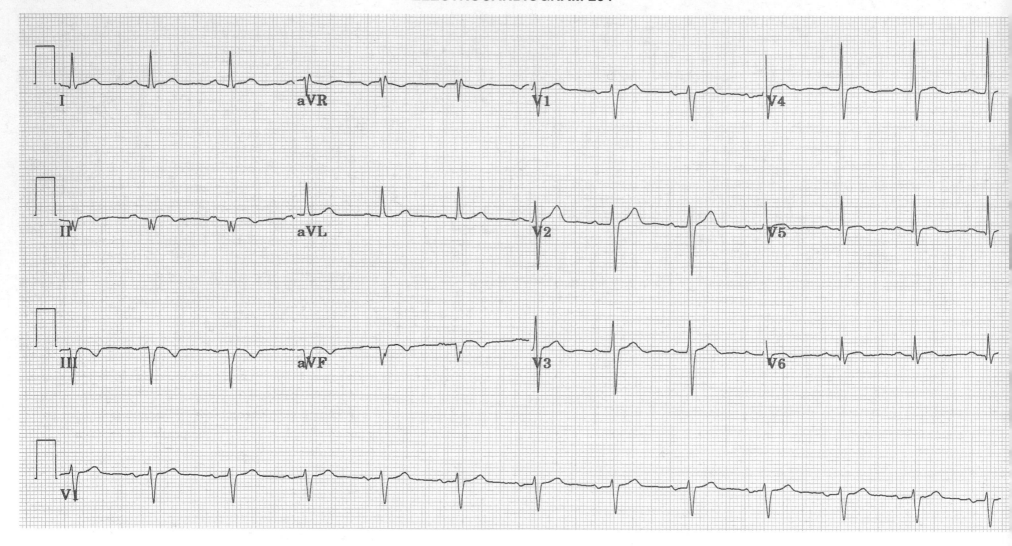

Interpretation Notes: _____

_____

ECG 204 Fifty-six year old gentleman status post an inferior myocardial infarction two years prior to this electrocardiogram subsequently followed by a cardiac catheterization and multi-vessel coronary artery bypass graft surgery. He is presently without symptoms. His past medical history includes hypercholesterolemia. Medications at the time of this electrocardiogram included lovastatin and aspirin.

ELECTROCARDIOGRAM 205

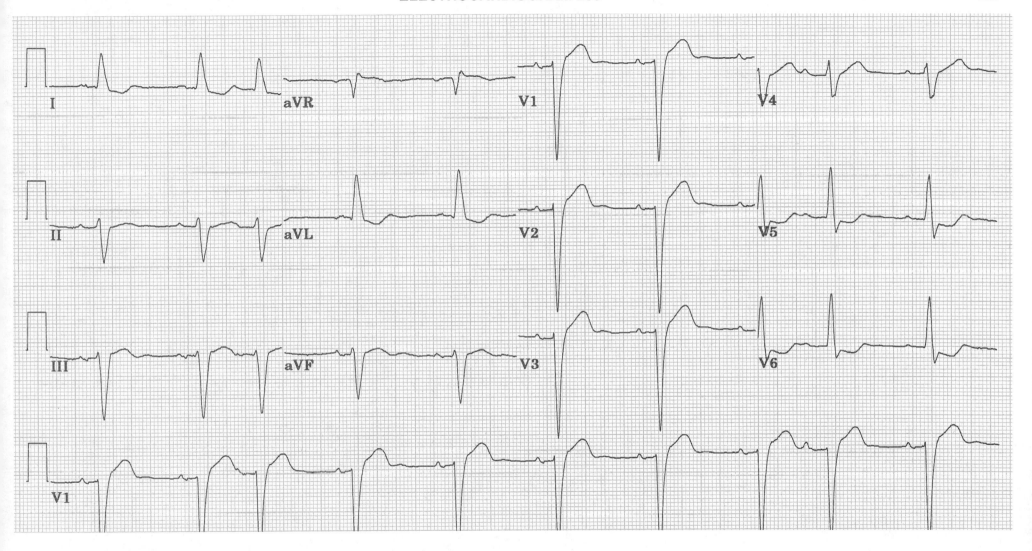

I aVR V1 V4

II aVL V2 V5

III aVF V3 V6

V1

Interpretation Notes: _____

ECG 205 Seventy-three year old gentleman who is being seen in the cardiology outpatient clinic at the time of this electrocardiogram. His past cardiac history includes severe global left ventricular systolic dysfunction, severe mitral insufficiency, and mild tricuspid insufficiency in the setting of mild coronary artery disease. Co-morbid conditions include chronic obstructive pulmonary disease and paroxysmal atrial fibrillation. Medications at the time of this electrocardiogram included enalapril, digoxin, furosemide, and amiodarone.

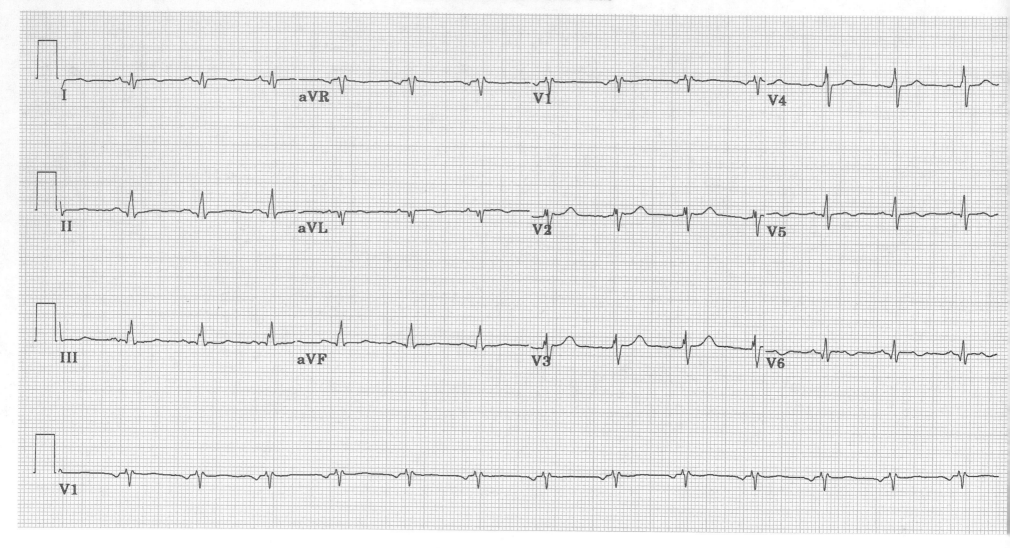

I aVR V1 V4
II aVL V2 V5
III aVF V3 V6
V1

Interpretation Notes: _____

_____

_____

ECG 206 Seventy-two year old gentleman with a history of non-insulin requiring diabetes mellitus and a recent left circumflex coronary artery territory myocardial infarction who underwent this electrocardiogram prior to anticipated coronary artery bypass graft surgery. Medications at the time of this electrocardiogram included intravenous heparin, atenolol, ranitidine, and intravenous nitroglycerin.

ELECTROCARDIOGRAM 207

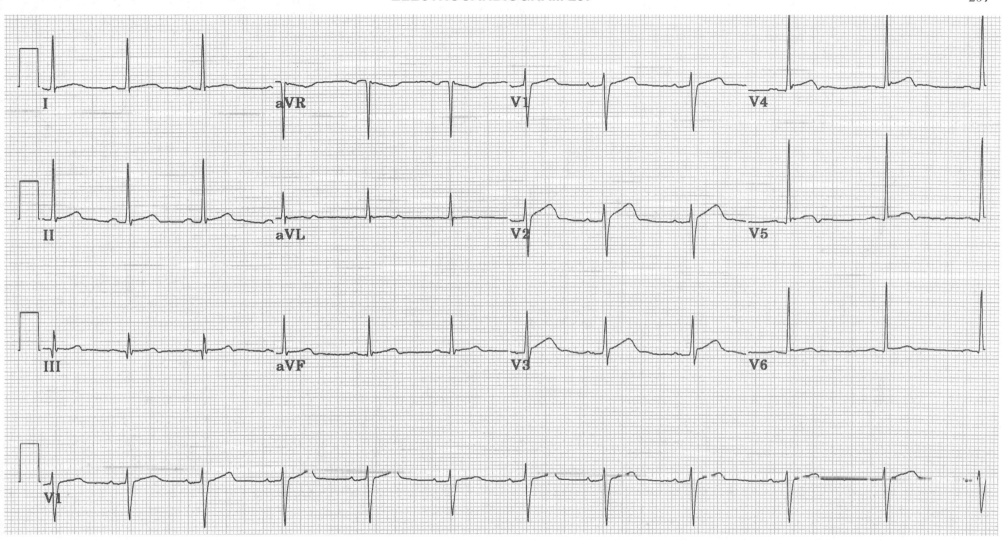

Interpretation Notes: _____

_____

ECG 207 Thirty year old African-American gentleman who is being evaluated in the pre-surgical department prior to inguinal hernia repair. He has no known prior cardiac history. An echocardiogram was normal without evidence of structural heart disease.

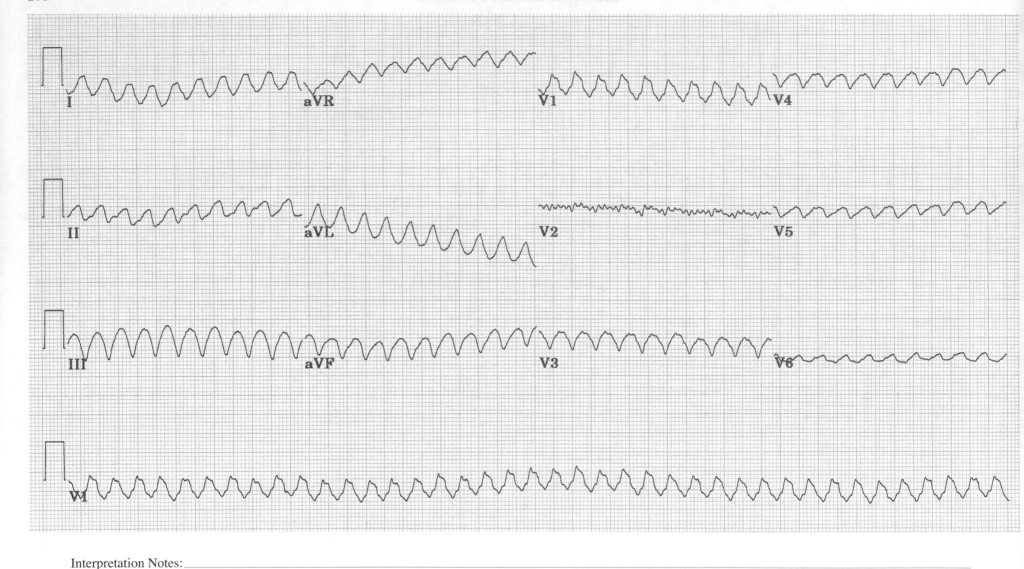

I aVR V1 V4

II aVL V2 V5

III aVF V3 V6

V1

Interpretation Notes: _____

ECG 208 Sixty-five year old gentleman resting comfortably on a left ventricular assist device with severe left ventricular systolic dysfunction awaiting cardiac transplantation. He has severe ischemic left ventricular systolic dysfunction. The patient underwent successful cardiac transplantation.

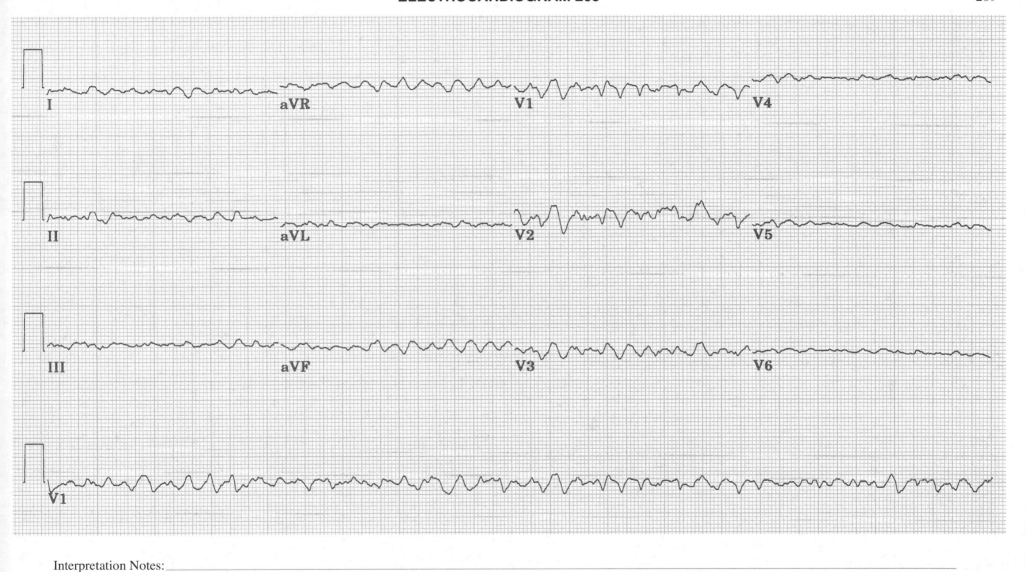

I aVR V1 V4

II aVL V2 V5

III aVF V3 V6

V1

Interpretation Notes: _____

_____

ECG 209 Sixty-five year old gentleman with advanced coronary artery disease and resultant severe left ventricular systolic dysfunction who is awaiting cardiac transplantation. This electrocardiogram was obtained while the patient was fully conscious and dependent on a left ventricular assist device. The patient underwent successful cardiac transplantation surgery.

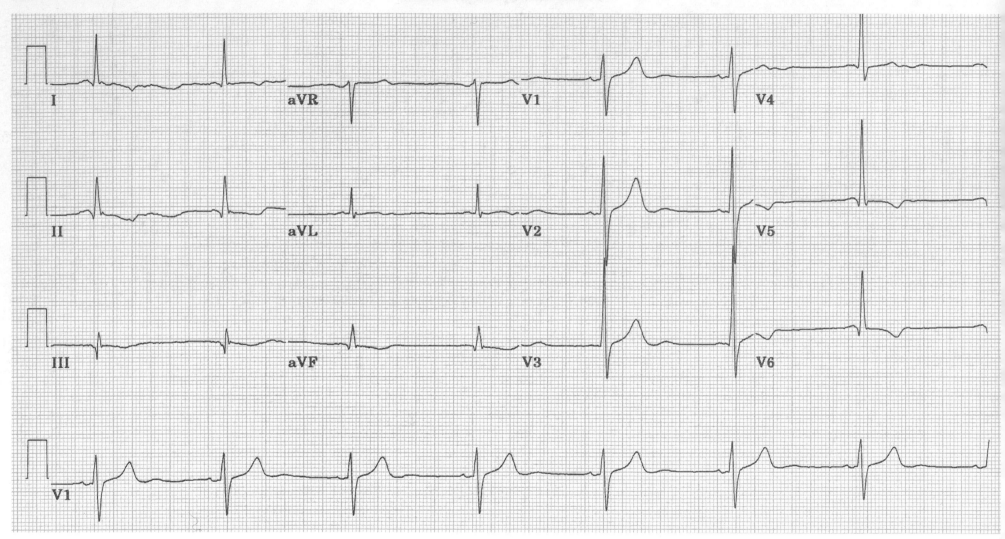

Interpretation Notes: _____

ECG 210 Sixty-three year old gentleman with an inferoposterior myocardial infarction six years prior to this electrocardiogram who is admitted to the hospital for evaluation of recurrent ventricular dysrhythmias. The patient is on no current medications. A recent echocardiogram demonstrated moderate regional left ventricular systolic dysfunction with inferoposterior segment akinesis.

ELECTROCARDIOGRAM 211

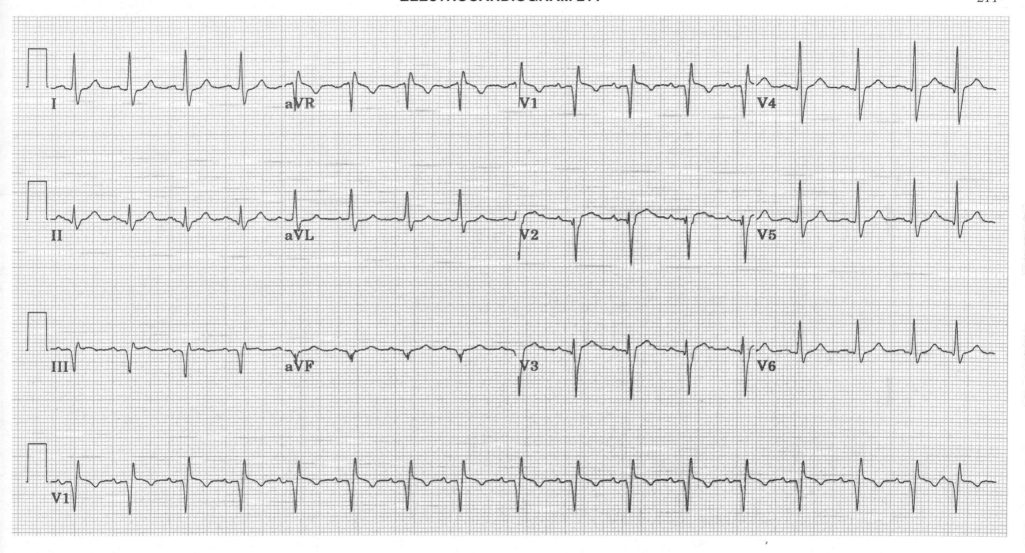

Interpretation Notes: _____

_____

_____

ECG 211 Sixty-eight year old gentleman status post recent coronary artery bypass graft surgery who returns for postoperative cardiac follow-up. His past cardiac history includes an anterior myocardial infarction one year prior to this electrocardiogram followed by a percutaneous transluminal coronary angioplasty of the left anterior descending coronary artery. His medications at the time of this tracing included metformin, diltiazem, procainamide, metoprolol, and simvastatin.

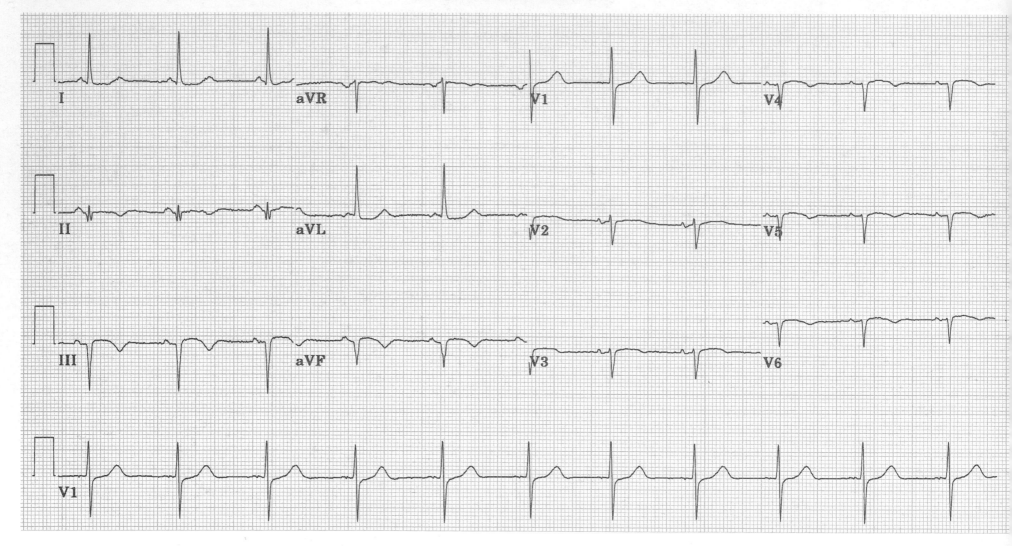

Interpretation Notes: _____

ECG 212 Seventy-nine year old woman with a history of non-insulin requiring diabetes mellitus who was referred to the emergency room from her private physician's office in the setting of acute onset bilateral shoulder discomfort, shortness of breath, and nausea. A cardiac catheterization was performed four days after her initial presentation and demonstrated advanced disease in the right coronary artery. This was successfully treated with percutaneous transluminal coronary angioplasty. Medications at the time of this electrocardiogram included aspirin, metoprolol, glyburide, intravenous nitroglycerin, and intravenous heparin.

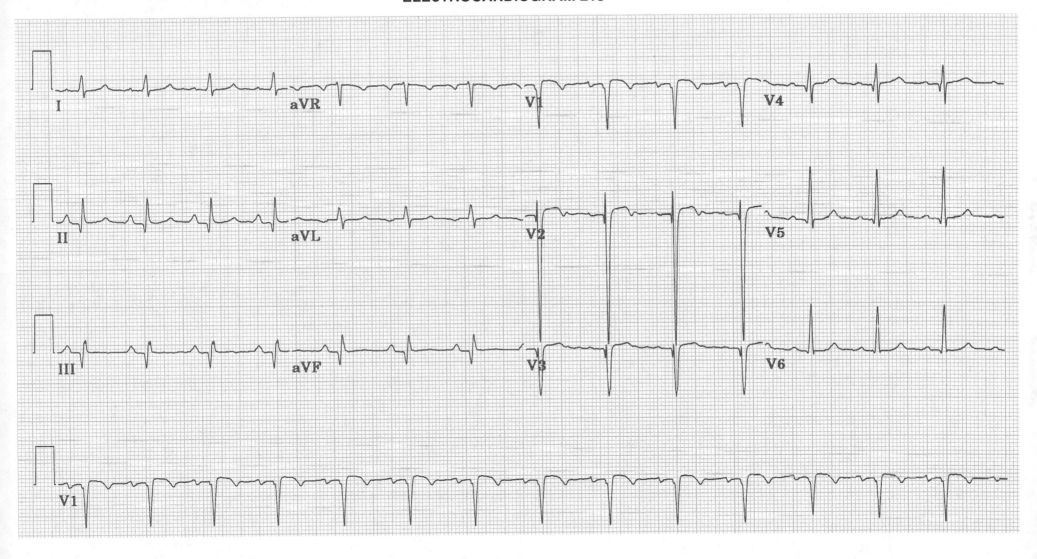

Interpretation Notes: _____

_____

ECG 213 Thirty-two year old gentleman with coronary artery disease who returns for a six month follow-up examination. A cardiac catheterization performed at the time of this electrocardiogram demonstrated severe coronary artery disease, moderate left ventricular systolic dysfunction, and evidence of prior inferior and anterior myocardial infarctions. Medications at the time of this electrocardiogram included isosorbide dinitrate, diltiazem, captopril, and aspirin.

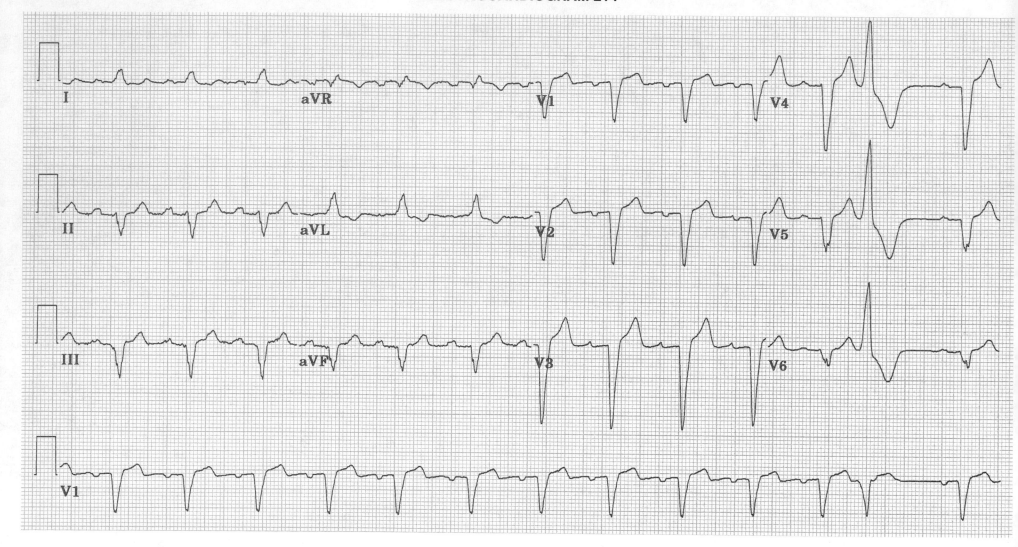

I aVR V1 V4

II aVL V2 V5

III aVF V3 V6

V1

Interpretation Notes: _____

_____

ECG 214 Seventy-three year old woman with long-standing hypertension who presents for evaluation of recent onset dyspnea upon exertion. Co-morbidities include obesity and insulin requiring diabetes mellitus.

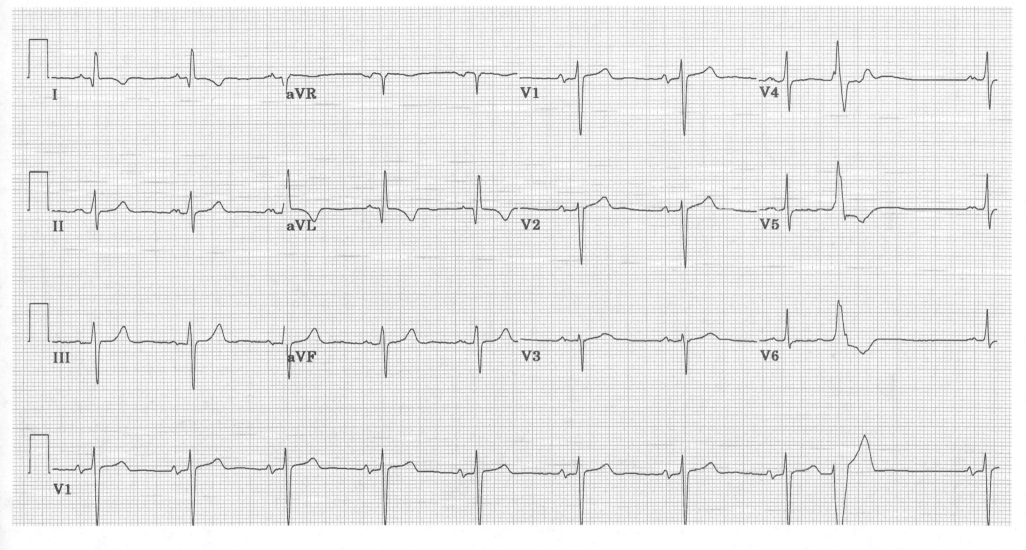

Interpretation Notes:_____

_____

ECG 215 Sixty-five year old gentleman with a myocardial infarction five years prior to this electrocardiogram referred for coronary artery bypass graft surgery. A recent cardiac catheterization demonstrated a 100% occlusion of the first diagonal branch of the left anterior descending coronary artery which was felt to reflect his prior high lateral myocardial infarction.

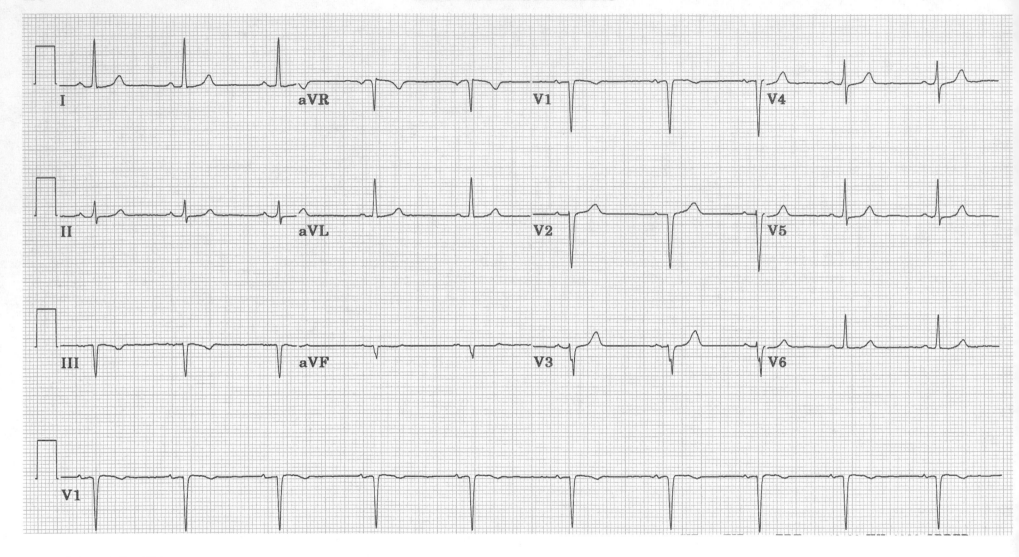

Interpretation Notes: _____
_____
_____

ECG 216 Fifty-three year old woman seen in preoperative anesthesia clearance prior to elective cosmetic surgery. She is currently healthy. Her medications include estrogen replacement. She has no cardiac history.

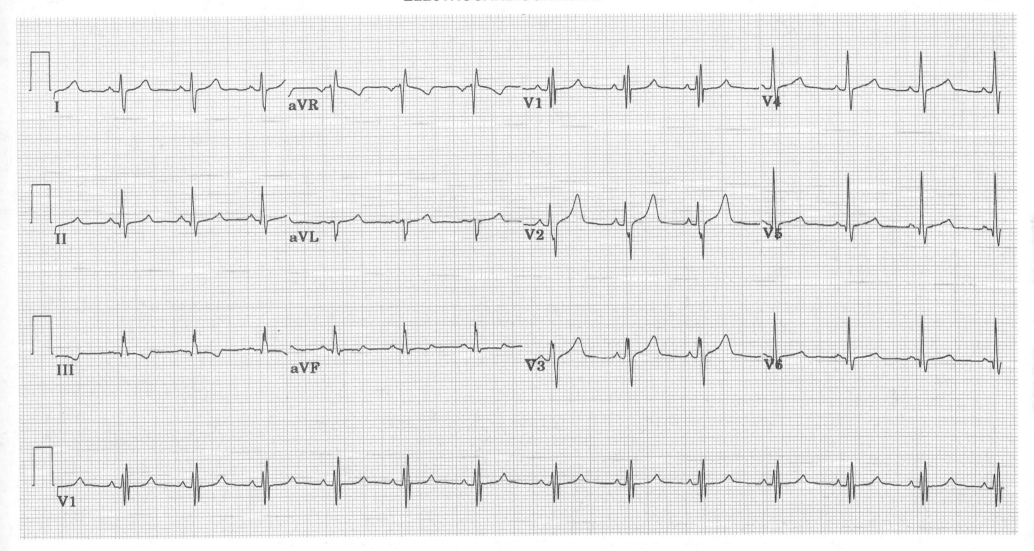

ECG 217 Nineteen year old gentleman seen preoperatively prior to intended ostium secundum atrial septal defect repair. A recent echocardiogram demonstrated a moderate sized ostium secundum atrial septal defect with left to right shunt flow, a dilated right ventricle with normal right ventricular systolic function, and moderate pulmonary hypertension.

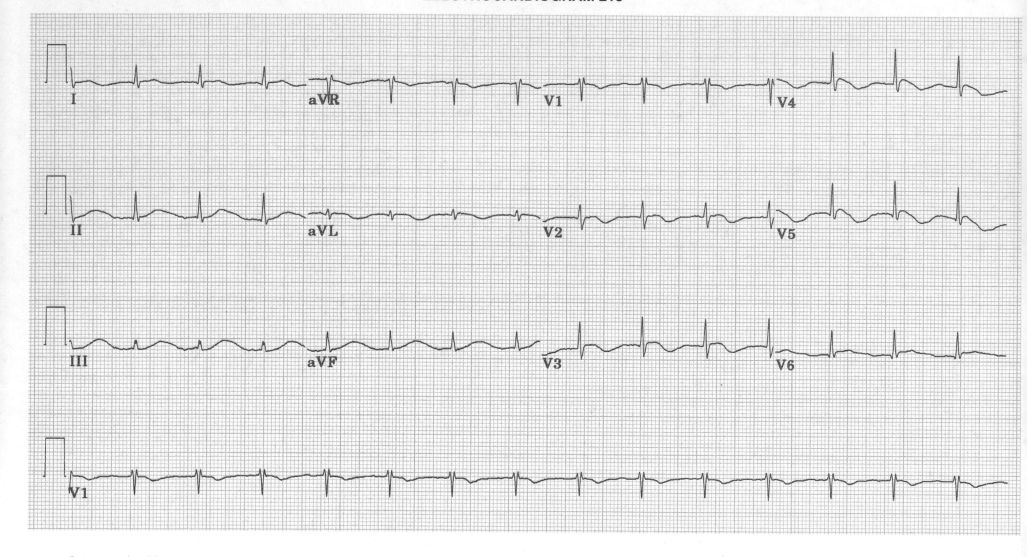

Interpretation Notes: _____

_____

_____

ECG 218 Sixty-three year old gentleman with a non-ischemic dilated cardiomyopathy status post cardiac transplantation.

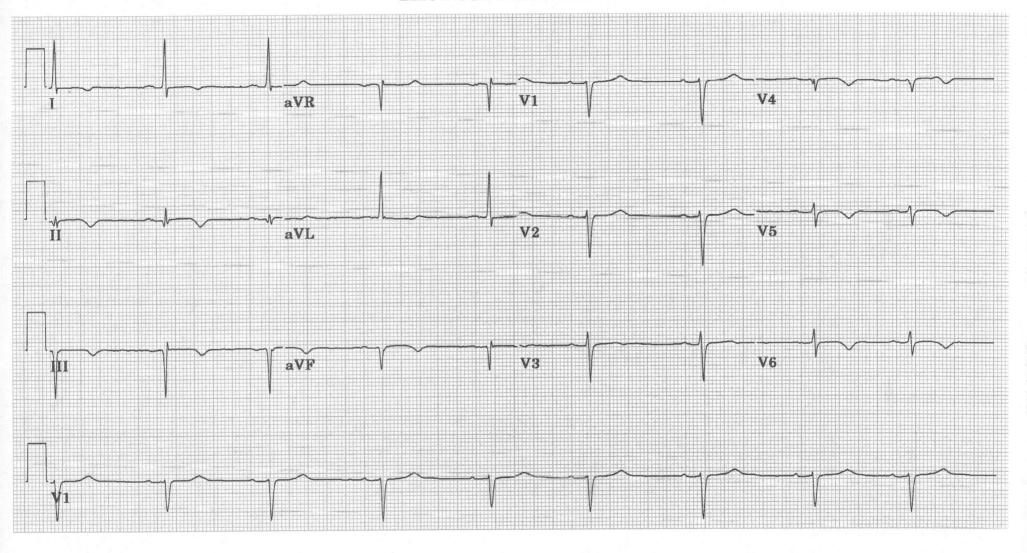

Interpretation Notes: _____

ECG 219 Sixty-five year old woman with a recent myocardial infarction of unknown location accepted in transfer from an outside hospital with symptoms of angina pectoris. A cardiac catheterization demonstrated an 80% proximal left anterior descending coronary artery stenosis and a 90% mid right coronary artery stenosis. The patient was subsequently referred for coronary artery bypass graft surgery.

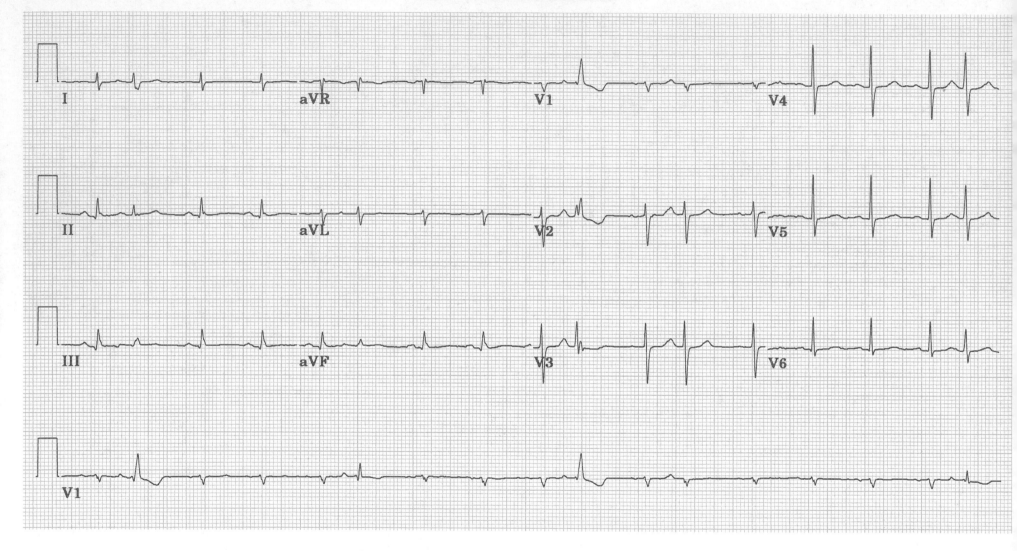

I   aVR   V1   V4

II   aVL   V2   V5

III   aVF   V3   V6

V1

Interpretation Notes: _____

_____

ECG 220 Sixty-six year old gentleman who presented with an acute chest discomfort syndrome. Serial cardiac enzymes documented a non-Q wave myocardial infarction. Subsequently coronary arteriography was performed demonstrating a severe obstruction in the left circumflex coronary artery. This was followed by successful coronary artery stent placement. Medications at the time of this electrocardiogram included ticlodipine, intravenous heparin, nebulized inhalers, and aspirin.

ELECTROCARDIOGRAM 221

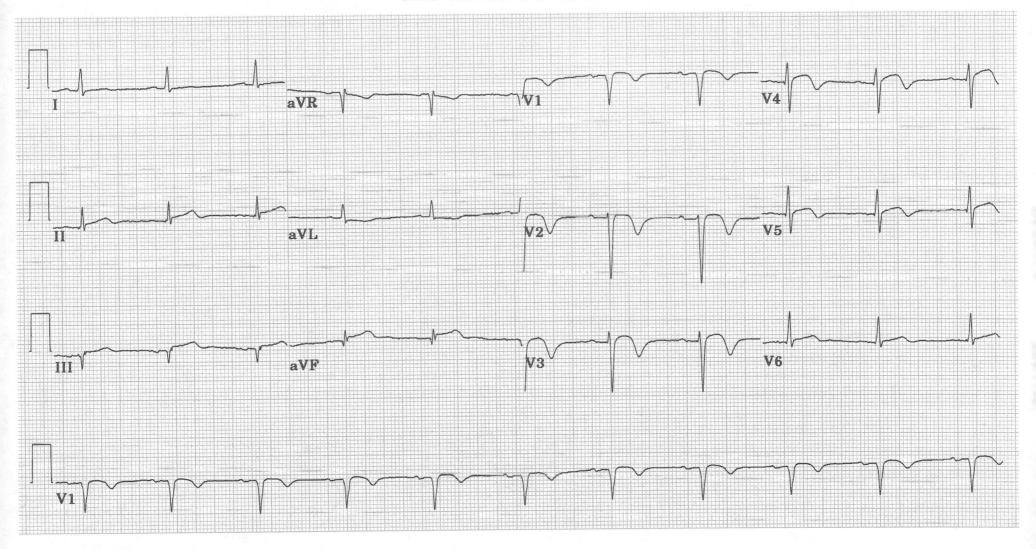

Interpretation Notes: _____

ECG 221 Sixty-eight year old gentleman with a history of coronary artery disease status post coronary artery bypass graft surgery four years prior to this electrocardiogram who presents with a one hour history of acute chest discomfort. He was stabilized with intravenous nitroglycerin and intravenous heparin.

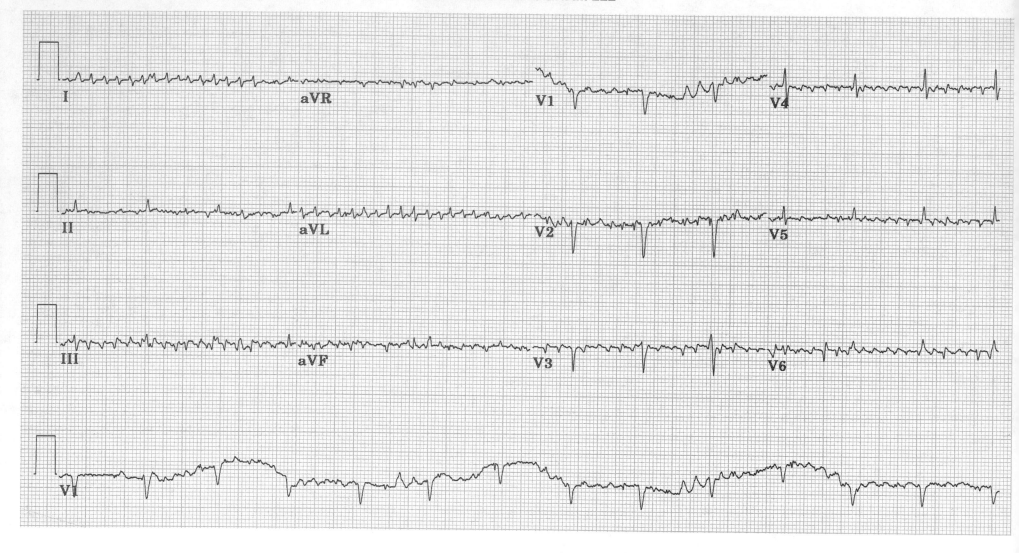

Interpretation Notes: _____

_____

ECG 222 Sixty-two year old woman admitted with fevers and chills of two days duration with suspected sepsis. Co-morbid conditions include rheumatoid arthritis and chronic obstructive lung disease.

ELECTROCARDIOGRAM 223

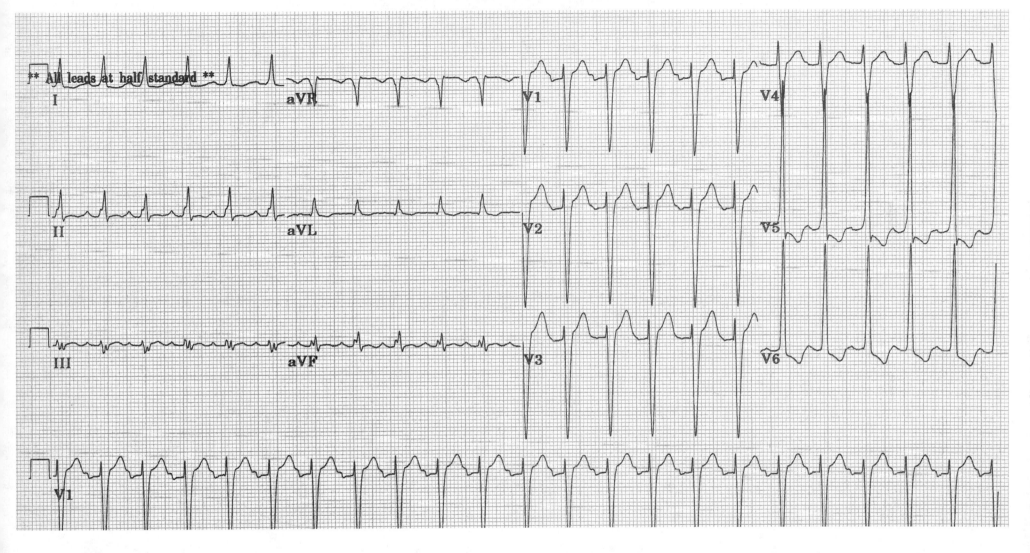

** All leads at half standard **

I   aVR   V1   V4

II   aVL   V2   V5

III   aVF   V3   V6

V1

Interpretation Notes: _____

ECG 223 Forty-five year old woman with a non-ischemic dilated cardiomyopathy who returns for an outpatient cardiac evaluation. Her medications included bumetanide, potassium, captopril, digoxin, warfarin, and amiodarone.

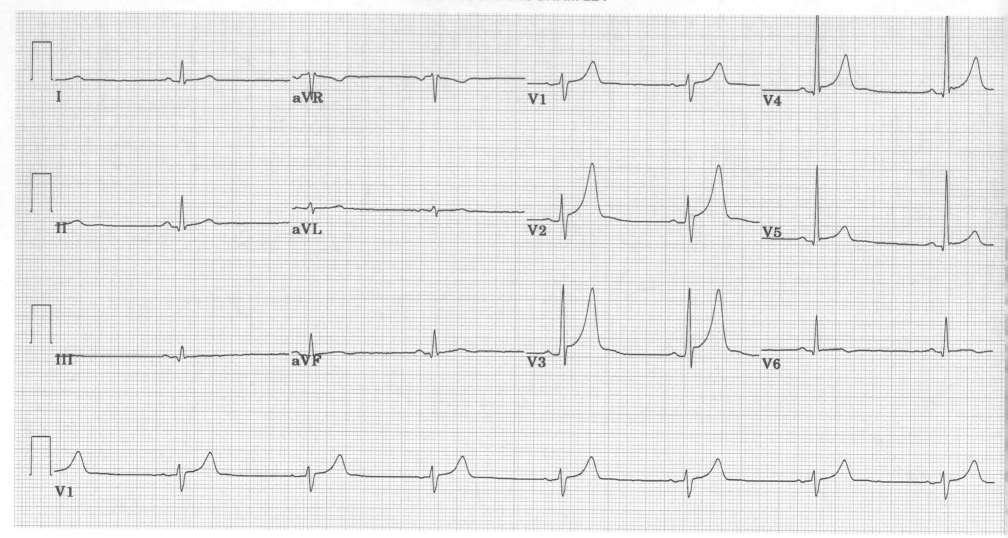

Interpretation Notes: _____

ECG 224 Thirty-nine year old gentleman referred for a cardiac catheterization in the setting of acute chest discomfort onset and suspected acute myocardial injury. His cardiac catheterization demonstrated an advanced stenosis of the right coronary artery. The patient underwent successful percutaneous transluminal rotational atherectomy of the distal right coronary artery. The electrocardiogram remained unchanged both before and after the procedure.

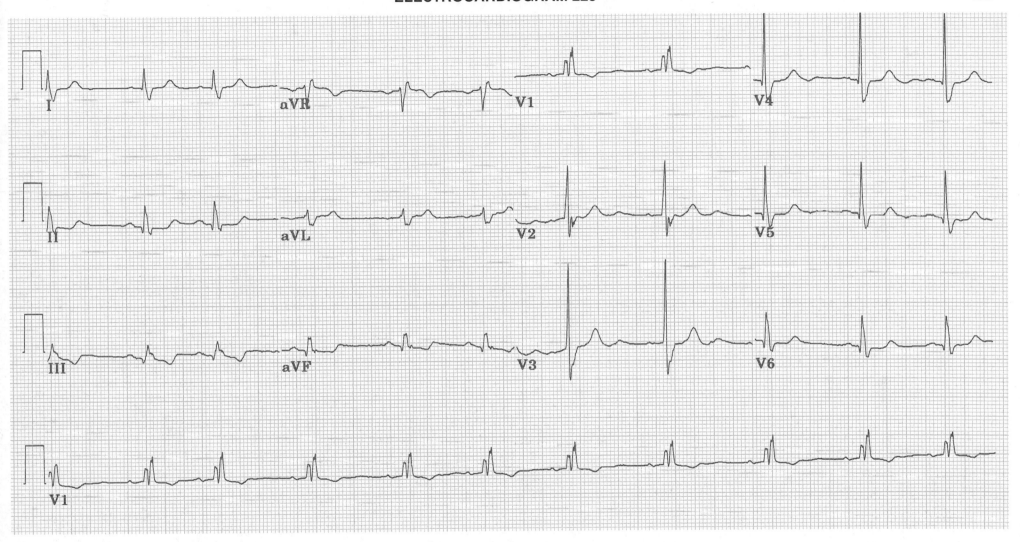

I aVR V1 V4

II aVL V2 V5

III aVF V3 V6

V1

Interpretation Notes: _____

ECG 225 Eighty year old woman being seen in preoperative anesthesia clearance prior to spinal stenosis surgical repair. Her cardiac health has been excellent without a known prior myocardial infarction. She is on no current medications.

ELECTROCARDIOGRAM 226

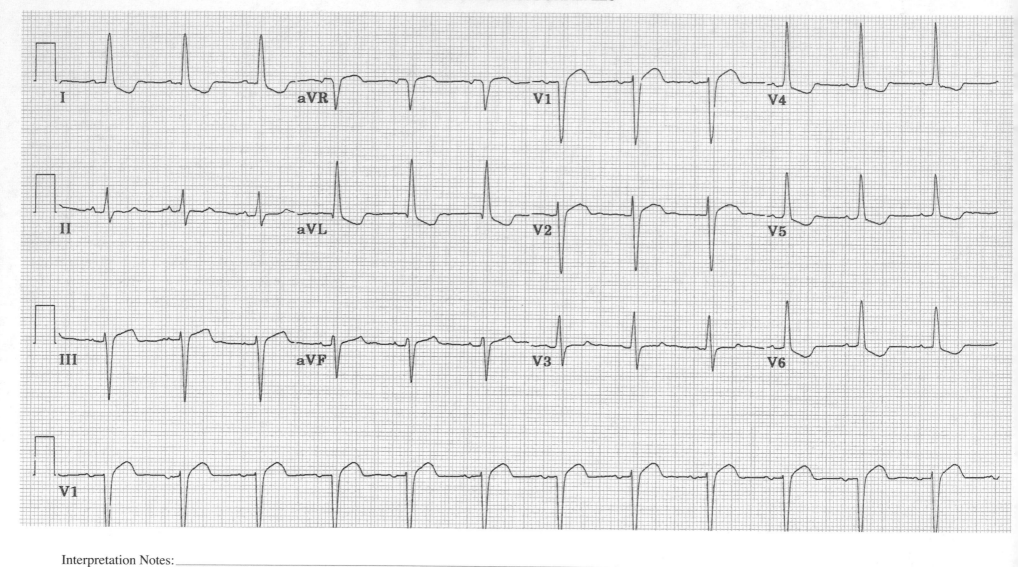

Interpretation Notes: _____

ECG 226 Seventy-four year old woman with a four year history of shortness of breath in the setting of a recent cardiac catheterization demonstrating multi-vessel coronary artery disease and severe aortic insufficiency. The patient recently underwent coronary artery bypass graft surgery and aortic valve replacement. Her medications included metoprolol and aspirin.

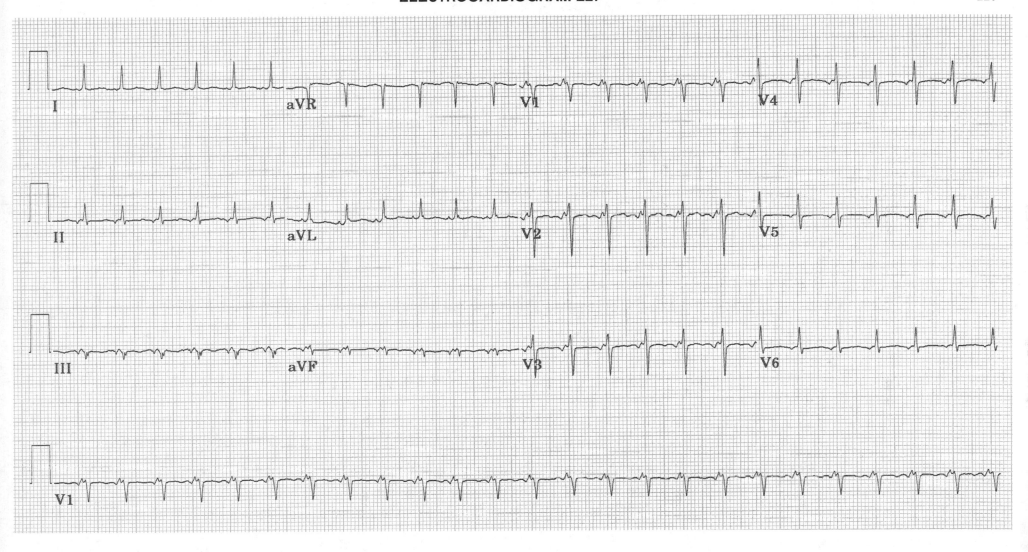

Interpretation Notes: _____

_____

ECG 227 Eighty-four year old woman with a history of hypertension and spinal stenosis who was noted to have a sudden onset tachycardia during preoperative evalua-tion. The patient received intravenous verapamil at which time she converted to normal sinus rhythm. Extended release verapamil was continued without further dysrhyth-mia recurrence.

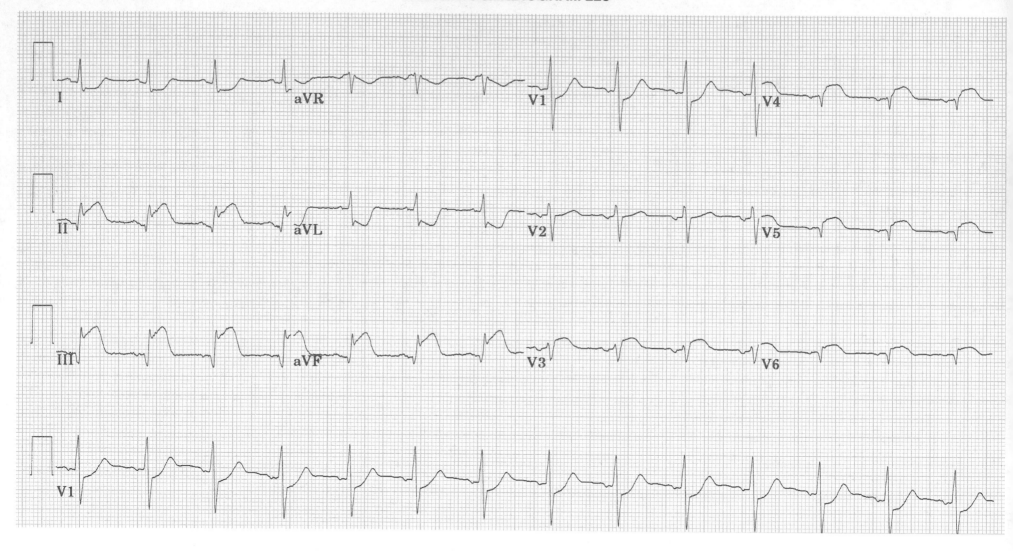

Interpretation Notes: _____

ECG 228 Forty-six year old gentleman accepted in hospital transfer two days after the sudden onset of severe anterior chest discomfort with radiation to both arms. Medications at the time of this tracing included metoprolol, intravenous heparin, and aspirin. The patient underwent a cardiac catheterization demonstrating a severe proximal right coronary artery stenosis and subsequent successful percutaneous transluminal coronary angioplasty.

ELECTROCARDIOGRAM 229

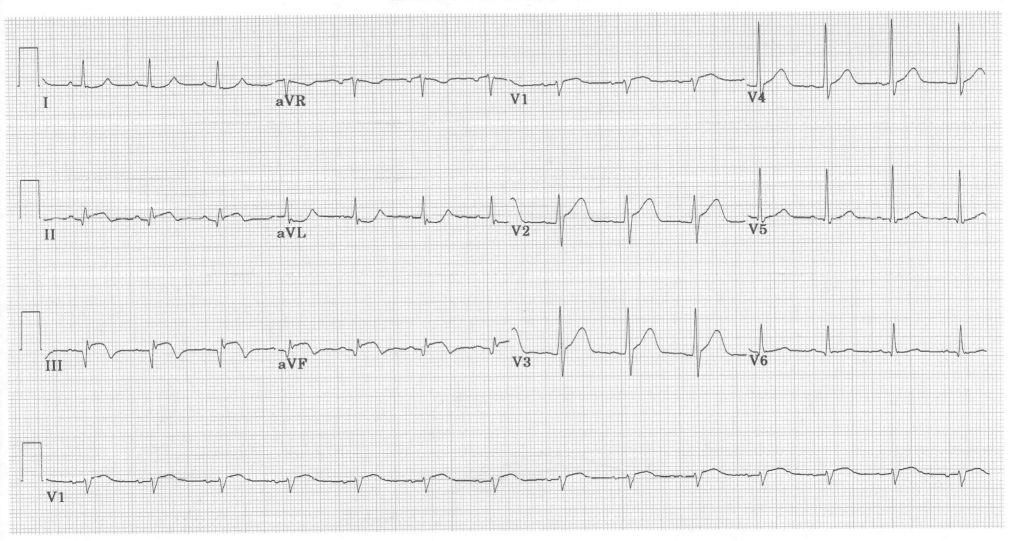

I aVR V1 V4

II aVL V2 V5

III aVF V3 V6

V1

Interpretation Notes: _____

ECG 229 Forty-six year old gentleman accepted in hospital transfer two days after the sudden onset of severe anterior chest discomfort with radiation to both arms. The patient received urgent intravenous thrombolytic therapy. Serial cardiac enzyme serum analysis confirmed a large myocardial infarction. Medications at the time of this electrocardiogram included metoprolol, intravenous heparin, and aspirin. The patient underwent a cardiac catheterization demonstrating a severe proximal right coronary artery stenosis and subsequent successful percutaneous transluminal coronary angioplasty.

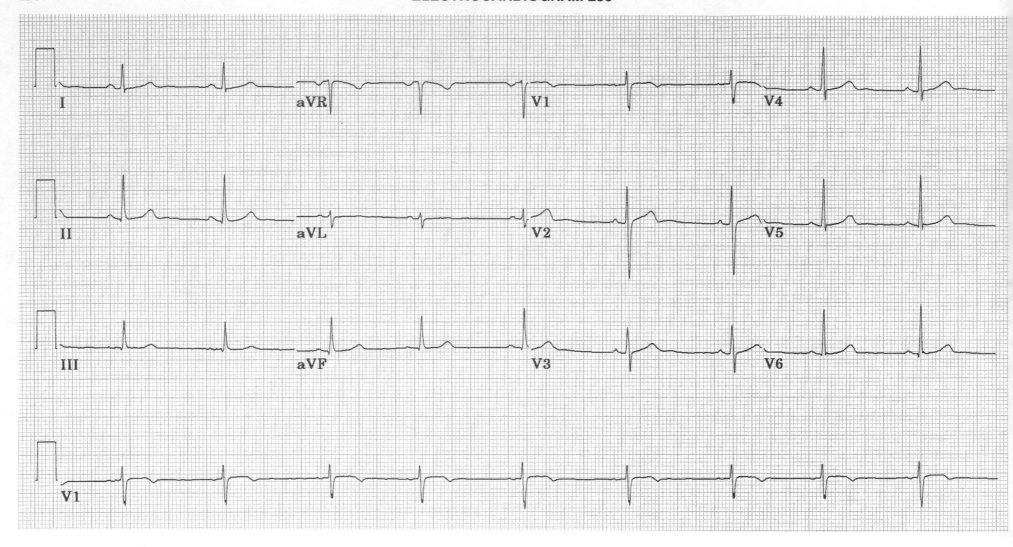

Interpretation Notes: _____

_____

ECG 230 Twenty-six year old woman with supraventricular tachycardia who subsequently underwent electrophysiology study and radiofrequency ablation of the slow atrio-ventricular nodal pathway with resolution of atrioventricular nodal re-entry tachycardia.

ELECTROCARDIOGRAM 231

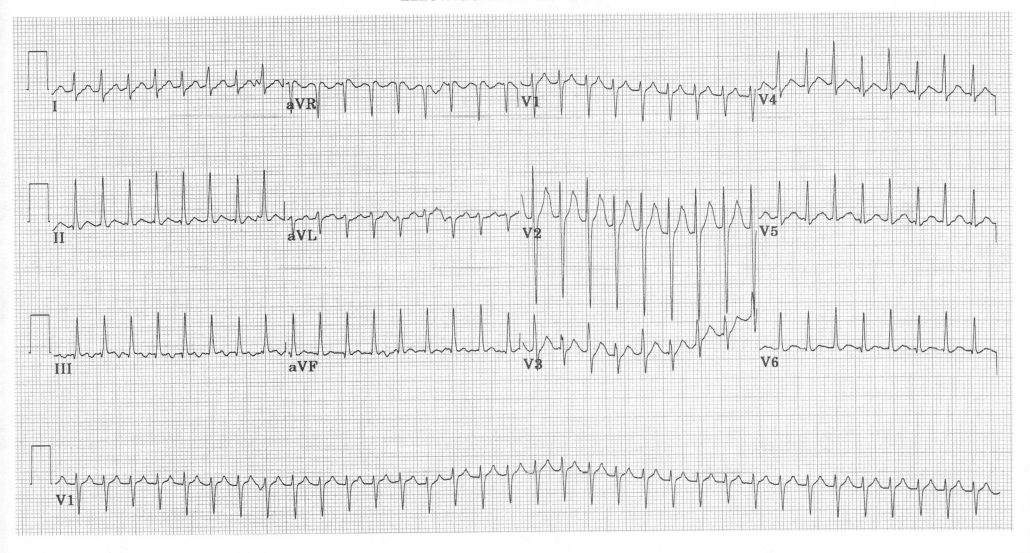

Interpretation Notes:_____

_____

ECG 231 Twenty-six year old woman with recurrent palpitations who proceeded to undergo a successful radiofrequency ablation of the slow atrioventricular nodal pathway with resolution of atypical atrioventricular nodal re-entrant tachycardia confirmed at the time of electrophysiology study.

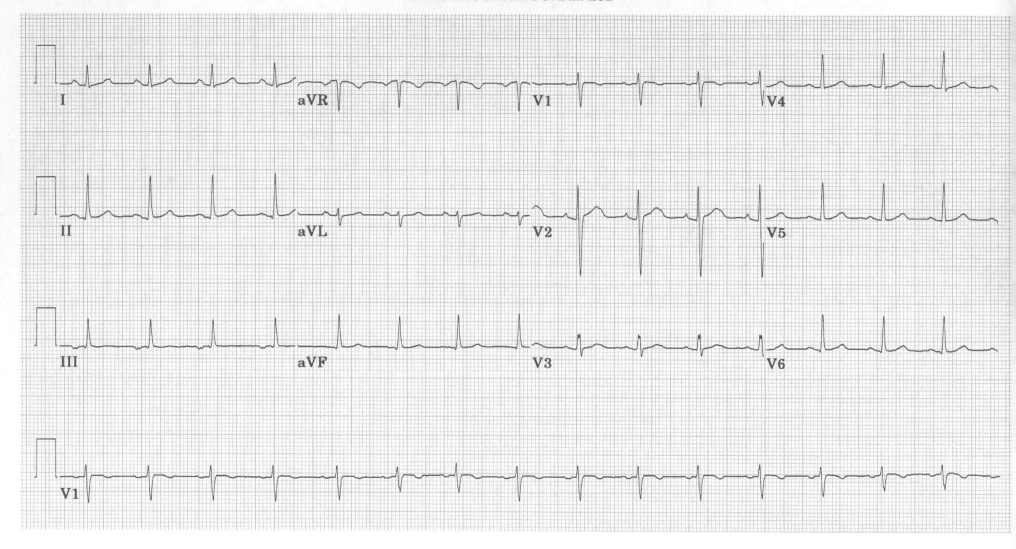

I aVR V1 V4

II aVL V2 V5

III aVF V3 V6

V1

Interpretation Notes: _____

_____

ECG 232 Twenty-six year old woman with supraventricular tachycardia who underwent an electrophysiology study and radiofrequency ablation of the slow atrioventricular nodal pathway with resolution of atypical atrioventricular nodal re-entry tachycardia. This electrocardiogram was obtained in a hospitalized setting after her recent radiofrequency ablation procedure.

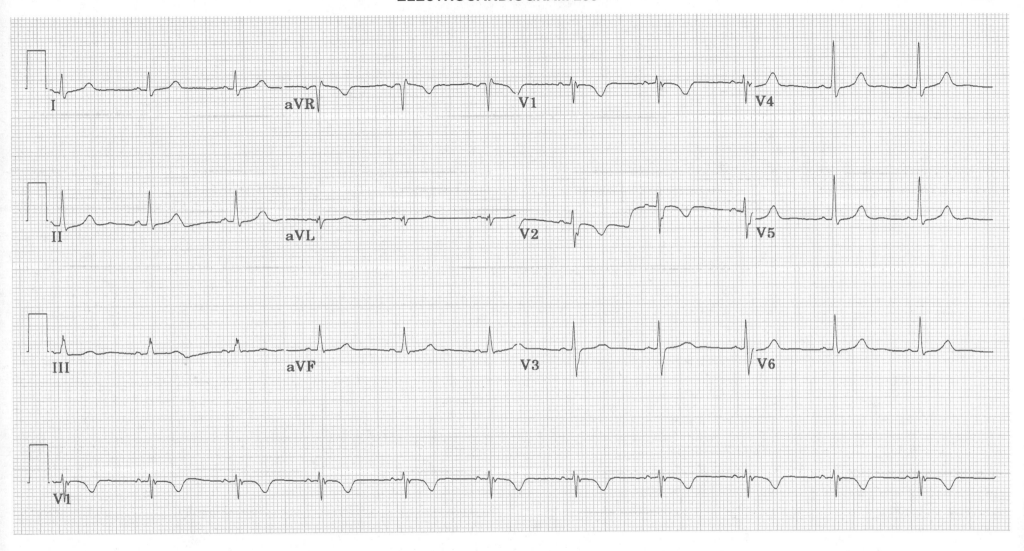

Interpretation Notes: _____

ECG 233 Forty year old woman who returns for outpatient follow-up after undergoing an ostium secundum atrial septal defect repair one year prior to this electrocardiogram. She currently feels well without cardiac symptomatology. Medications at the time of this electrocardiogram included antidepressants.

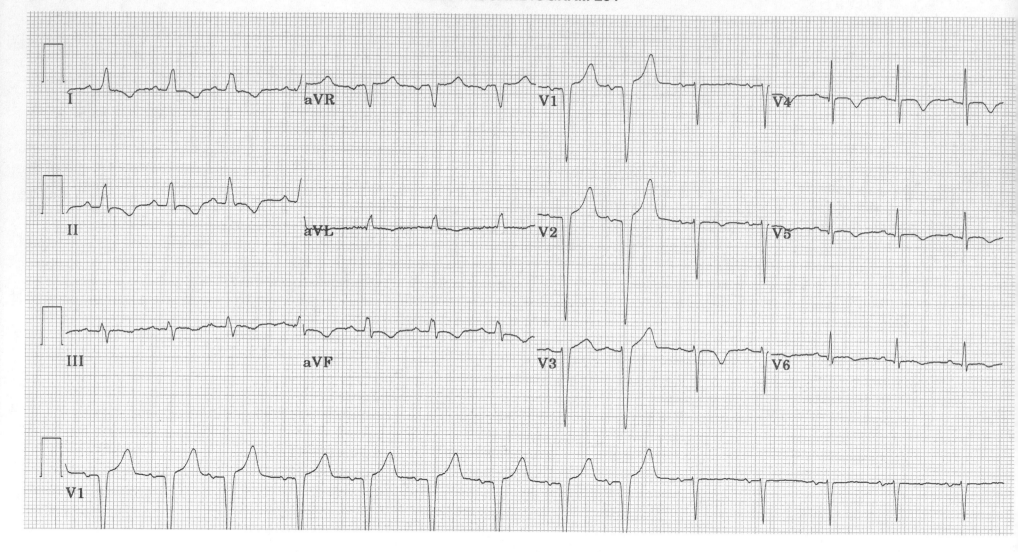

Interpretation Notes:

ECG 234 Seventy-six year old woman with coronary artery disease who underwent multi-vessel coronary artery bypass graft surgery one year prior to this electrocardiogram. She now presents for evaluation of a recent syncopal episode.

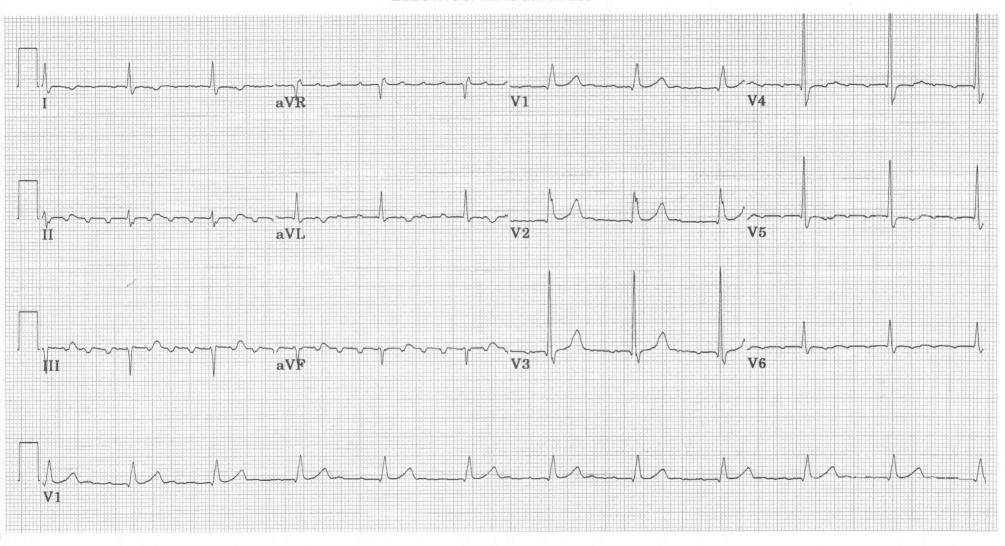

I aVR V1 V4

II aVL V2 V5

III aVF V3 V6

V1

Interpretation Notes: _____

ECG 235 Seventy-eight year old gentleman status post remote aortic valve replacement, coronary artery bypass graft surgery, and recurrent transitional cell carcinoma of the bladder who developed this cardiac dysrhythmia during the intravenous administration of a chemotherapeutic medication.

ELECTROCARDIOGRAM 236

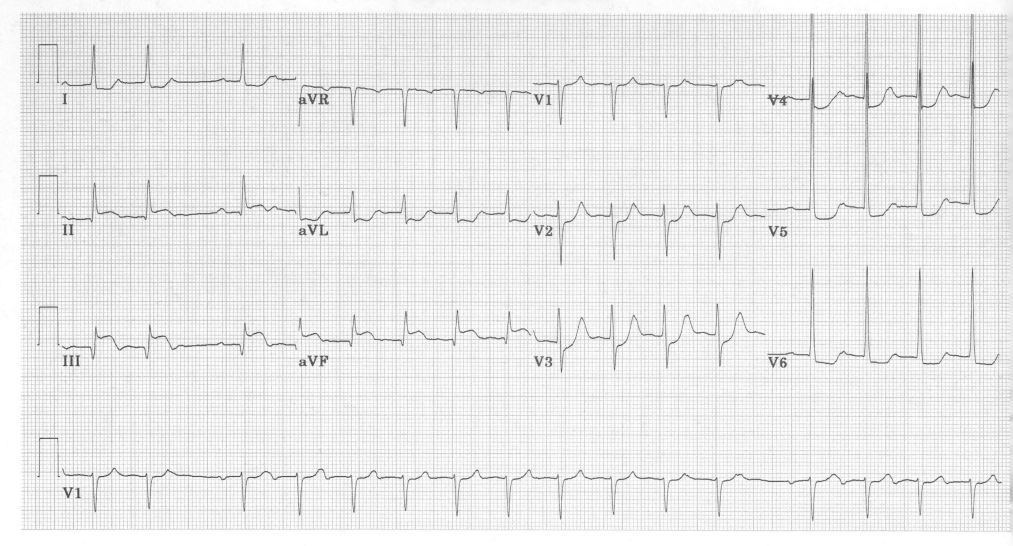

Interpretation Notes: _____

_____

ECG 236 Seventy-four year old woman who was accepted in hospital transfer after presenting earlier the same day with acute onset chest discomfort consistent with acute myocardial injury. Serial cardiac enzymes documented an acute myocardial infarction. She continued to demonstrate post-infarction angina and was transferred for cardiac catheterization. Her cardiac catheterization demonstrated severe right coronary artery disease and a successful angioplasty was performed.

ELECTROCARDIOGRAM 237

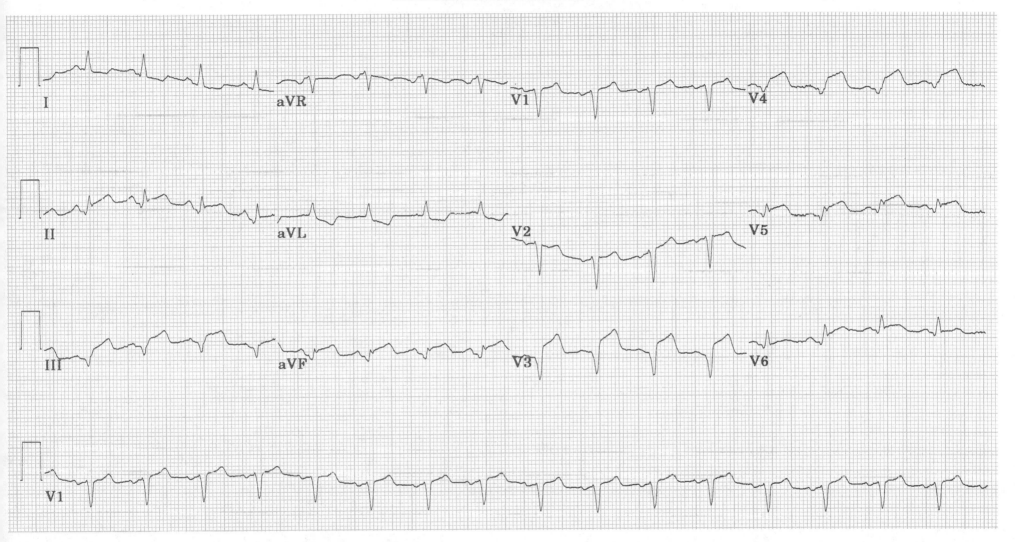

Interpretation Notes: _____

_____

_____

ECG 237 Fifty-eight year old woman who presented to an outside medical center with three hours of acute onset chest discomfort. An acute myocardial infarction was confirmed by serial cardiac enzyme analysis. Recurrent post-infarction angina pectoris culminated in a left heart catheterization demonstrating advanced multi-vessel coronary artery disease and severe left ventricular systolic dysfunction.

ELECTROCARDIOGRAM 238

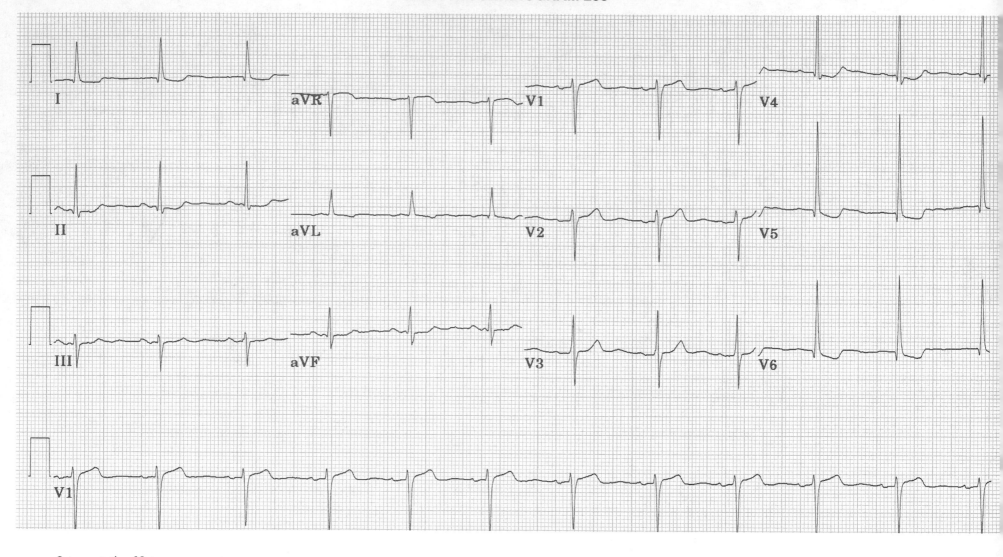

I aVR V1 V4

II aVL V2 V5

III aVF V3 V6

V1

Interpretation Notes: _____

_____

ECG 238 Seventy-six year old woman with coronary artery disease who underwent an angioplasty to the right coronary artery ten years prior to this tracing. She now returns for cardiology outpatient follow-up in the setting of recurrent angina pectoris. Her past medical history includes an embolic cerebral vascular accident, paroxysmal atrial fibrillation, hypertension, and diabetes mellitus. Her cardiac medications included nifedipine, digoxin, and sublingual nitroglycerin.

ELECTROCARDIOGRAM 239

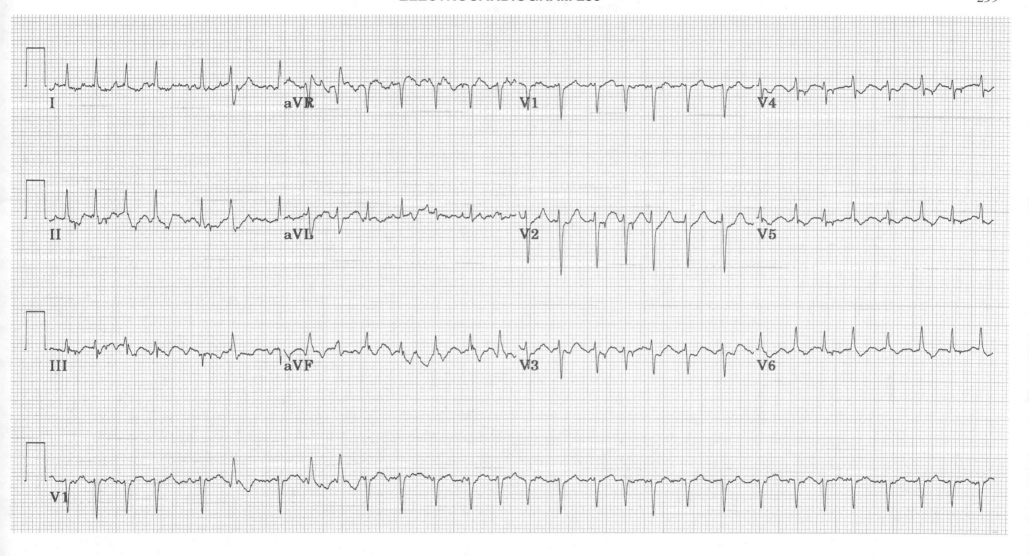

Interpretation Notes: _____

_____

_____

ECG 239 Forty-six year old woman admitted to the hospital with acute pneumonia and recent onset perceived rapid heart beating. Her pertinent past medical history includes steroid-dependent polymyositis. A cardiac catheterization performed one year before this electrocardiogram demonstrated normal coronary arteries.

ELECTROCARDIOGRAM 240

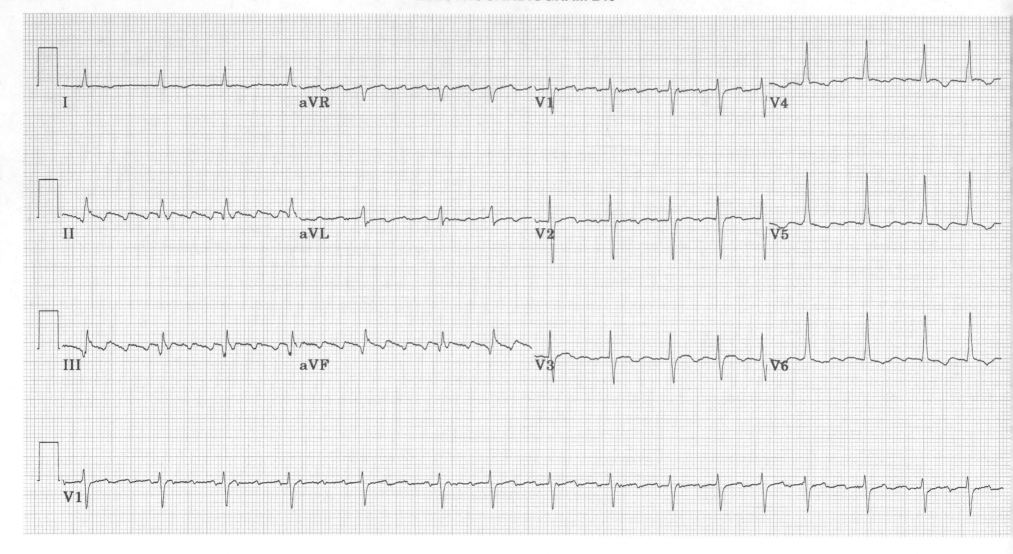

Interpretation Notes:

ECG 240 Seventy-seven year old gentleman with moderate left ventricular systolic dysfunction status post two coronary artery bypass grafting procedures admitted to the hospital with recurrent congestive heart failure and newly discovered atrial flutter.

ELECTROCARDIOGRAM 241

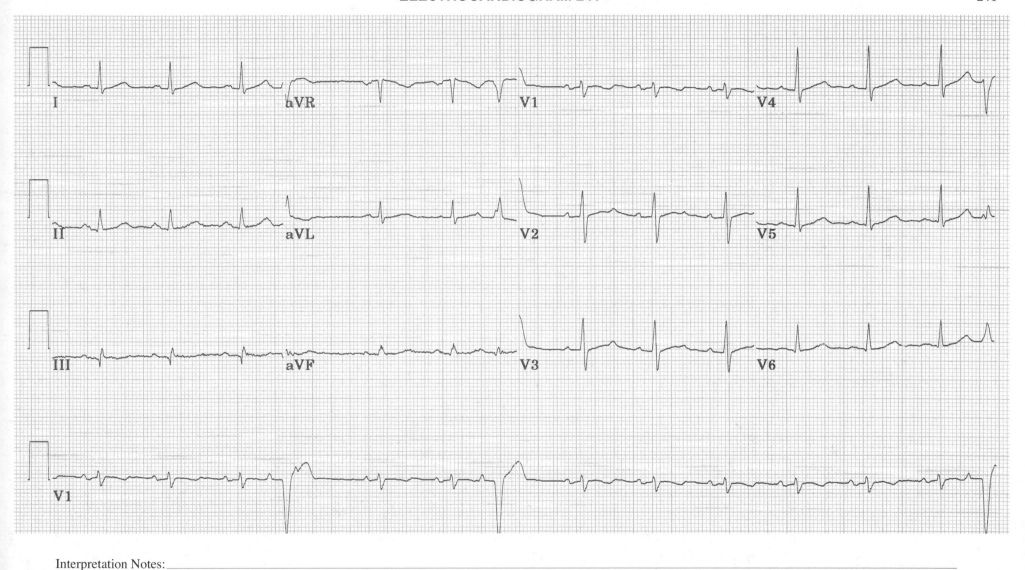

Interpretation Notes:_____

_____

_____

ECG 241 Sixty-four year old gentleman admitted to the hospital for evaluation of prostate cancer. His past medical history includes paroxysmal atrial fibrillation. His medications at the time of this electrocardiogram included atenolol and warfarin.

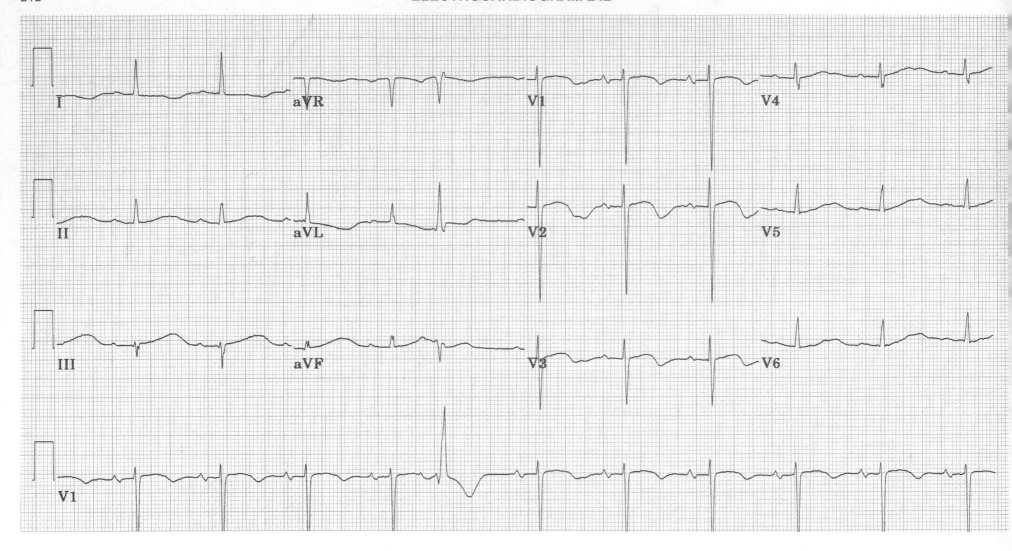

Interpretation Notes:

ECG 242 Seventy-four year old woman with a febrile illness. She was diagnosed with aortic valve endocarditis and underwent recent aortic valve homograft placement.

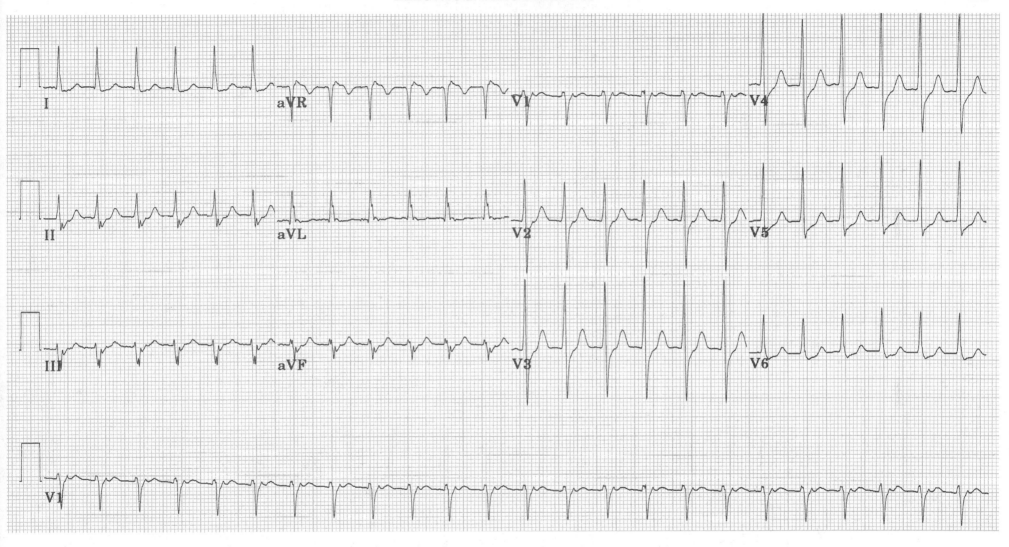

Interpretation Notes: _____

_____

ECG 243 Seventy-four year old woman with a history of breast cancer who is status post mastectomy and chemotherapy administration. This is a routine post-chemotherapy electrocardiogram.

ELECTROCARDIOGRAM 244

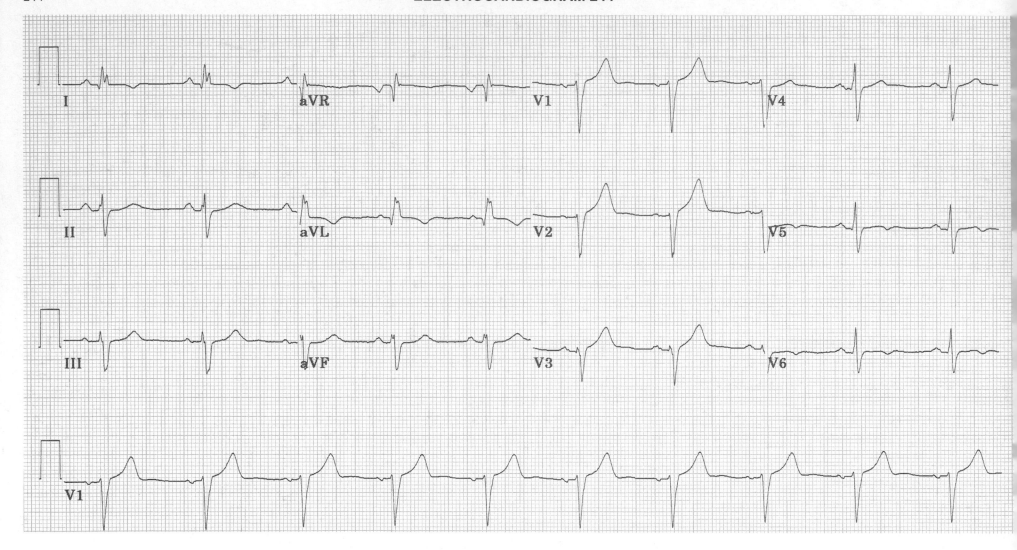

I   aVR   V1   V4

II   aVL   V2   V5

III   aVF   V3   V6

V1

Interpretation Notes:_____

_____

ECG 244 Sixty-eight year old gentleman with recent symptoms of accelerating angina pectoris in the setting of previously diagnosed coronary artery disease. He suffered a myocardial infarction of unknown location twenty-one years prior to this electrocardiogram. A subsequent cardiac catheterization six years prior to this tracing demonstrated an occluded left anterior descending coronary artery with the remainder of the coronary arteries demonstrating diffuse moderate obstruction. The patient was managed medically and at the time of this electrocardiogram was taking aspirin and isosorbide mononitrate.

ELECTROCARDIOGRAM 245

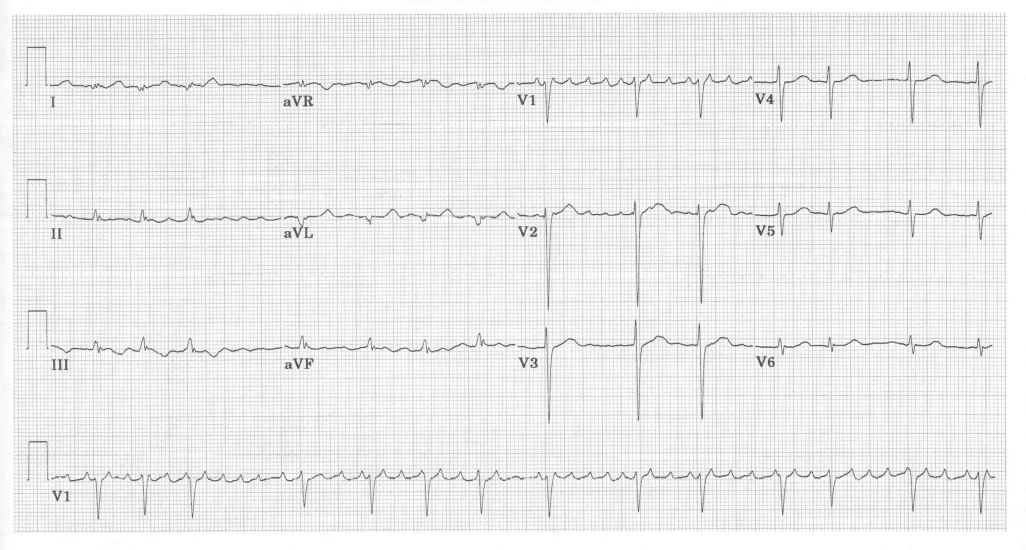

I	aVR	V1	V4
II	aVL	V2	V5
III	aVF	V3	V6

V1

Interpretation Notes: _____

ECG 245 Seventy-four year old gentleman admitted for evaluation of recurrent syncope. His past medical history is notable for hypertrophic obstructive cardiomyopathy and coronary artery disease. He is status post angioplasty to his left anterior descending coronary artery one year prior to this tracing. He also experienced a prior myocardial infarction in the left circumflex coronary artery distribution.

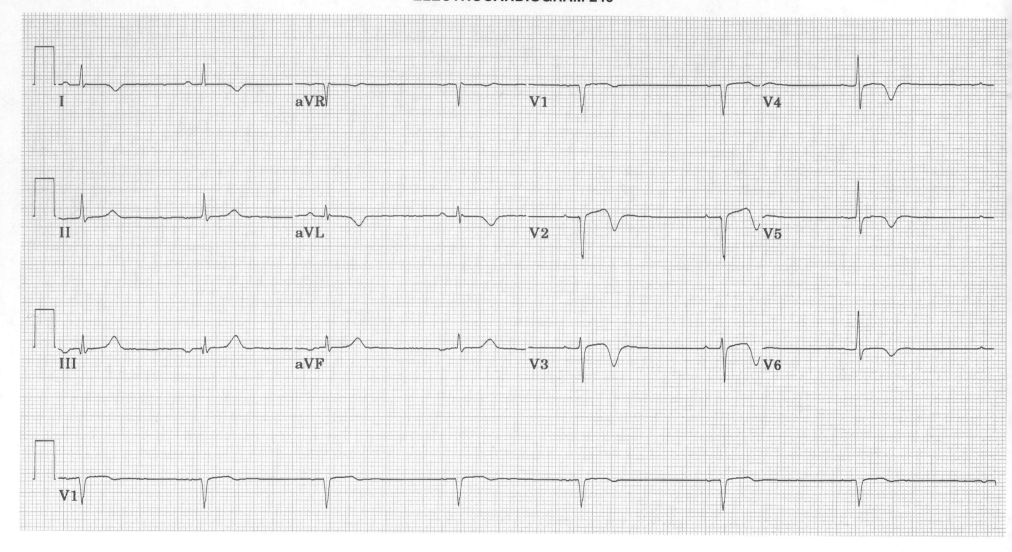

I   aVR   V1   V4

II   aVL   V2   V5

III   aVF   V3   V6

V1

Interpretation Notes:

ECG 246 Forty-two year old gentleman who three days prior to this electrocardiogram awoke early in the morning with acute onset chest discomfort. He was accepted in transfer from an outside hospital for cardiac evaluation. Cardiac enzymes confirmed the presence of acute myocardial injury and a subsequent cardiac catheterization demonstrated severe multi-vessel coronary artery disease. Medications at the time of this electrocardiogram included aspirin, atenolol, atorvastatin, isosorbide mononitrate, and captopril.

ELECTROCARDIOGRAM 247

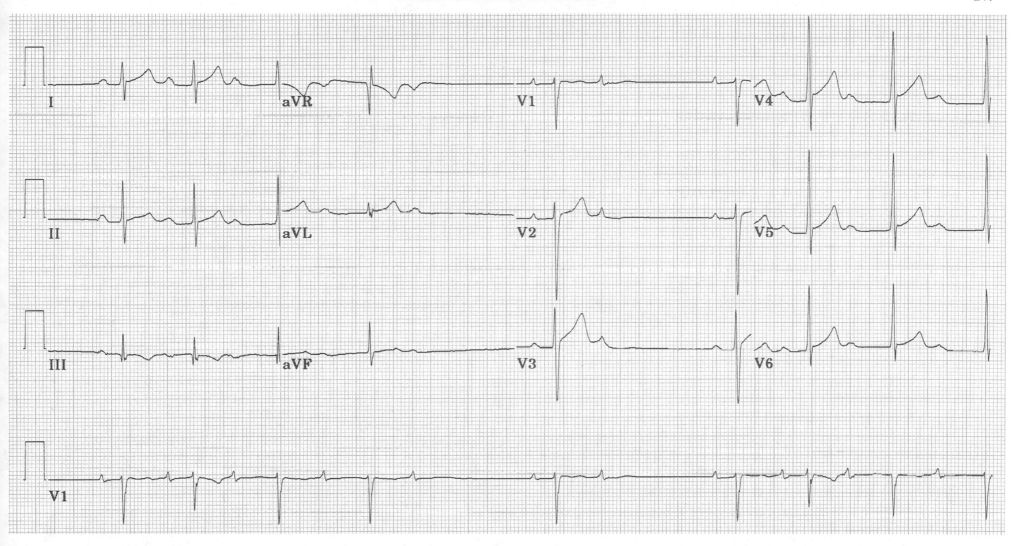

Interpretation Notes: _____

_____

_____

ECG 247 Twenty-four year old professional basketball player who is being evaluated for a pre-season physical examination. He has no known cardiac history or complaints.

LEVEL II

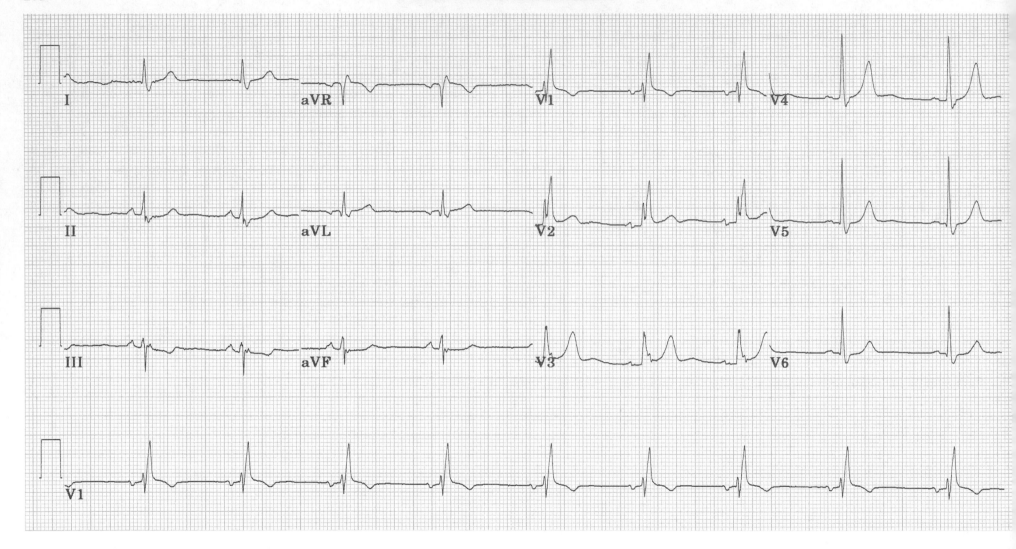

Interpretation Notes: _____

_____

ECG 248 Sixty-two year old woman undergoing preoperative assessment prior to a breast biopsy. She has no known cardiac disease.

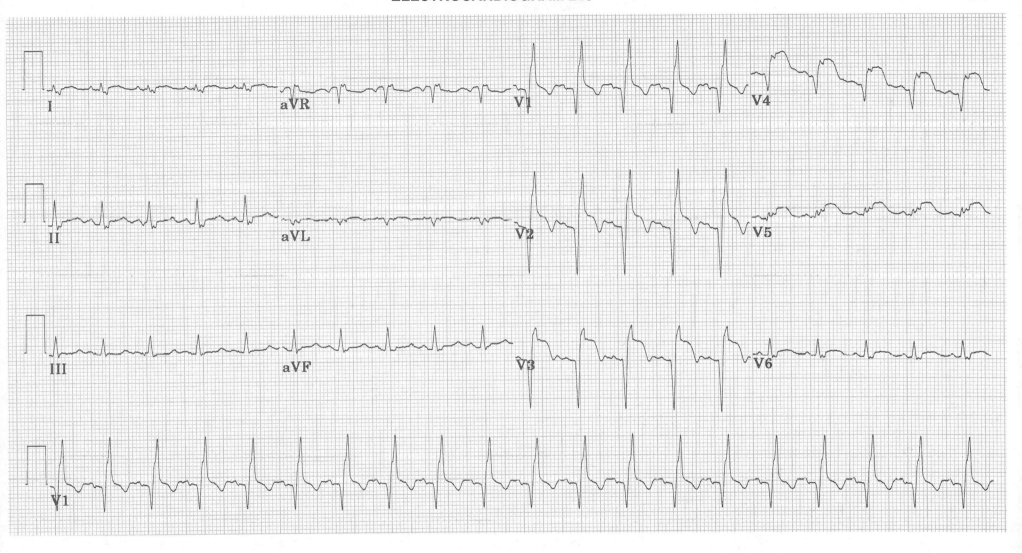

Interpretation Notes: _____

_____

ECG 249 Seventy-four year old gentleman with a history of hypertension, non-insulin requiring diabetes mellitus, and hyperlipidemia who presented urgently to the hospital with severe anterior precordial chest discomfort and the above electrocardiogram. The patient underwent an urgent cardiac catheterization and percutaneous transluminal coronary angioplasty of the left anterior descending coronary artery.

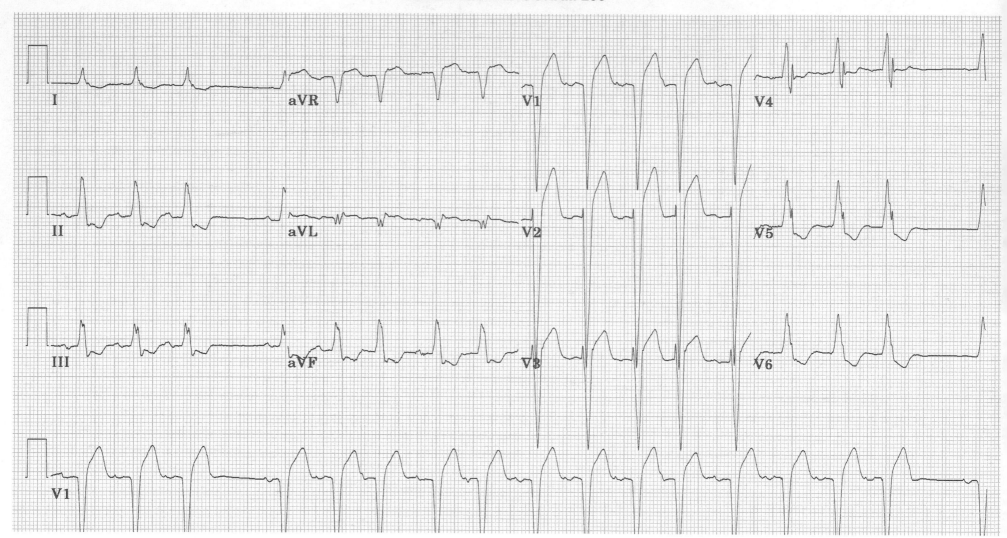

Interpretation Notes:_____

ECG 250 Seventy-six year old gentleman with two prior coronary artery bypass graft surgeries and moderate left ventricular systolic dysfunction who returns for outpatient cardiology follow-up. The patient is being seen preoperatively prior to a planned carotid endarterectomy. His co-morbid conditions include severe chronic obstructive pulmonary disease, paroxysmal atrial fibrillation, and chronic renal insufficiency. His medications included prednisone, digoxin, enalapril, furosemide, and warfarin.

ELECTROCARDIOGRAM 251

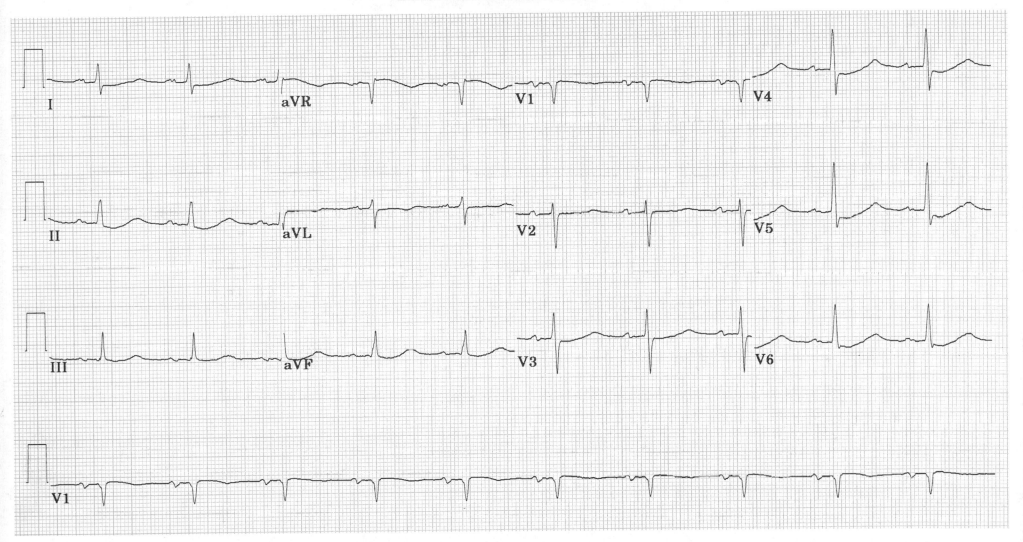

Interpretation Notes: _____

ECG 251 Seventy-two year old gentleman with advanced peripheral vascular disease who is admitted to the hospital for a semi-elective below the knee amputation. His past medical history includes chronic obstructive pulmonary disease, a remote myocardial infarction, and prior pacemaker placement. His medications included quinidine and digoxin.

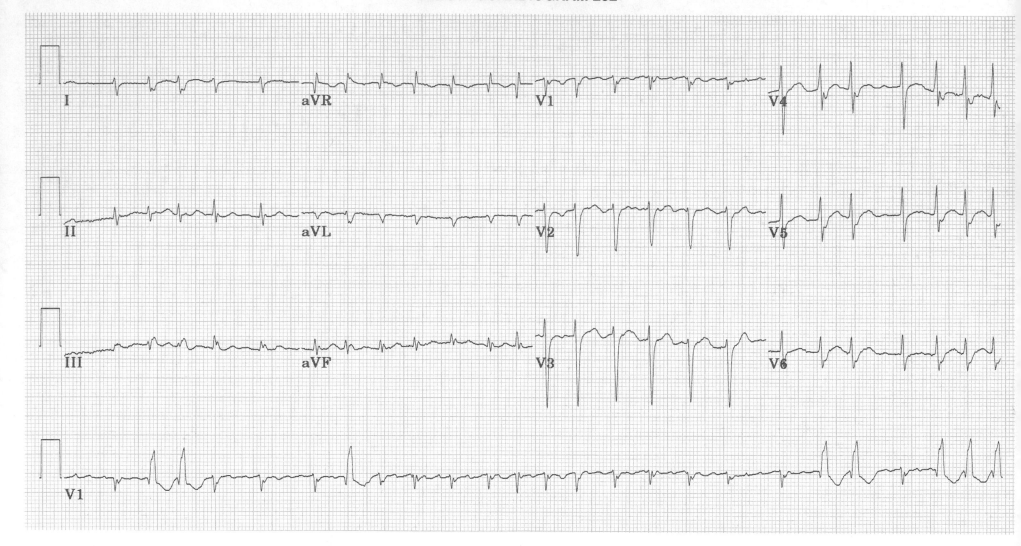

Interpretation Notes: _____

ECG 252 Sixty-seven year old gentleman with laryngeal carcinoma admitted urgently to the hospital with upper airway bleeding and new onset rapid atrial fibrillation.

ELECTROCARDIOGRAM 253

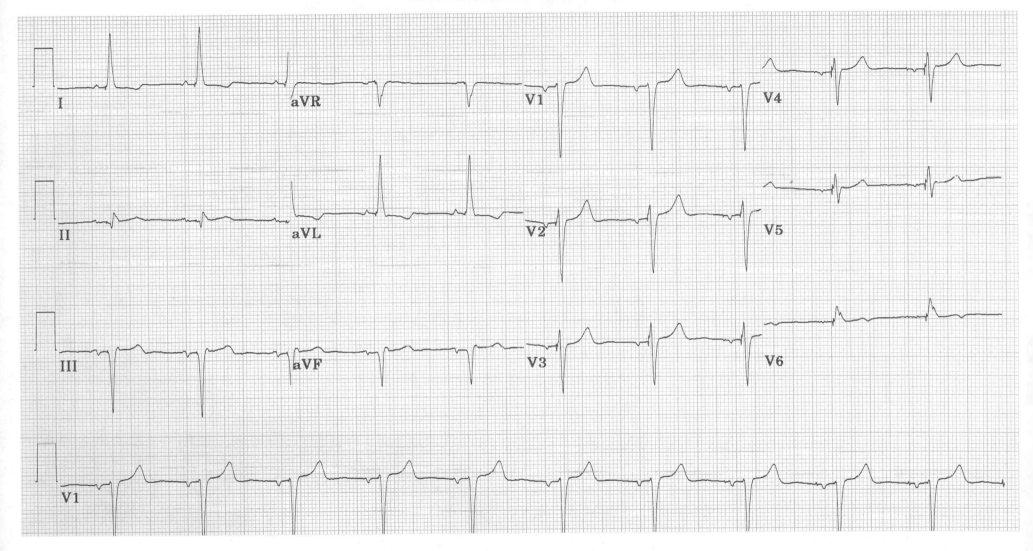

Interpretation Notes: _____

ECG 253 Seventy year old gentleman with coronary artery disease and moderately severe left ventricular systolic dysfunction who is status post coronary artery bypass graft surgery in the remote past. He returns for cardiology and pacemaker follow-up. He also has a history of ventricular tachycardia and is status post implantable cardiac defibrillator placement. His medications at the time of this electrocardiogram included captopril, aspirin, metoprolol, furosemide, warfarin, and topical nitroglycerin.

LEVEL II

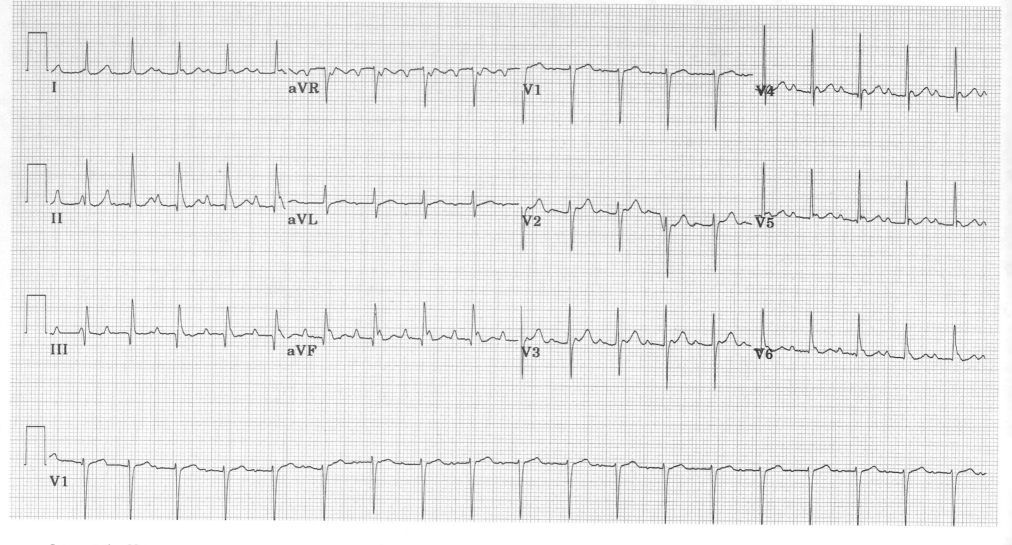

Interpretation Notes: _____

ECG 254 Seventy-seven year old woman status post an acute left middle cerebral artery occlusion and urokinase administration who is now experiencing recurrent atrial arrhythmias. Medications at the time of this electrocardiogram included diltiazem, topical nitroglycerin, and isosorbide mononitrate. An echocardiogram performed during this hospitalization demonstrated moderate left atrial enlargement and normal left ventricular systolic function without evidence of a prior myocardial infarction.

ELECTROCARDIOGRAM 255

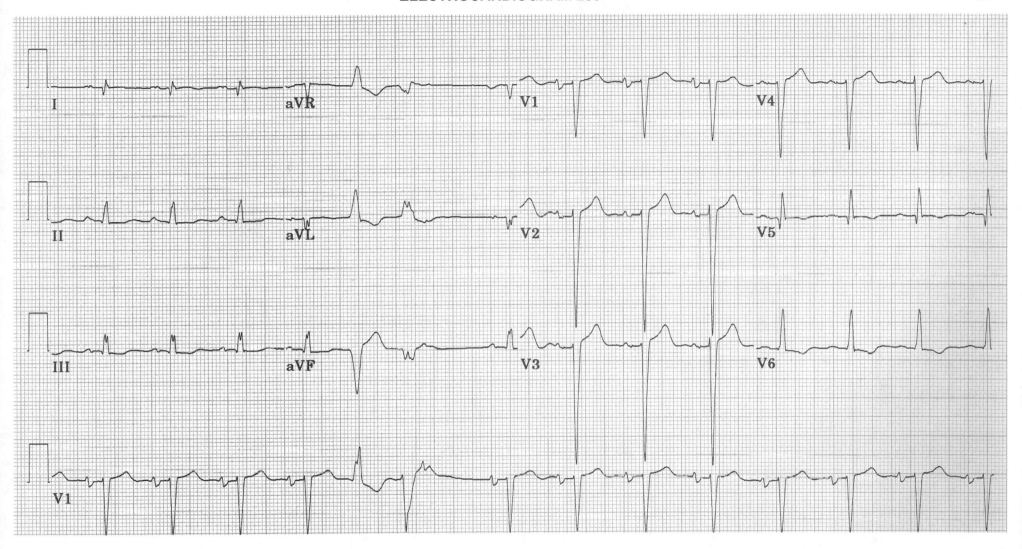

Interpretation Notes: _____

_____

ECG 255 Sixty-one year old gentleman with coronary artery disease and a myocardial infarction six years prior to this electrocardiogram who returns for outpatient internal medicine follow-up. Co-morbid conditions include hypertension, insulin requiring diabetes mellitus, and carotid vascular disease. His medications included captopril, isosorbide dinitrate, insulin, aspirin, digoxin, and furosemide.

LEVEL II

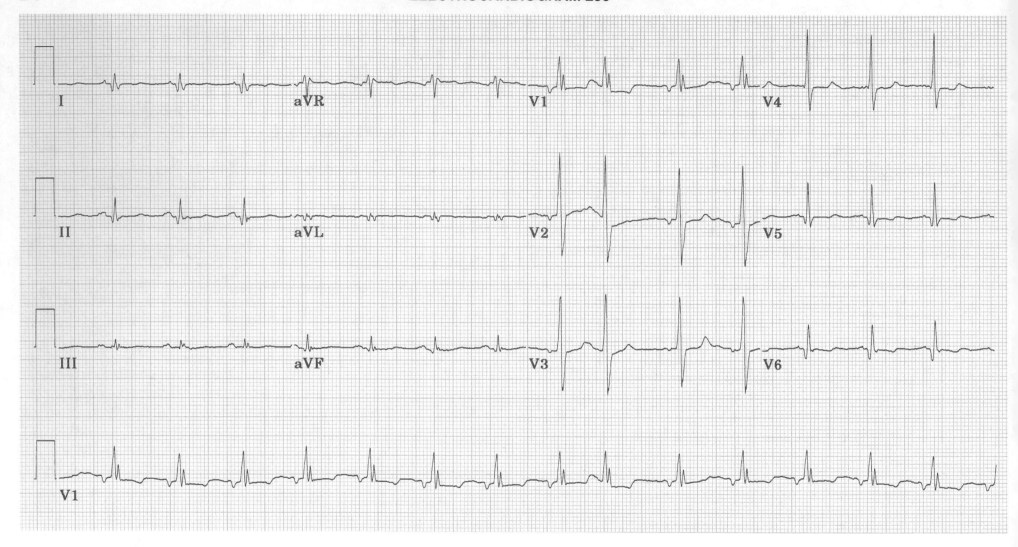

Interpretation Notes: _____

_____

ECG 256 Sixty-six year old gentleman status post recent coronary artery bypass graft surgery, paroxysmal atrial fibrillation, and a cerebrovascular accident who returns for a follow-up evaluation after his bypass surgery. Other co-morbidities include hypertension, non-insulin requiring diabetes mellitus, and hyperlipidemia.

ELECTROCARDIOGRAM 257

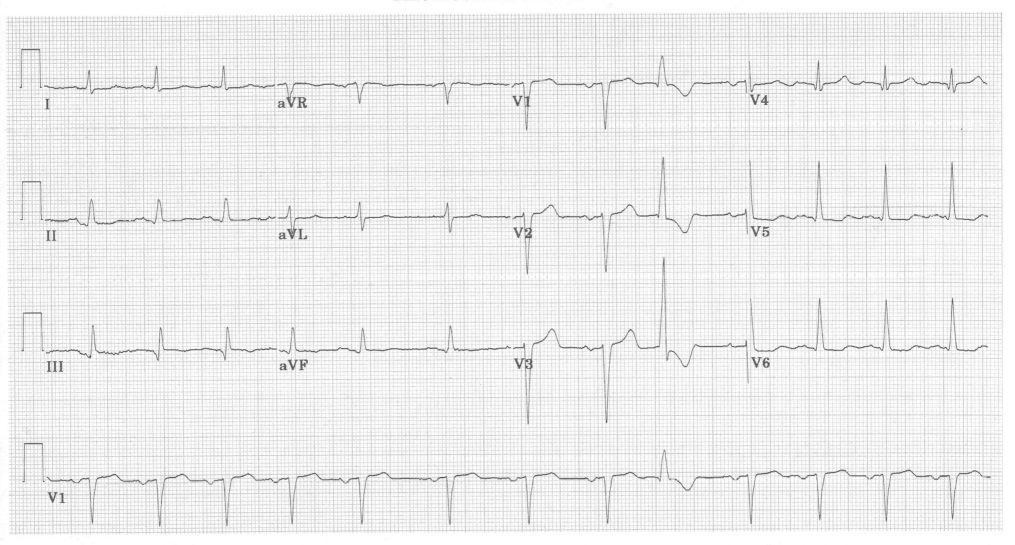

Interpretation Notes: _____

_____

_____

ECG 257 Seventy-one year old woman with recurrent congestive heart failure accepted in hospital transfer for further evaluation. A recent cardiac catheterization demonstrated severe diffuse atherosclerotic coronary disease, moderately severe left ventricular systolic dysfunction with remote anterior, apical, and inferior wall myocardial infarctions. Medications at the time of this electrocardiogram included amlodipine, enalapril, furosemide, prazosin, and metolazone.

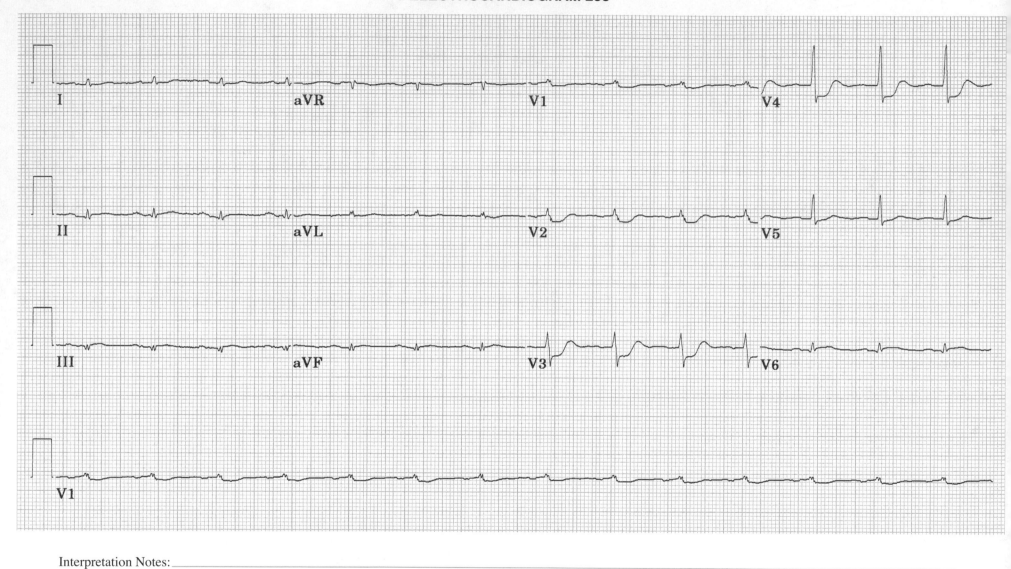

I aVR V1 V4

II aVL V2 V5

III aVF V3 V6

V1

Interpretation Notes: _____

ECG 258 Seventy-six year old woman status post aorto-femoral bypass surgery one day prior to this electrocardiogram who suffered an acute myocardial infarction and cardiogenic shock. She had a successful percutaneous transluminal coronary angioplasty to a large left circumflex coronary artery. She developed interval pneumonia, acute renal failure, and an anoxic encephalopathy. She ultimately expired during the same hospitalization.

ELECTROCARDIOGRAM 259

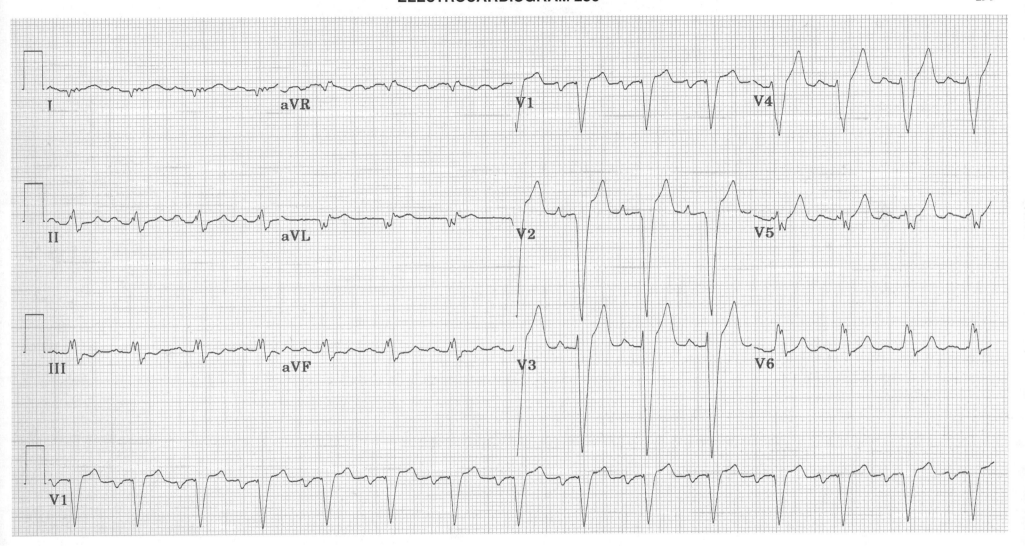

I   aVR   V1   V4

II   aVL   V2   V5

III   aVF   V3   V6

V1

Interpretation Notes: _____

ECG 259 Fifty-six year old woman with ischemic left ventricular systolic dysfunction and symptoms of advanced congestive heart failure who presents for further outpatient cardiology evaluation. Her medications included digoxin, warfarin, lisinopril, furosemide, potassium, and thyroxine.

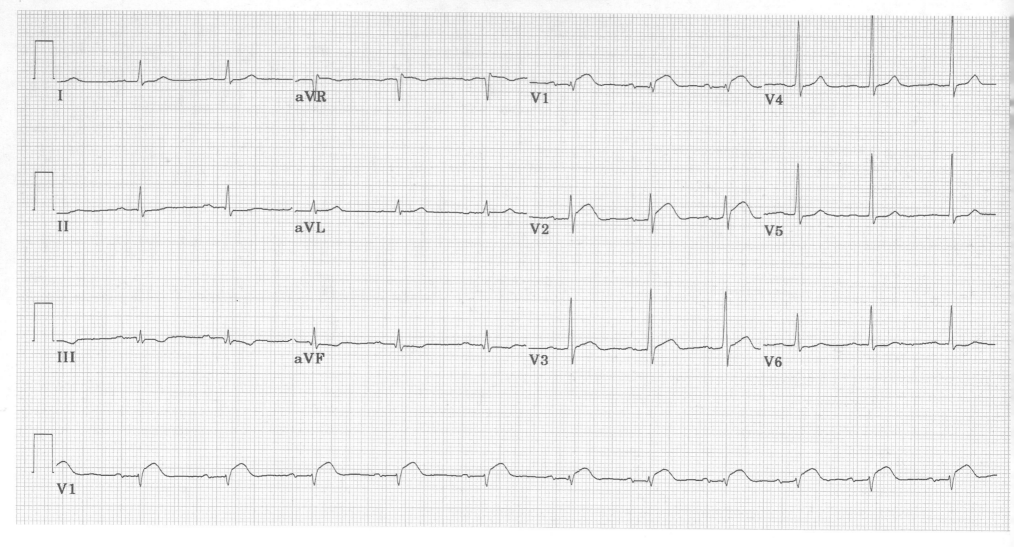

Interpretation Notes: _____

_____

_____

ECG 260 Fifty year old gentleman who presents to the hospital with a clinical syndrome consistent with crescendo angina. A cardiac catheterization demonstrated a subtotal proximal occlusion of the left anterior descending coronary artery. This stenosis was successfully angioplastied. The patient subsequently presented to the hospital with recurrent chest pain and this electrocardiogram. A repeat cardiac catheterization demonstrated a patent PTCA site, however a new 90% stenosis of the right coronary artery was found and successfully angioplastied. The patient suffered a small inferior myocardial infarction as serial serum cardiac enzymes were elevated.

ELECTROCARDIOGRAM 261

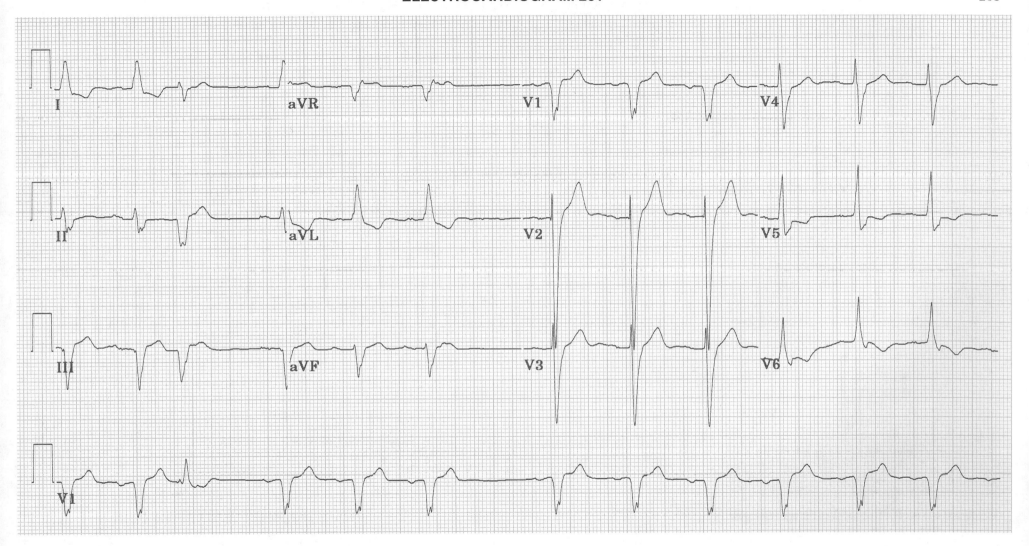

Interpretation Notes: _____

_____

_____

ECG 261 Eighty-two year old gentleman with coronary artery disease status post remote coronary artery bypass graft surgery and a prior myocardial infarction who is accepted in transfer from an outside hospital with signs and symptoms consistent with an acute myocardial infarction. The patient received intravenous thrombolytic therapy and at the time of this electrocardiogram was awaiting cardiac catheterization. An echocardiogram performed six years prior to this electrocardiogram demonstrated moderate regional left ventricular systolic dysfunction consistent with his prior myocardial infarction.

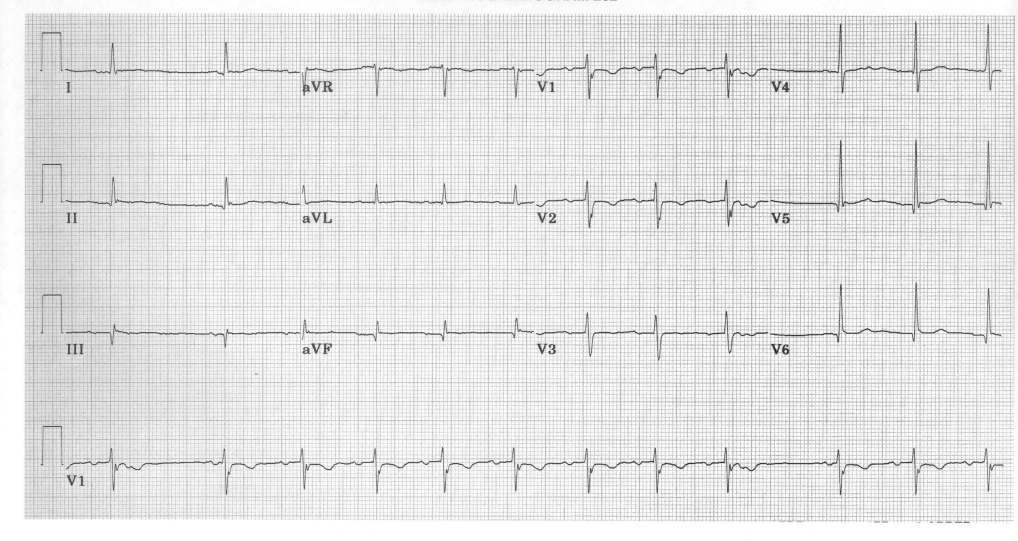

Interpretation Notes: _____

_____

ECG 262 Seventy-four year old gentleman status post coronary artery bypass surgery several days prior to this electrocardiogram. Co-morbidities include hypertension, hyperlipidemia, and postoperative paroxysmal atrial fibrillation. Medications at the time of this electrocardiogram included aspirin and atenolol.

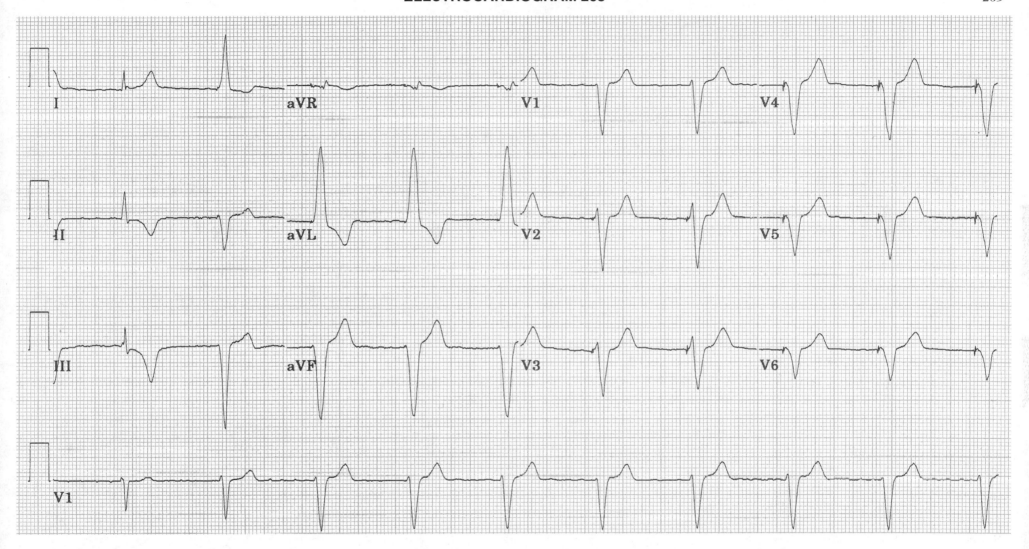

Interpretation Notes:_____

_____

ECG 263 Seventy-five year old gentleman with a recent history of syncope and permanent pacemaker implantation. Co-morbidities include chronic atrial fibrillation and past coronary artery bypass graft surgery.

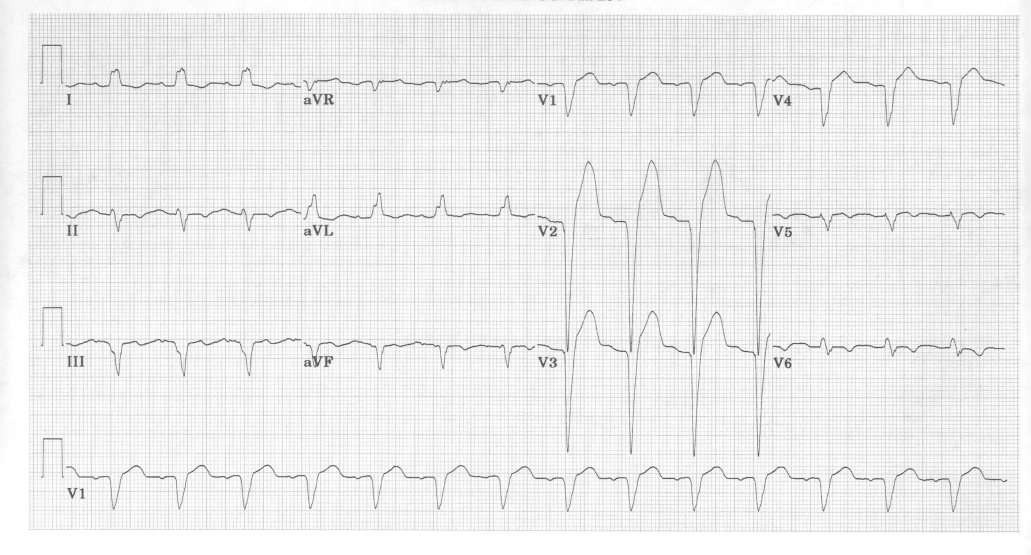

I aVR V1 V4

II aVL V2 V5

III aVF V3 V6

V1

Interpretation Notes: _____

_____

ECG 264 Seventy year old gentleman who is recently status post bioprosthetic aortic valve replacement for severe aortic stenosis and multi-vessel coronary artery bypass graft surgery.

ELECTROCARDIOGRAM 265

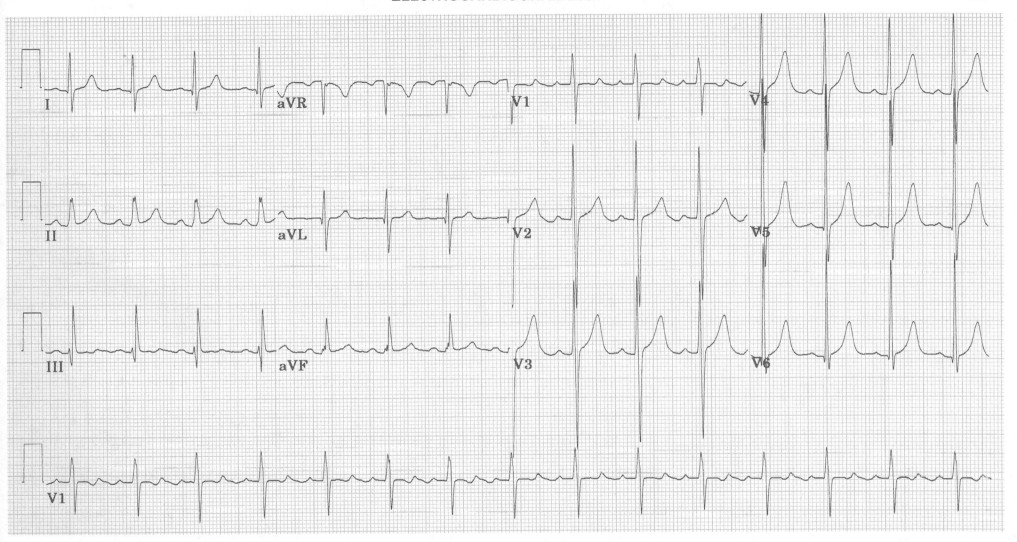

Interpretation Notes: _____

_____

ECG 265 Twenty-three year old gentleman with surgically unrepaired Tetralogy of Fallot including a right ventricular outflow tract obstruction and a large ventricular septal defect with bi-directional shunting. He is admitted for evaluation and treatment of acute pulmonic valve endocarditis.

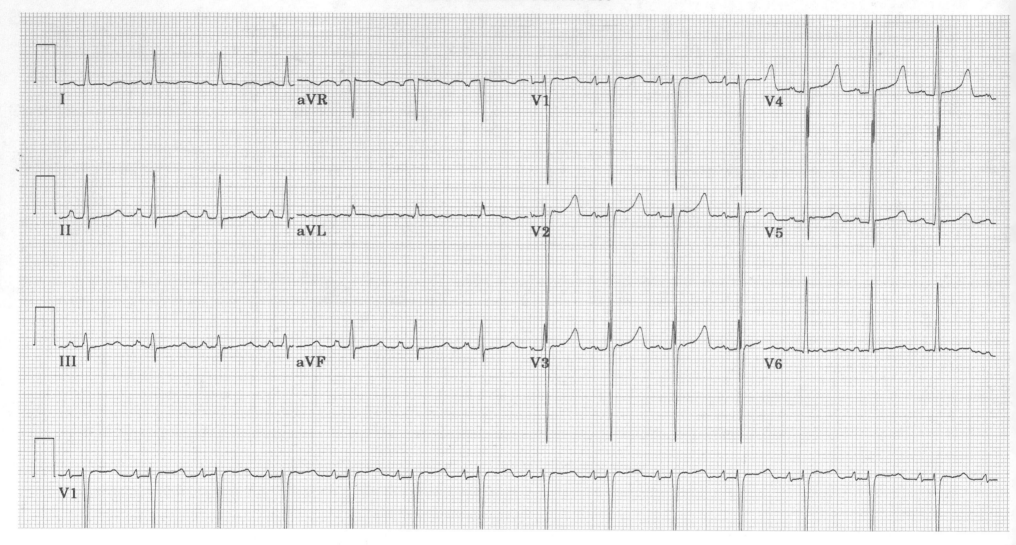

Interpretation Notes:_____

ECG 266 Thirty year old gentleman with dialysis requiring renal failure of unknown etiology who presents with leg pain and tingling, a serum calcium of 4.9 mg/dl, and a serum potassium of 6.2 meq/L. Co-morbidities include hypertension and a seizure disorder.

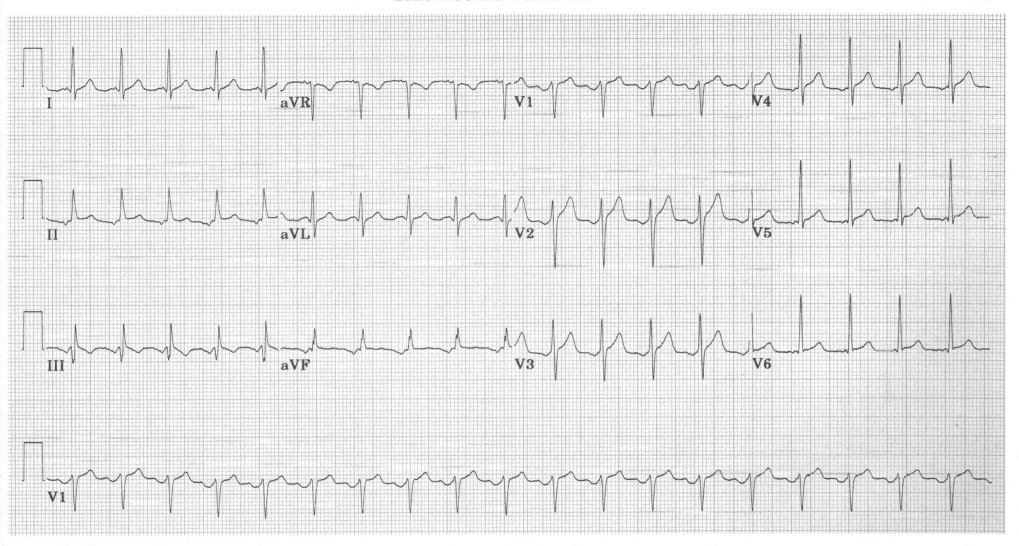

Interpretation Notes: _____

_____

ECG 267 Forty-four year old gentleman who is status post radiofrequency ablation who returns with recurrent palpitations. An echocardiogram demonstrated mild to moderate left ventricular systolic dysfunction felt secondary to a tachycardia-induced cardiomyopathy. The patient underwent a successful repeat radiofrequency ablation of an ectopic atrial tachycardia site originating from the posterior right atrium.

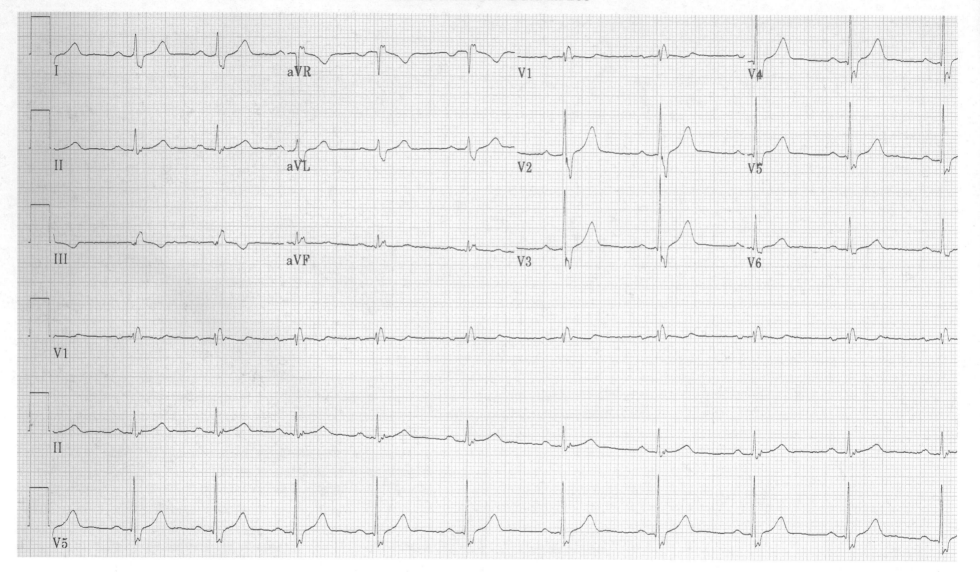

Interpretation Notes: _____

_____

ECG 268 Forty year old gentleman with a history of "an enlarged heart" since a young age who seeks a cardiac evaluation. A prior echocardiogram demonstrated evidence of Ebstein's anomaly.

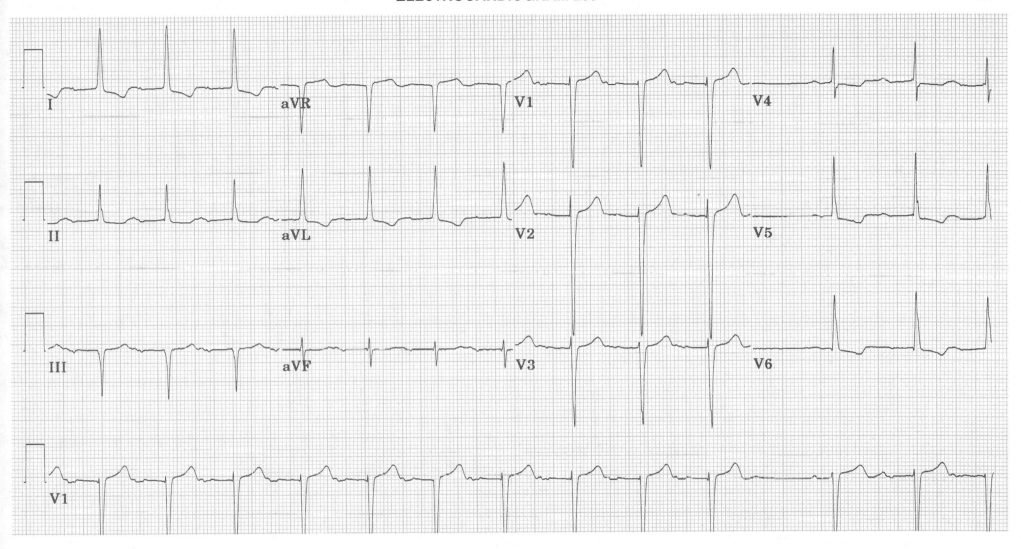

Interpretation Notes: _____

ECG 269 Seventy-seven year old woman with hypertension, hyperlipidemia, and angina pectoris who returns for routine cardiac follow-up in the setting of atherosclerotic coronary artery disease. She is status post a percutaneous revascularization procedure to her left circumflex coronary artery, mitral valve replacement, and a remote myocardial infarction of unknown location. Her medications included ticlodipine, prilosec, and aspirin.

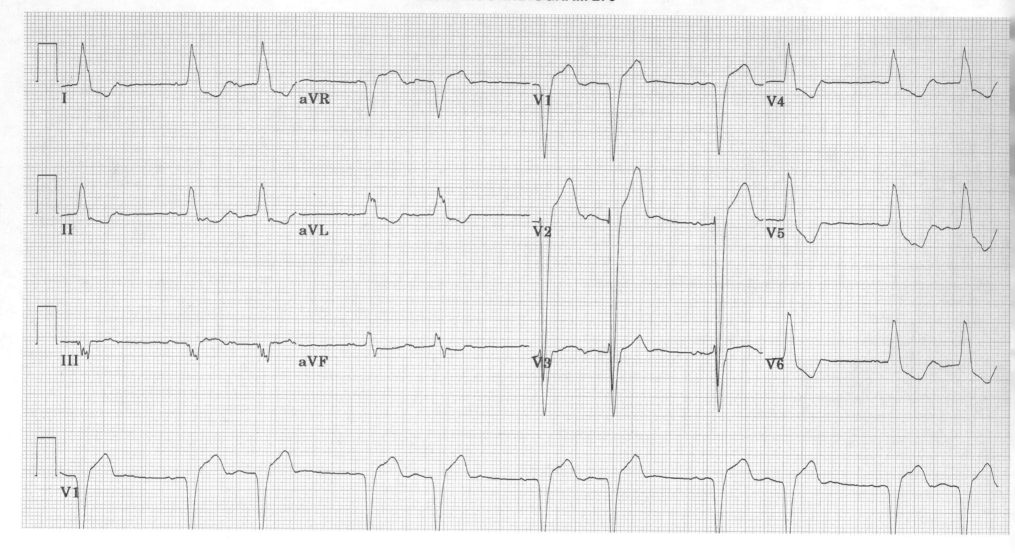

Interpretation Notes: _____

ECG 270 Seventy-five year old woman with coronary artery disease status post angioplasty and coronary artery bypass graft surgery who is currently being seen in the outpatient cardiology clinic. Other co-morbidities include non-insulin requiring diabetes mellitus and hypertension. This patient developed progressive heart block shortly after this electrocardiogram and permanent pacemaker implantation was undertaken. Medications at the time of this electrocardiogram included captopril, diltiazem, furosemide, aspirin, topical nitrates, and simvastatin.

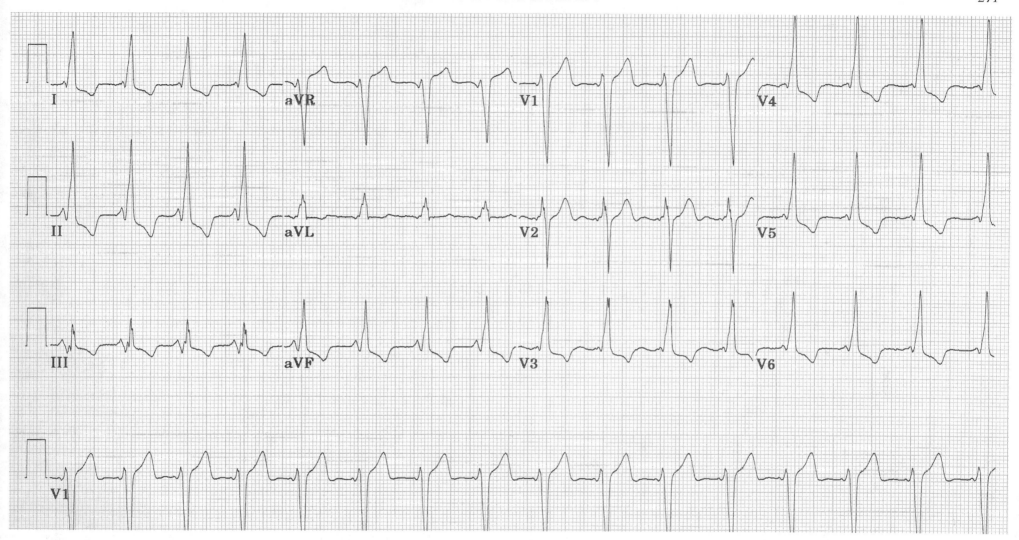

I aVR V1 V4

II aVL V2 V5

III aVF V3 V6

V1

Interpretation Notes: _____

_____

_____

ECG 271 Asymptomatic 18-year old woman with Wolff-Parkinson-White syndrome referred for further evaluation and possible treatment.

LEVEL II

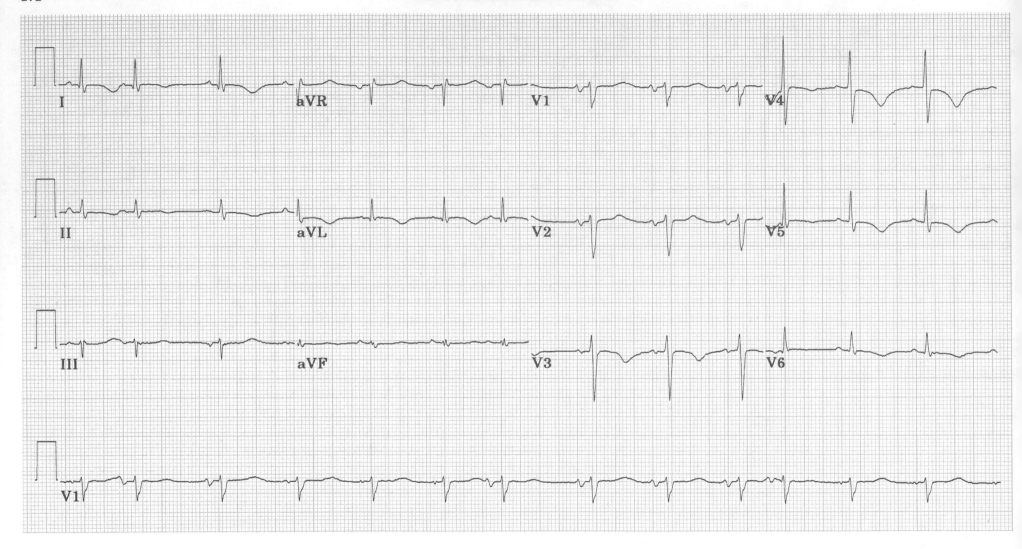

I aVR V1 V4

II aVL V2 V5

III aVF V3 V6

V1

Interpretation Notes: _____

_____

_____

ECG 272 Seventy-three year old gentleman with Hodgkin's lymphoma hospitalized for further evaluation and treatment. His past medical history includes hypertension. The patient has no known past cardiac history. His medications included hydralazine, lisinopril, and chemotherapeutic agents. His serum potassium level was 4.0 meq/L at the time of this tracing.

ELECTROCARDIOGRAM 273

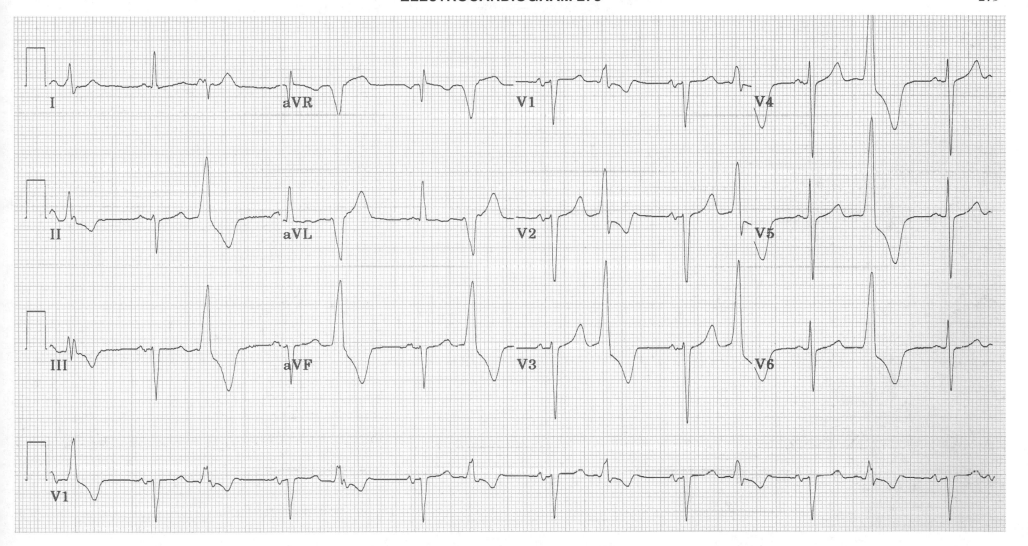

Interpretation Notes: _____

ECG 273 Sixty-eight year old gentleman with coronary artery disease status post coronary artery bypass graft surgery two years prior to this electrocardiogram who re-presents for evaluation of aortic insufficiency. Medications at the time of this electrocardiogram included captopril, furosemide, potassium, and aspirin.

ELECTROCARDIOGRAM 274

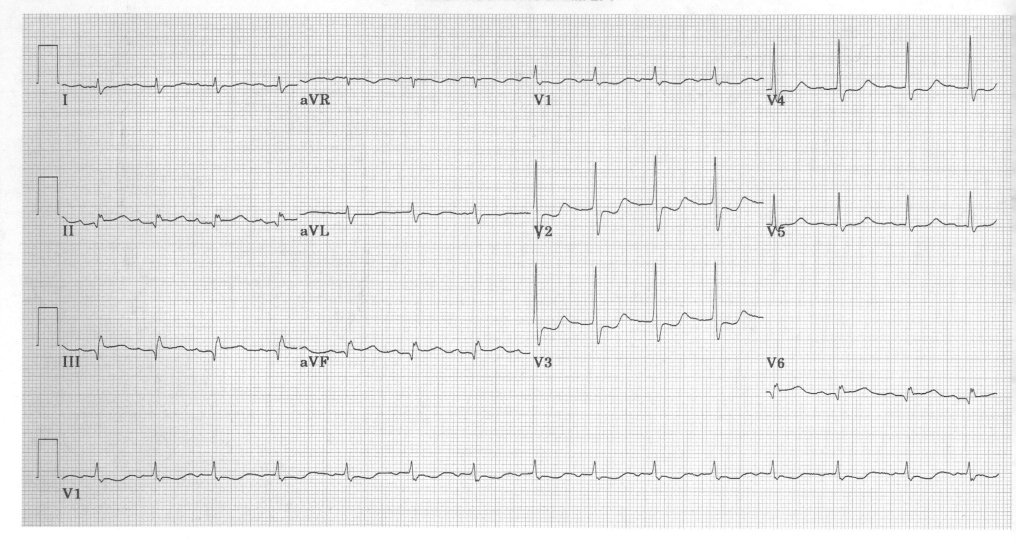

Interpretation Notes: _____

_____

_____

ECG 274 Seventy-five year old gentleman who underwent unsuccessful percutaneous transluminal coronary angioplasty of his right coronary artery referred immediately for coronary artery bypass graft surgery.

ELECTROCARDIOGRAM 275

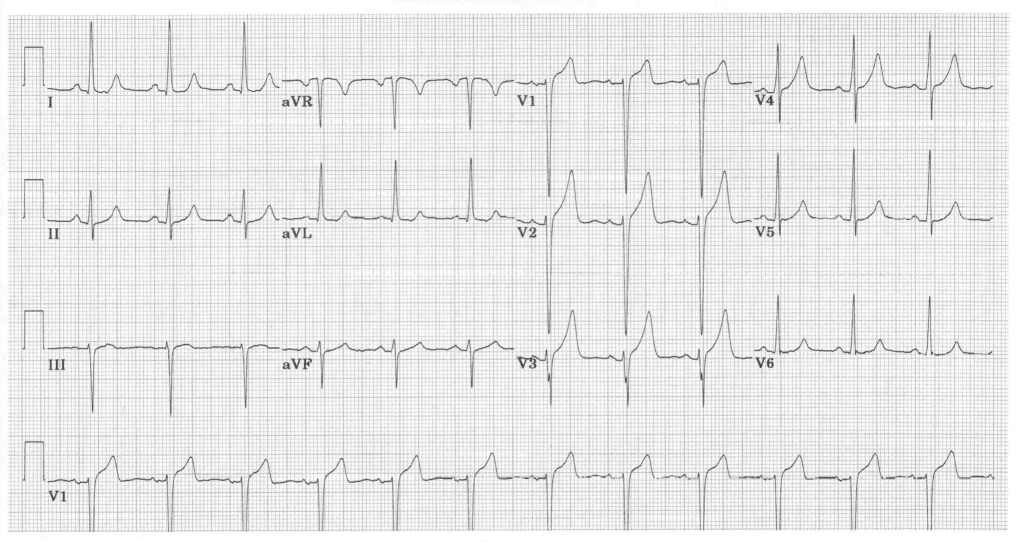

Interpretation Notes: _____

_____

_____

ECG 275 Twenty-nine year old gentleman with hypertrophic obstructive cardiomyopathy. The patient eventually underwent surgical myectomy with symptomatic improvement.

ELECTROCARDIOGRAM 276

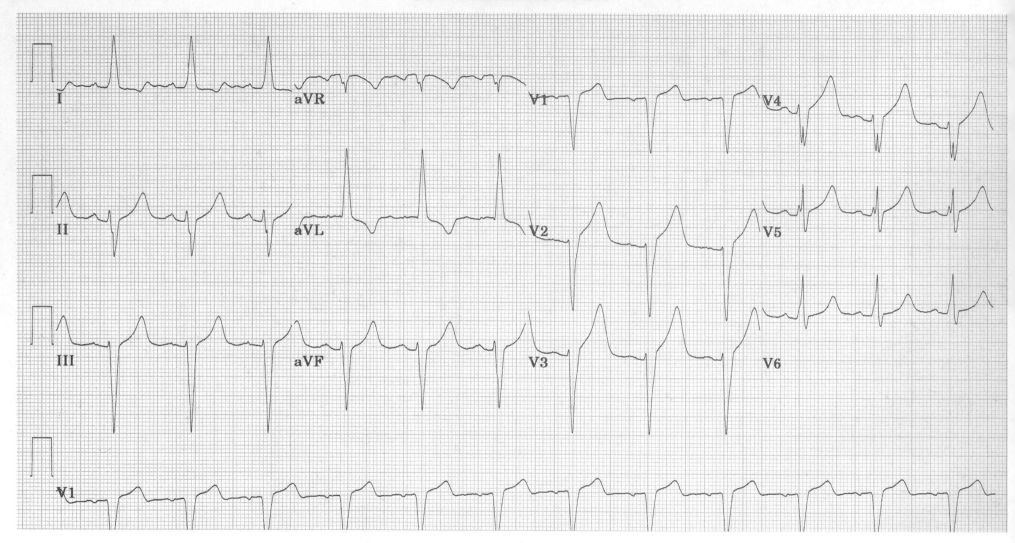

Interpretation Notes: _____

_____

_____

ECG 276 Twenty-nine year old gentleman with hypertrophic obstructive cardiomyopathy status post recent surgical myectomy.

ELECTROCARDIOGRAM 277

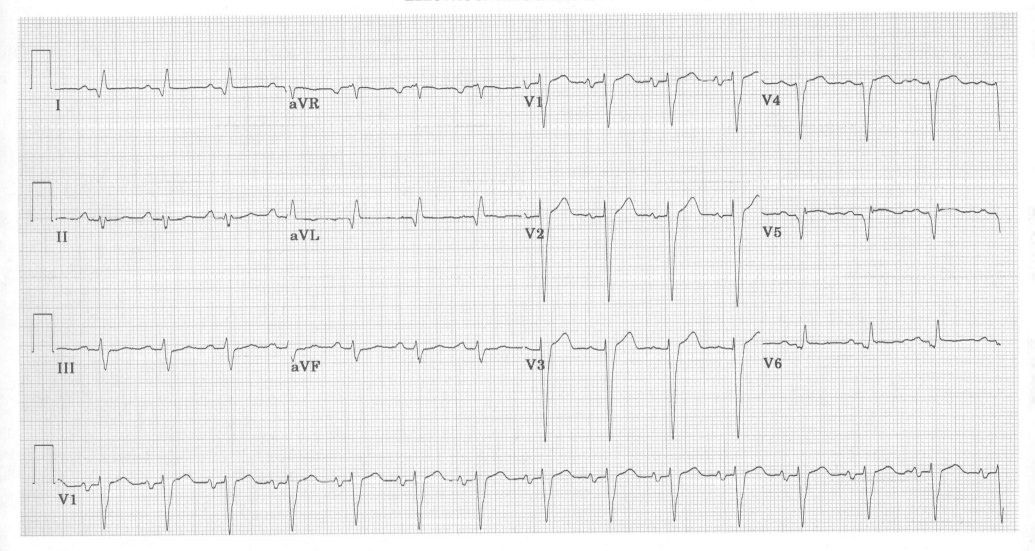

Interpretation Notes: _____

_____

ECG 277 Forty-eight year old gentleman with multiple prior myocardial infarctions who was admitted recently to the hospital with severe congestive heart failure. The patient subsequently expired.

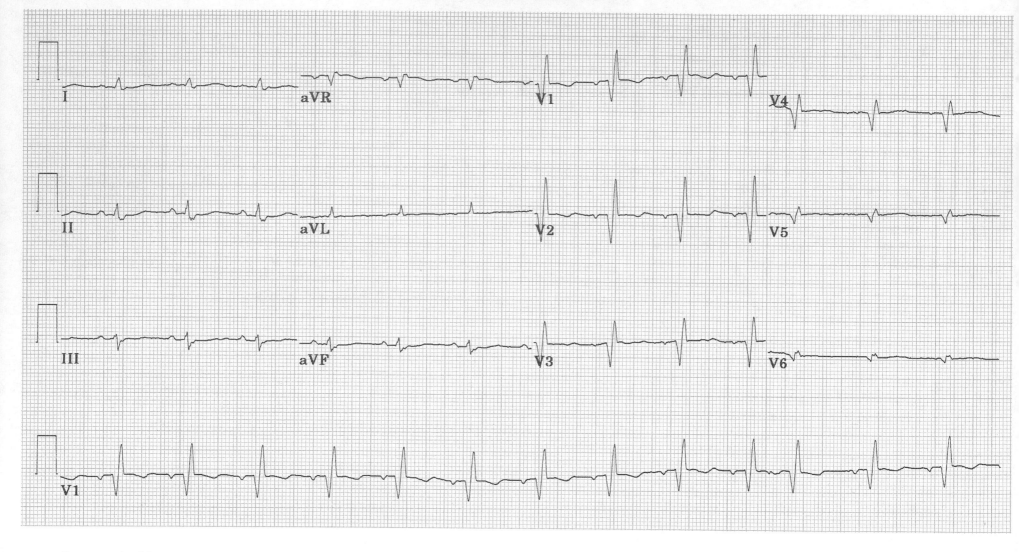

I   aVR   V1   V4
II   aVL   V2   V5
III   aVF   V3   V6
V1

Interpretation Notes:

ECG 278 Seventy-five year old gentleman status post a remote anterolateral myocardial infarction and percutaneous transluminal coronary angioplasty of the left anterior descending coronary artery who re-presents with recurrent angina pectoris. Medications at the time of this electrocardiogram included intravenous nitroglycerin, intravenous heparin, metoprolol, and aspirin.

ELECTROCARDIOGRAM 279

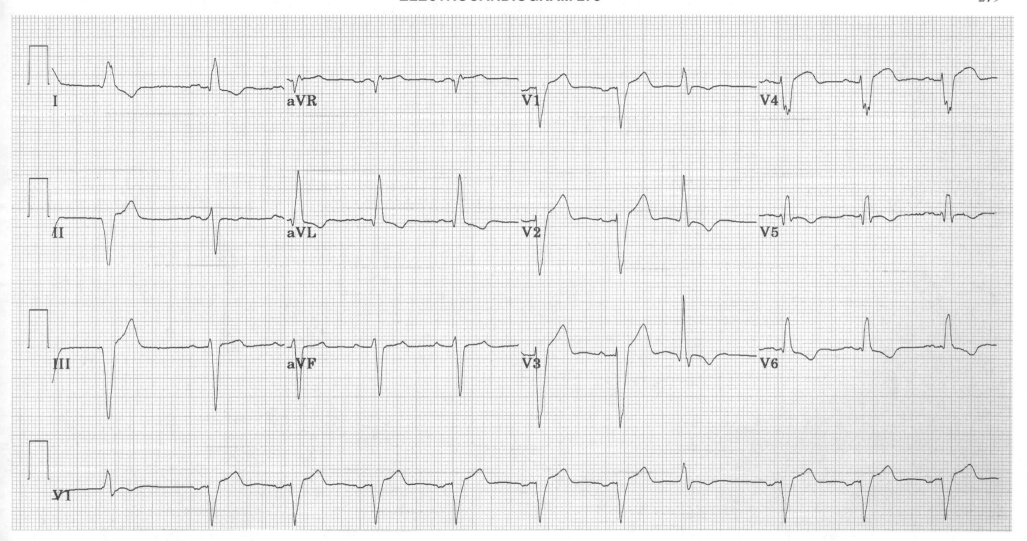

I	aVR	V1	V4
II	aVL	V2	V5
III	aVF	V3	V6

V1

Interpretation Notes: _____

_____

_____

ECG 279 Eighty-eight year old gentleman with severe multi-vessel coronary artery disease and severe left ventricular systolic dysfunction who is being evaluated for coronary artery bypass graft surgery. His medications included aspirin, digoxin, furosemide, captopril, and amiodarone.

ELECTROCARDIOGRAM 280

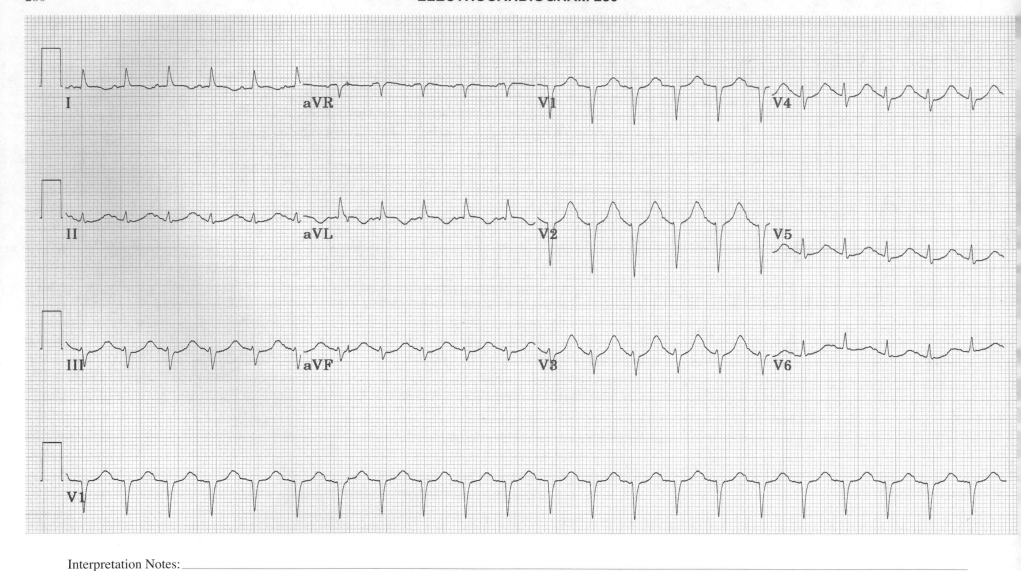

Interpretation Notes: _____

_____

_____

ECG 280 Fifty-three year old woman admitted to the coronary intensive care unit with a two hour history of chest discomfort. She has a history of hypertension, diabetes, and severe peripheral vascular disease. Serial cardiac enzymes confirmed acute myocardial injury and the patient underwent a subsequent cardiac catheterization demonstrating advanced left circumflex coronary artery disease.

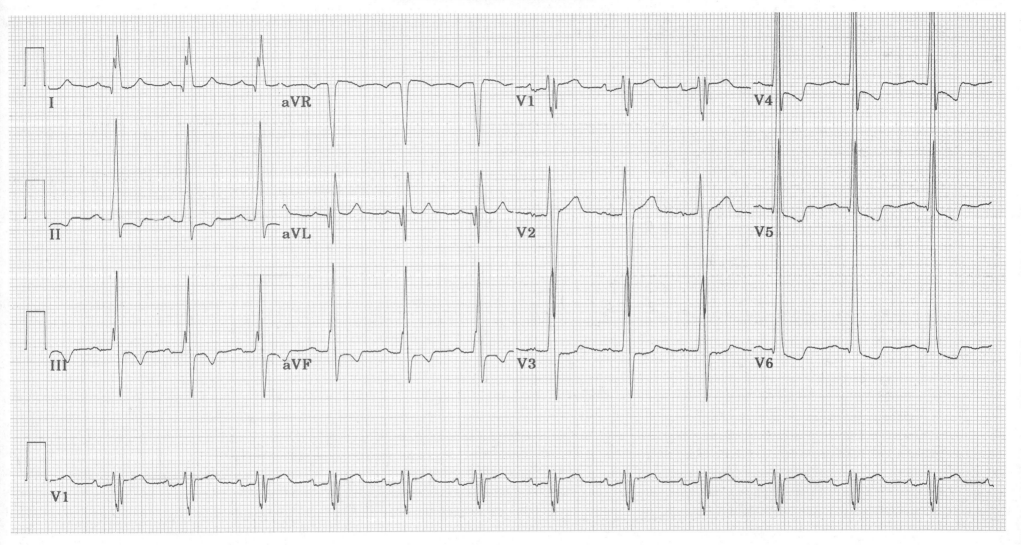

Interpretation Notes: _____

_____

ECG 281 Asymptomatic thirty-two year old gentleman currently seen in the outpatient department for routine follow-up. He does have a pertinent past cardiac history including a ventricular septal defect repair ten years previous to this electrocardiogram. A recent echocardiogram demonstrated severe biventricular systolic dysfunction and severe four chamber cardiac enlargement.

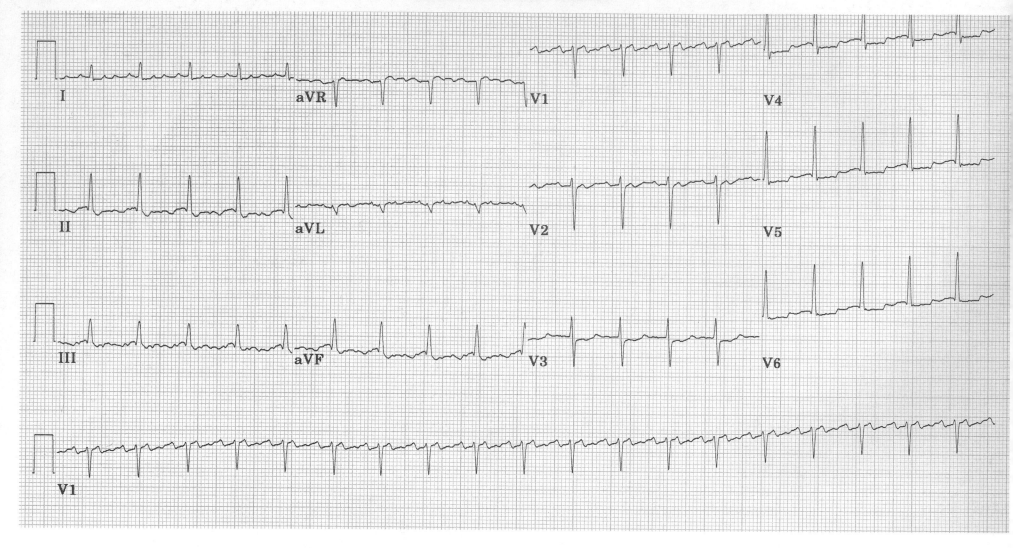

Interpretation Notes: _____

_____

ECG 282 Fifty-six year old woman with a history of rheumatic valvular heart disease including mitral stenosis and aortic stenosis who is recently status post two valve replacement surgery. She has a history of paroxysmal atrial arrhythmias. Her medications included amiodarone, atenolol, furosemide, and warfarin.

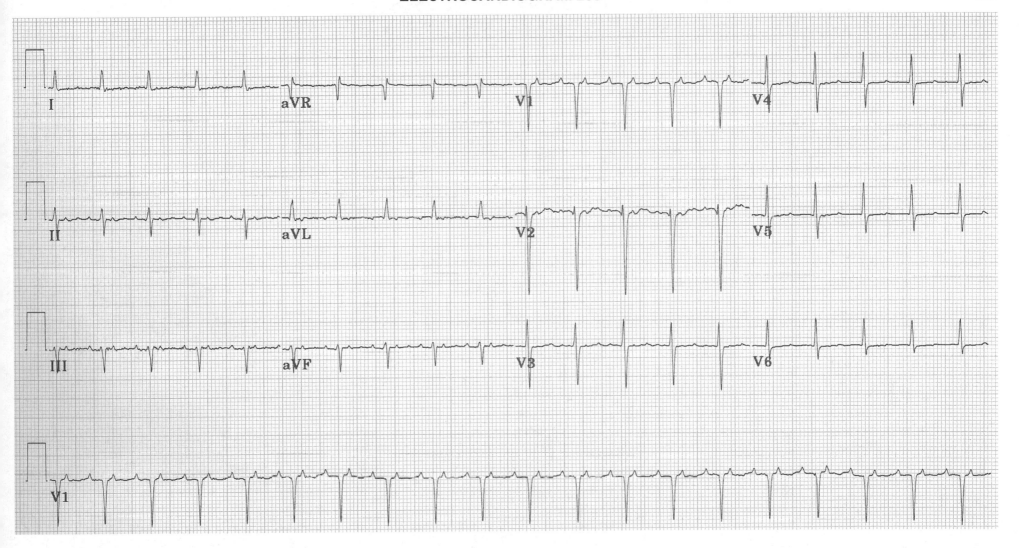

ECG 283 Ninety-five year old woman with a history of hypertension, anemia, and advanced peripheral vascular disease who underwent this electrocardiogram prior to a lower extremity revascularization procedure.

Interpretation Notes: _____

_____

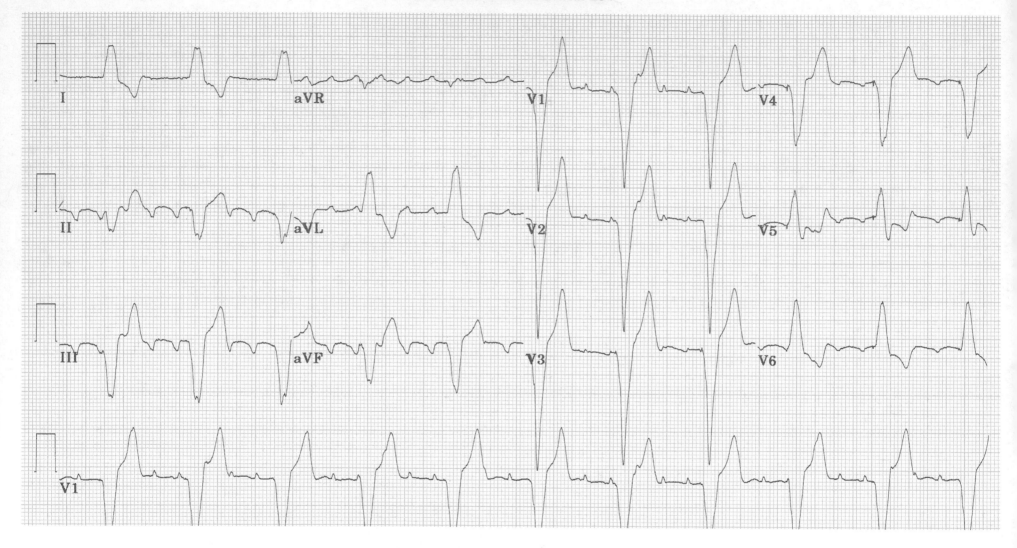

I   aVR   V1   V4

II   aVL   V2   V5

III   aVF   V3   V6

V1

Interpretation Notes:_____

_____

_____

ECG 284 Sixty-six year old gentleman with a long-standing history of atrial dysrhythmias who is status post aortic valve replacement for endocarditis. He returns for an outpatient cardiology follow-up evaluation. Complete heart block ensued necessitating permanent pacemaker placement.

ELECTROCARDIOGRAM 285

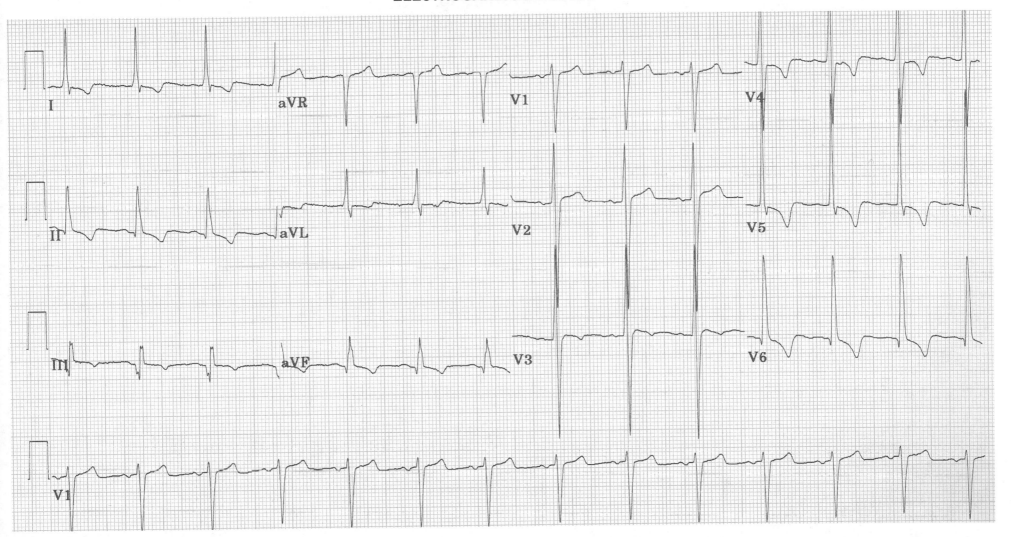

Interpretation Notes: _____

_____

ECG 285 Sixty-three year old gentleman with a history of rheumatic fever at a young age who was transferred for surgical evaluation of advanced coronary artery obstructive disease and severe aortic insufficiency. The patient underwent successful coronary artery bypass graft surgery and aortic valve replacement.

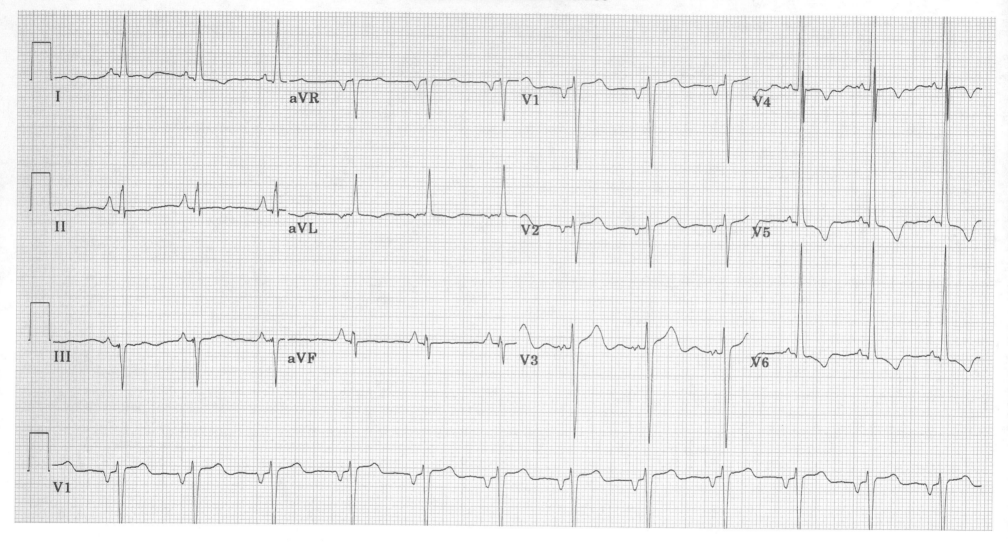

Interpretation Notes: _____

_____

ECG 286 Sixty-three year old gentleman with an approximate twenty-five year history of hypertension who presents to the hypertension clinic for further evaluation. He has noticed recent dyspnea upon exertion. Medications at the time of this tracing included lisinopril.

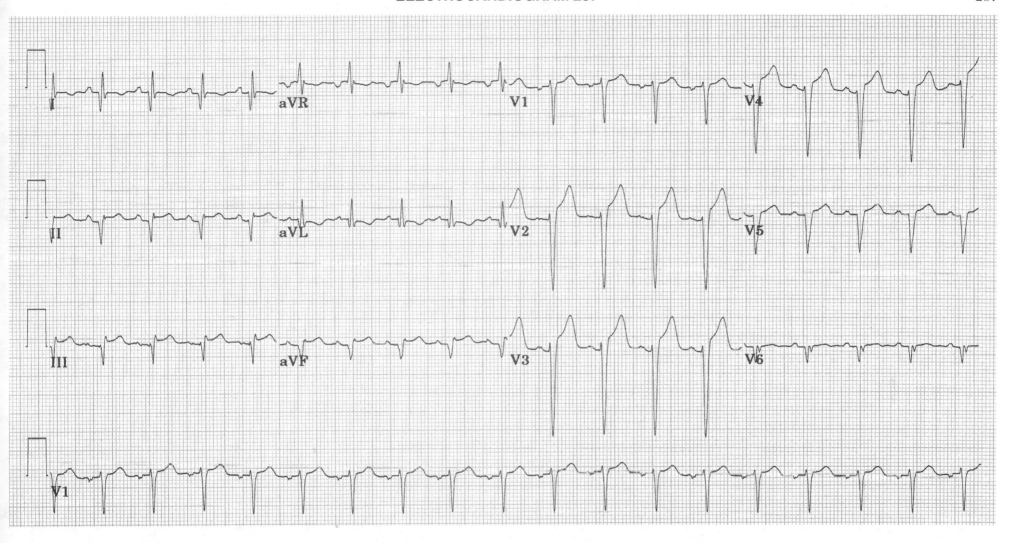

Interpretation Notes: _____

_____

ECG 287 Forty-one year old gentleman who suffered a remote inferolateral myocardial infarction with recurrent angina pectoris and severe native coronary artery disease. The patient underwent recent coronary artery bypass graft surgery. This electrocardiogram represents a routine postoperative tracing.

ELECTROCARDIOGRAM 288

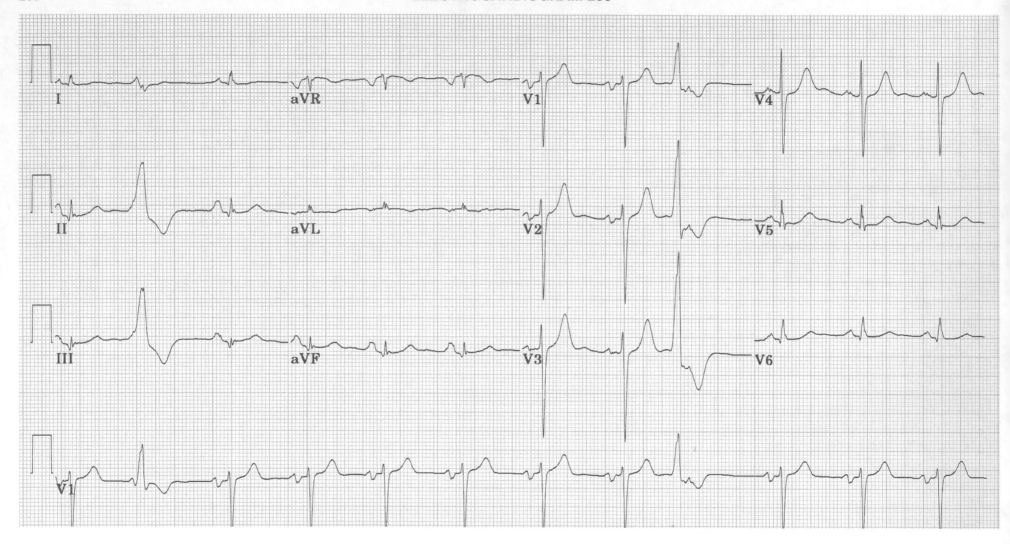

Interpretation Notes: _____

_____

ECG 288 Sixty-six year old gentleman with hypertrophic obstructive cardiomyopathy, severe mitral insufficiency, and normal coronary arteries referred for preoperative evaluation prior to planned septal myectomy and mitral valve repair.

ELECTROCARDIOGRAM 289

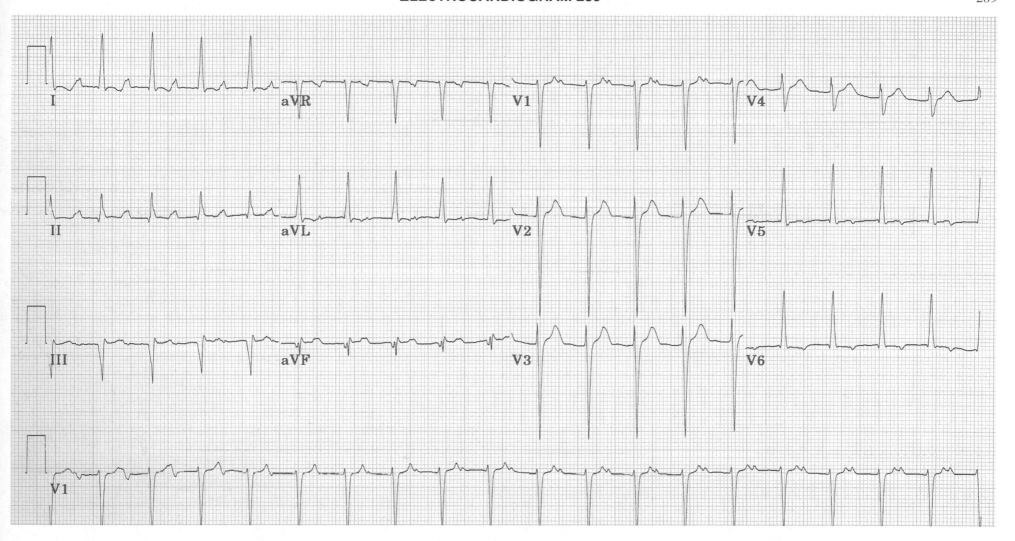

Interpretation Notes: _____

_____

ECG 289 Sixty year old gentleman with long-standing hypertension and dialysis requiring renal failure who presents for an elective cardiac catheterization. A recent echocardiogram demonstrated moderately severe left ventricular systolic dysfunction. The cardiac catheterization demonstrated severe diffuse coronary artery disease. Medications at the time of this electrocardiogram included captopril, nitroglycerin, and allopurinol.

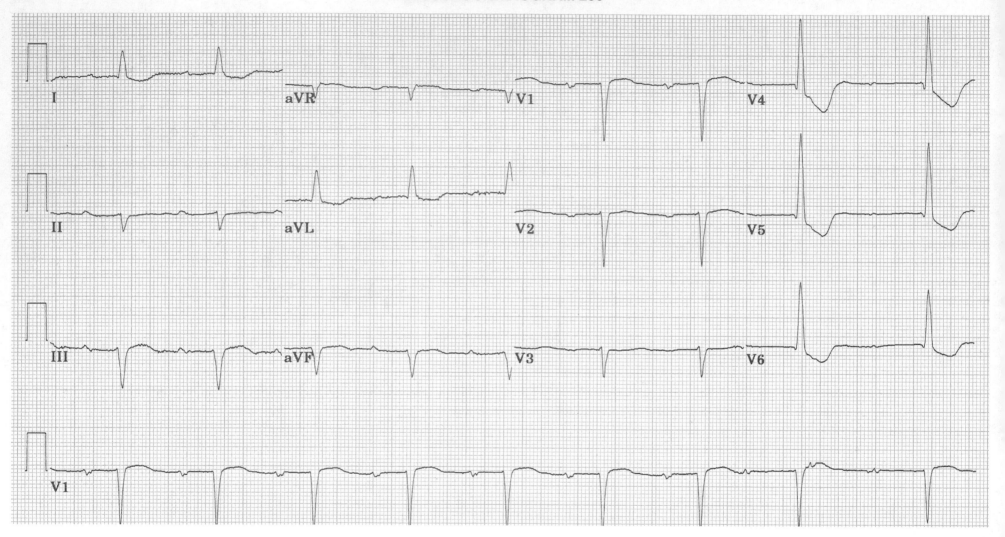

Interpretation Notes: _____

_____

_____

ECG 290 Eighty year old gentleman with coronary artery disease and severe left ventricular systolic dysfunction admitted for evaluation of sustained ventricular dysrhythmias. His past history includes chronic renal insufficiency, congestive heart failure, and severe mitral insufficiency. His medications included amiodarone, furosemide and digoxin.

ELECTROCARDIOGRAM 291

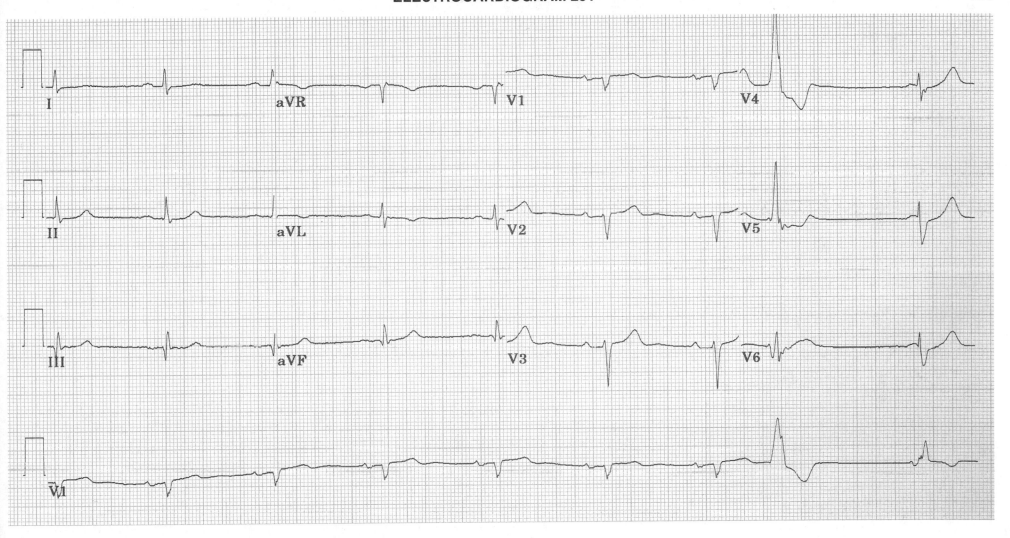

I
aVR
V1
V4

II
aVL
V2
V5

III
aVF
V3
V6

V1

Interpretation Notes: _____

ECG 291 Seventy-four year old gentleman with a history of a remote inferior myocardial infarction and non-sustained ventricular tachycardia who returns for follow-up out-patient cardiac evaluation. His medications included metoprolol, aspirin, and isosorbide mononitrate.

ELECTROCARDIOGRAM 292

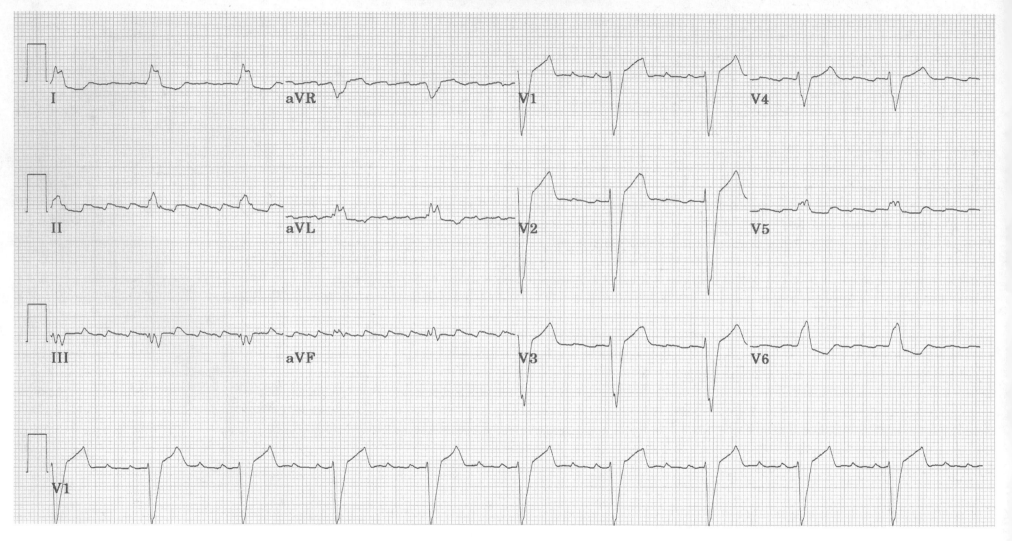

I   aVR   V1   V4

II   aVL   V2   V5

III   aVF   V3   V6

V1

Interpretation Notes: _____

_____

_____

ECG 292 Fifty-five year old gentleman who presents for cardiology clinic follow-up in the setting of a non-ischemic dilated cardiomyopathy. His past medical history includes non-insulin requiring diabetes mellitus. His medications included furosemide, lisinopril, digoxin, atenolol, quinidine, glyburide, and ranitidine.

ELECTROCARDIOGRAM 293

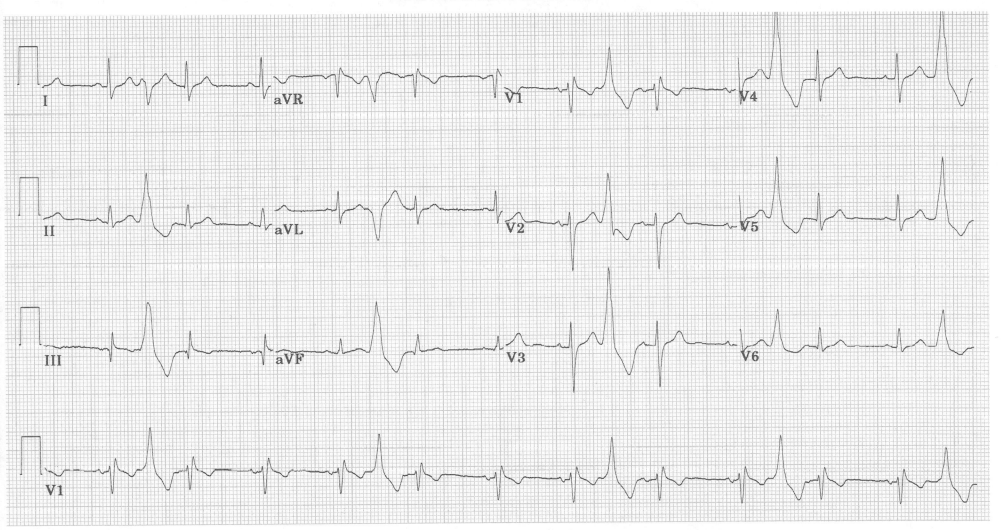

Interpretation Notes:_____

ECG 293 Thirty-four year old woman who is status post ventricular septal defect repair who returns for a right shoulder injury evaluation. Her medications included thyroxine. A cardiac catheterization performed prior to her heart surgery was without obstructive coronary disease.

LEVEL II

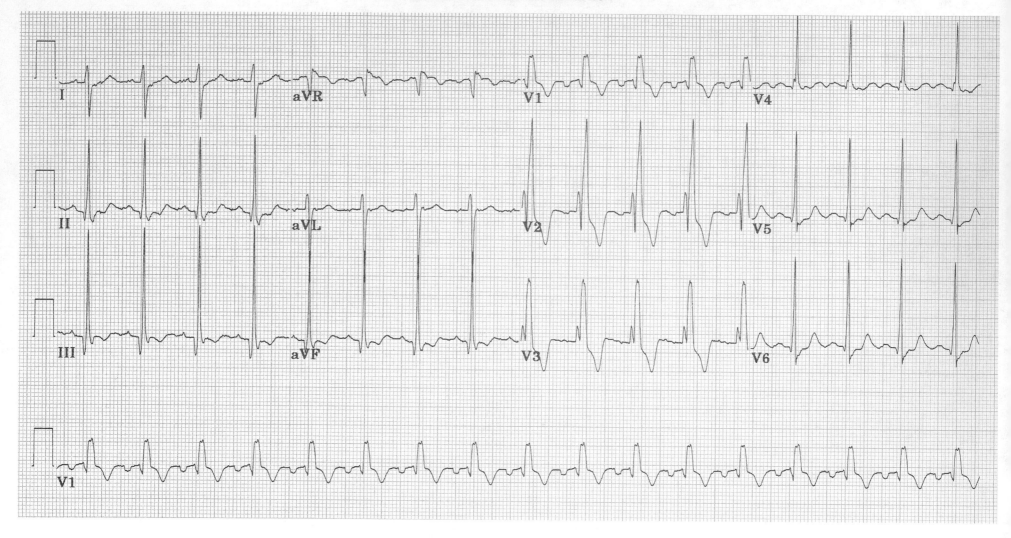

Interpretation Notes: _____

_____

_____

ECG 294 Forty-four year old woman with rheumatic heart disease status post bioprosthetic aortic and mitral valve replacements three years prior to this electrocardiogram who returns for outpatient cardiology follow-up evaluation. Co-morbidities include hypertension and a seizure disorder. Her medications included furosemide, potassium, warfarin, enalapril, carbamazepine, and digoxin.

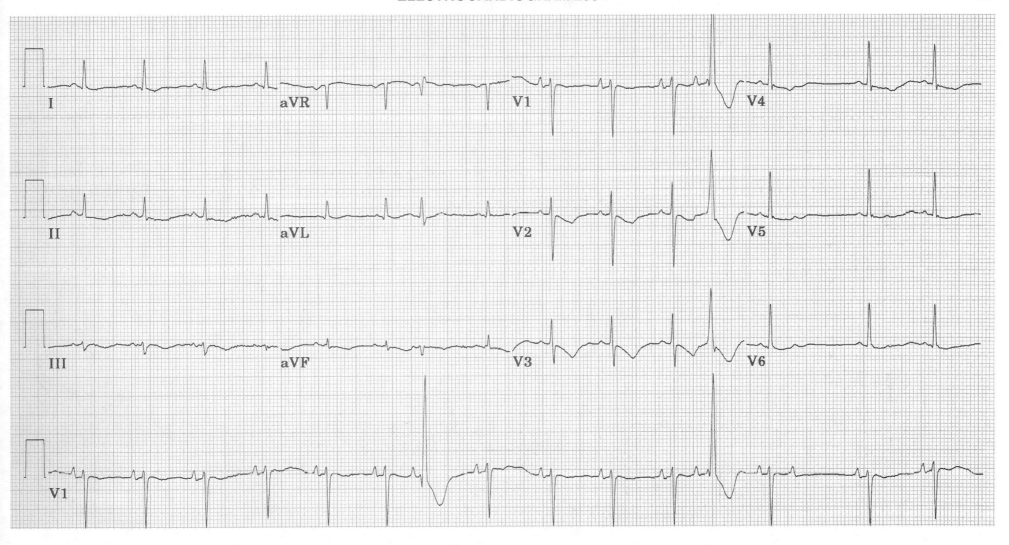

I aVR V1 V4

II aVL V2 V5

III aVF V3 V6

V1

Interpretation Notes:

ECG 295 Seventy-three year old gentleman with a history of pneumonia two years prior to this electrocardiogram who was admitted for a recurrent pleural effusion and an empyema. His medications included digoxin. His past medical history includes paroxysmal atrial fibrillation and long-standing tobacco use.

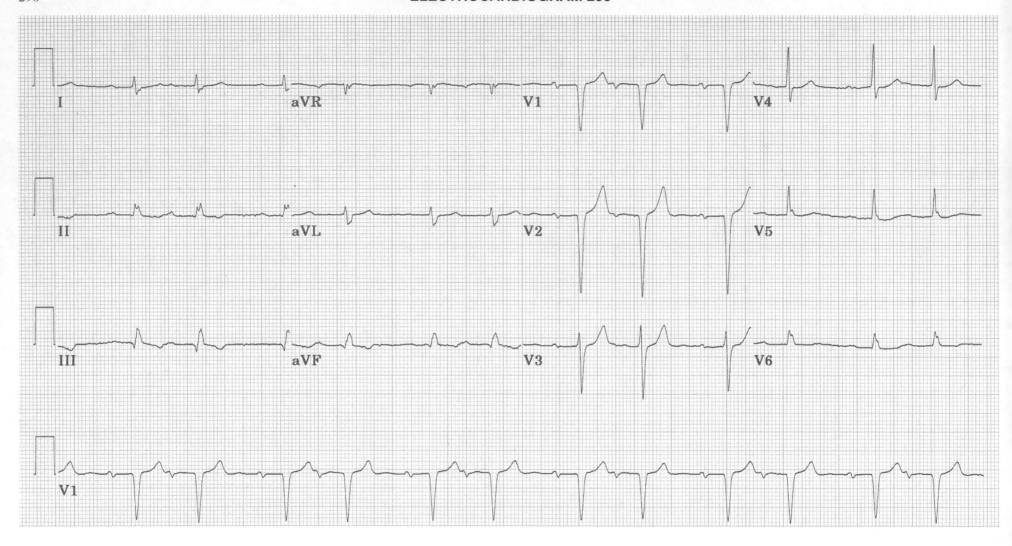

Interpretation Notes: _____

_____

_____

ECG 296 Sixty-nine year old gentleman status post two prior coronary artery bypass grafting procedures, the most recent two years prior to this electrocardiogram, who returns for an outpatient cardiac follow-up evaluation. His past cardiac history also includes an inferior myocardial infarction documented by echocardiography one year before this tracing.

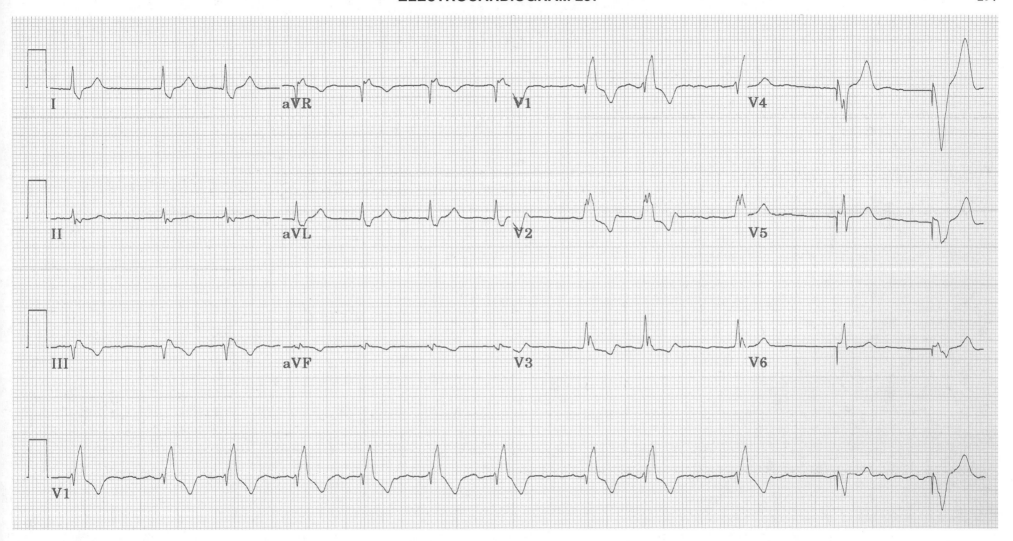

I aVR V1 V4

II aVL V2 V5

III aVF V3 V6

V1

Interpretation Notes:_____

_____

_____

ECG 297 Eighty-one year old gentleman with a history of tachycardia/bradycardia syndrome requiring permanent pacemaker implantation. Co-morbidities include chronic atrial fibrillation and long-standing hypertension.

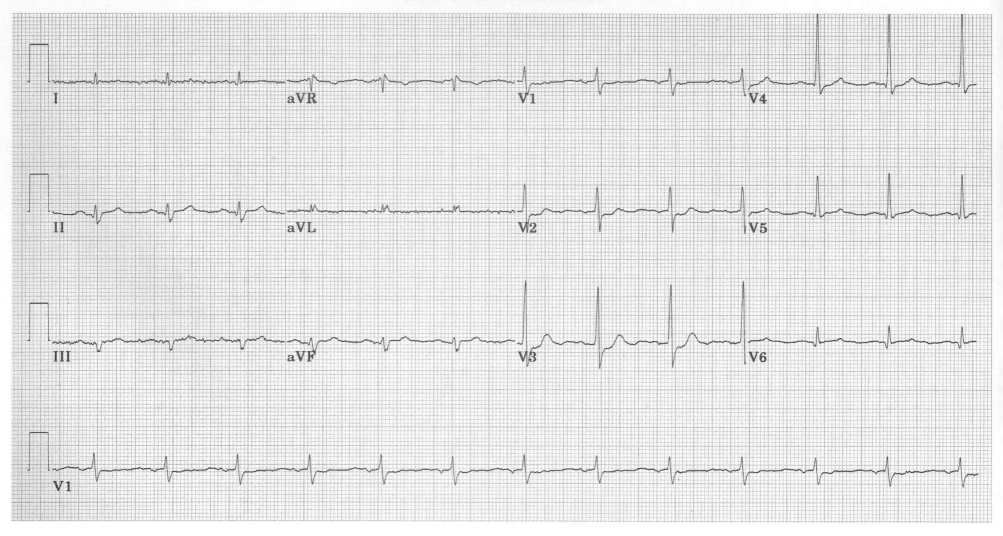

Interpretation Notes: _____

_____

_____

ECG 298 Eighty-nine year old gentleman with no known prior cardiac history who is undergoing preoperative evaluation prior to intended eye surgery. Co-morbid conditions include hypertension and non-insulin requiring diabetes mellitus. His medications included digoxin, captopril, and ranitidine.

ELECTROCARDIOGRAM 299

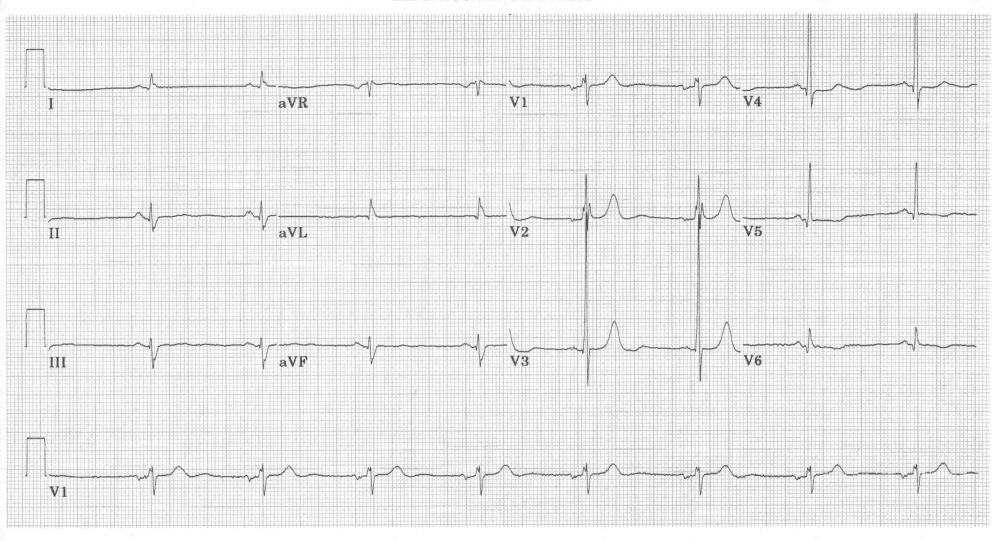

Interpretation Notes: _____

_____

ECG 299 Sixty-three year old gentleman with progressive exertional angina pectoris who is referred for a cardiac catheterization. A recent thallium stress test demonstrated an inferolateral myocardial infarction with peri-infarction myocardial ischemia. His medications included isosorbide mononitrate. A cardiac catheterization demonstrated moderately severe left ventricular systolic dysfunction and three-vessel coronary artery disease.

ELECTROCARDIOGRAM 300

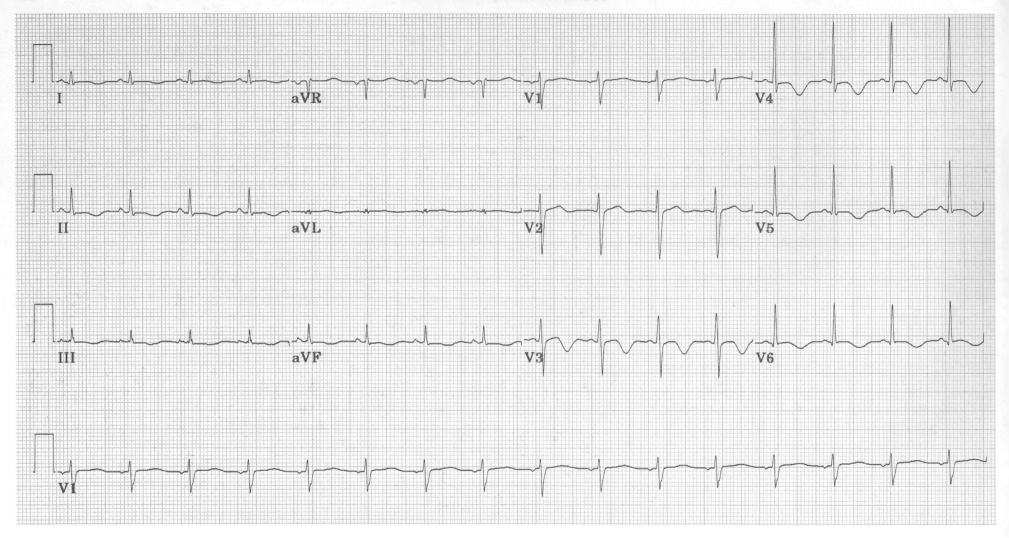

I aVR V1 V4

II aVL V2 V5

III aVF V3 V6

V1

Interpretation Notes: _____

_____

_____

ECG 300 Eighteen year old gentleman hospitalized with intractable seizures and suspected elevated intracranial pressure. The patient's serum potassium at the time of this electrocardiogram was 6.2 meq/L.

ELECTROCARDIOGRAM 301

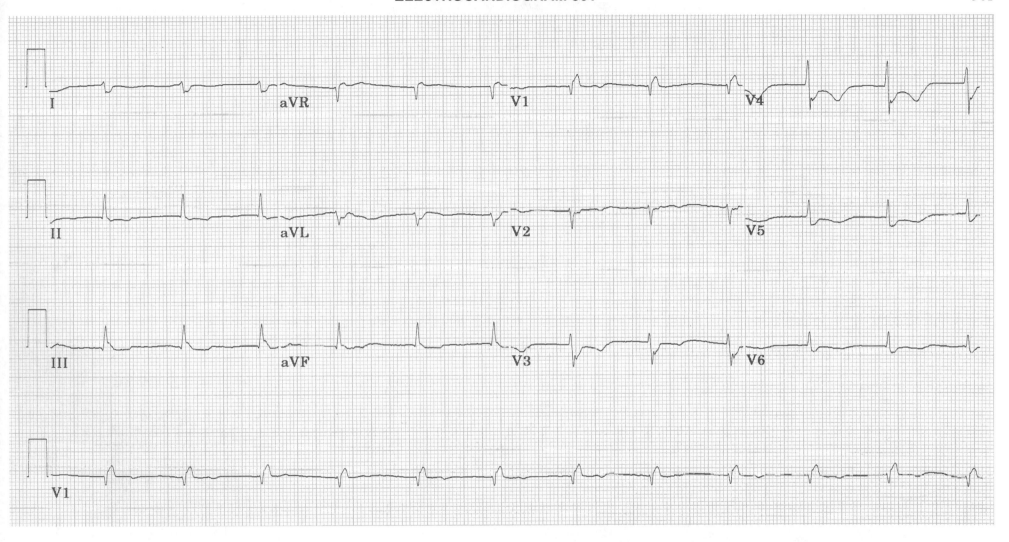

Interpretation Notes: _____

_____

ECG 301 Eighteen year old gentleman with a congenital brain abnormality hospitalized with intractable seizure activity and abrupt elevation of his serum potassium level in the setting of rhabdomyolysis.

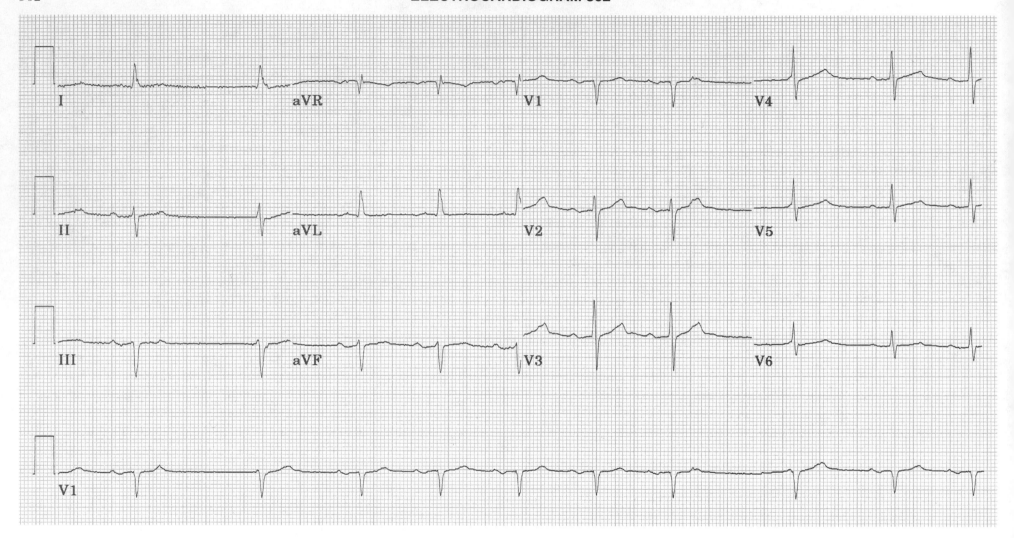

Interpretation Notes: _____

ECG 302 Seventy-nine year old gentleman admitted to the hospital acutely with an asthma exacerbation. His past medical history includes paroxysmal atrial flutter and atrial fibrillation, non-insulin requiring diabetes mellitus, and benign prostatic hypertrophy. His medications at the time of this electrocardiogram included aspirin, verapamil, procainamide, amitriptyline, and numerous inhalers.

ELECTROCARDIOGRAM 303

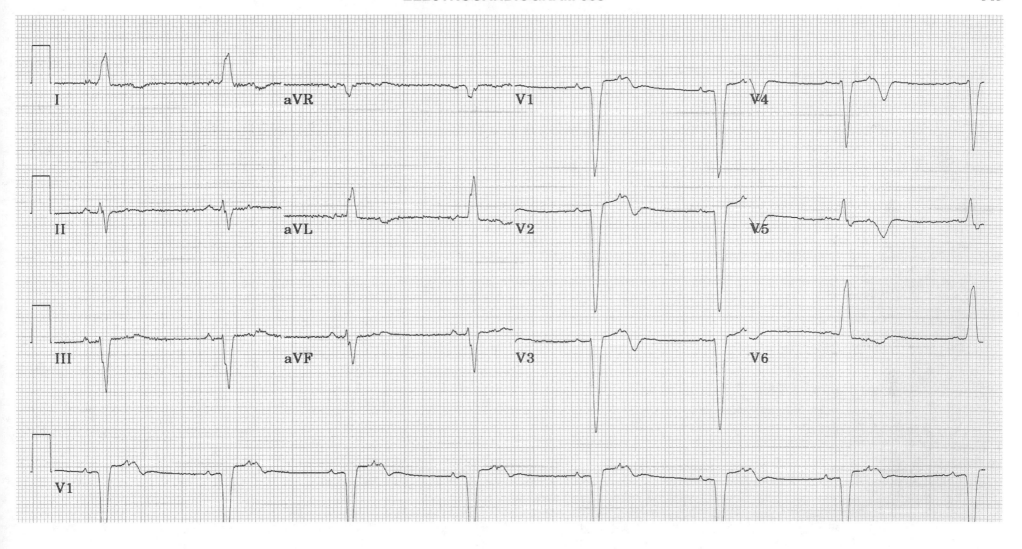

Interpretation Notes: _____

ECG 303 Ninety-two year old woman with an accelerating pattern of angina pectoris. A recent heart catheterization demonstrated normal coronary arteries and severe aortic stenosis.

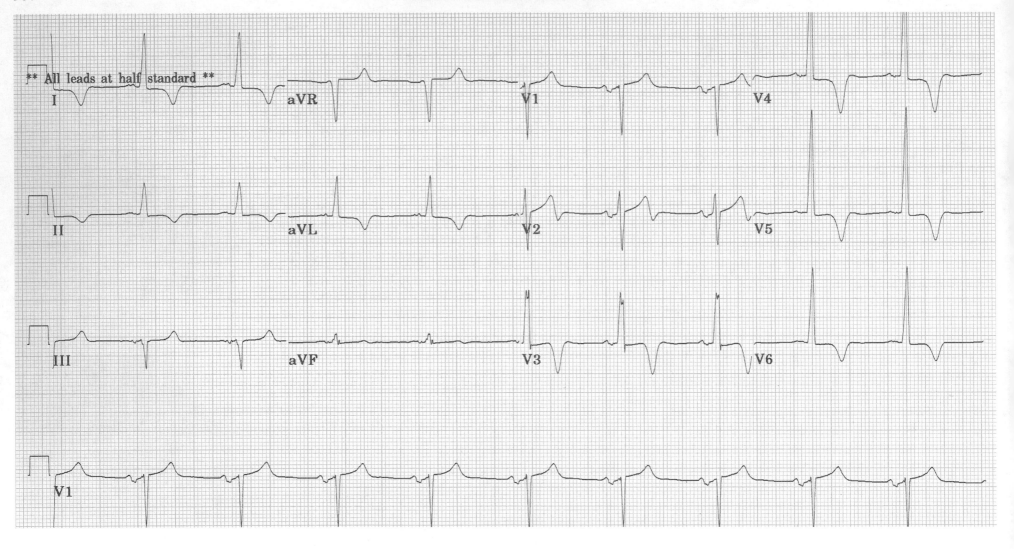

** All leads at half standard **

I aVR V1 V4

II aVL V2 V5

III aVF V3 V6

V1

Interpretation Notes:

ECG 304 Seventy-two year old woman who is seen in cardiology follow-up as an outpatient. She has a known history of hypertrophic obstructive cardiomyopathy as diagnosed by both heart catheterization and transthoracic echocardiogram. At the time of her heart catheterization approximately fifteen years prior to this electrocardiogram the patient had a measurable left ventricular outflow tract gradient of 50 mm Hg.

ELECTROCARDIOGRAM 305

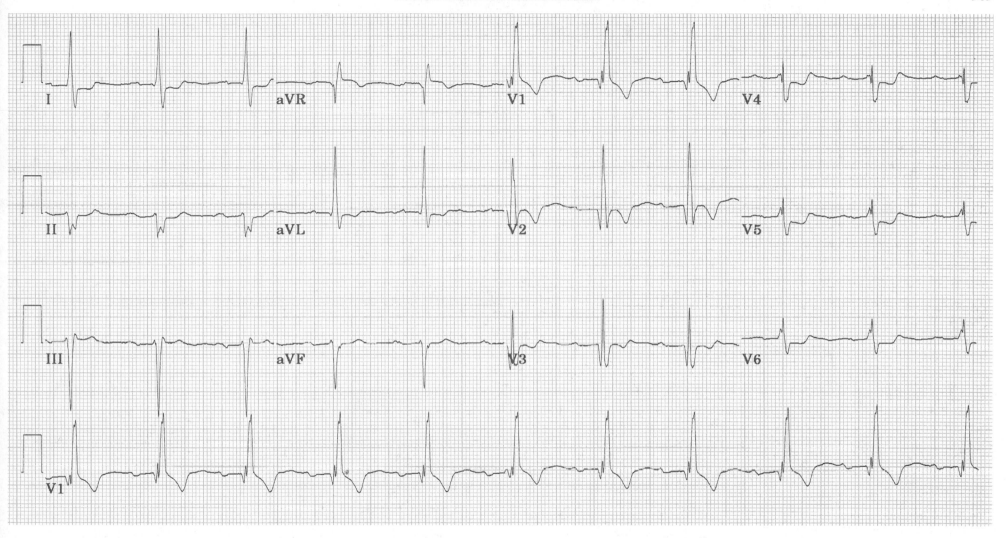

Interpretation Notes: _____

_____

ECG 305 Sixty-nine year old gentleman with an acute chest discomfort syndrome in the setting of a prior coronary artery bypass graft procedure. Emergency cardiac catheterization was undertaken with a successful angioplasty and stent to the right coronary artery. This procedure was complicated by oliguric renal failure, pulmonary edema, and obtundation. The patient expired several days after the coronary intervention.

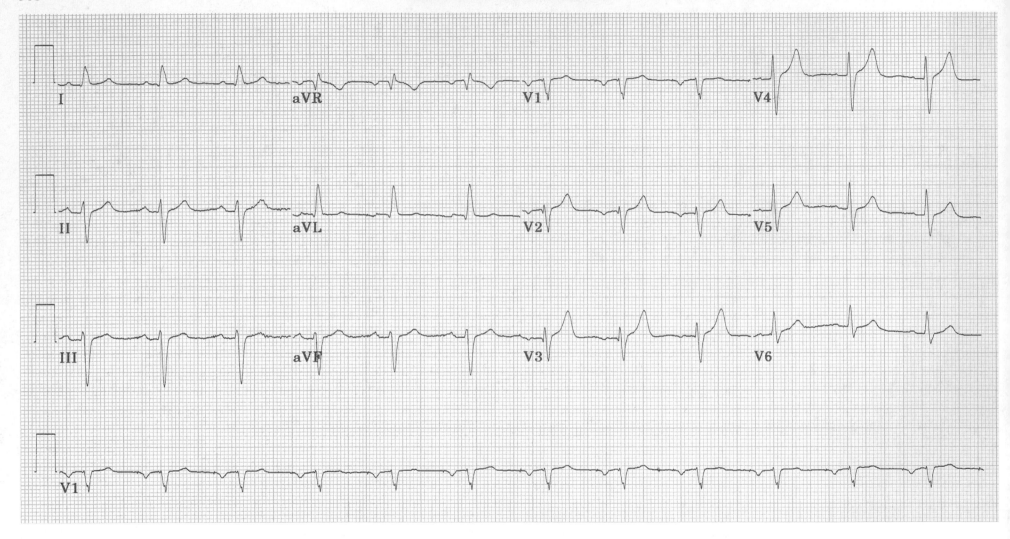

I   aVR   V1   V4

II   aVL   V2   V5

III   aVF   V3   V6

V1

Interpretation Notes:_____

_____

_____

ECG 306 Eighty-one year old gentleman with coronary artery disease and coronary artery bypass graft surgery four years prior to this electrocardiogram who returns for outpatient cardiac evaluation and pacemaker follow-up. A recent heart catheterization documented patent bypass grafts and normal left ventricular systolic function without evidence of a prior myocardial infarction. Pertinent co-morbidities included peripheral vascular disease, hypertension, and paroxysmal atrial fibrillation. Medications at the time of this electrocardiogram included metoprolol, diltiazem, and aspirin.

ELECTROCARDIOGRAM 307

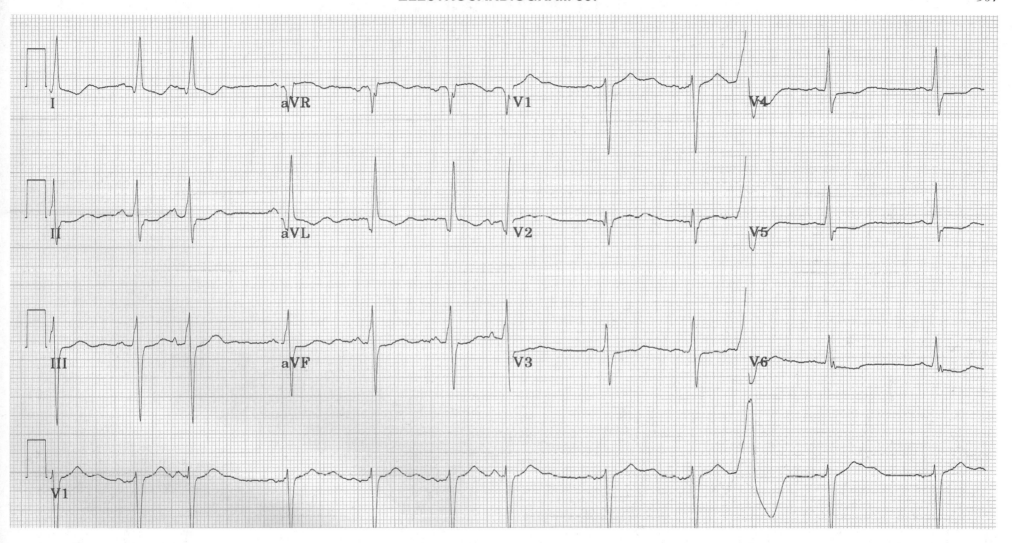

I aVR V1 V4

II aVL V2 V5

III aVF V3 V6

V1

Interpretation Notes: _____

_____

ECG 307 Fifty-six year old gentleman with atherosclerotic coronary artery disease and a history of an anterior myocardial infarction three years prior to this electrocardiogram who re-presents with symptoms of angina pectoris. Medications at the time of this electrocardiogram included metolazone, isosorbide mononitrate, captopril, potassium, and furosemide.

ELECTROCARDIOGRAM 308

308

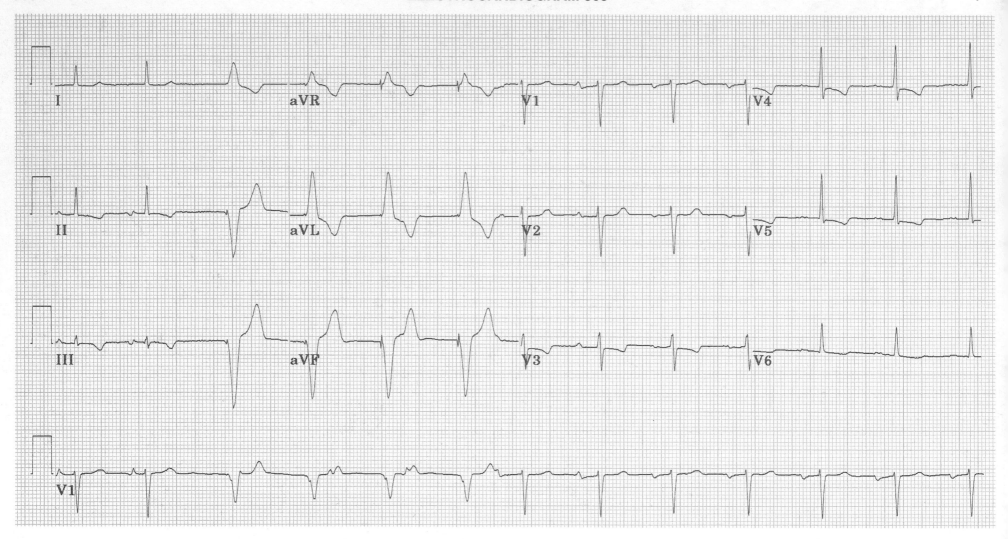

I   aVR   V1   V4

II   aVL   V2   V5

III   aVF   V3   V6

V1

Interpretation Notes:_____

ECG 308 Eighty-one year old woman with a history of near syncope and advanced heart block who returns for clinical follow-up and pacemaker reassessment. Her past medical history includes hyperlipidemia. Medications at the time of this electrocardiogram included metolazone.

ELECTROCARDIOGRAM 309

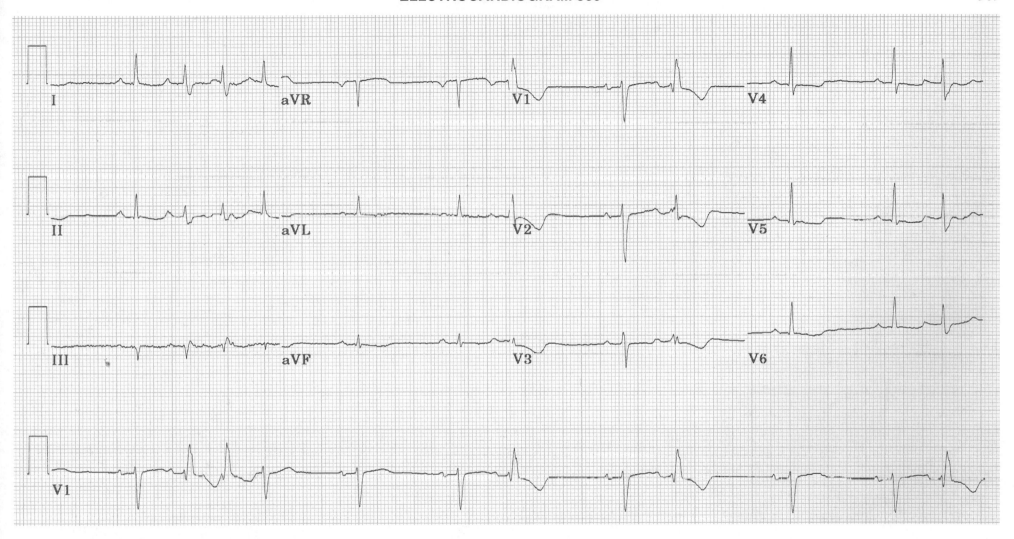

Interpretation Notes: _____

_____

_____

ECG 309 Seventy-eight year old woman with a normal resting echocardiogram who returns for a follow-up appointment in the setting of paroxysmal supraventricular tachy-cardia. Her medications included digoxin and flecainide.

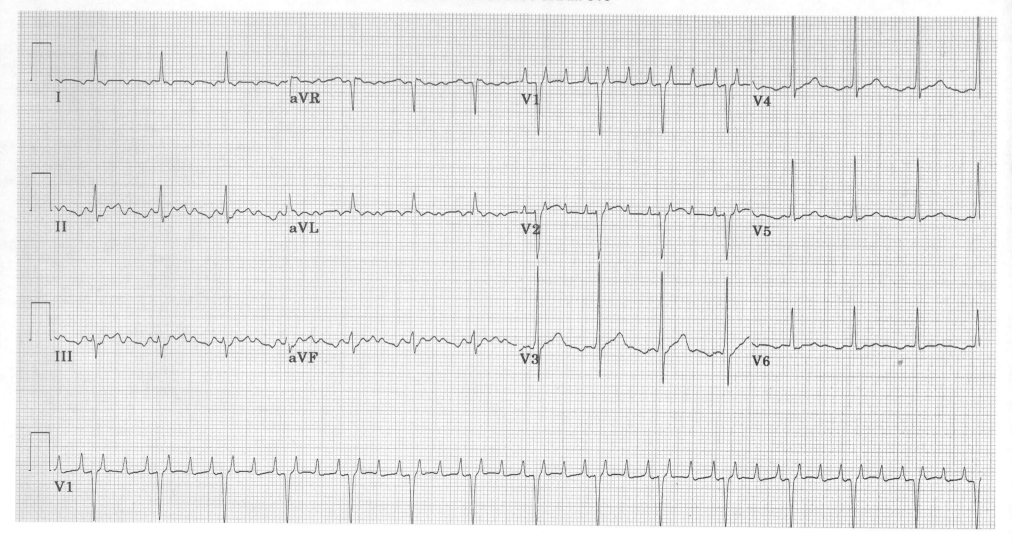

Interpretation Notes: _____

_____

ECG 310 Fifty-nine year old woman with rheumatic heart disease status post mitral valve replacement two years prior to this electrocardiogram. She returns for evaluation of recurrent atrial arrhythmias. Her medications at the time of this electrocardiogram included diltiazem, furosemide, glucotrol, prednisone, and warfarin.

ELECTROCARDIOGRAM 311

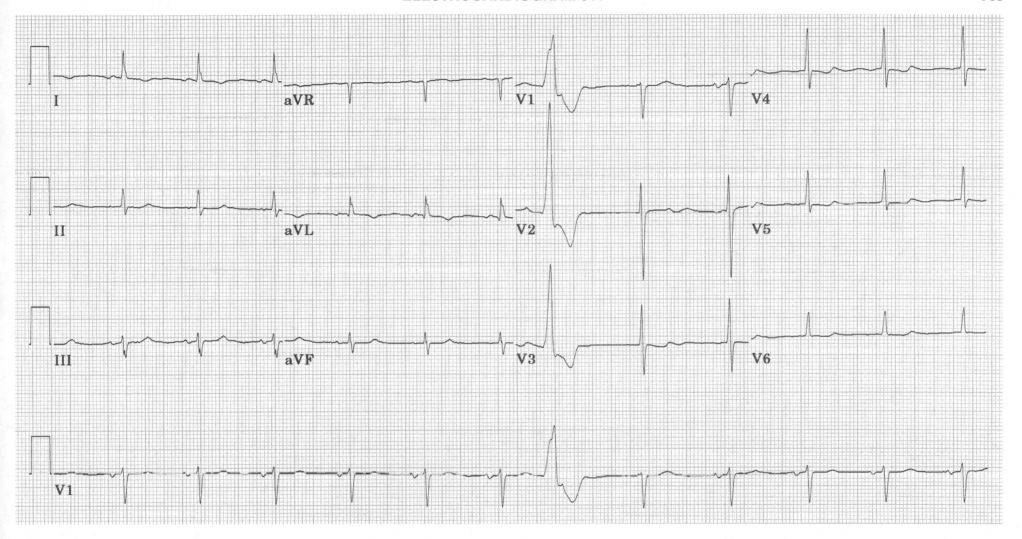

I aVR V1 V4

II aVL V2 V5

III aVF V3 V6

V1

Interpretation Notes: _____

_____

ECG 311 Fifty-eight year old woman with insulin requiring diabetes mellitus, chronic renal insufficiency, and congestive heart failure of unknown etiology who returns for evaluation of an ischemic left foot ulcer. Her medications included ranitidine, isosorbide dinitrate, digoxin, and hydralazine.

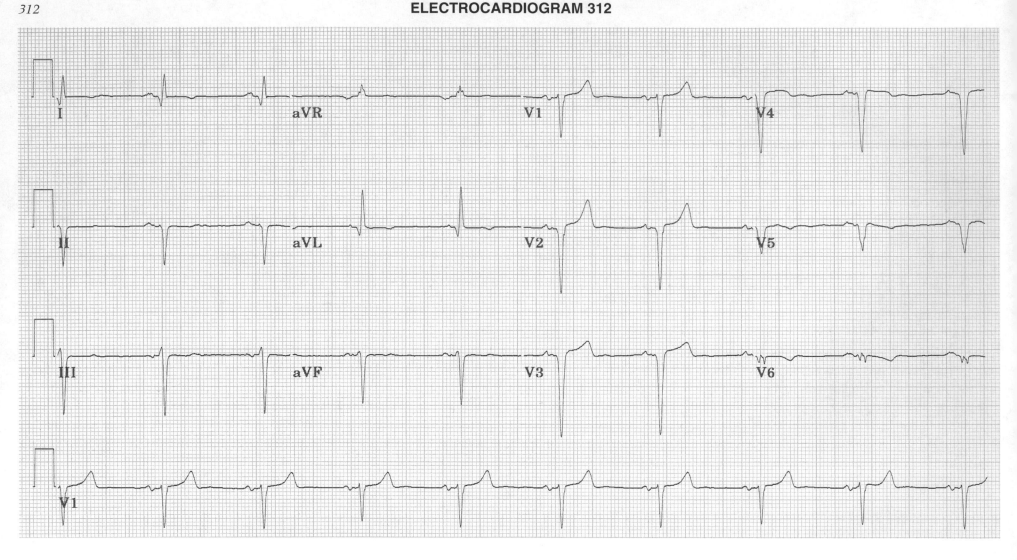

Interpretation Notes: _____

_____

_____

ECG 312 Sixty-three year old gentleman with a large anterior myocardial infarction four years prior to this electrocardiogram who presents for further evaluation. A cardiac catheterization demonstrated apical and anterior dyskinesia and multi-vessel coronary artery obstructions. The patient was subsequently referred for coronary artery by-pass graft surgery.

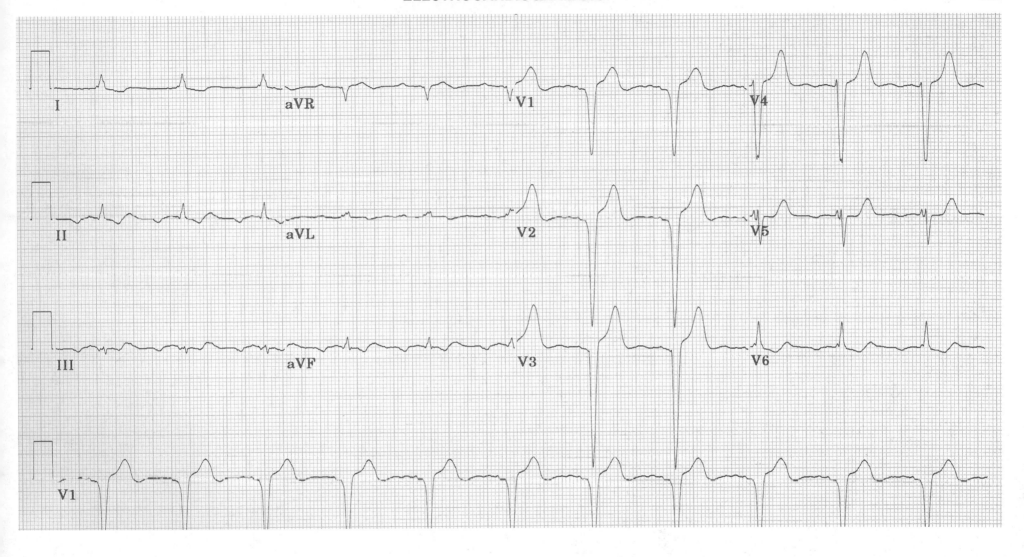

I

aVR

V1

V4

II

aVL

V2

V5

III

aVF

V3

V6

V1

Interpretation Notes: _____

_____

ECG 313 Sixty-six year old gentleman who presents for a cardiac catheterization in the setting of stable angina pectoris and progressive dyspnea upon exertion. His past medical history includes chronic renal insufficiency. Medications at the time of this electrocardiogram included amiodarone. The cardiac catheterization findings included severe aortic stenosis, severe pulmonary hypertension, and minimal coronary artery obstructive disease.

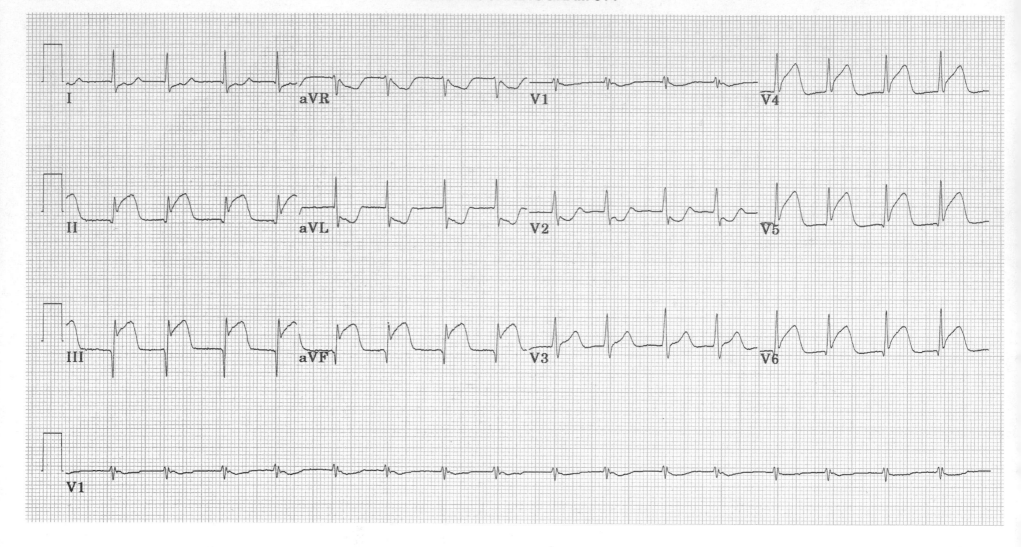

I aVR V1 V4

II aVL V2 V5

III aVF V3 V6

V1

Interpretation Notes: _____

_____

_____

ECG 314 Seventy-eight year old gentleman transferred by helicopter from an outside hospital after the sudden onset of severe chest discomfort awakening him from sleep. This electrocardiogram was performed prior to an urgent cardiac catheterization demonstrating an advanced occlusion of the right coronary artery.

ELECTROCARDIOGRAM 315

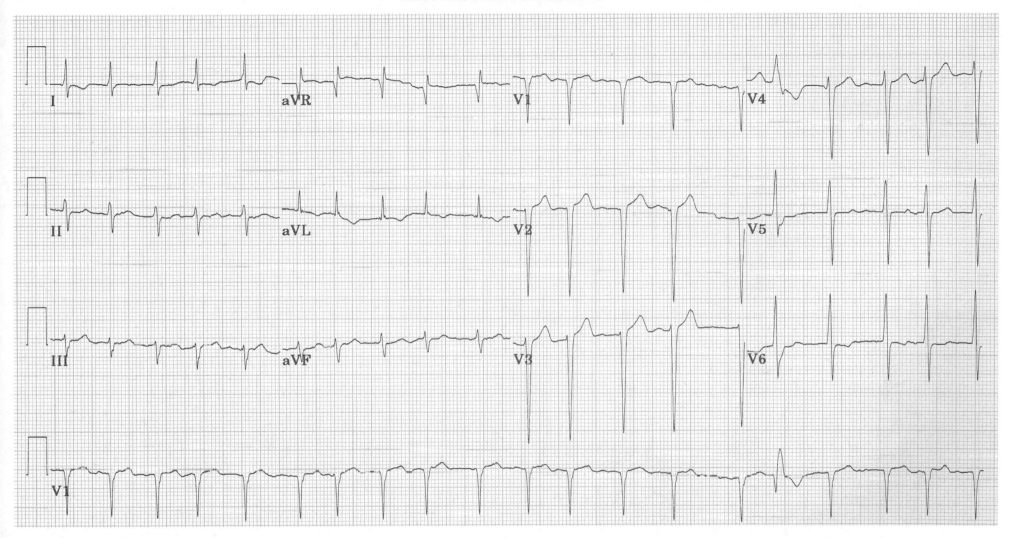

Interpretation Notes: _____

_____

ECG 315 Sixty-seven year old gentleman admitted acutely to the hospital for evaluation and treatment of new onset atrial fibrillation. His past medical history includes emphysema, long-standing tobacco and alcohol use, and an abdominal aortic aneurysm repair. Medications at the time of this electrocardiogram included inhalers and lisinopril.

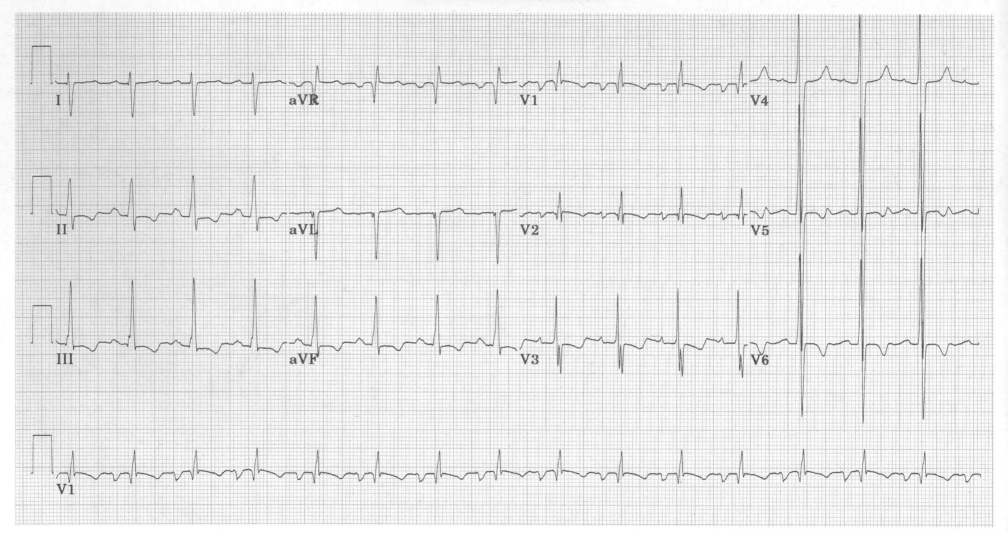

I aVR V1 V4

II aVL V2 V5

III aVF V3 V6

V1

Interpretation Notes: _____

_____

ECG 316 Thirty-six year old woman with primary pulmonary hypertension admitted with signs and symptoms of right-sided congestive heart failure. Her medications included nifedipine, furosemide, potassium, and warfarin. A subsequent echocardiogram demonstrated a dilated right ventricle with severe systolic dysfunction and a small left ventricle with mild systolic dysfunction. An atrial septal defect was present with a right-to-left interatrial shunt.

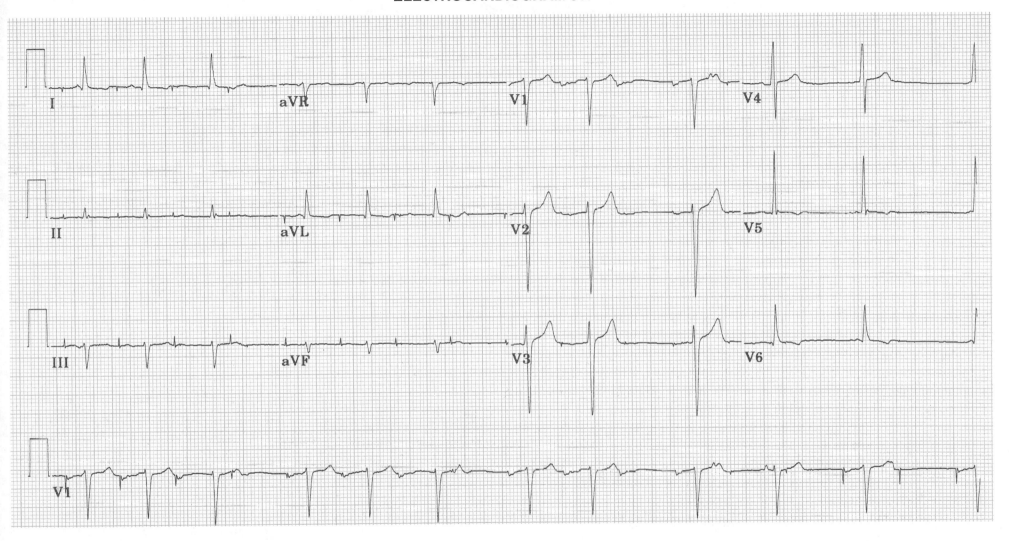

I aVR V1 V4
II aVL V2 V5
III aVF V3 V6
V1

Interpretation Notes: _____

ECG 317 Seventy-seven year old gentleman with a recurrent history of congestive heart failure who is referred for coronary artery bypass grafting and mitral valve repair secondary to mitral insufficiency. He also has a long-standing history of atrial fibrillation. His medications at the time of this electrocardiogram included lisinopril, furosemide, digoxin, and warfarin.

ELECTROCARDIOGRAM 318

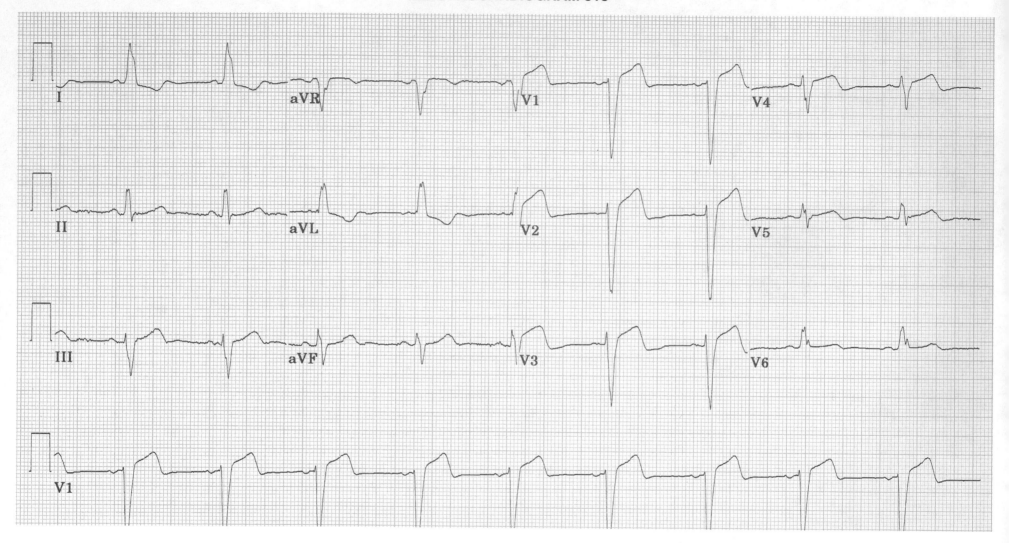

Interpretation Notes: _____

ECG 318 Sixty-seven year old woman who presents to the hospital with a several hour history of nausea and substernal chest discomfort. The patient was treated with intravenous nitroglycerin and heparin in addition to beta-blockers and aspirin. A near future cardiac catheterization demonstrated evidence of an antero-apical myocardial infarction and an 85% mid left anterior descending coronary artery stenosis.

ELECTROCARDIOGRAM 319

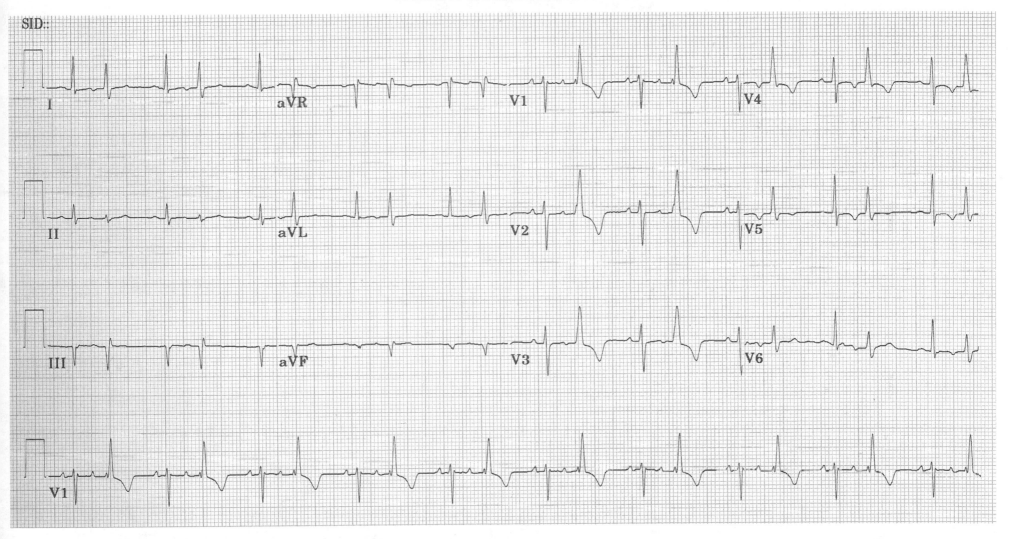

I aVR V1 V4

II aVL V2 V5

III aVF V3 V6

V1

Interpretation Notes: _____

_____

ECG 319 Sixty-two year old gentleman with two prior coronary artery bypass graft surgeries who is awaiting cardiac transplantation. He has severe left ventricular systolic dysfunction.

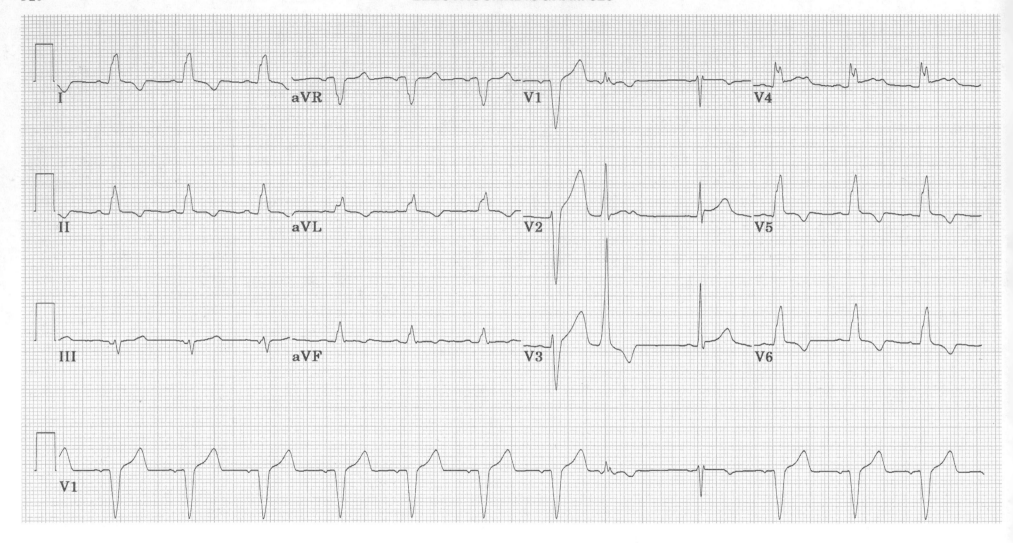

Interpretation Notes: _____

_____

ECG 320 Seventy-seven year old gentleman with recent accelerating angina pectoris referred for coronary artery bypass graft surgery in the setting of multi-vessel coronary artery obstructive disease. The patient is recently status post open heart surgery.

ELECTROCARDIOGRAM 321

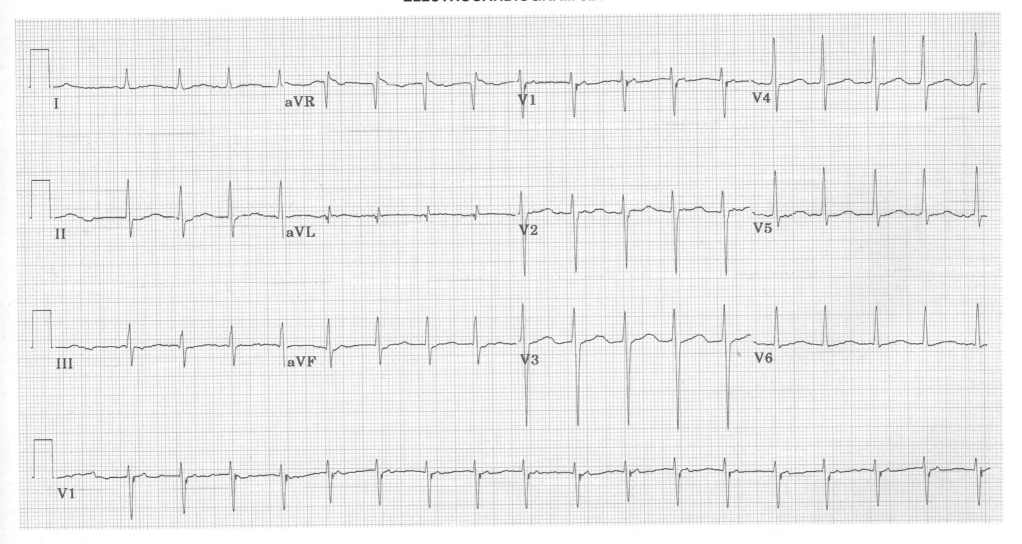

Interpretation Notes: _____

ECG 321 Sixty-four year old woman with severe mitral stenosis who returns for an outpatient cardiac evaluation and consideration for mitral valve surgery. She has a history of paroxysmal supraventricular dysrhythmias. Co-morbid conditions include hyperlipidemia and hypertension. Her medications included amiodarone, enalapril, bumetanide, thyroxine, warfarin, and potassium.

LEVEL II

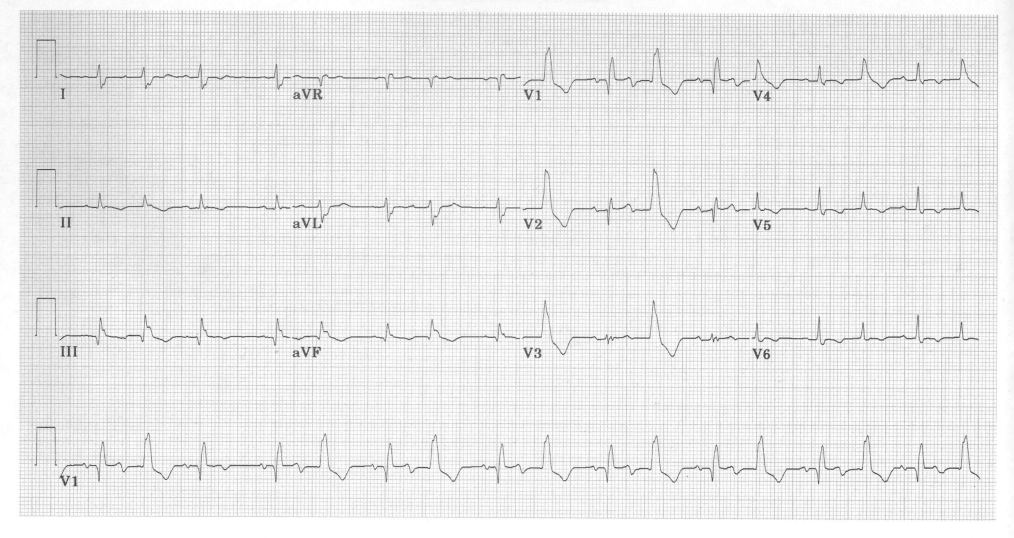

Interpretation Notes:_____

_____

ECG 322 Fifty year old gentleman status post recent cardiac transplantation complicated by sepsis, bacteremia, and an inferior myocardial infarction.

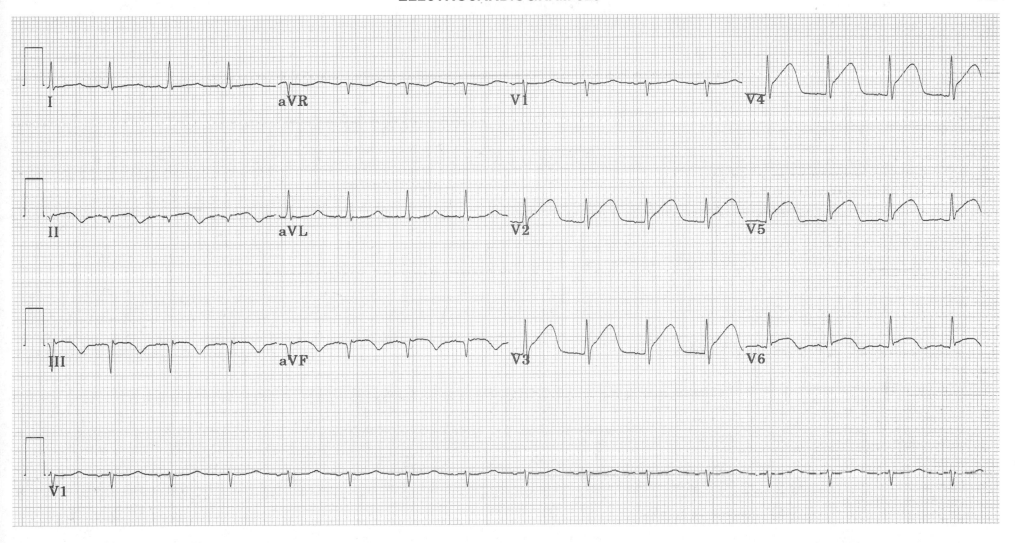

Interpretation Notes: _____

_____

_____

ECG 323 Sixty-three year old woman who underwent coronary artery bypass graft surgery and an ascending aorta repair of a Type I aortic dissection who had this electrocardiogram performed as a routine postoperative tracing. Acute myocardial injury was suspected. A subsequent echocardiogram and serial cardiac enzymes confirmed acute myocardial injury.

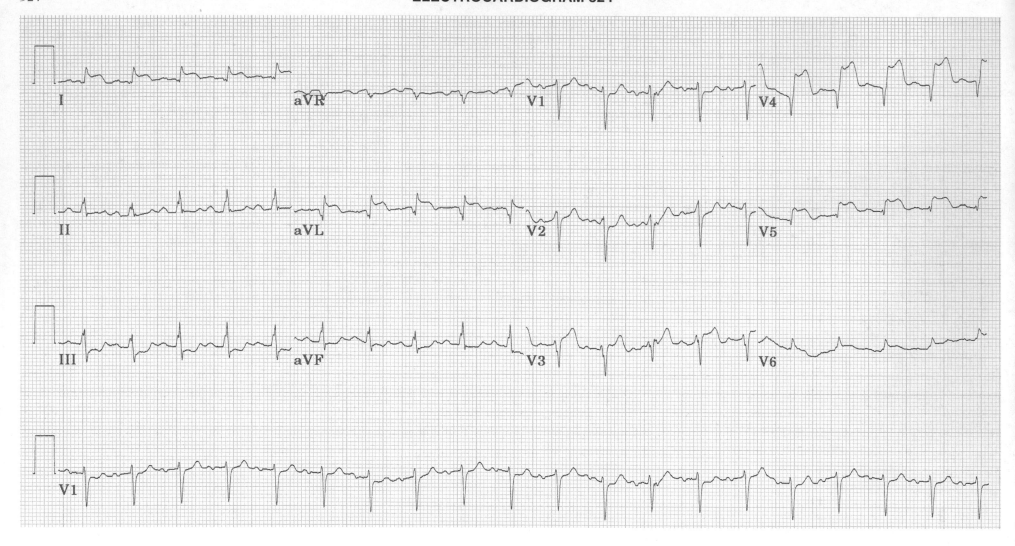

Interpretation Notes: _____

_____

_____

ECG 324 Fifty-four year old gentleman who presented to the emergency room two hours after the acute onset of substernal chest pressure. He is known to suffer from hypertension, diabetes, and lymphoma. Serial electrocardiograms and cardiac enzyme serum analysis confirmed an acute myocardial infarction.

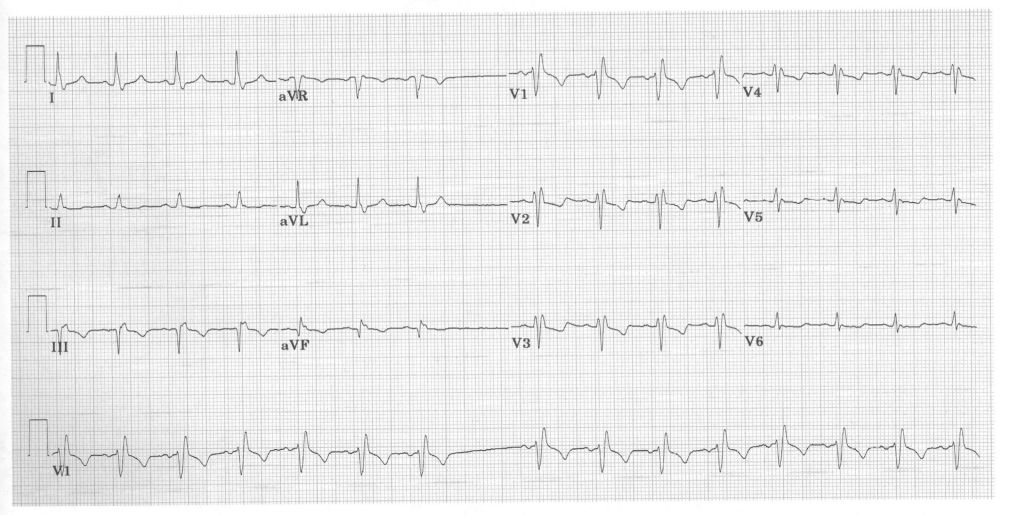

Interpretation Notes: _____

ECG 325 Fifty-one year old gentleman with a recently positive thallium stress test referred for coronary arteriography. The cardiac catheterization demonstrated single vessel coronary artery disease with a 90% proximal left anterior descending coronary artery obstruction. The patient underwent successful angioplasty. The patient subsequently re-presented with restenosis of the prior angioplasty site and progressive coronary artery obstructions including the right coronary artery and underwent coronary artery bypass graft surgery.

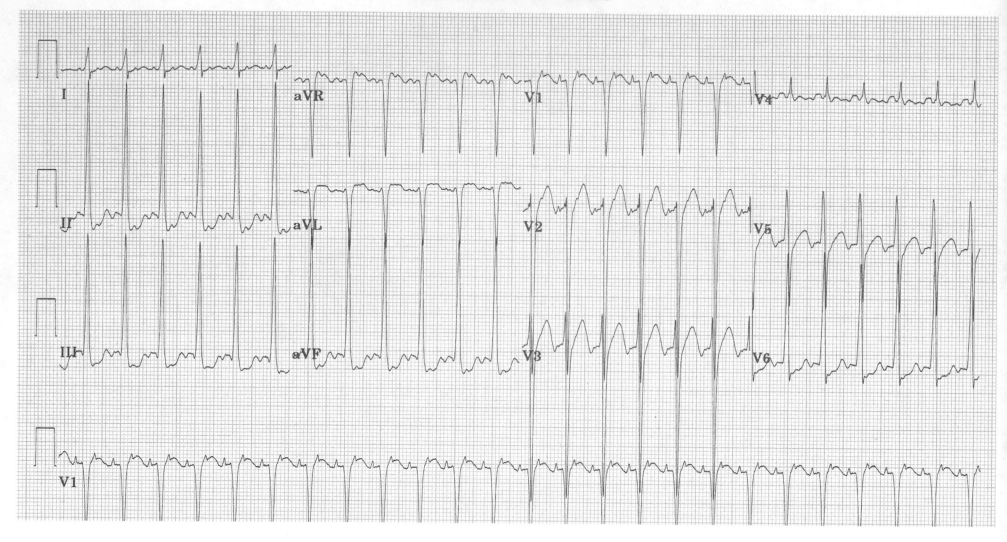

Interpretation Notes: _____

_____

_____

ECG 326 Fifty-two year old gentleman with long-standing hypertension, renal insufficiency, and severe peripheral vascular disease who is seen in the cardiology outpatient clinic. He has coronary artery obstructive disease undergoing a left heart catheterization in the past. Medical therapy of his coronary artery disease has been successfully initiated. Medications at the time of this electrocardiogram included captopril, warfarin, and fluoxetine.

ELECTROCARDIOGRAM 327

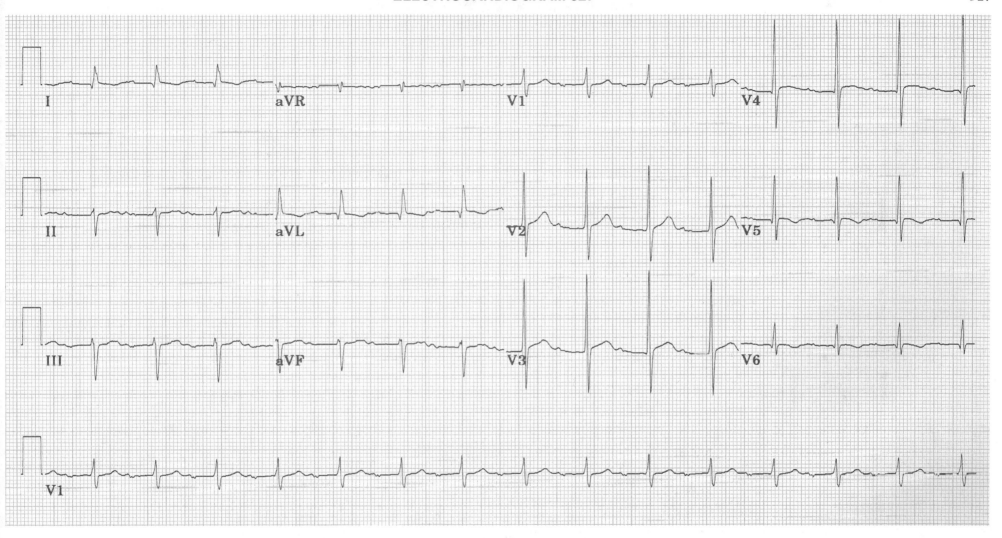

Interpretation Notes:_____

_____

_____

ECG 327 Sixty-seven year old gentleman accepted in hospital transfer for evaluation of coronary artery disease and severe aortic stenosis. He is experiencing increasing dyspnea on exertion and recurrent syncope. A recent cardiac catheterization demonstrated a 70% right coronary artery stenosis and diffuse severe disease in the left cir-cumflex coronary artery system. The patient underwent subsequent aortic valve replacement and coronary artery bypass graft surgery.

ELECTROCARDIOGRAM 328

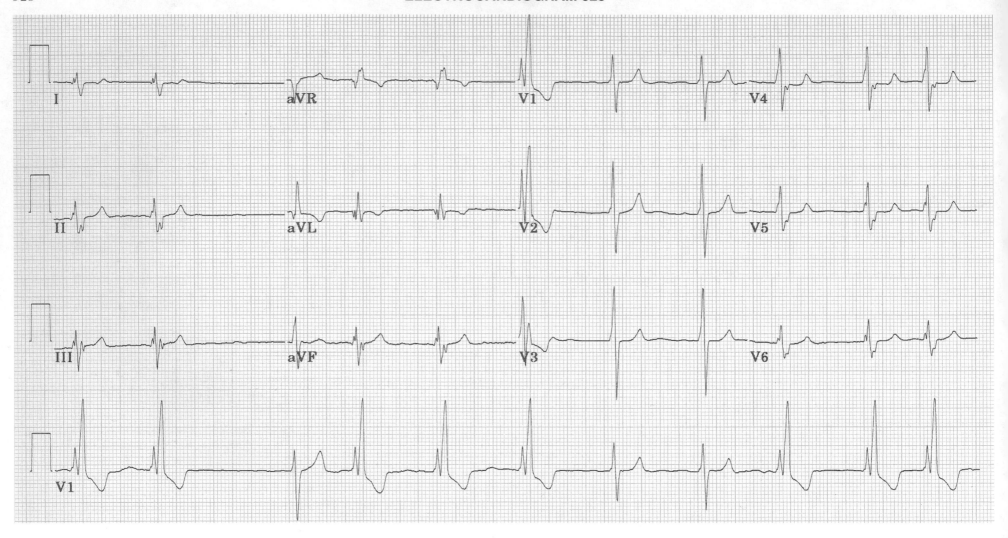

Interpretation Notes:_____

_____

_____

ECG 328 Forty-seven year old gentleman with a history of aortic stenosis status post prior aortic valve replacement who re-presents with perivalvular moderately severe aortic insufficiency and congestive heart failure. Co-morbid conditions include insulin requiring diabetes mellitus and a recently repaired rectal fistula. His medications included insulin, potassium, metolazone, metoprolol, captopril, and digoxin.

ELECTROCARDIOGRAM 329

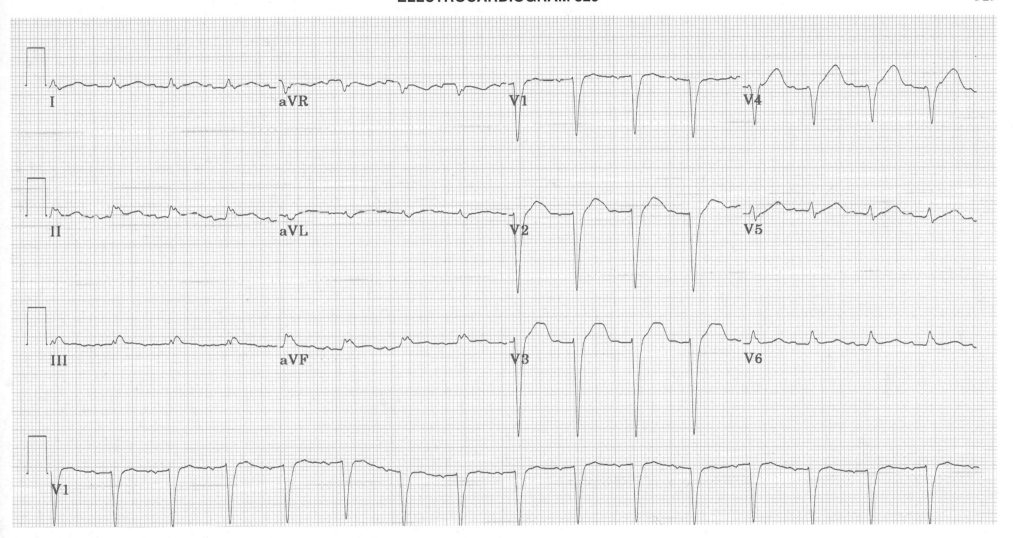

Interpretation Notes: _____

ECG 329 Fifty-four year old gentleman with recurrent congestive heart failure and severe left ventricular systolic dysfunction who is status post recent coronary artery by-pass surgery.

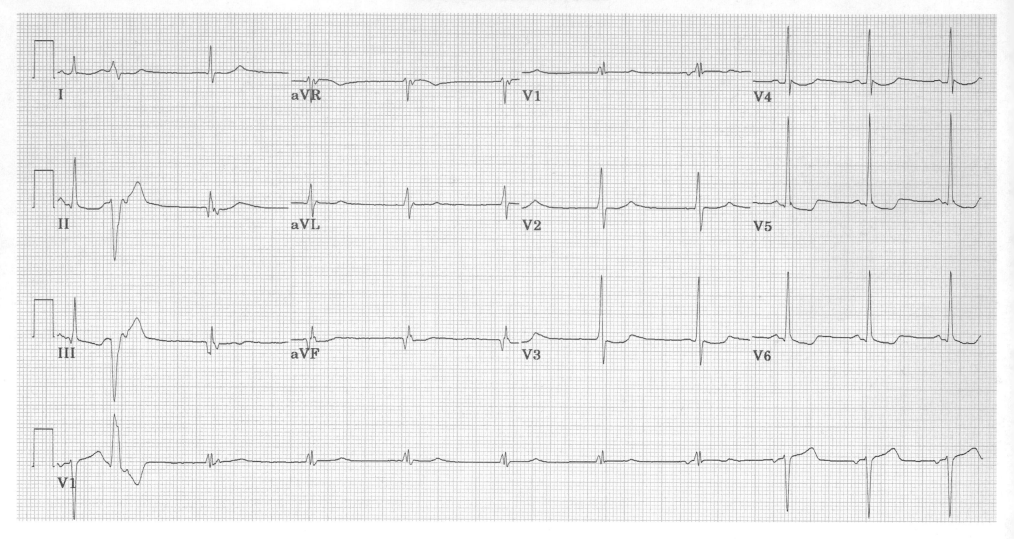

Interpretation Notes: _____

_____

ECG 330 Sixty-two year old gentleman with recent symptoms of accelerating angina pectoris with a subsequent cardiac catheterization demonstrating severe multi-vessel coronary artery disease. This electrocardiogram was obtained prior to anticipated near future coronary artery bypass graft surgery. His cardiac catheterization demonstrated evidence of an age indeterminate inferior myocardial infarction. Medications at the time of this electrocardiogram included metoprolol, furosemide, digoxin, topical nitroglycerin, and captopril.

ELECTROCARDIOGRAM 331

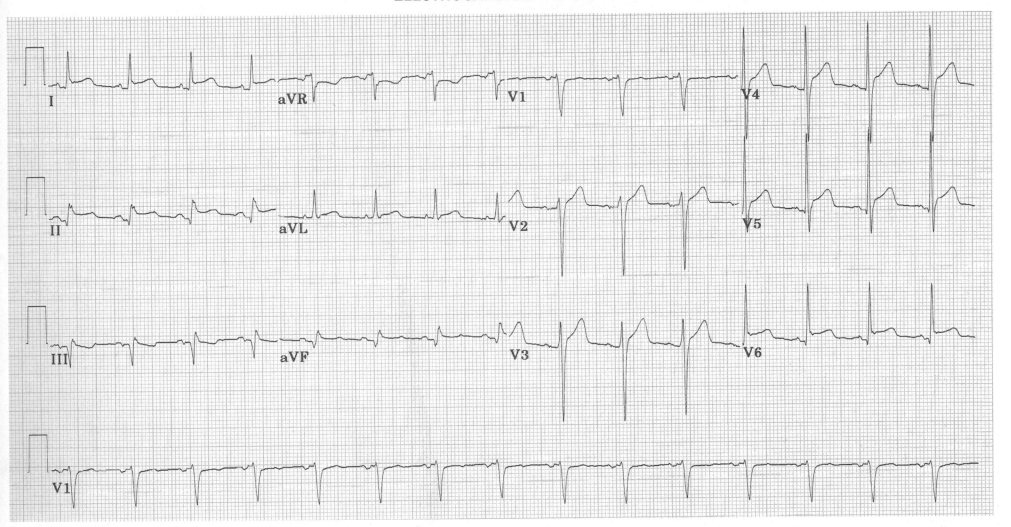

I   aVR   V1   V4

II   aVL   V2   V5

III   aVF   V3   V6

V1

Interpretation Notes: _____

_____

ECG 331 Seventy-five year old gentleman with a remote inferior myocardial infarction who presents for follow-up cardiac evaluation in the setting of a recently abnormal stress test. A subsequent cardiac catheterization demonstrated multi-vessel coronary artery obstructions and the patient was referred for coronary artery bypass graft surgery. This electrocardiogram was obtained immediately after open heart surgery.

ELECTROCARDIOGRAM 332

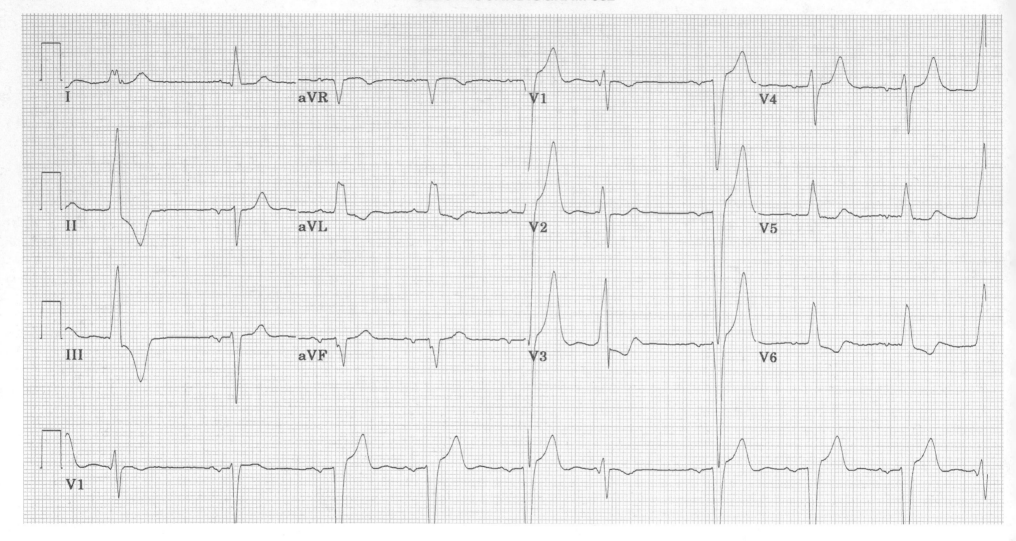

Interpretation Notes: _____

_____

_____

ECG 332 Fifty-two year old woman who presents for a general physical examination. Her past medical history includes hypertension. Her medications included hydrochlorothiazide.

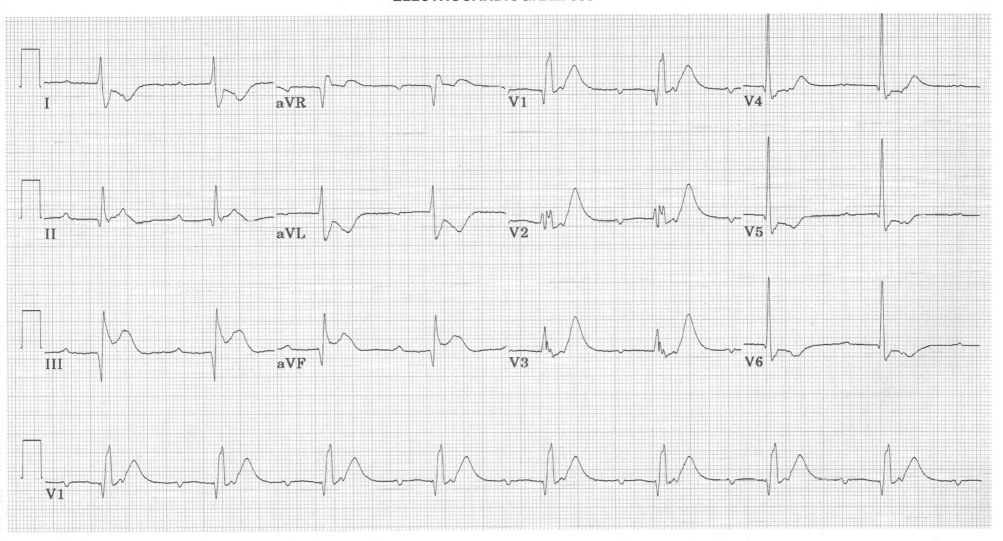

I aVR V1 V4

II aVL V2 V5

III aVF V3 V6

V1

Interpretation Notes: _____

ECG 333 Seventy year old gentleman status post coronary artery bypass graft surgery nine years prior to this electrocardiogram who presents with a one hour history of acute chest discomfort. A cardiac catheterization demonstrated an advanced stenosis in the right coronary artery. The patient subsequently demonstrated complete heart block requiring permanent pacemaker placement.

ELECTROCARDIOGRAM 334

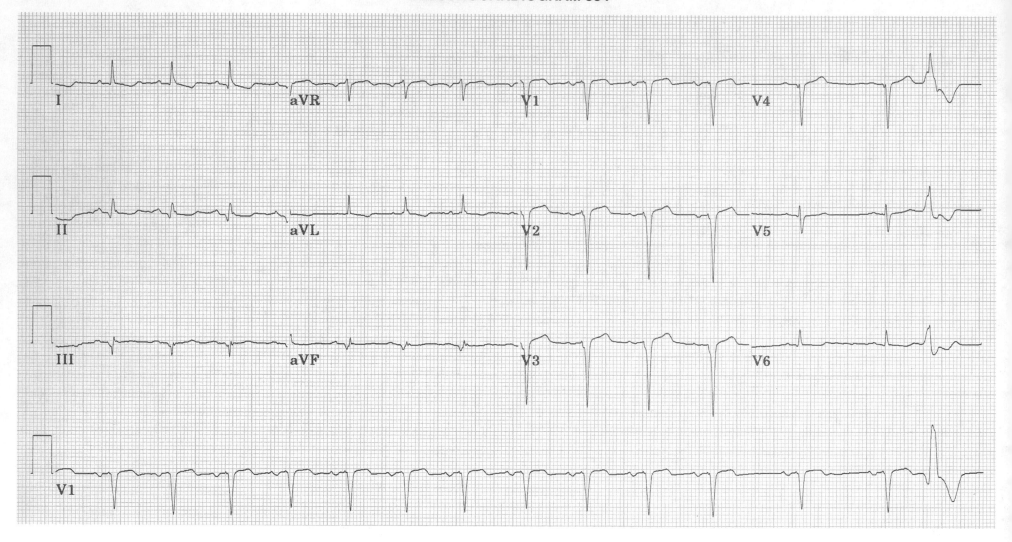

I aVR V1 V4

II aVL V2 V5

III aVF V3 V6

V1

Interpretation Notes: _____

_____

_____

ECG 334 Forty-four year old gentleman who presents with increasing symptoms of angina in the setting of a recent echocardiogram demonstrating moderate left ventricular systolic dysfunction. Co-morbid conditions include hyperlipidemia, hypertension, and long-standing tobacco use. His medications included furosemide, enalapril, topical nitroglycerin, digoxin, and aspirin. A subsequent cardiac catheterization demonstrated multi-vessel coronary artery disease and the patient was referred for successful coronary artery bypass graft surgery.

ELECTROCARDIOGRAM 335

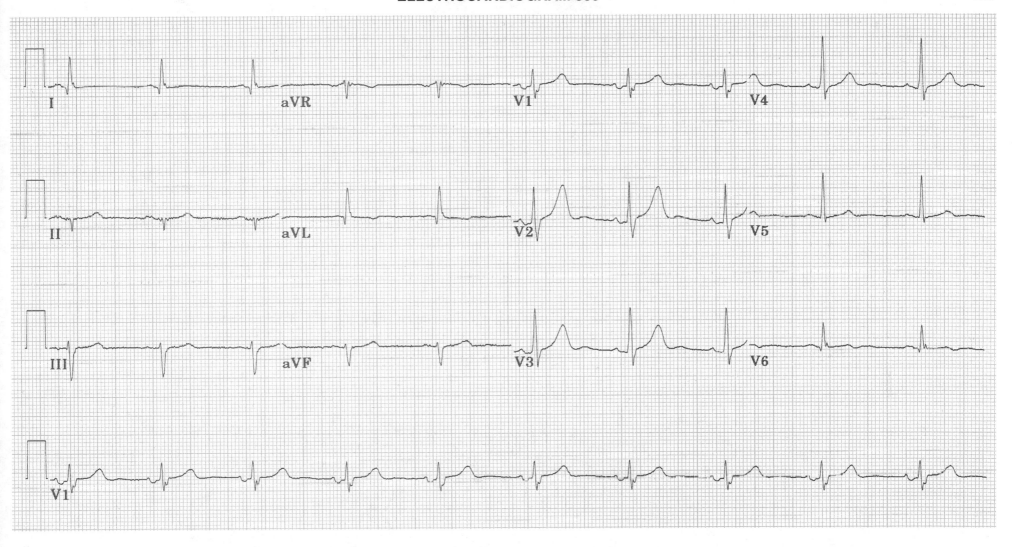

Interpretation Notes: _____

_____

ECG 335 Sixty-eight year old gentleman with recurrent angina pectoris in the setting of a remote myocardial infarction who underwent an urgent cardiac catheterization. The cardiac catheterization demonstrated severe inferior hypokinesis with an estimated ejection fraction of 40%, a subtotal occlusion of the left circumflex coronary artery, and a 90% proximal stenosis of the right coronary artery. The patient underwent successful stent placement to the right coronary artery.

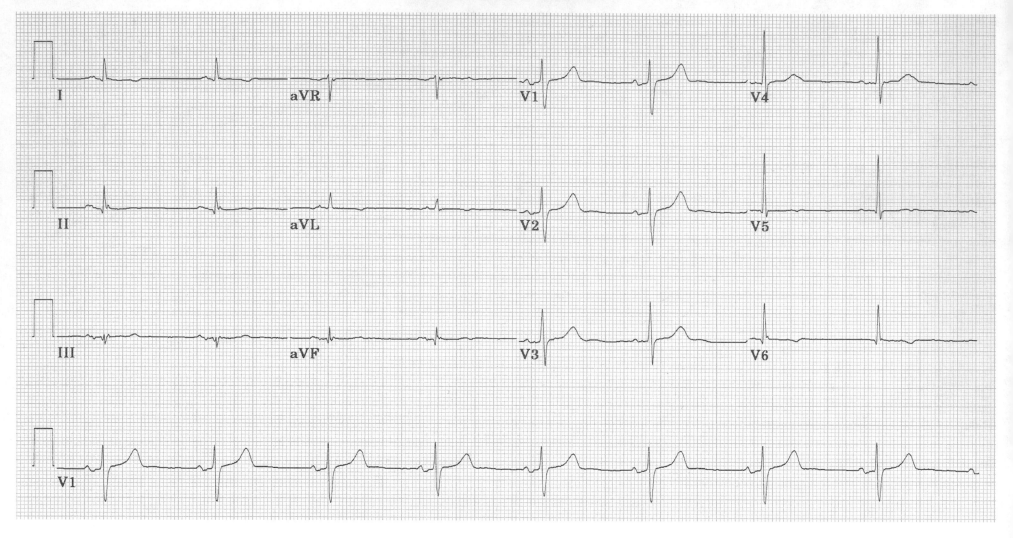

Interpretation Notes:_____

_____

_____

ECG 336 Seventy-two year old gentleman with a history of an age indeterminate inferior myocardial infarction who returns for cardiology follow-up and cardiac stress testing. Medications at the time of this electrocardiogram included lovastatin, diltiazem, and aspirin.

ELECTROCARDIOGRAM 337

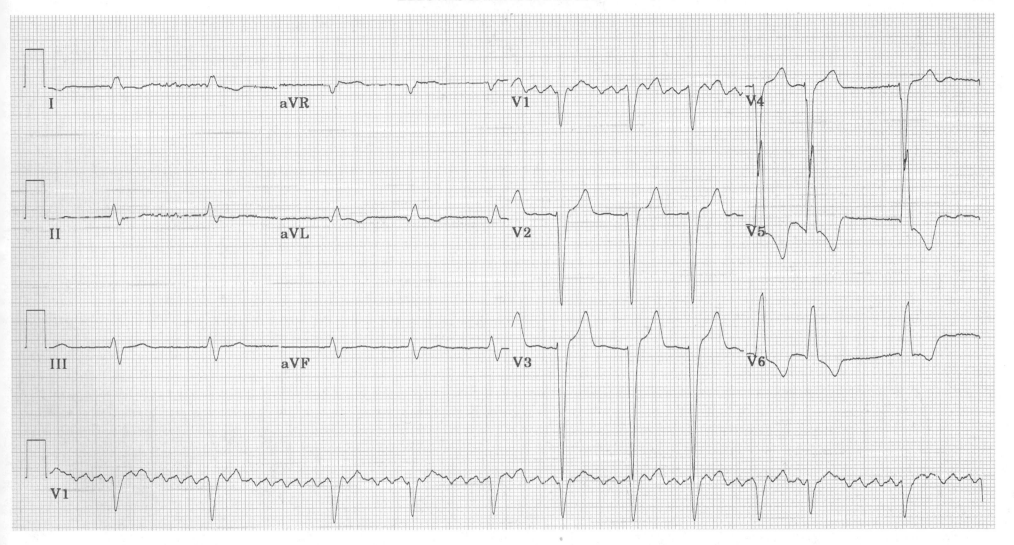

ECG 337 Eighty-two year old gentleman status post a bioprosthetic aortic and mitral valve replacement twelve years prior to this electrocardiogram who returns for out-patient cardiology follow-up. The patient has chronic atrial fibrillation, hypertension, and known mild coronary artery disease. His medications included warfarin, digoxin, and triamterene/hydrochlorothiazide.

Interpretation Notes: _____

_____

_____

ELECTROCARDIOGRAM 338

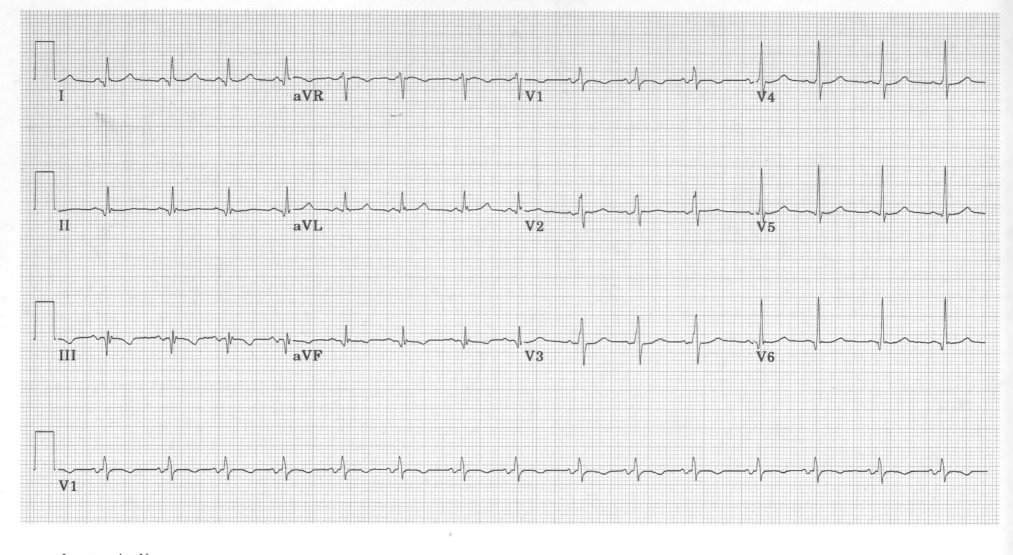

I   aVR   V1   V4

II   aVL   V2   V5

III   aVF   V3   V6

V1

Interpretation Notes: _____

_____

ECG 338 Eighty-seven year old gentleman with a history of gastritis and benign prostatic hypertrophy admitted to the hospital with acute onset abdominal pain. The patient subsequently underwent an exploratory laparotomy for a small bowel obstruction. His past medical history is notable for a myocardial infarction twenty-six years prior to this electrocardiogram.

ELECTROCARDIOGRAM 339

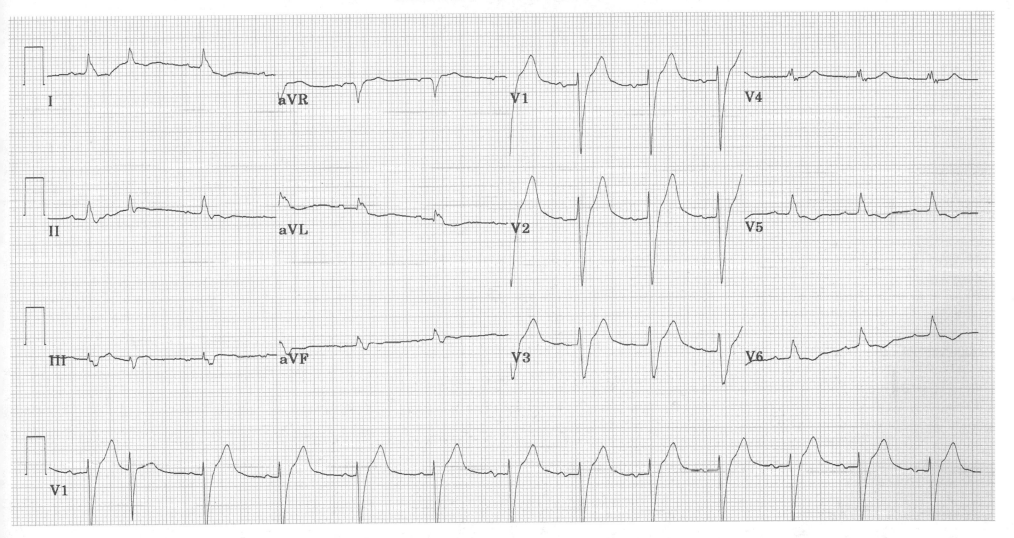

I aVR V1 V4

II aVL V2 V5

III aVF V3 V6

V1

Interpretation Notes: _____

_____

ECG 339 Sixty-six year old gentleman status post recent repeat coronary artery bypass graft surgery recovering in the hospital at the time of this electrocardiogram. Co-morbidities include a prior myocardial infarction, mitral insufficiency, and hypercholesterolemia.

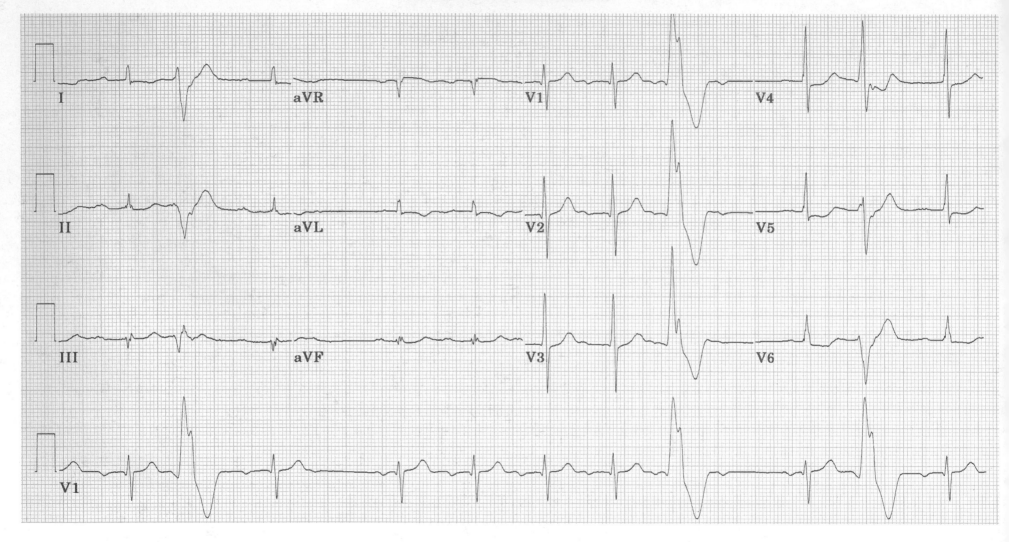

Interpretation Notes: _____

ECG 340 Seventy-one year old gentleman with ischemic heart disease status post coronary artery bypass graft surgery eight years prior to this electrocardiogram who returns for cardiology follow-up. Co-morbidities include bilateral carotid artery stenoses. His medications included amlodipine, simvastatin, lisinopril, triamterene/hydrochlorothiazide, and multi-vitamins.

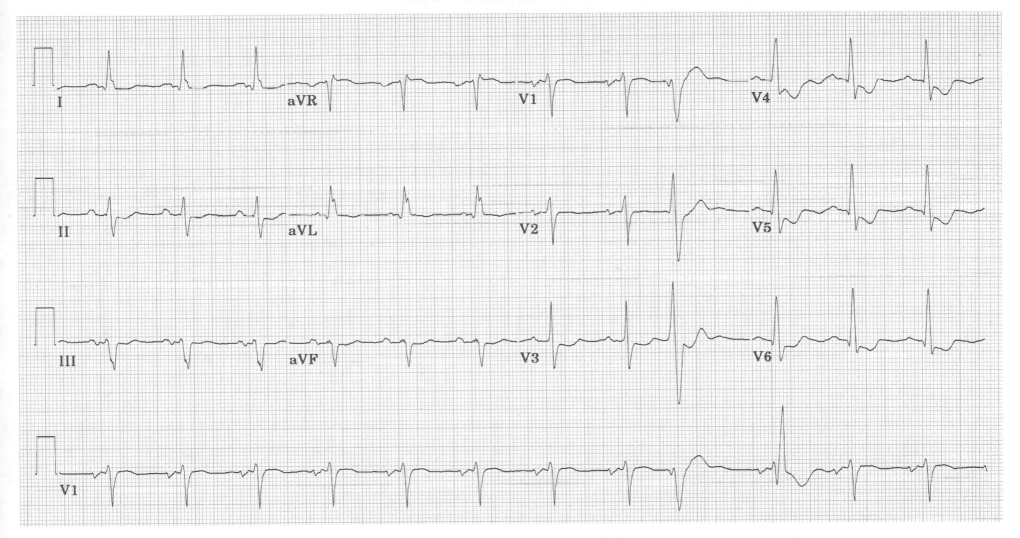

I aVR V1 V4
II aVL V2 V5
III aVF V3 V6
V1

Interpretation Notes:_____

ECG 341 Seventy-one year old gentleman with coronary artery disease and moderately severe left ventricular systolic dysfunction who is accepted in transfer from an out-side hospital after suffering a cardiac arrest. His medications at the time of this tracing included intravenous lidocaine, intravenous heparin, metolazone, gemfibrozil, hy-dralazine, metoprolol, insulin, and aspirin.

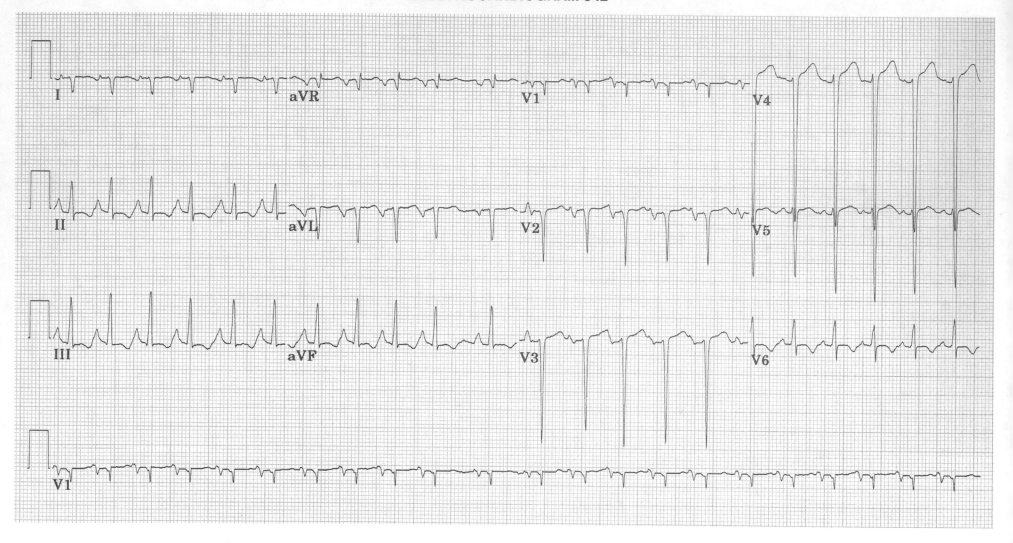

Interpretation Notes: _____

_____

ECG 342 Twenty-three year old gentleman with a non-ischemic idiopathic cardiomyopathy and recurrent atrial dysrhythmias referred for radiofrequency ablation. At electrophysiology study an ectopic atrial tachycardia was identified and successfully ablated. The ectopic atrial tachycardia originated from the right atrium. Medications at the time of this electrocardiogram included digoxin, aspirin, and captopril.

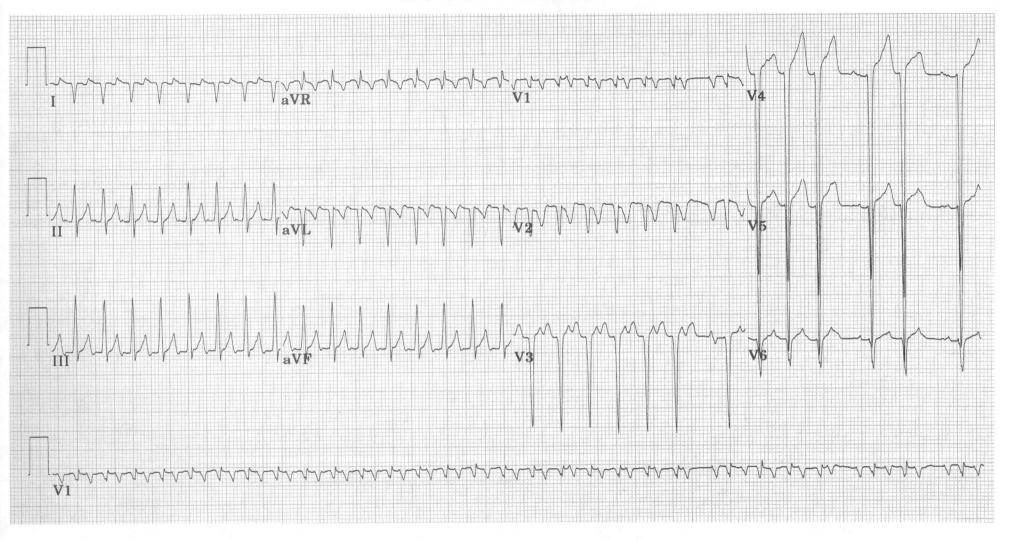

Interpretation Notes: _____

_____

ECG 343 Twenty-three year old gentleman with a non-ischemic idiopathic cardiomyopathy and recurrent atrial dysrhythmias referred for radiofrequency ablation. At electrophysiology study an ectopic atrial tachycardia was identified and successfully ablated. The ectopic atrial tachycardia originated from the right atrium. Medications at the time of this electrocardiogram included digoxin, aspirin, and captopril.

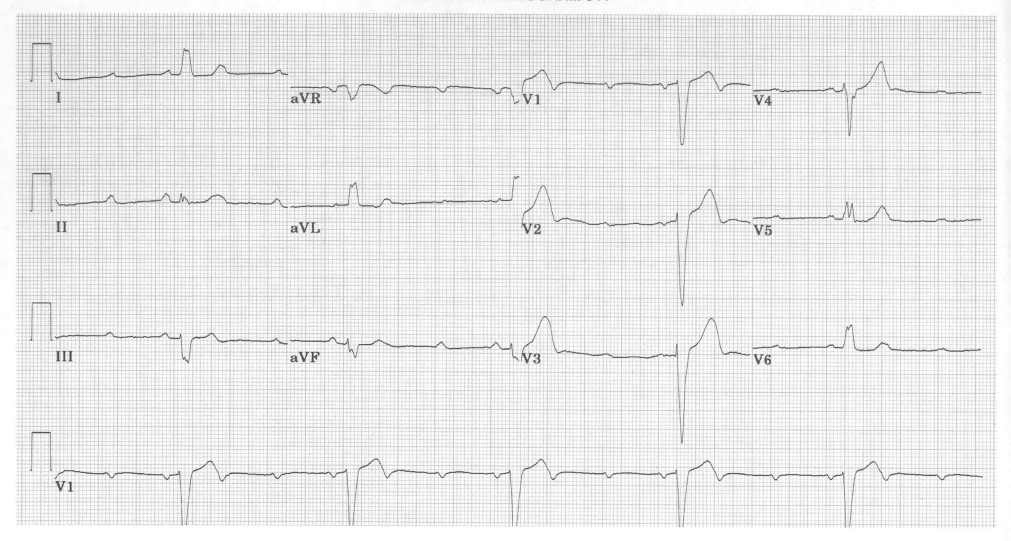

Interpretation Notes: _____

_____

ECG 344 Sixty-nine year old gentleman with coronary artery disease admitted for permanent pacemaker placement in the setting of recent syncope. His medications included topical nitroglycerin, thyroxine, and aspirin. A recent heart catheterization demonstrated mild left ventricular systolic dysfunction with severe inferolateral hypokinesis, an 80 percent left circumflex coronary artery stenosis, and a 60 percent mid-left anterior descending coronary artery stenosis.

ELECTROCARDIOGRAM 345

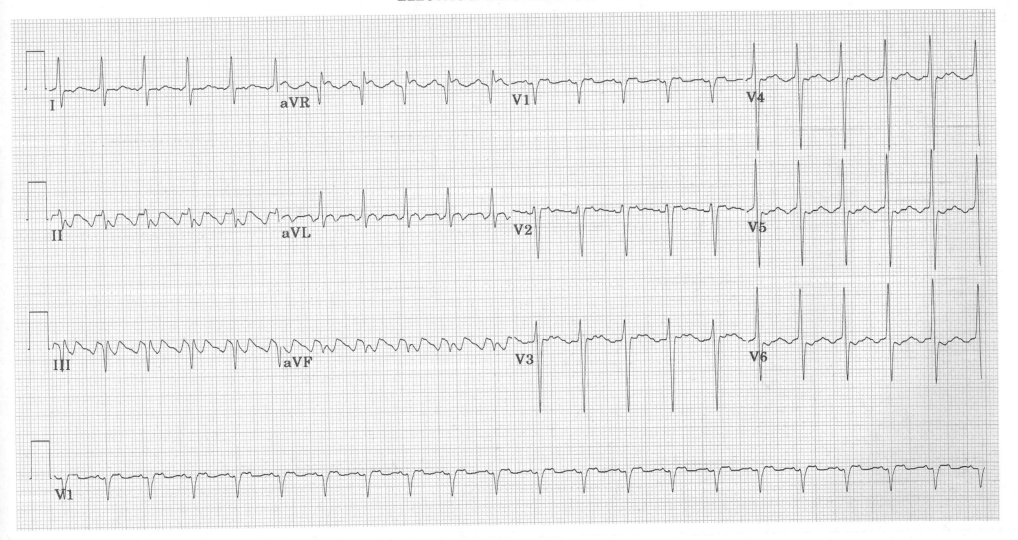

Interpretation Notes: _____

ECG 345 Sixty-one year old gentleman with coronary artery disease, a prior myocardial infarction, and resultant severe left ventricular systolic dysfunction who returns to the outpatient clinic for evaluation of drug refractory atrial dysrhythmias. Medications at the time of this electrocardiogram included quinidine, verapamil, and warfarin.

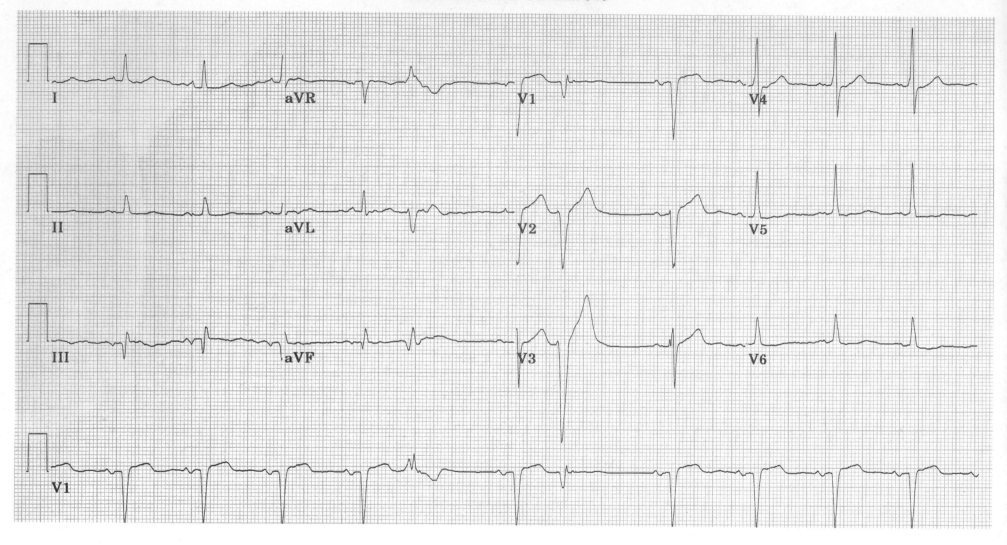

Interpretation Notes:_____

_____

_____

ECG 346 Seventy-nine year old gentleman with prostate cancer undergoing evaluation for radiation proctitis. The patient also has recent onset chest discomfort but no known coronary artery disease. A subsequent dobutamine stress echocardiogram demonstrated myocardial ischemia in the left anterior descending and left circumflex coronary artery territories and a prior myocardial infarction in the right coronary artery territory.

ELECTROCARDIOGRAM 347

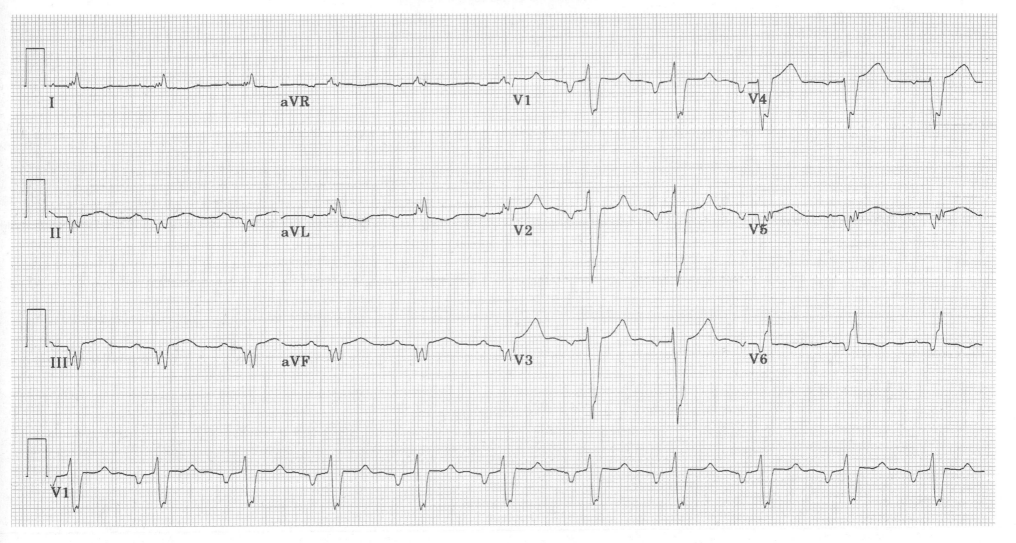

Interpretation Notes: _____

_____

_____

ECG 347 Fifty-five year old gentleman with coronary artery disease and a remote history of coronary artery bypass graft surgery who presented to a local emergency room with a wide complex tachycardia felt to represent ventricular tachycardia. The patient was accepted in hospital transfer and underwent an eventual electrophysiology study demonstrating inducible ventricular tachycardia. Successful implantable cardiac defibrillator placement was undertaken.

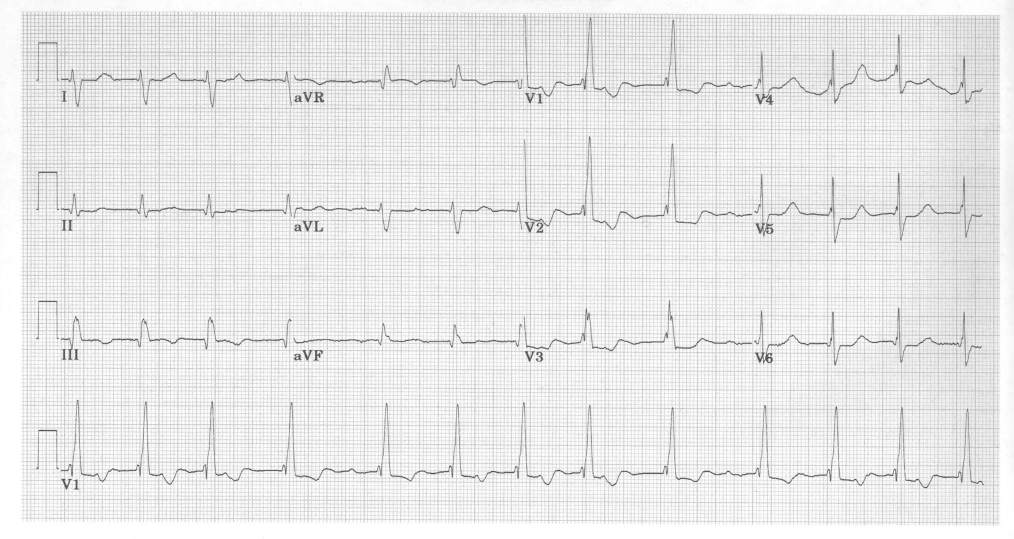

Interpretation Notes: _____

ECG 348 Sixty-six year old gentleman with coronary artery disease status post coronary artery bypass surgery four years prior to this electrocardiogram who presents with signs and symptoms of progressive congestive heart failure. Co-morbid conditions include diabetes mellitus, hypertension, and a prior cerebrovascular accident with residual left-sided hemiparesis.

ELECTROCARDIOGRAM 349

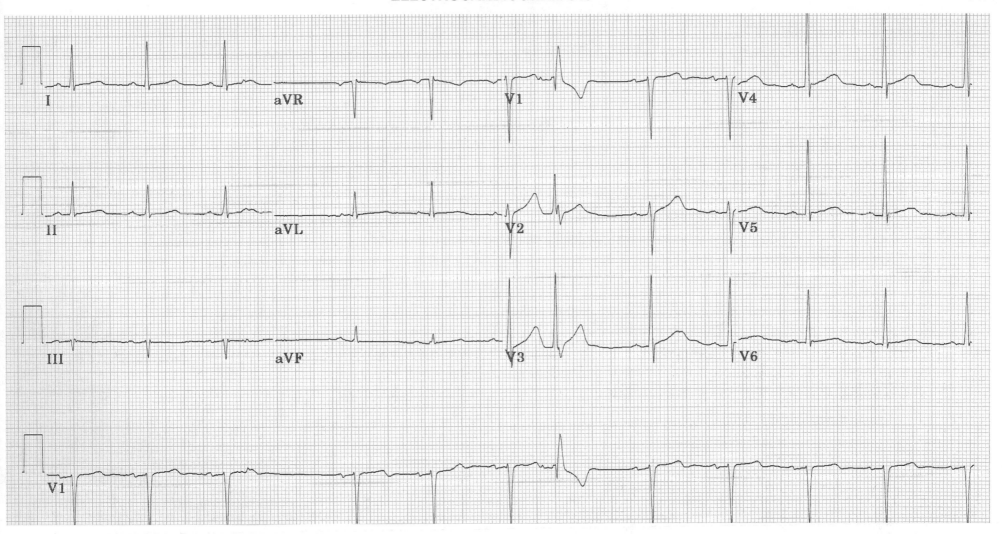

Interpretation Notes: _____

_____

_____

ECG 349 Previously healthy forty year old gentleman who presented to the hospital with acute onset left-sided hemiplegia and sensory loss. He was on no medications. He was diagnosed with an acute cerebrovascular accident.

ELECTROCARDIOGRAM 350

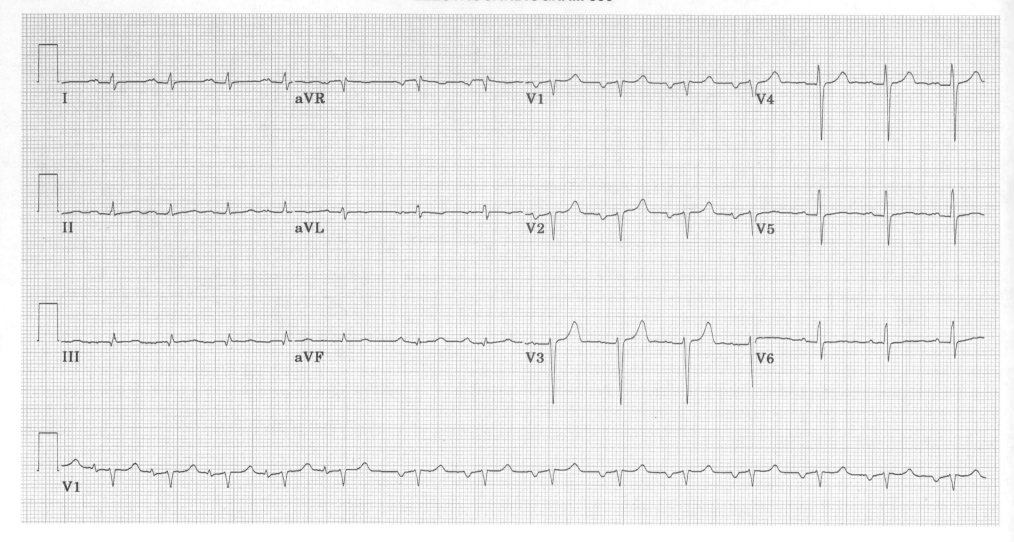

I   aVR   V1   V4

II   aVL   V2   V5

III   aVF   V3   V6

V1

Interpretation Notes: _____

_____

_____

ECG 350 Seventy-one year old gentleman with increasing dyspnea over the past three weeks admitted to the hospital with a congestive heart failure exacerbation. His medications included allopurinol, furosemide, and amlodipine. His past medical history includes hypertension. A recent echocardiogram demonstrated moderately severe left ventricular hypertrophy and moderately severe left atrial abnormality. He had normal left ventricular systolic function without evidence of a prior myocardial infarction.

ELECTROCARDIOGRAM 351

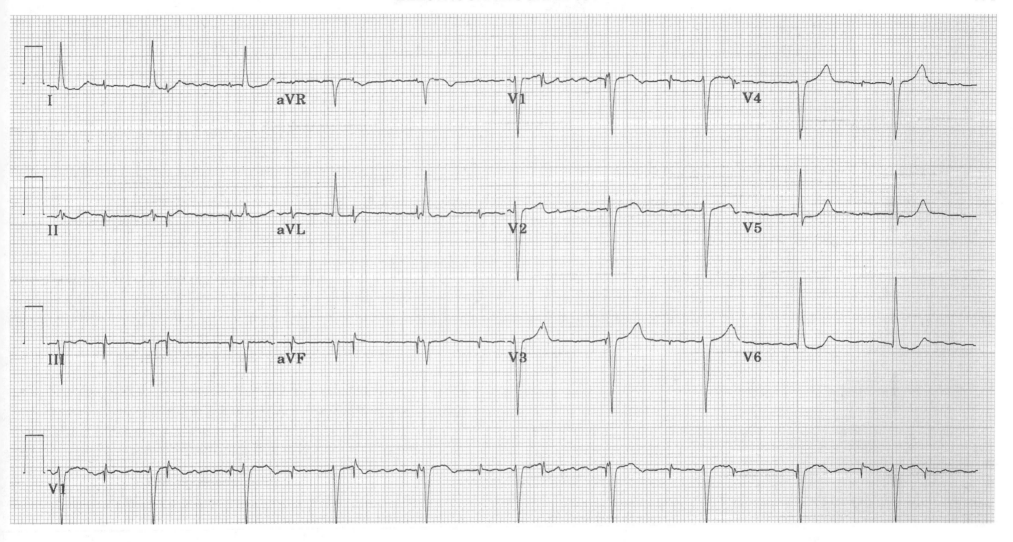

Interpretation Notes: _____

_____

ECG 351 Seventy-two year old woman with advanced atrioventricular block necessitating prior permanent pacemaker placement who returns for pacemaker follow-up. Co-morbid conditions include coronary artery disease, hypertension, and hyperlipidemia. Medications at the time of this electrocardiogram included metoprolol, aspirin, digoxin, and simvastatin.

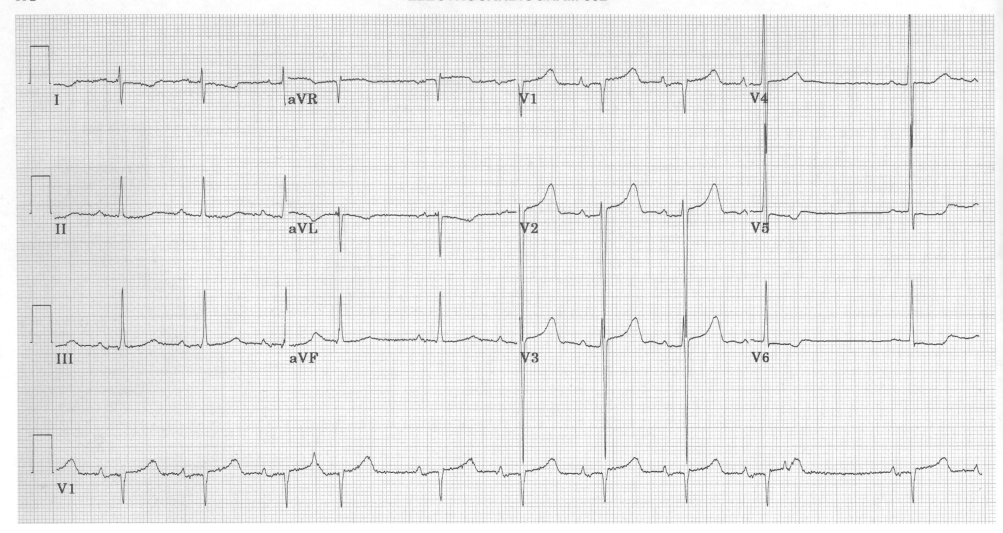

Interpretation Notes: _____

_____

ECG 352 Eighty-two year old gentleman who was found at home disoriented and confused. An inpatient evaluation including a CT scan of the head demonstrated an acute cerebrovascular accident. Co-morbidities include long-standing hypertension with a recent echocardiogram demonstrating moderately severe left ventricular hypertrophy and moderate left ventricular systolic dysfunction. The patient was on no medications at the time of this electrocardiogram.

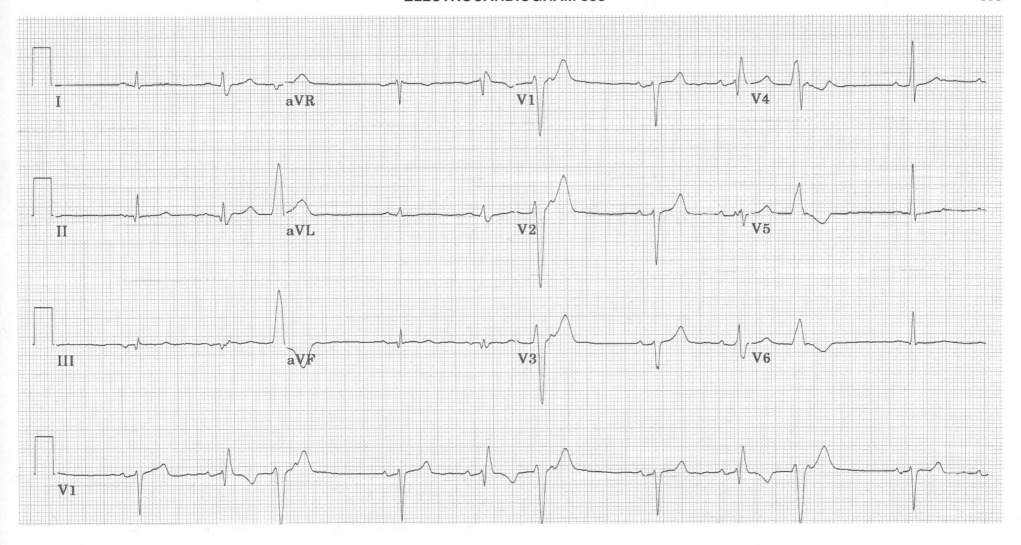

Interpretation Notes: _____

_____

_____

ECG 353 Sixty-five year old gentleman with coronary artery disease status post both inferior and anterior myocardial infarctions approximately two years prior to this electrocardiogram who returns for follow-up examination. Co-morbidities include recurrent monomorphic ventricular tachycardia and hypertension. Medications at the time of this electrocardiogram included mexiletine, atenolol, enalapril, and aspirin.

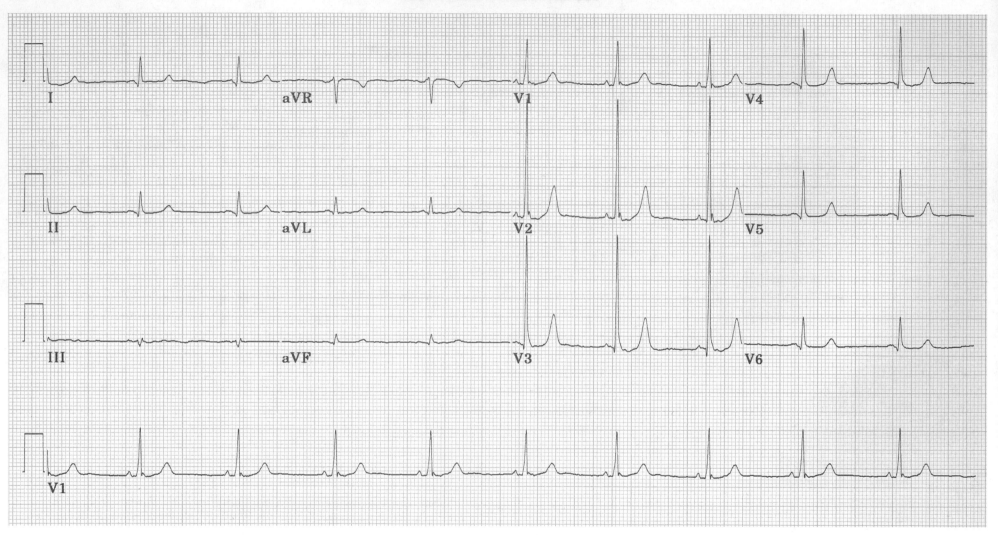

Interpretation Notes: _____

ECG 354 Fifty-five year old gentleman hospitalized with acute onset lower gastrointestinal bleeding. His hospitalization was complicated by a lower extremity deep venous thrombosis. He has no known cardiac diagnoses and remained asymptomatic from a cardiac standpoint. His medications included famotidine, allopurinol, and warfarin.

ELECTROCARDIOGRAM 355

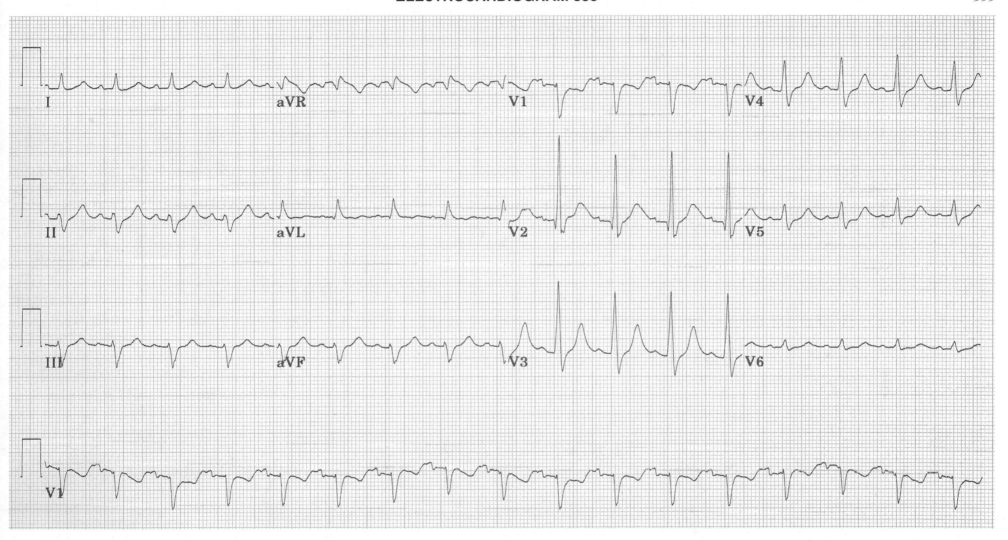

Interpretation Notes: _____

_____

ECG 355 Forty-nine year old gentleman with alcoholic cirrhosis and advanced liver dysfunction admitted to the hospital for evaluation and treatment of suspected spontaneous bacterial peritonitis. His past medical history includes non-insulin requiring diabetes mellitus and hepatitis C. A serum potassium was not available at the time of this electrocardiogram.

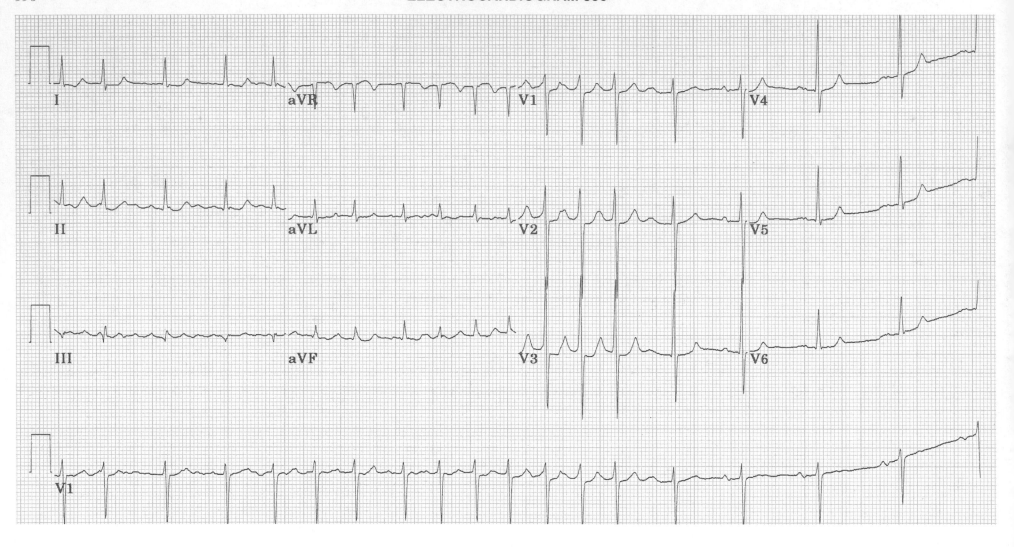

Interpretation Notes: _____

ECG 356 Sixty-nine year old woman with coronary artery disease status post percutaneous transluminal coronary angioplasty of her right coronary artery three years prior to this electrocardiogram who presents in follow-up to the outpatient cardiology clinic. Co-morbidities include diffuse peripheral vascular disease, hypertension, and hypercholesterolemia. Medications at the time of this electrocardiogram included aspirin, lisinopril, thyroxine, diltiazem, and atenolol.

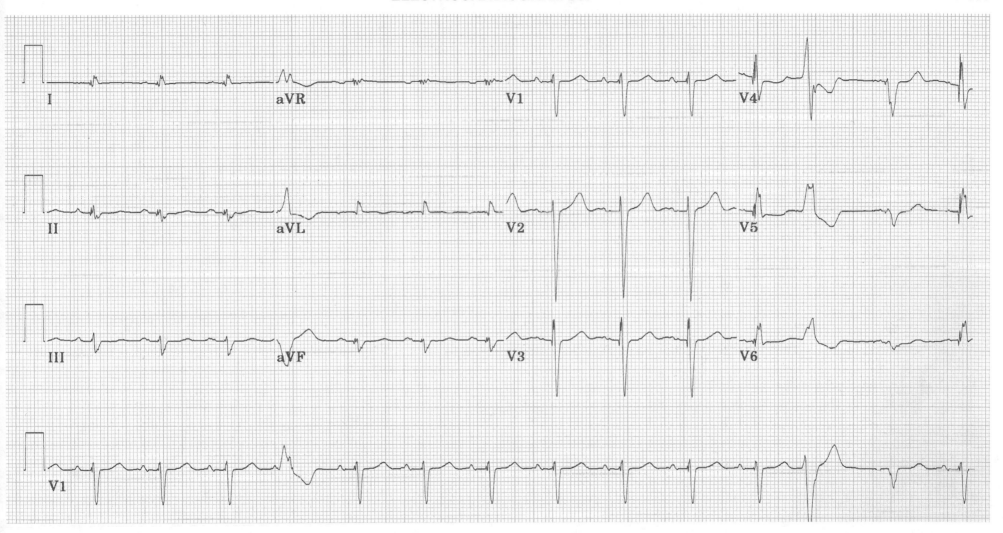

Interpretation Notes: _____

_____

_____

ECG 357 Seventy-two year old gentleman with a remote history of coronary artery bypass graft surgery, insulin requiring diabetes mellitus, and chronic obstructive pulmonary disease who is admitted to the hospital for further evaluation of fever and shortness of breath. He has a suspected pneumonia. He is status post permanent pacemaker placement two years prior to this electrocardiogram. Medications at the time of this electrocardiogram included furosemide, isosorbide dinitrate, insulin, ranitidine, and intravenous antibiotics.

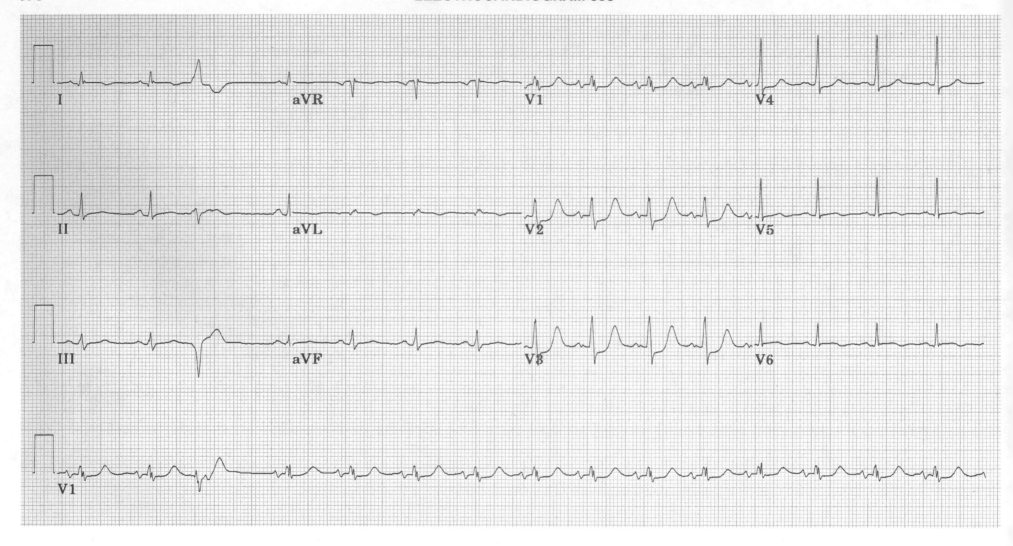

Interpretation Notes: _____

_____

ECG 358 Sixty-seven year old woman accepted in hospital transfer after the sudden onset of acute chest discomfort and the accompanying electrocardiogram. A cardiac catheterization performed five days following this electrocardiogram demonstrated a severe proximal left circumflex coronary artery stenosis with an ulcerated plaque. This was successfully dilated by percutaneous transluminal coronary angioplasty.

ELECTROCARDIOGRAM 359

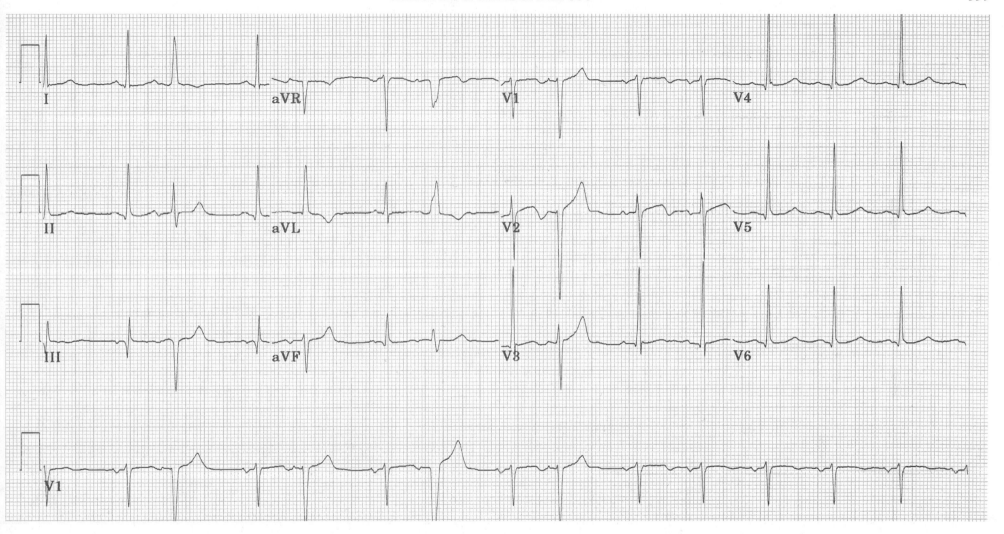

Interpretation Notes:_____
_____
_____

ECG 359 Sixty-six year old gentleman with acute myelogenous leukemia admitted to the hospital for induction chemotherapy. Co-morbidities include hypertension and glaucoma.

ELECTROCARDIOGRAM 360

360

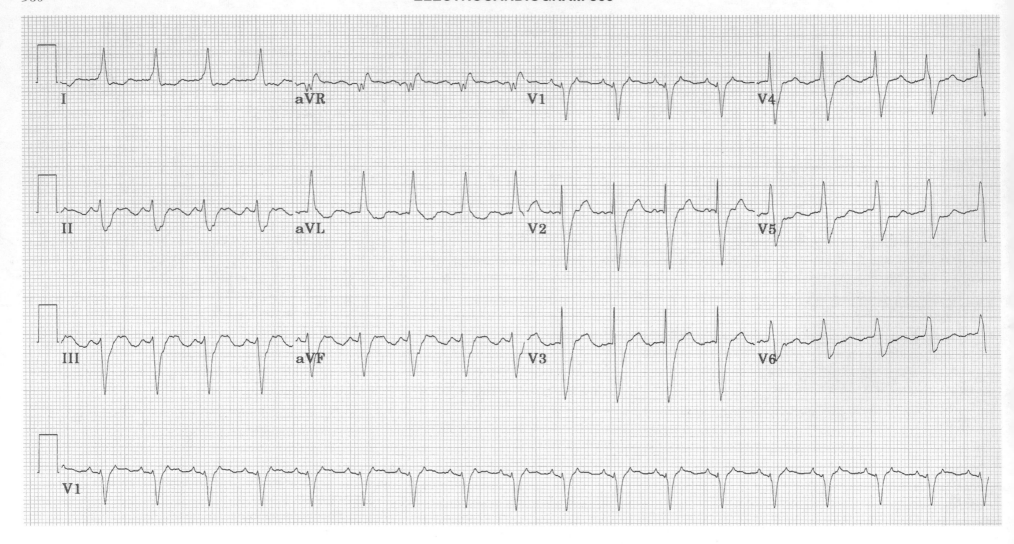

Interpretation Notes:_____

_____

ECG 360 Eighty-two year old gentleman with diabetes mellitus, chronic renal insufficiency, and recurrent paroxysmal atrial arrhythmias who is admitted via the emergency room with a serum potassium level of 6.8 meq/L.

ELECTROCARDIOGRAM 361

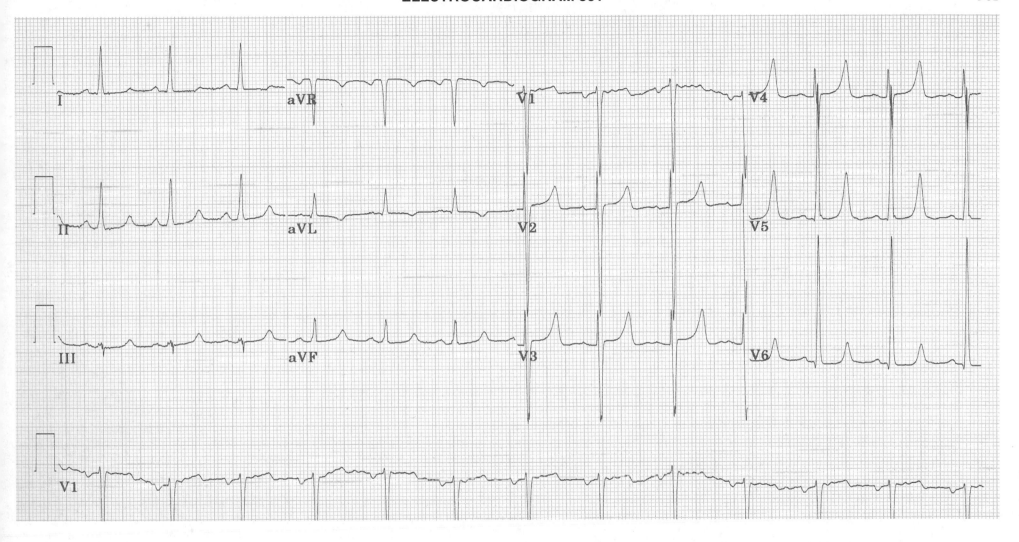

Interpretation Notes: _____

_____

_____

ECG 361 Forty-seven year old woman with dialysis requiring renal failure secondary to long-standing hypertension who at the time of this electrocardiogram presented to the hospital with recent onset shortness of breath. Her serum calcium level was 7.4 mg/dl and her serum potassium level was 6.4 meq/L.

ELECTROCARDIOGRAM 362

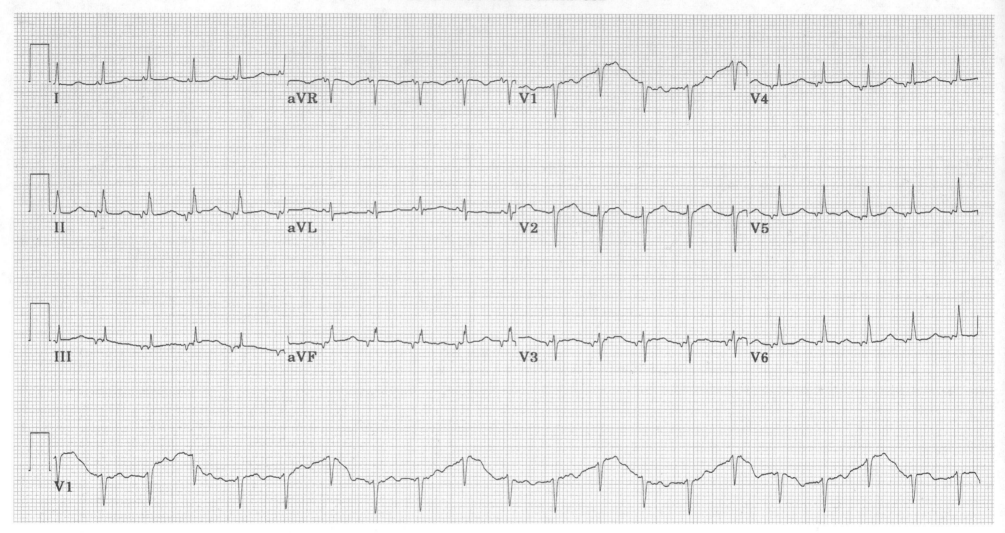

Interpretation Notes: _____

ECG 362 Seventy-four year old woman with a history of colon cancer status post partial colectomy who presents to the hospital with a three day history of progressive shortness of breath and chest discomfort. Her medications included insulin, lisinopril, and aspirin.

ELECTROCARDIOGRAM 363

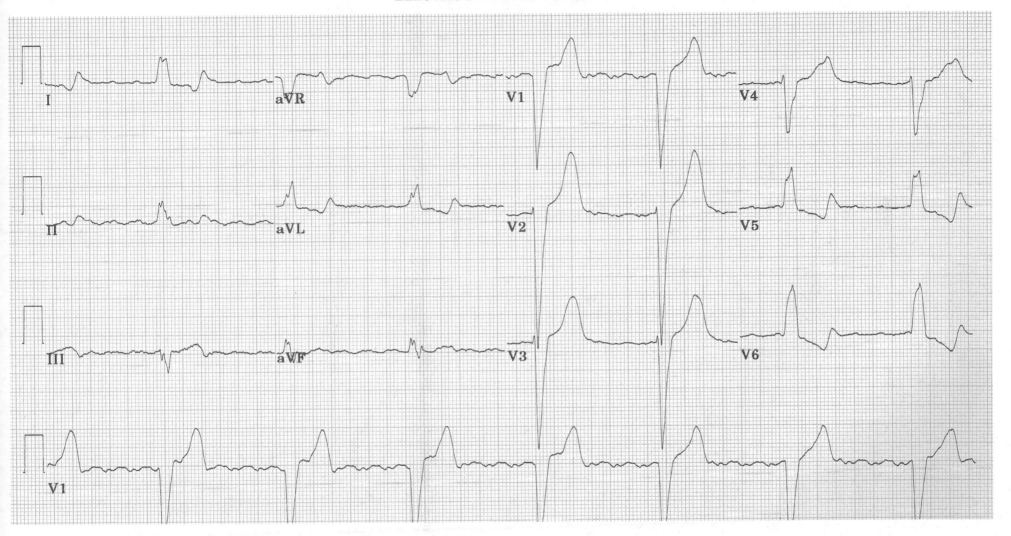

I   aVR   V1   V4

II   aVL   V2   V5

III   aVF   V3   V6

V1

Interpretation Notes: _____

_____

ECG 363 Sixty-six year old gentleman with a long-standing history of atrial dysrhythmias and recent endocarditis who is status post aortic valve replacement. He returns for outpatient cardiology follow-up. He subsequently re-developed bacterial endocarditis and complete heart block ensued necessitating permanent pacemaker placement. He has no known coronary artery obstructive disease.

ELECTROCARDIOGRAM 364

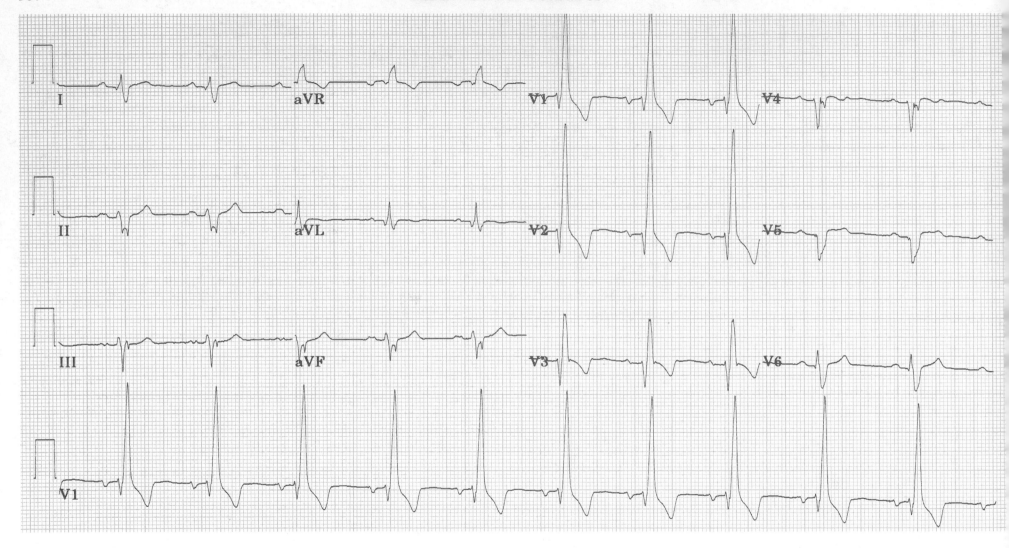

I   aVR   V1   V4

II   aVL   V2   V5

III   aVF   V3   V6

V1

Interpretation Notes: _____

ECG 364 Fifty-seven year old gentleman with insulin requiring diabetes mellitus and coronary artery disease who is status post coronary artery bypass graft surgery four years prior to this electrocardiogram. He now returns for cardiology follow-up. He has severe left ventricular systolic dysfunction and is currently on the cardiac transplantation waiting list. His medications included isosorbide dinitrate, digoxin, captopril, furosemide, insulin, and potassium.

ELECTROCARDIOGRAM 365

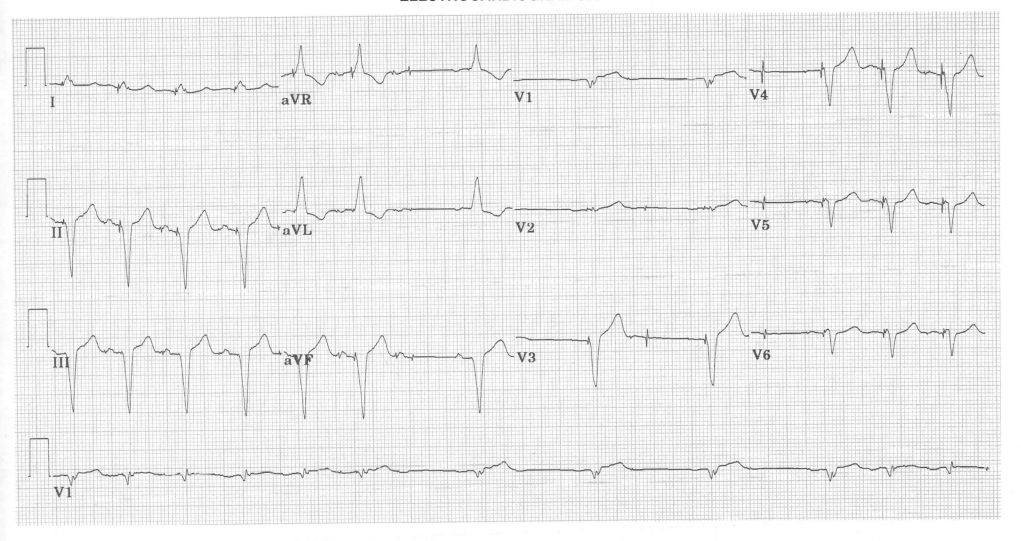

Interpretation Notes: _____

ECG 365 Seventy-seven year old woman with a history of paroxysmal atrial fibrillation who returns for routine cardiac assessment and pacemaker interrogation. Her medications included amiodarone, digoxin, and furosemide.

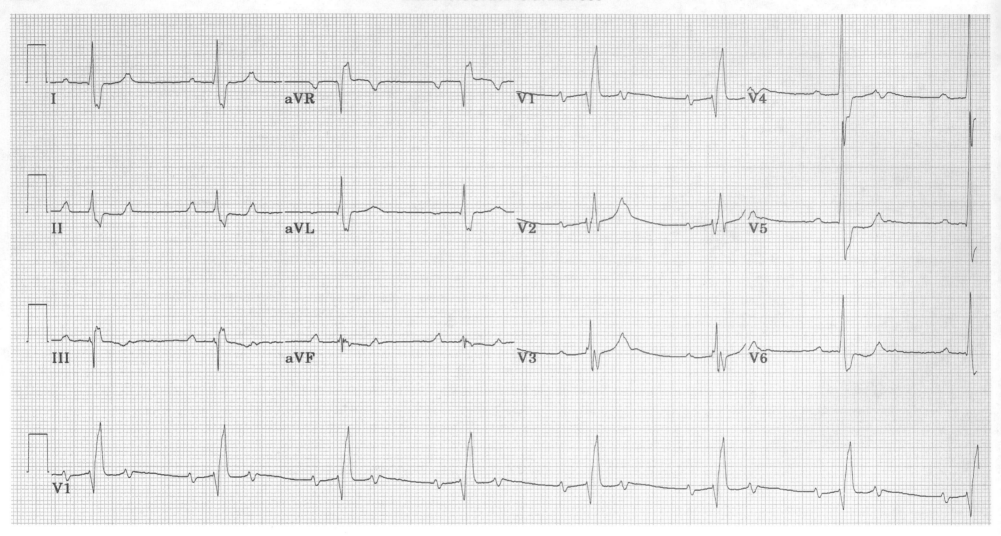

Interpretation Notes: _____

_____

_____

ECG 366 Thirty-four year old gentleman with a prior history of congestive heart failure referred for a cardiac catheterization. His medications included furosemide and captopril. A subsequent cardiac catheterization demonstrated a dilated non-ischemic cardiomyopathy.

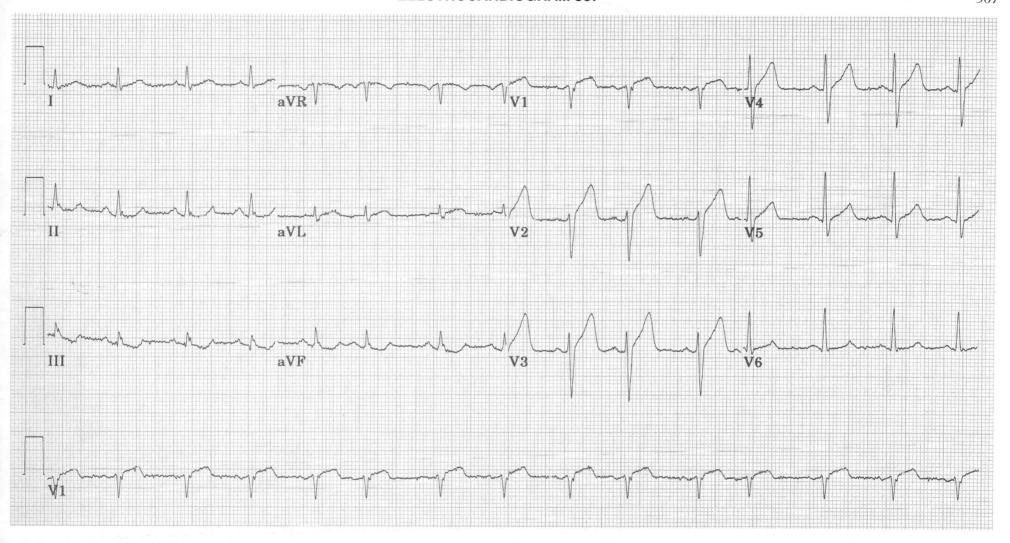

Interpretation Notes: _____

ECG 367 Sixty-seven year old gentleman with progressive angina pectoris who underwent elective percutaneous transluminal coronary angioplasty and rotoblator of a proximal left anterior descending coronary artery obstruction. The procedure was complicated by coronary artery dissection and acute closure. This electrocardiogram was obtained during the peri-procedure complication. Two stents were urgently placed with a satisfactory result with no detectable myocardial injury by serial cardiac enzyme analysis.

ELECTROCARDIOGRAM 368

368

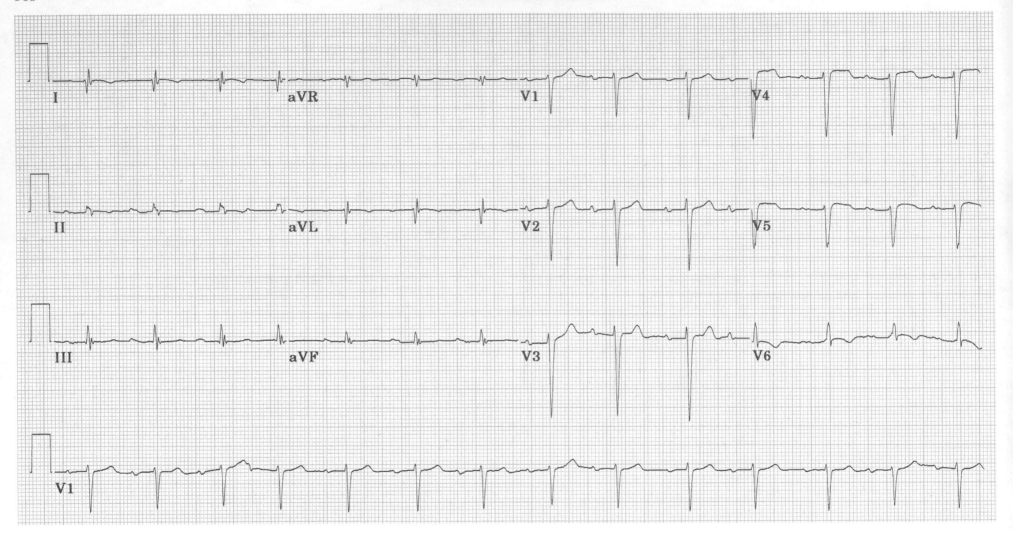

Interpretation Notes: _____

ECG 368 Seventy-four year old woman with coronary artery disease, a prior anterior myocardial infarction, and percutaneous transluminal coronary angioplasty to the left anterior descending coronary artery who presents to the hospital with an altered mental status. Co-morbidities include hypertension, a remote cerebrovascular accident, and diabetes mellitus. Medications at the time of this electrocardiogram included furosemide, insulin, captopril, and digoxin.

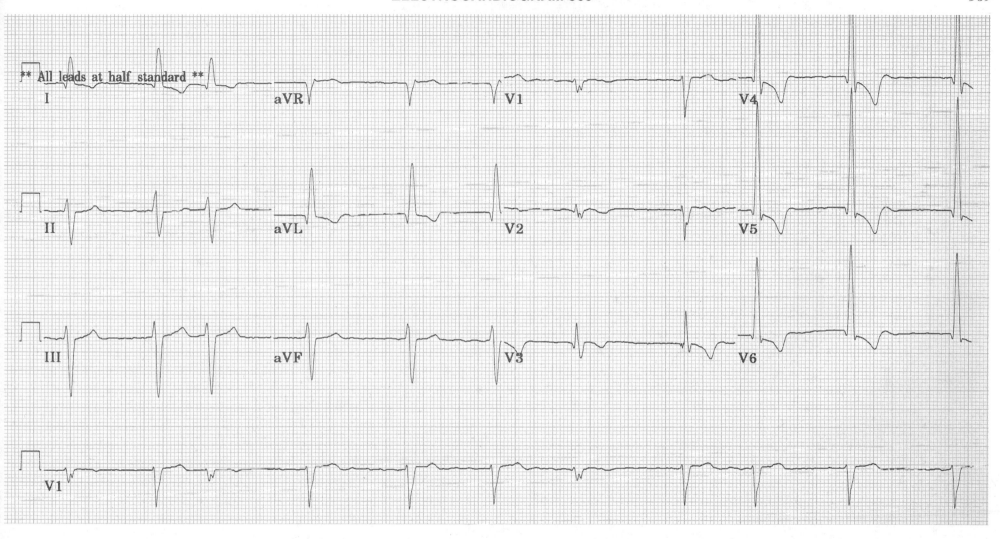

** All leads at half standard **

I   aVR   V1   V4

II   aVL   V2   V5

III   aVF   V3   V6

V1

Interpretation Notes:_____

_____

ECG 369 Eighty-five year old gentleman status post bioprosthetic aortic valve replacement who re-presents with peri-prosthetic moderately severe aortic insufficiency.

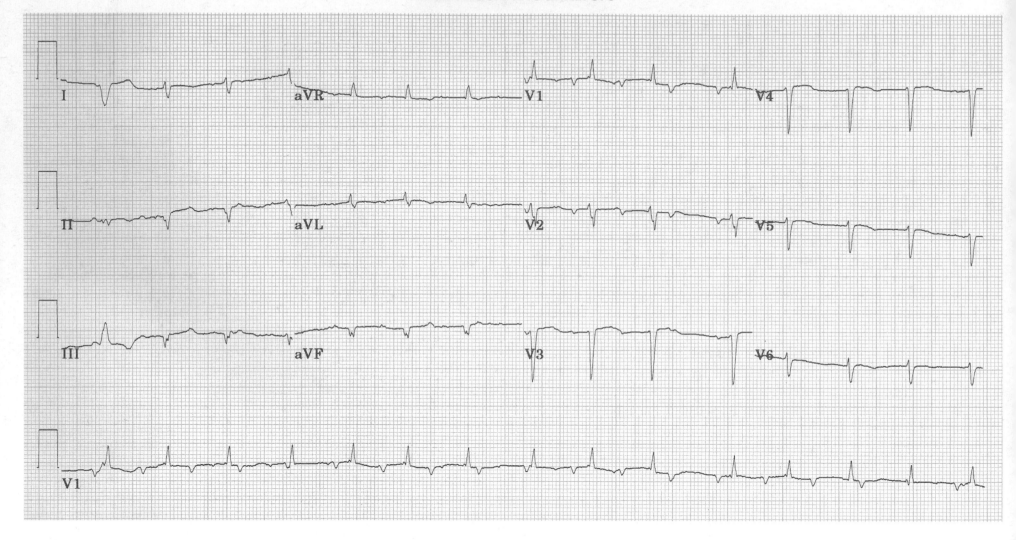

Interpretation Notes: _____

_____

_____

ECG 370 Sixty-one year old gentleman status post cardiac transplantation who has developed severe ischemic post transplantation vasculopathy. He is known to have suffered both inferior and anterior myocardial infarctions since his transplantation. His medications at the time of this electrocardiogram included cyclosporine, prednisone, azathioprine, nifedipine, and famotidine.

ELECTROCARDIOGRAM 371

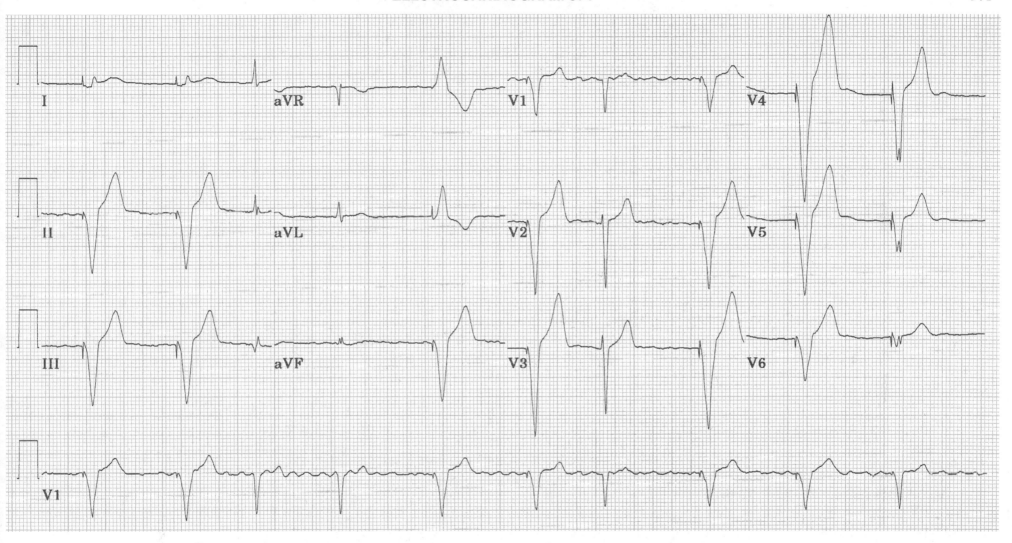

Interpretation Notes: _____

_____

ECG 371 Seventy year old gentleman with a history of hypertension, chronic atrial fibrillation, and syncope who re-presents to the hospital after three recent syncopal episodes. The patient recently underwent ventricular pacemaker implantation and this electrocardiogram represents a post-implantation tracing. He has no known history of coronary artery disease or a prior myocardial infarction.

372

ELECTROCARDIOGRAM 372

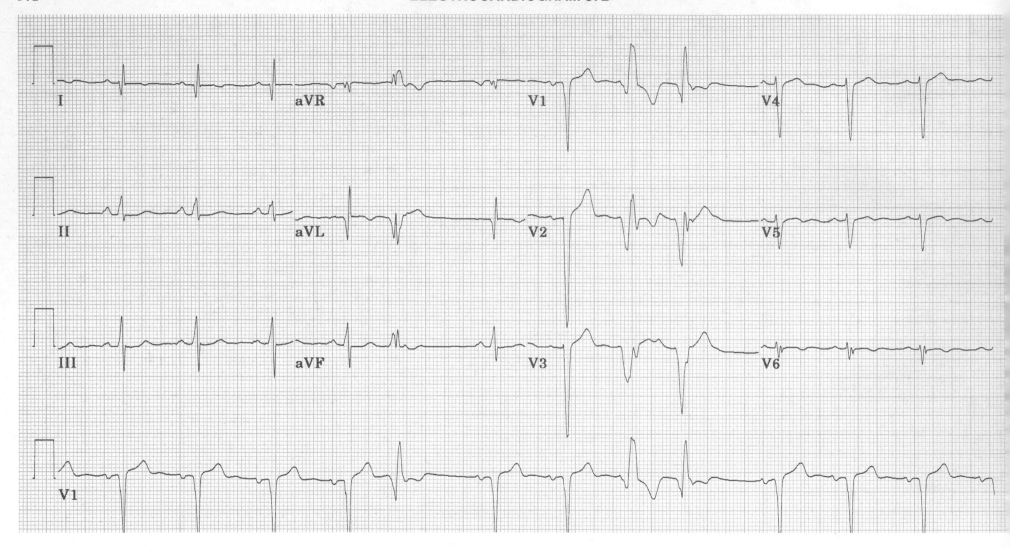

Interpretation Notes: _____

ECG 372 Forty-seven year old gentleman with coronary artery disease who is status post an antero-apical myocardial infarction and resultant aneurysm formation. He has severe left ventricular systolic dysfunction and now returns to the hospital for evaluation of recurrent angina pectoris. This electrocardiogram was obtained prior to a repeat cardiac catheterization. Medications at the time of this electrocardiogram included warfarin, topical nitroglycerin, enalapril, and lovastatin.

ELECTROCARDIOGRAM 373

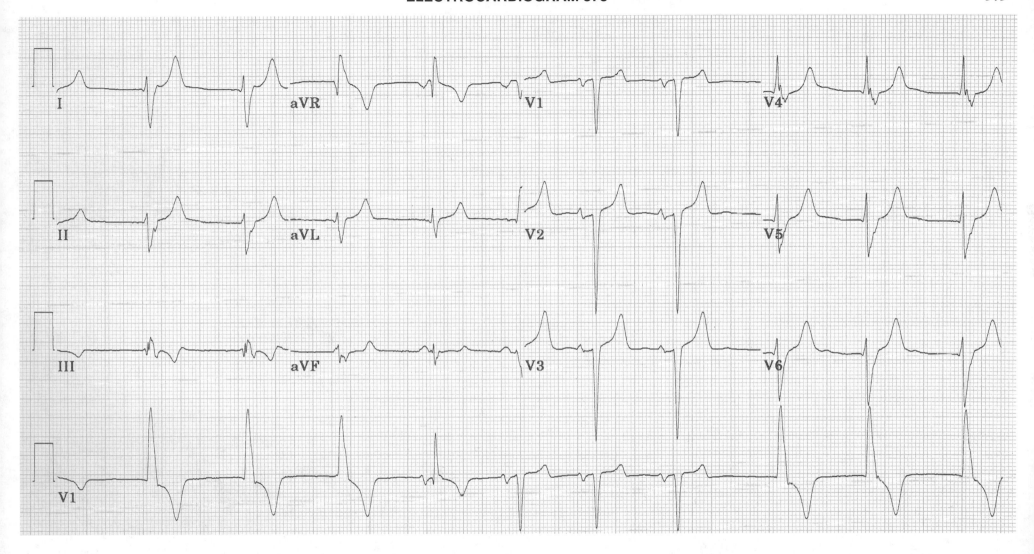

Interpretation Notes: _____

ECG 373 Forty-six year old woman with severe hypertension status post cadaveric renal transplantation one year prior to this electrocardiogram referred to the cardiology clinic for evaluation of recent onset palpitations and a suspected slow heart rate. A cardiac catheterization several months prior to this electrocardiogram demonstrated near normal coronary arteries with advanced left ventricular hypertrophy. The patient was on numerous medications at the time of this electrocardiogram including diltiazem, clonidine, doxazosin, and immunosuppressive agents for her renal transplant. Her serum potassium was normal.

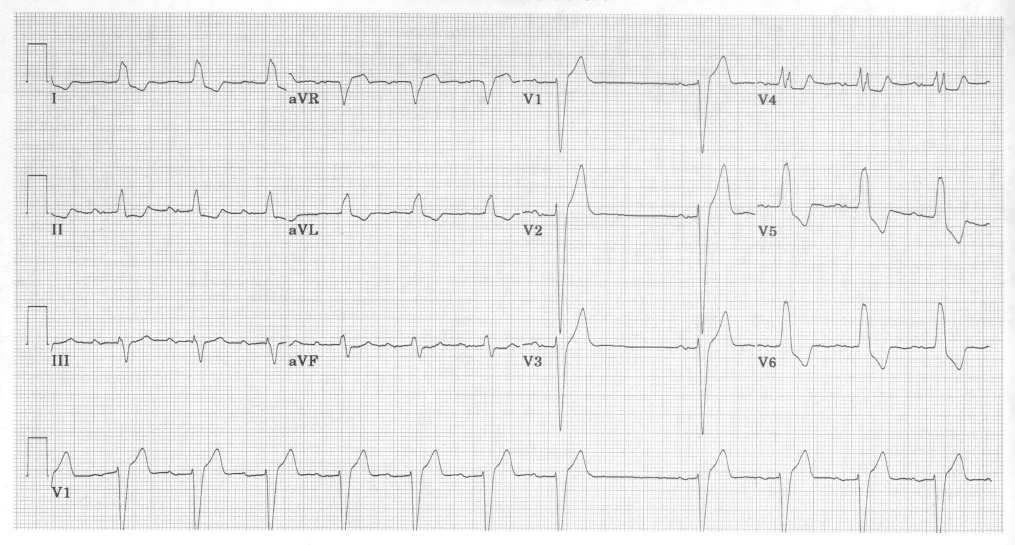

Interpretation Notes: _____

_____

ECG 374 Eighty-four year old gentleman who is being seen preoperatively prior to a colon mass resection. He has coronary artery disease status post prior angioplasties to both the left anterior descending and left circumflex coronary arteries. He also has a history of paroxysmal supraventricular tachycardia. His medications included diltiazem, potassium, and aspirin.

ELECTROCARDIOGRAM 375

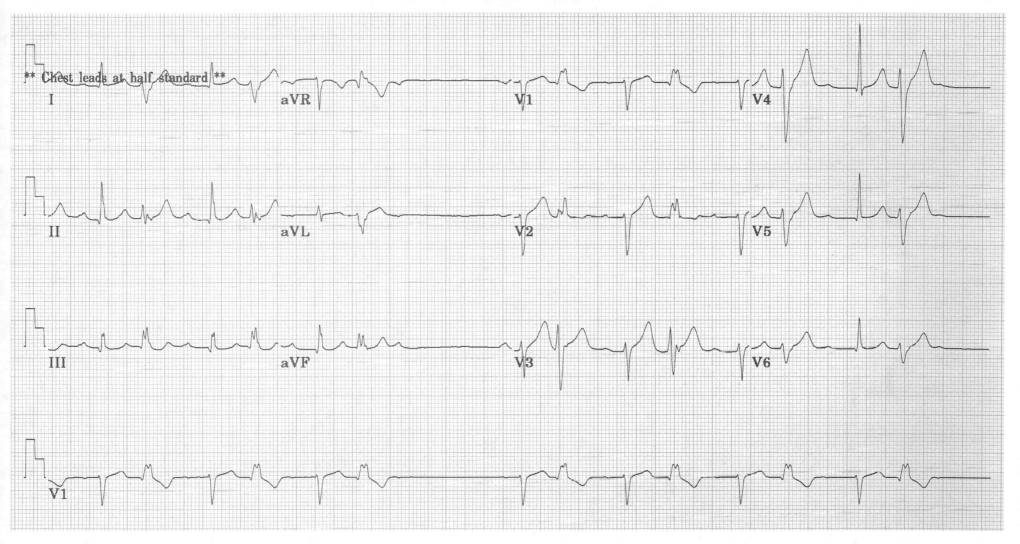

** Chest leads at half standard **

I aVR V1 V4

II aVL V2 V5

III aVF V3 V6

V1

Interpretation Notes: _____

_____

ECG 375 Sixty-seven year old gentleman with a history of coronary artery disease who presents to the hospital with recent onset palpitations and retrosternal chest discomfort. His medications included atenolol and aspirin.

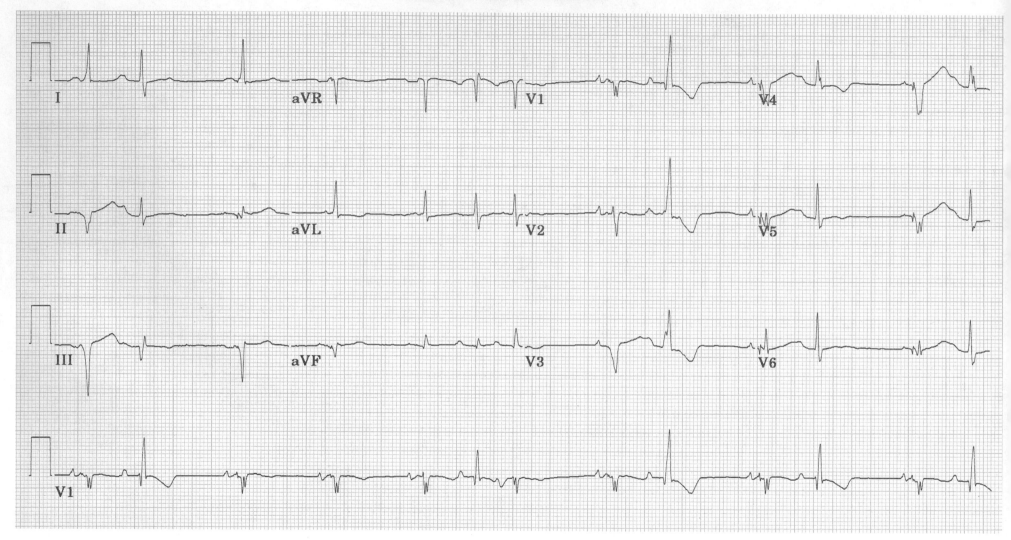

I   aVR   V1   V4

II   aVL   V2   V5

III   aVF   V3   V6

V1

Interpretation Notes: _____

_____

_____

ECG 376 Seventy year old gentleman referred for coronary artery bypass graft surgery in the setting of advanced coronary artery obstructive disease and recent symptoms of congestive heart failure. His past medical history includes diabetes mellitus and permanent pacemaker placement. Medications at the time of this electrocardiogram included aspirin, digoxin, glyburide, furosemide, and ticlodipine.

ELECTROCARDIOGRAM 377

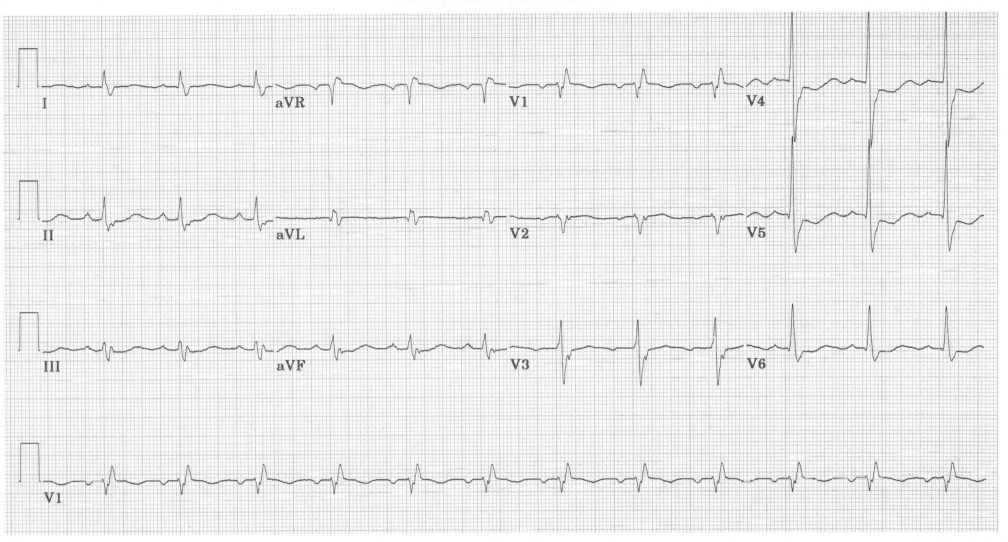

Interpretation Notes: _____

_____

ECG 377 Seventy-one year old man admitted to the hospital with a history of acute onset chest discomfort three hours prior to his presentation. Cardiac risk factors include ongoing tobacco use and hypertension. His medications included hydrochlorothiazide and verapamil. A subsequent cardiac catheterization demonstrated moderate left ventricular systolic dysfunction and severe three vessel coronary artery disease. His serum potassium level was 3.2 meq/l.

ELECTROCARDIOGRAM 378

378

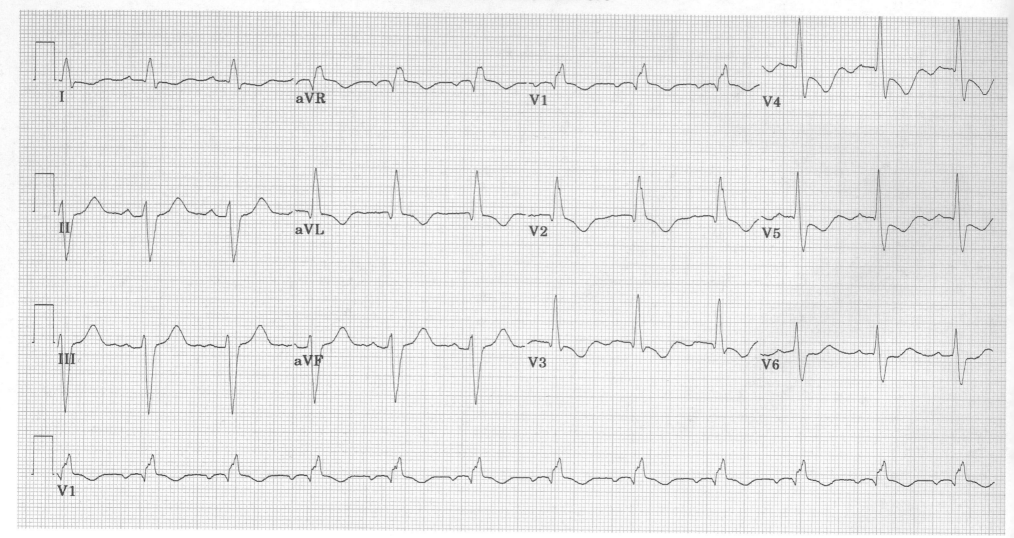

Interpretation Notes: _____

ECG 378 Seventy-one year old man admitted to the hospital with a history of acute onset chest discomfort three hours prior to his presentation. Cardiac risk factors include tobacco use and hypertension. His medications included hydrochlorothiazide and verapamil. A subsequent cardiac catheterization demonstrated moderate left ventricular systolic dysfunction and severe three vessel coronary artery disease.

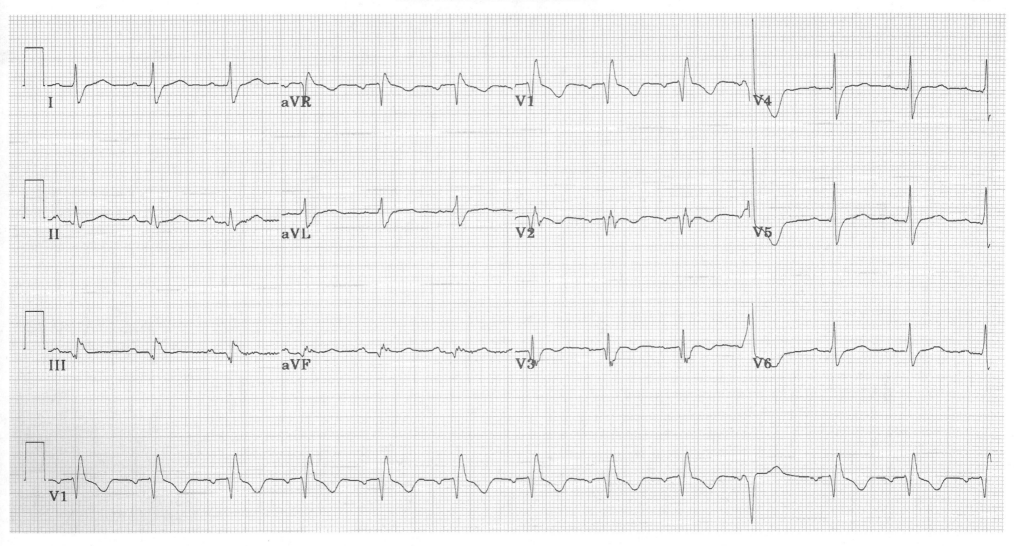

Interpretation Notes: _____

_____

ECG 379 Sixty-one year old gentleman status post two prior coronary artery bypass graft operations who presents for an outpatient follow-up evaluation after a recent hospitalization for congestive heart failure.

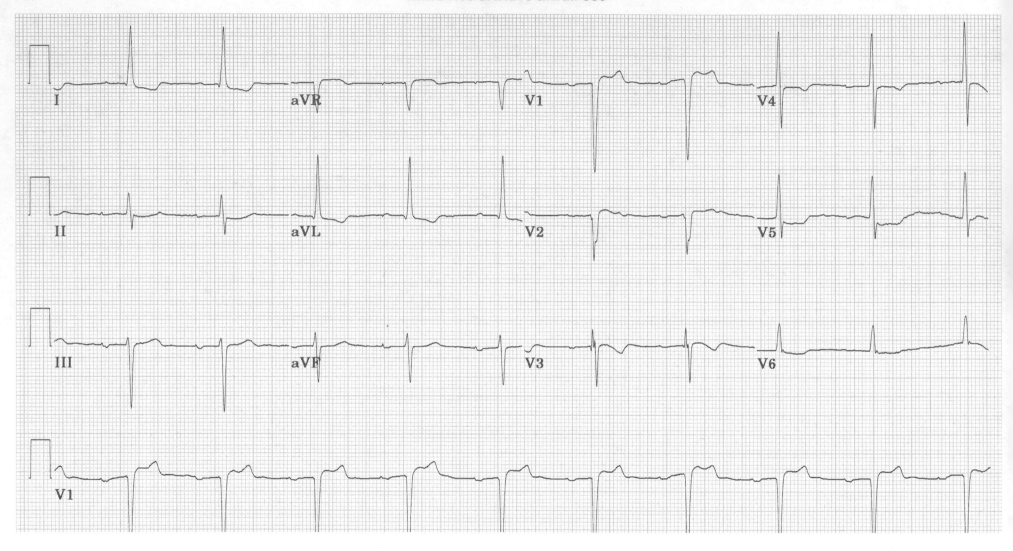

Interpretation Notes: _____

_____

_____

ECG 380 Seventy-five year old woman who was brought to the emergency room by family members with a several day history of shortness of breath. A chest x-ray demonstrated pulmonary edema. Her past medical history included Alzheimer's dementia, hypertension, non-insulin requiring diabetes mellitus, and chronic obstructive pulmonary disease. An echocardiogram demonstrated severe left ventricular systolic dysfunction. Serum cardiac enzymes confirmed the presence of acute myocardial injury.

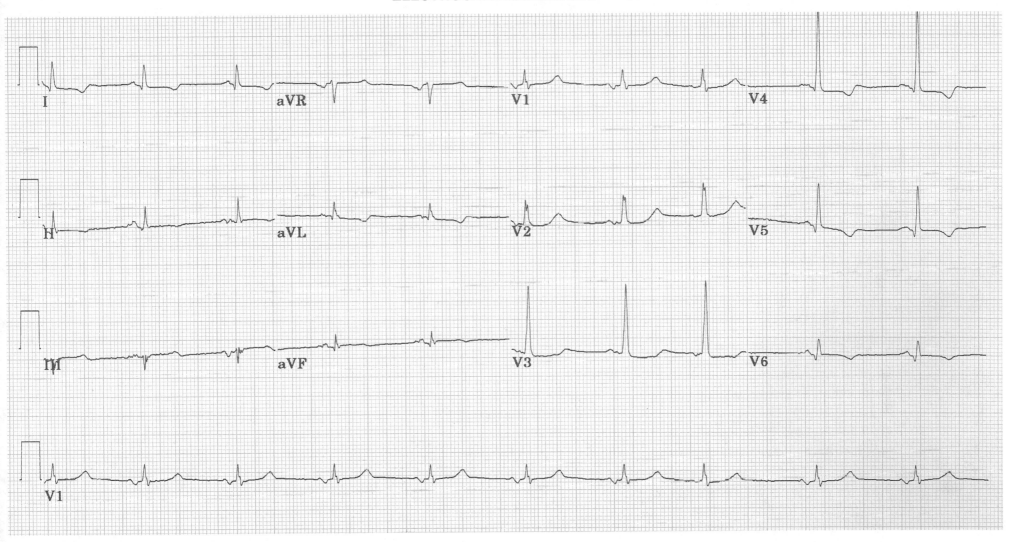

Interpretation Notes: _____

ECG 381 Sixty-seven year old gentleman admitted acutely to the hospital with progressive shortness of breath in the setting of coronary artery disease. He is status post a myocardial infarction nine years prior to this electrocardiogram. Co-morbid conditions include insulin requiring diabetes mellitus and severe hypertension. Medications at the time of this electrocardiogram included topical nitroglycerin, insulin, digoxin, and lisinopril.

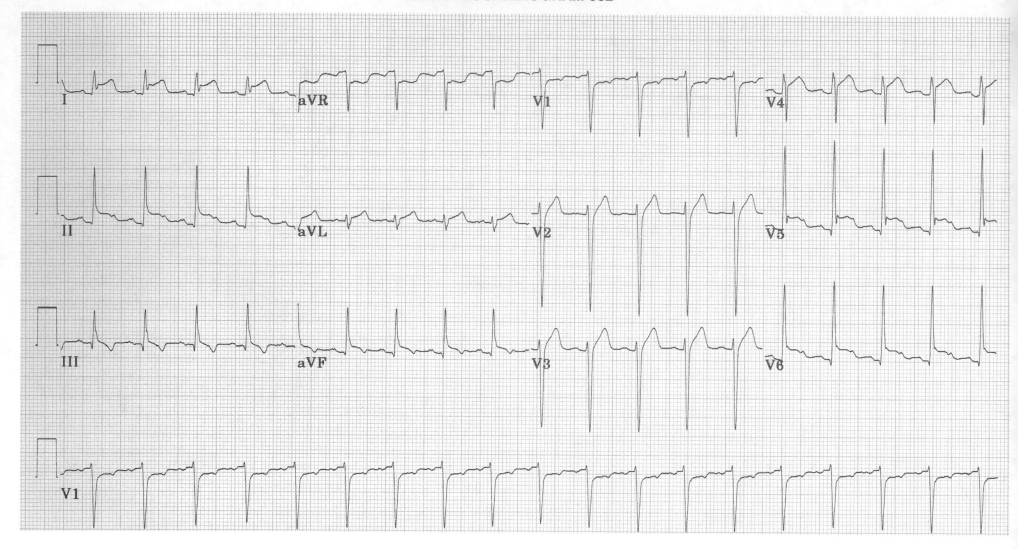

I   aVR   V1   V4

II   aVL   V2   V5

III   aVF   V3   V6

V1

Interpretation Notes: _____

_____

ECG 382 Eighteen year old gentleman recently status post open heart surgery including an aortic valve repair for moderately severe aortic insufficiency. The patient had a dilated left ventricle with normal left ventricular systolic function.

ELECTROCARDIOGRAM 383

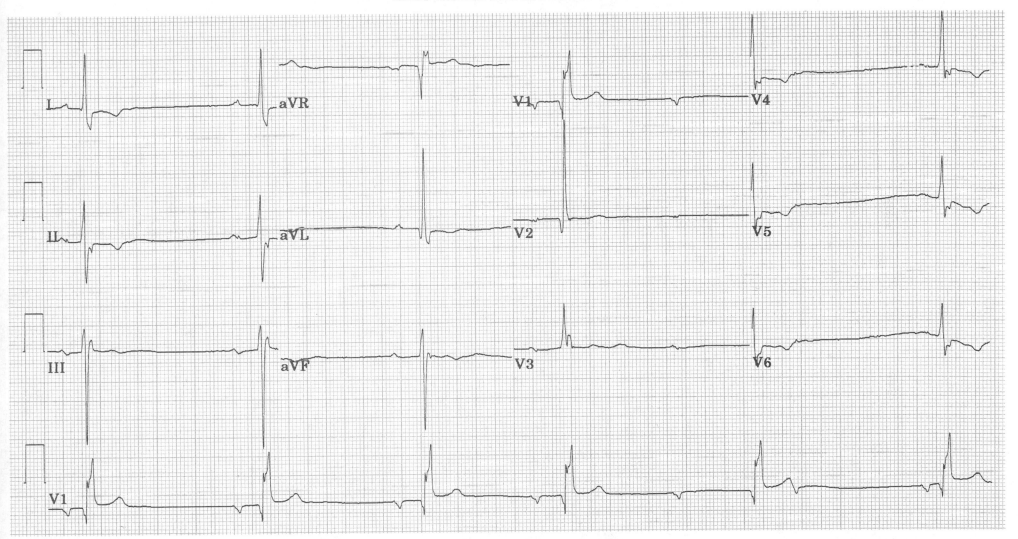

Interpretation Notes: _____

_____

ECG 383 Eighty-one year old woman who is seen in the outpatient geriatric clinic for a routine check-up. Her past medical history includes a deep venous thrombosis, hypertension, dementia, coronary artery disease, and anemia of chronic disease. Her medications included topical nitroglycerin, diltiazem, and prednisone.

ELECTROCARDIOGRAM 384

384

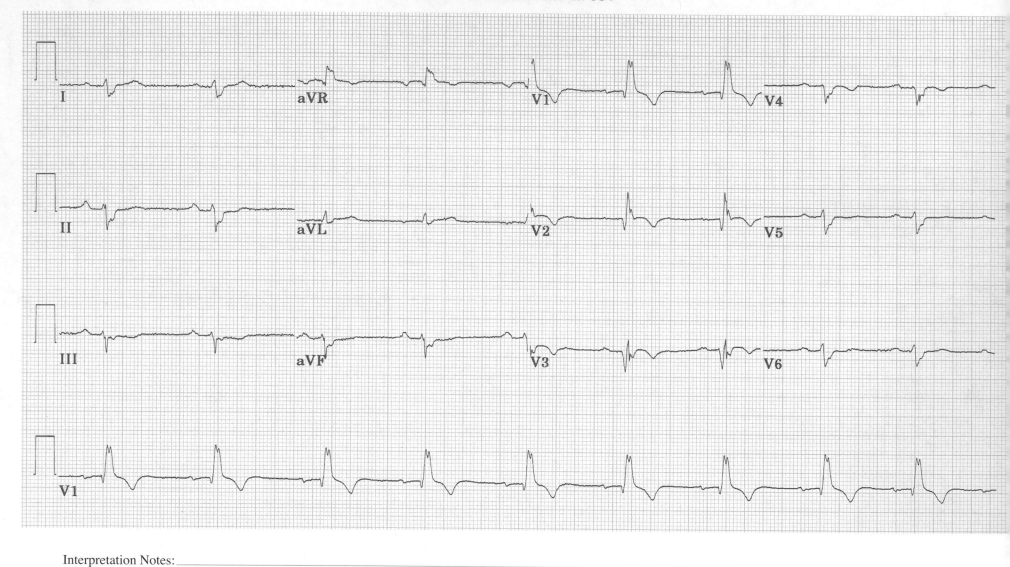

Interpretation Notes: _____

ECG 384 Sixty-six year old gentleman with recent symptoms of accelerating angina pectoris who underwent a five-vessel coronary artery bypass grafting procedure. This represents a preoperative tracing. A cardiac catheterization demonstrated moderate left ventricular systolic dysfunction with evidence of prior inferoposterior and septal myocardial infarctions. Medications at the time of this electrocardiogram included furosemide, nifedipine, aspirin, digoxin, procainamide, and metoprolol.

ELECTROCARDIOGRAM 385

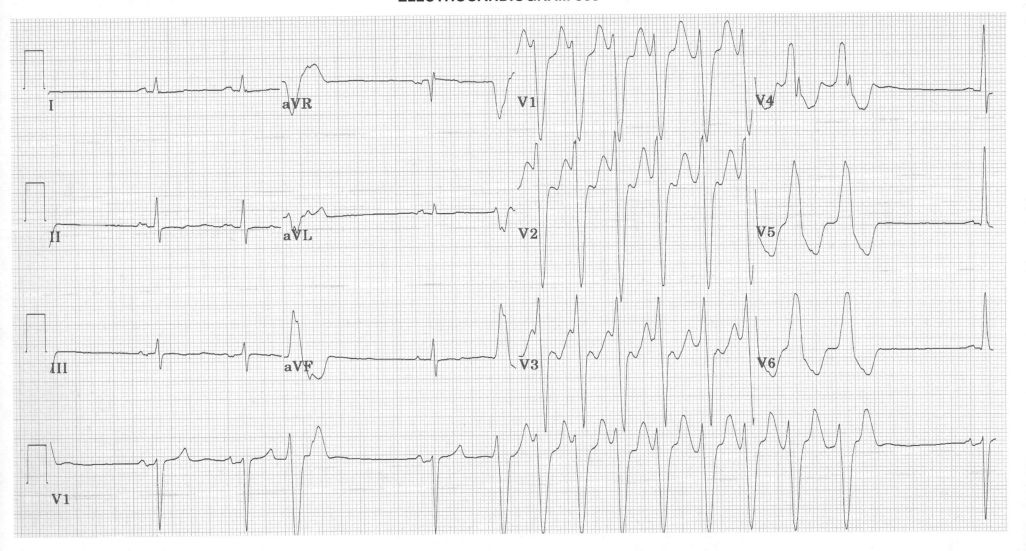

Interpretation Notes: _____

_____

ECG 385 Twenty year old gentleman with a presumed viral cardiomyopathy and resultant severe left ventricular systolic dysfunction admitted for evaluation of non-sustained ventricular tachycardia. The patient underwent an electrophysiology study demonstrating inducible sustained monomorphic ventricular tachycardia. Medications at the time of this electrocardiogram included warfarin, furosemide, digoxin, enalapril, and metoprolol.

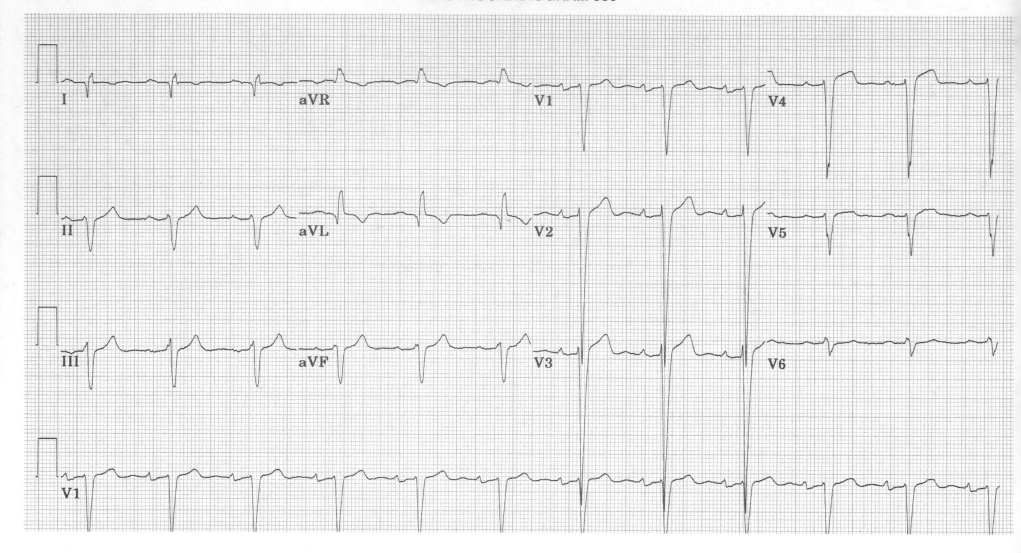

Interpretation Notes: _____

_____

ECG 386 Sixty-six year old gentleman with severe left ventricular systolic dysfunction in the setting of advanced coronary artery disease and prior coronary artery bypass graft surgery admitted to the hospital with a congestive heart failure exacerbation. Co-morbid conditions include peripheral vascular disease, diabetes mellitus and hypertension. His medications included digoxin, aspirin, enalapril, hydralazine, furosemide, and isosorbide mononitrate.

ELECTROCARDIOGRAM 387

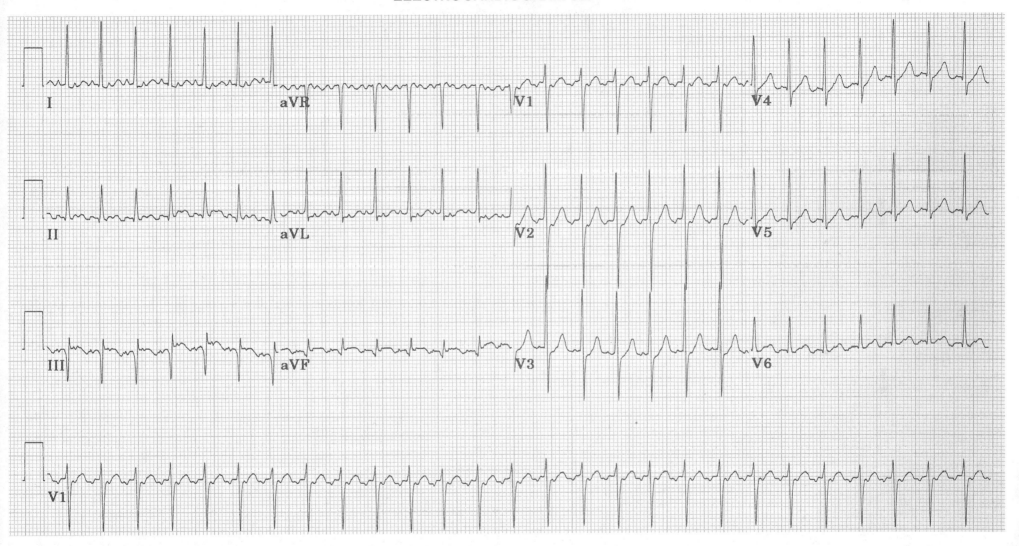

I   aVR   V1   V4

II   aVL   V2   V5

III   aVF   V3   V6

V1

Interpretation Notes: _____

_____

_____

ECG 387 Sixty year old gentleman who presents acutely to the hospital with a one hour history of severe chest discomfort. The patient was taken urgently to the cardiac catheterization laboratory where an acute occlusion of the right coronary artery with superimposed thrombus was found. Urgent successful angioplasty and stent placement to the right coronary artery was performed.

ELECTROCARDIOGRAM 388

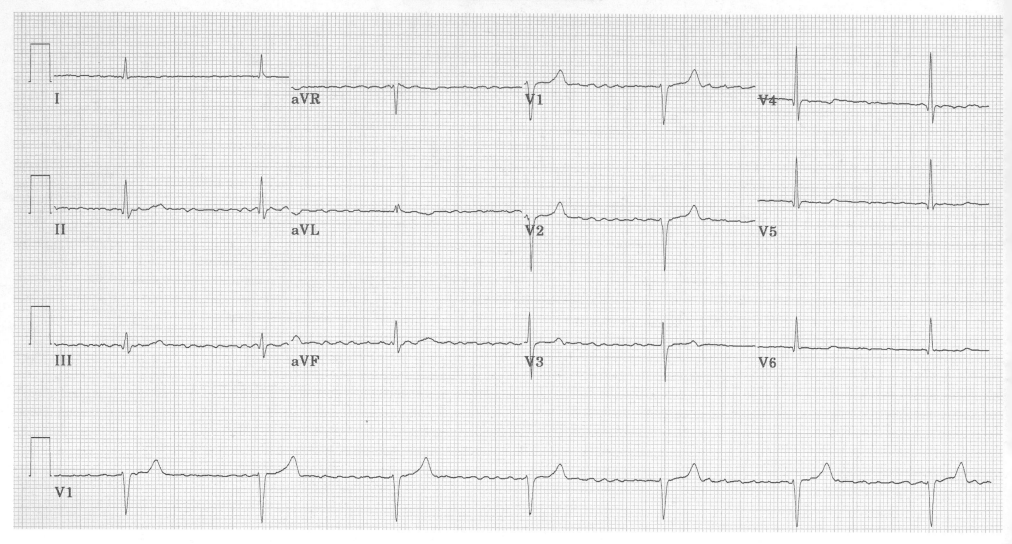

I   aVR   V1   V4

II   aVL   V2   V5

III   aVF   V3   V6

V1

Interpretation Notes:

ECG 388 Forty-seven year old gentleman with chronic atrial fibrillation who underwent an attempted radiofrequency ablation procedure resulting in complete heart block. Successful permanent pacemaker placement transpired.

ELECTROCARDIOGRAM 389

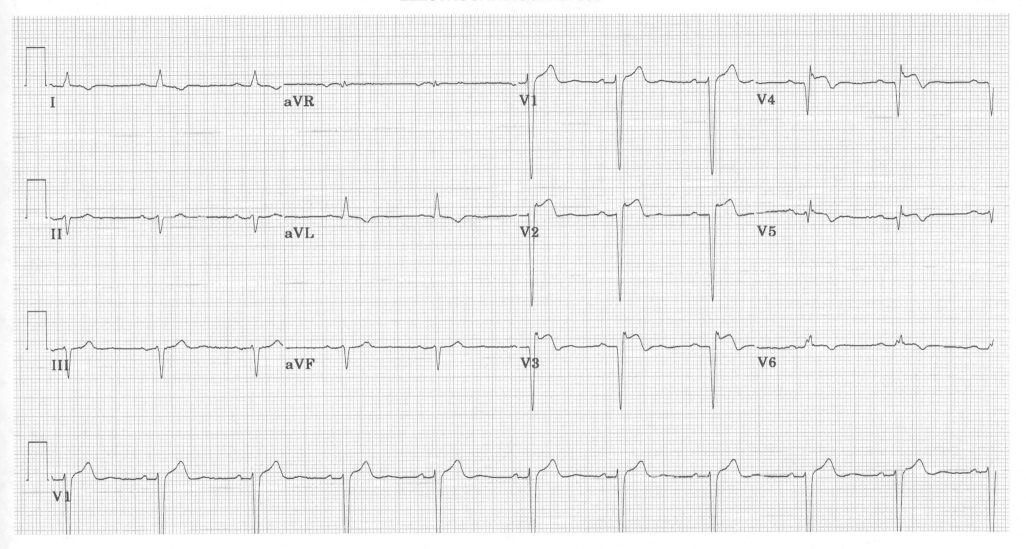

Interpretation Notes:_____

_____

_____

ECG 389 Seventy-six year old gentleman with a remote extensive anterolateral myocardial infarction and subsequent left ventricular aneurysm formation who returns for outpatient evaluation of his implantable cardiac defibrillator. He is presently asymptomatic. The patient has a past history of drug-refractory ventricular tachycardia and an abdominal aortic aneurysm repair. His medications at the time of this electrocardiogram included ethmozine, aspirin, digoxin, and nadolol.

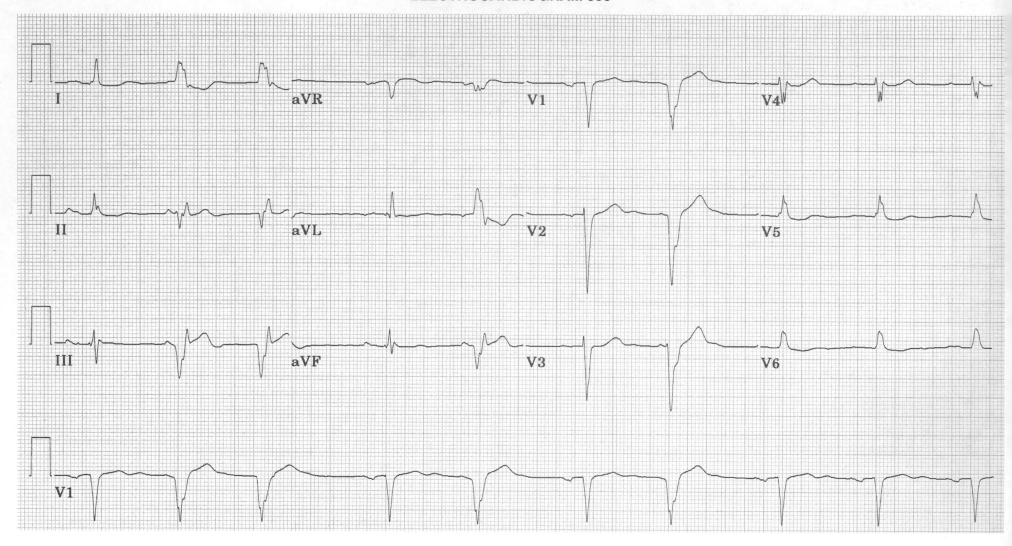

Interpretation Notes: _____

_____

ECG 390 Fifty-seven year old gentleman with advanced coronary artery disease status post a remote myocardial infarction of unknown location and coronary artery by-pass graft surgery. He is admitted for evaluation of suspected pneumonia. His medications at the time of this electrocardiogram included furosemide, warfarin, digoxin, lisinopril, and atorvastatin.

ELECTROCARDIOGRAM 391

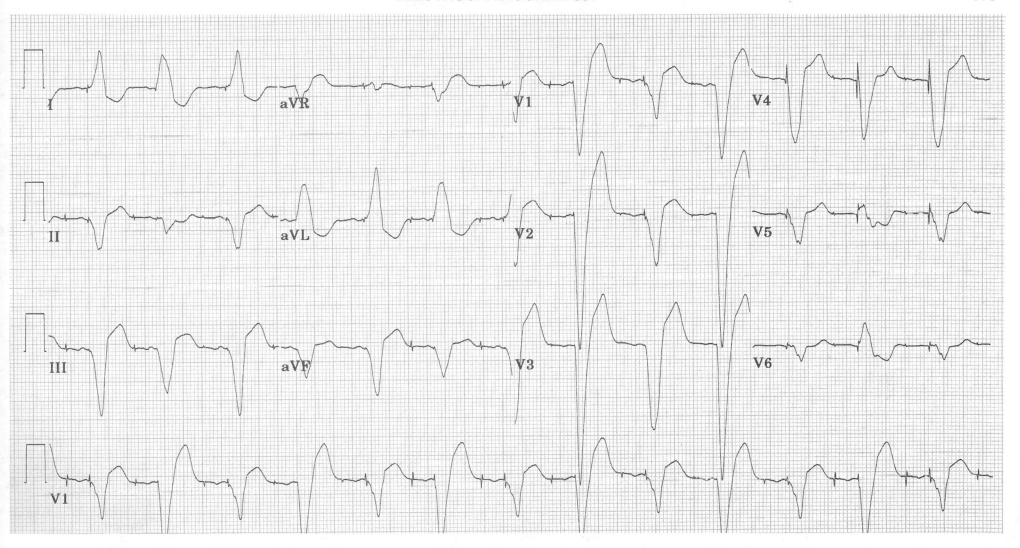

Interpretation Notes: _____

_____

_____

ECG 391 Fifty-four year old woman who is immediately postoperative bioprosthetic aortic valve replacement secondary to aortic stenosis. Co-morbid conditions include hypertension, non-insulin requiring diabetes mellitus, and dialysis requiring renal insufficiency.

ELECTROCARDIOGRAM 392

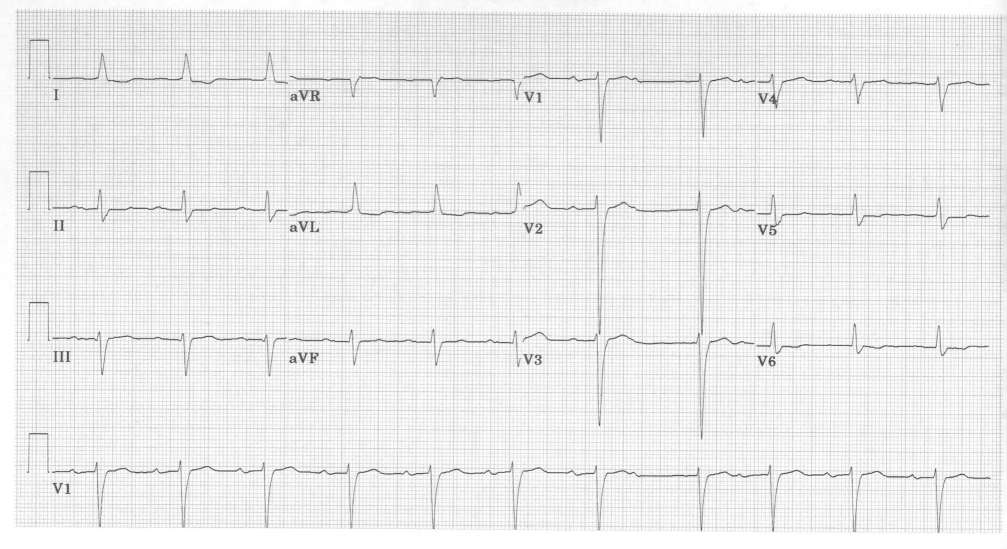

Interpretation Notes: _____

_____

ECG 392 Seventy-five year old gentleman with coronary artery disease who presents to the hospital with unstable angina. His past medical history includes insulin requiring diabetes mellitus, chronic renal insufficiency, and hypertension.

ELECTROCARDIOGRAM 393

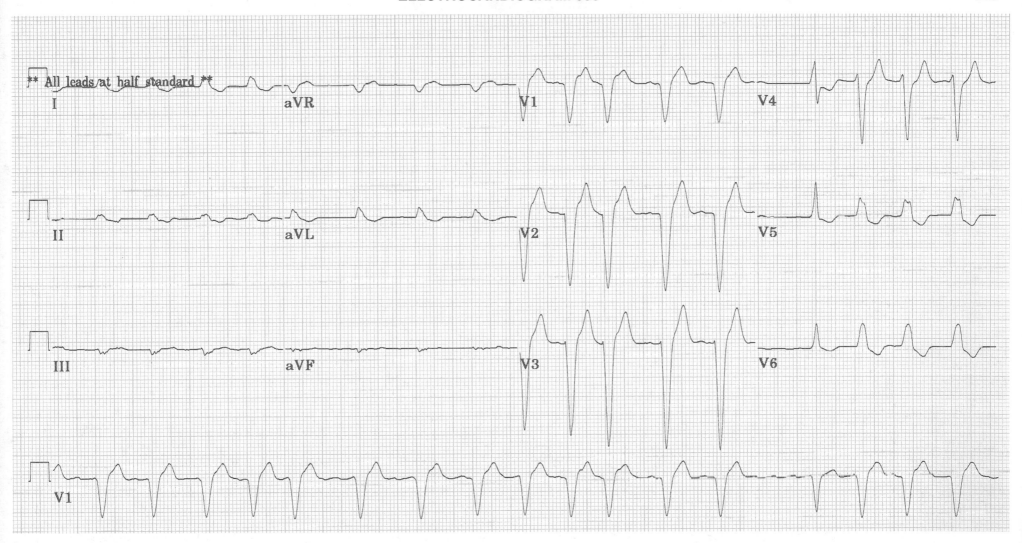

** All leads at half standard **

Interpretation Notes: _____

ECG 393 Seventy year old woman with a history of breast cancer status post a mastectomy who is readmitted to the hospital for evaluation of left-sided hydronephrosis. Her past cardiac history includes paroxysmal atrial fibrillation. Her medications included digoxin, famotidine, insulin, prednisone, and warfarin.

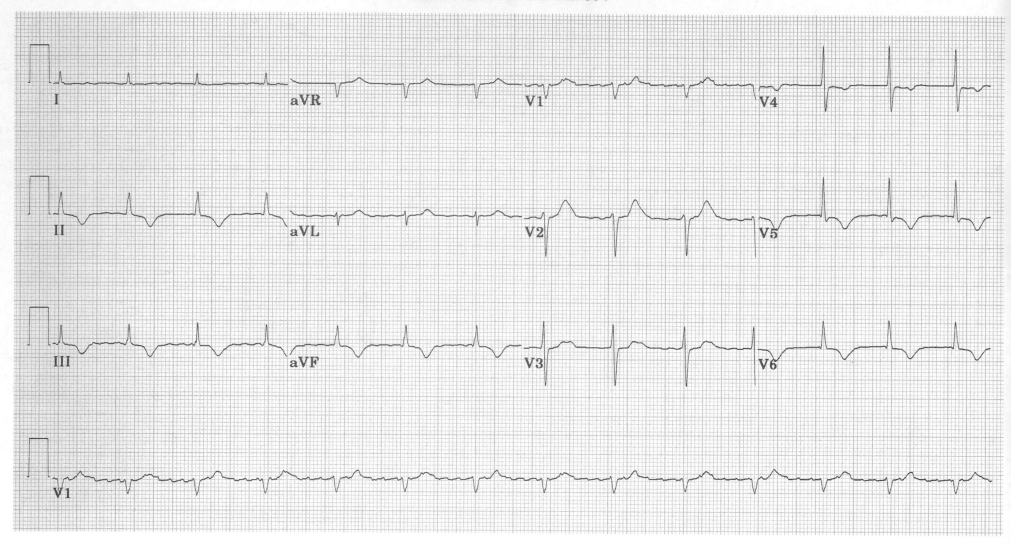

Interpretation Notes: _____

ECG 394 Seventy-three year old gentleman with severe ischemic left ventricular systolic dysfunction who is recently status post a second coronary artery bypass graft operation. Co-morbid conditions include hypertension, non-insulin requiring diabetes mellitus, and chronic atrial fibrillation.

ELECTROCARDIOGRAM 395

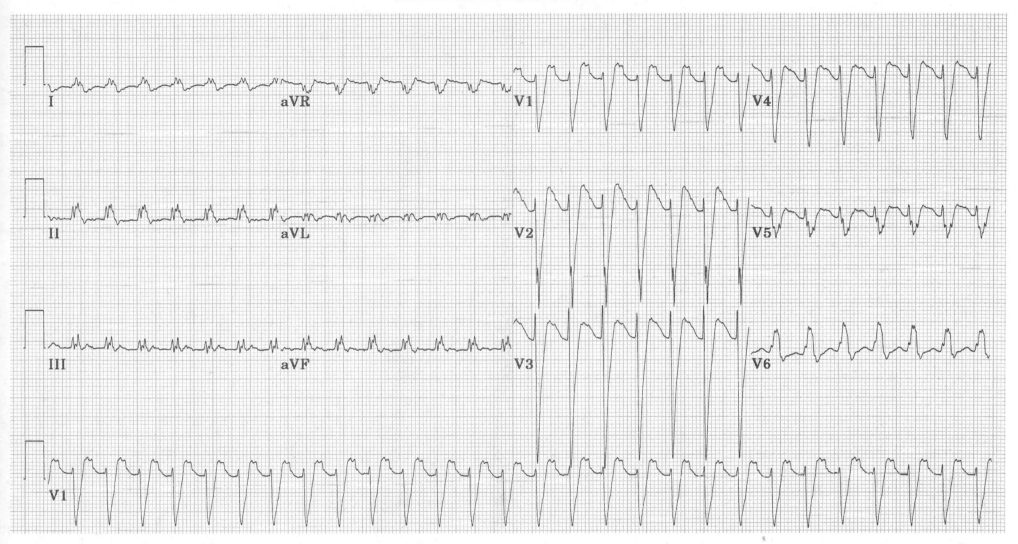

Interpretation Notes: _____

_____

ECG 395 Forty-seven year old woman with a history of Hodgkin's disease and mantle irradiation who is admitted to the hospital with severe congestive heart failure in the setting of a non-ischemic dilated cardiomyopathy. The patient subsequently underwent left ventricular assist device placement complicated by pneumonia and a large pericardial effusion.

ELECTROCARDIOGRAM 396

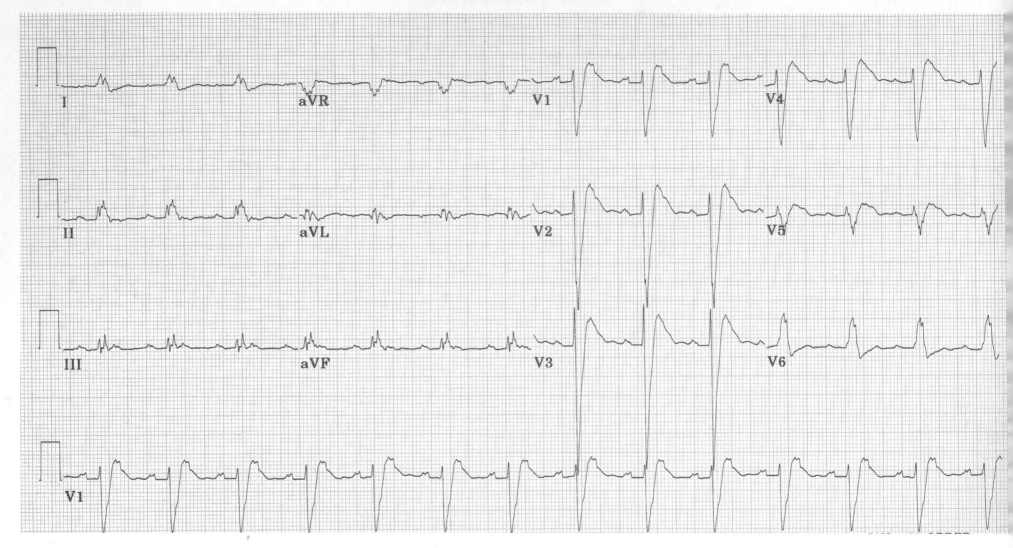

Interpretation Notes: _____

_____

ECG 396 Forty-seven year old woman with a history of Hodgkin's disease and mantle irradiation who is admitted to the hospital with severe congestive heart failure in the setting of a non-ischemic dilated cardiomyopathy. The patient subsequently underwent left ventricular assist device placement complicated by pneumonia and a large pericardial effusion.

ELECTROCARDIOGRAM 397

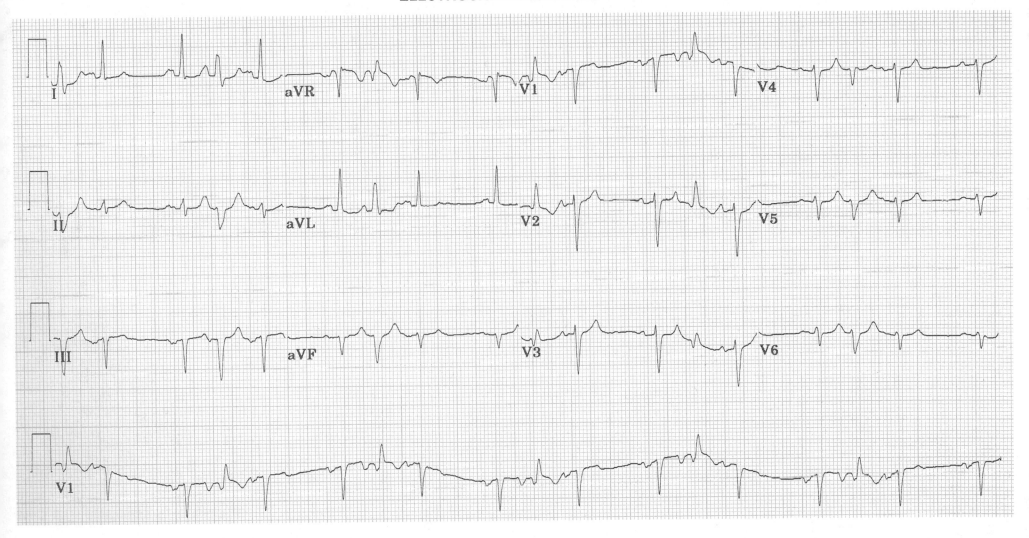

Interpretation Notes: _____

ECG 397 Sixty-four year old woman with paroxysmal atrial fibrillation, hypertension, and diabetes mellitus admitted to the hospital for evaluation of recent onset diarrhea. She has no known cardiac history.

ELECTROCARDIOGRAM 398

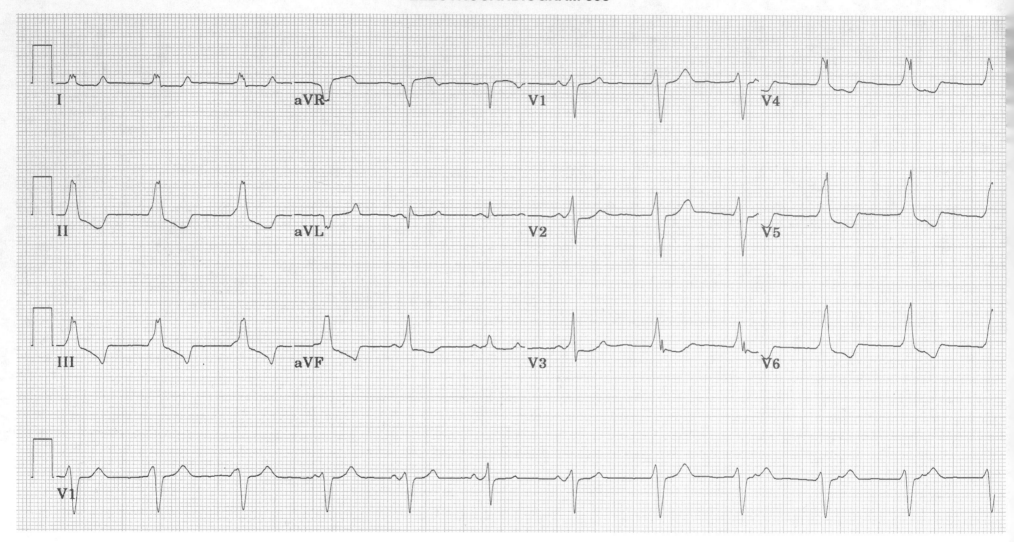

I aVR V1 V4

II aVL V2 V5

III aVF V3 V6

V1

Interpretation Notes: _____

_____

_____

ECG 398 Sixty year old gentleman with a history of paroxysmal supraventricular tachycardia who returns for a routine cardiology follow-up evaluation. His medications included acebutalol, aspirin, and vitamin E.

ELECTROCARDIOGRAM 399

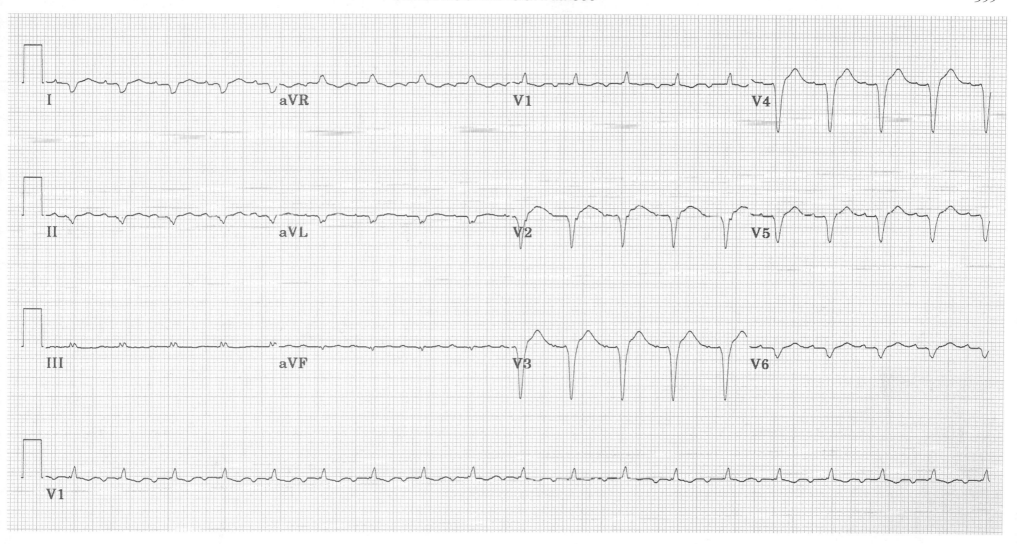

Interpretation Notes: _____

_____

ECG 399 Sixty-one year old gentleman who presented to the hospital with recent onset unstable angina. Serial cardiac enzyme analysis demonstrated acute myocardial injury. A cardiac catheterization demonstrated severe multi-vessel coronary artery disease and the patient was referred for successful coronary artery bypass graft surgery.

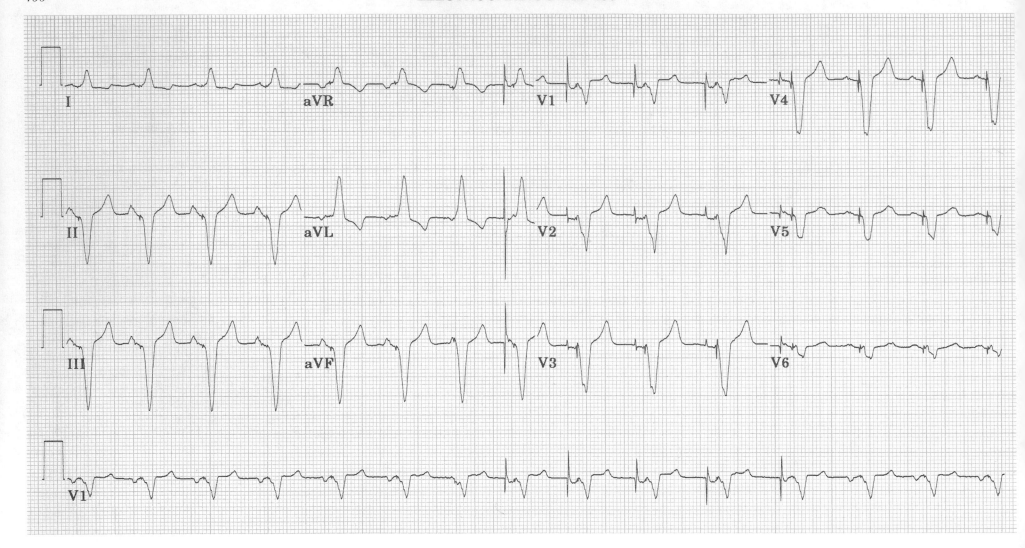

Interpretation Notes: _____

_____

_____

ECG 400 Fifty-nine year old gentleman with paroxysmal atrial fibrillation, hypertension, and peripheral vascular disease who presents to the cardiology clinic for clinical re-assessment and pacemaker interrogation. His medications at the time of this electrocardiogram included warfarin and simvastatin.

ELECTROCARDIOGRAM 401

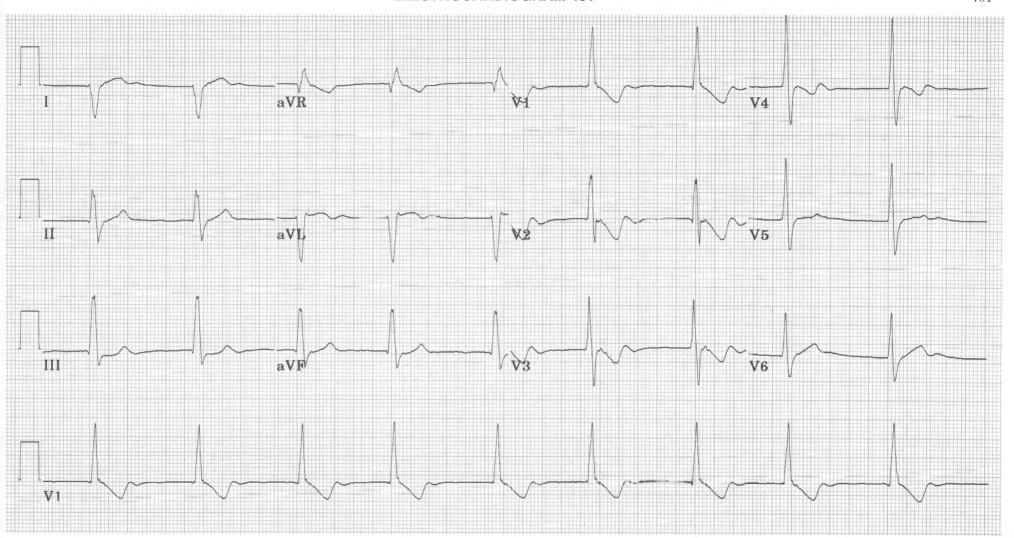

Interpretation Notes:_____

_____

ECG 401 Twenty-one year old gentleman with a history of transposition of the great arteries and a ventricular septal defect pericardial patch repair who is being seen in the outpatient cardiology clinic.

402

ELECTROCARDIOGRAM 402

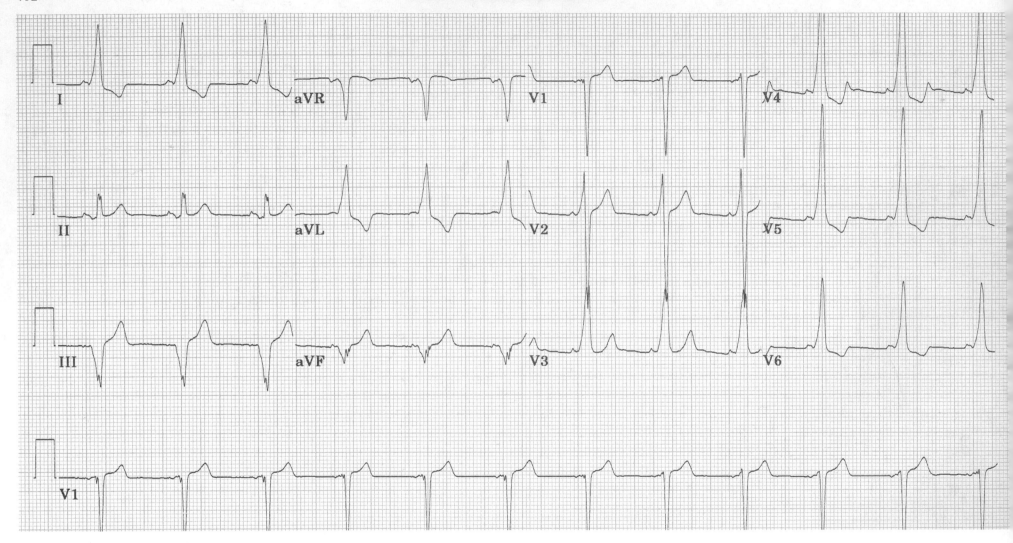

Interpretation Notes: _____

_____

_____

ECG 402 Forty-two year old gentleman who is being seen for a routine physical examination. He has no known cardiac disease and no history of cardiac dysrhythmias.

ELECTROCARDIOGRAM 403

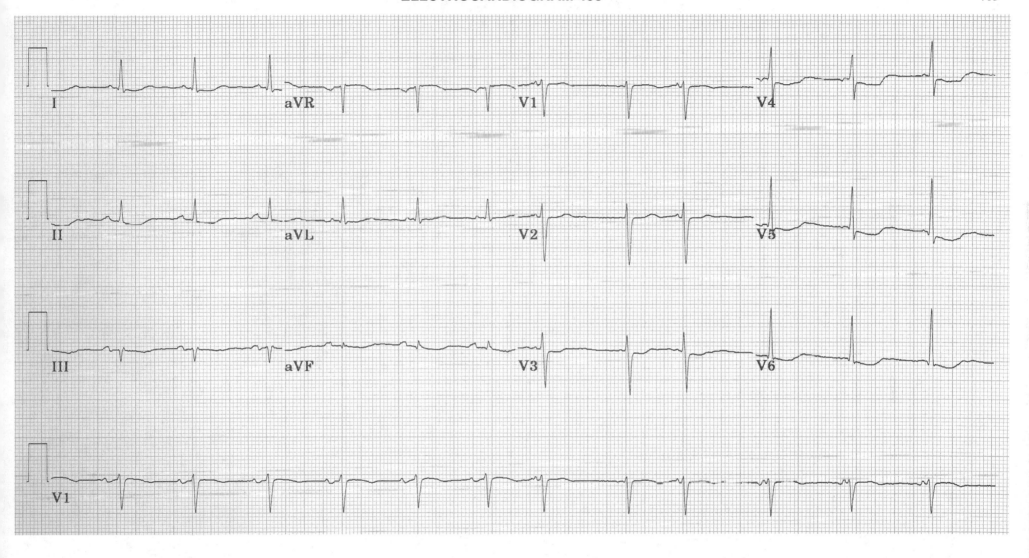

I aVR V1 V4

II aVL V2 V5

III aVF V3 V6

V1

Interpretation Notes: _____

_____

_____

ECG 403 Seventy year old woman with a long-standing history of hypertension, non-insulin requiring diabetes mellitus, and a remote pulmonary embolism who presented to the hospital with recent onset exertional chest pressure. Her medications included warfarin, theophylline, potassium, furosemide, captopril, isosorbide dinitrate, and digoxin. The patient subsequently underwent a stress echocardiogram which was normal.

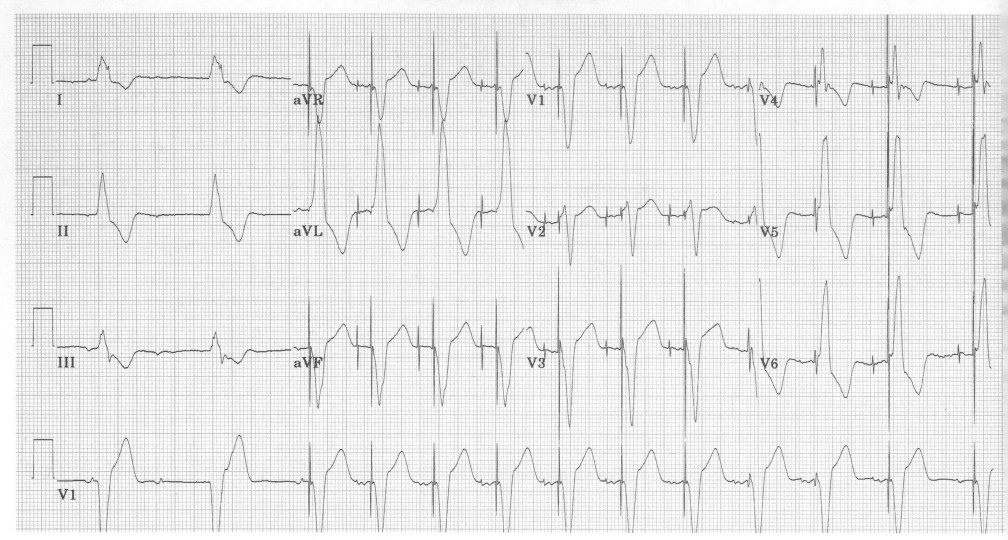

Interpretation Notes: _____

_____

ECG 404 Sixty-two year old gentleman admitted to the hospital with progressive shortness of breath. He has severe aortic stenosis and moderately severe aortic insufficiency. The patient underwent successful cardiac surgery including aortic valve replacement.

ELECTROCARDIOGRAM 405

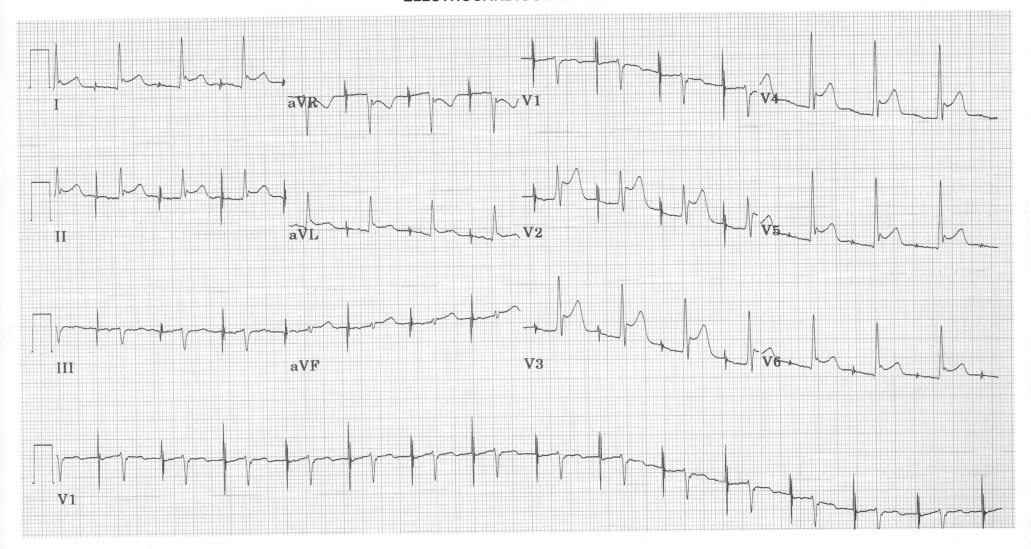

Interpretation Notes: _____

ECG 405 Seventy-four year old gentleman who presents for further evaluation of increasing chest discomfort felt to represent angina pectoris. Co-morbid conditions include hypercholesterolemia and hypertension. Medications at the time of this electrocardiogram included nifedipine and aspirin. The patient subsequently underwent a cardiac catheterization demonstrating multi-vessel coronary artery disease. This electrocardiogram was obtained shortly after open heart surgery.

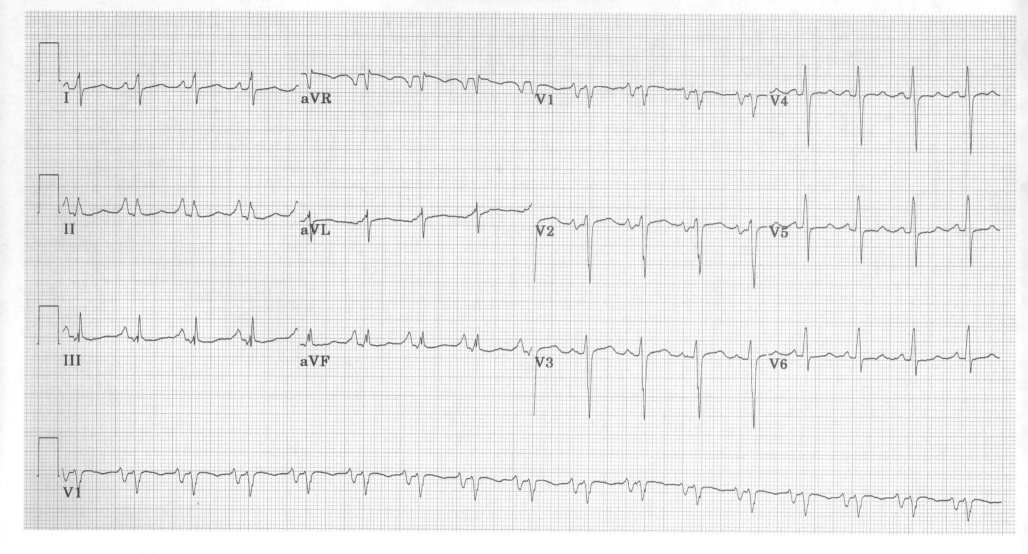

Interpretation Notes: _____

_____

ECG 406 Thirty-eight year old gentleman with a dilated cardiomyopathy and class III congestive heart failure who returns for a cardiology follow-up evaluation. His medications included lisinopril, digoxin, metolazone, aspirin, and potassium.

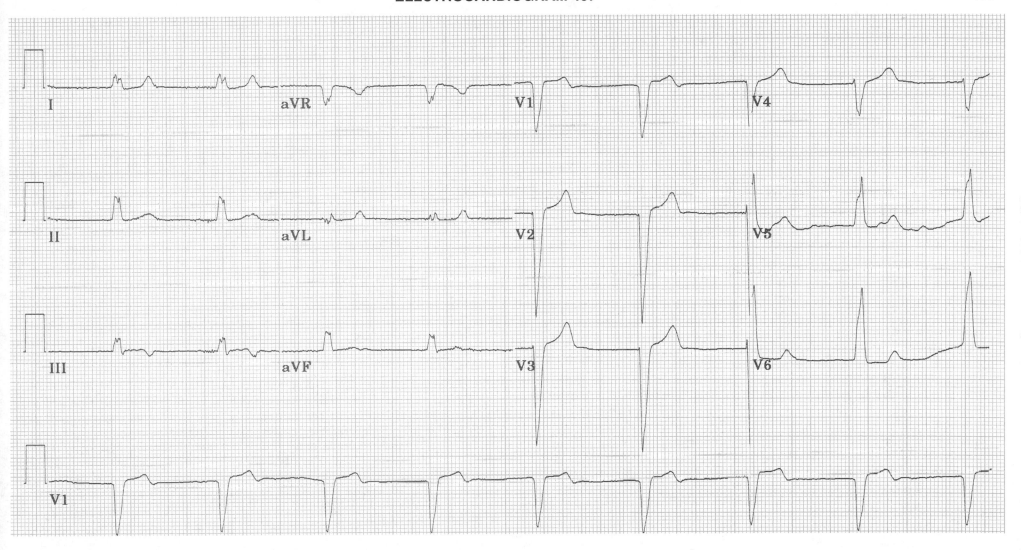

Interpretation Notes: _____

ECG 407 Seventy-five year old gentleman with coronary artery disease and recent symptoms of accelerating angina pectoris. This electrocardiogram was obtained shortly after coronary artery bypass graft surgery. His pertinent past history includes a recent echocardiogram demonstrating a left atrial myxoma. This was resected at the time of his bypass surgery. Preoperative left ventricular systolic function was moderately decreased with severe hypokinesis of the inferior segment.

ELECTROCARDIOGRAM 408

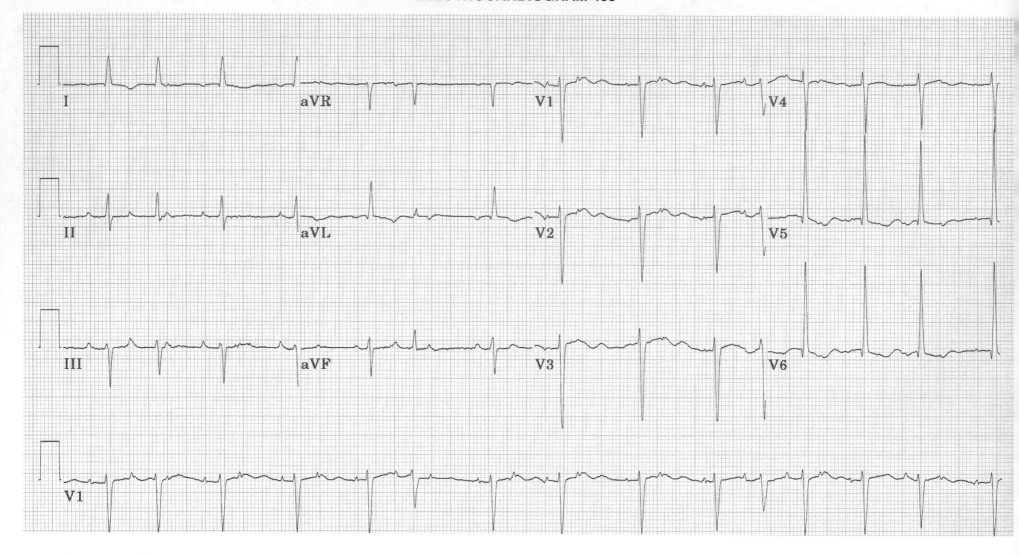

Interpretation Notes: _____

_____

ECG 408 Sixty-eight year old gentleman with severe chronic obstructive pulmonary disease, chronic renal insufficiency, and hypertension who presents to the hospital with severe weakness and dyspnea upon exertion. His medications included terazosin, diltiazem, insulin, ranitidine, and furosemide. He has a long history of tobacco use.

ELECTROCARDIOGRAM 409

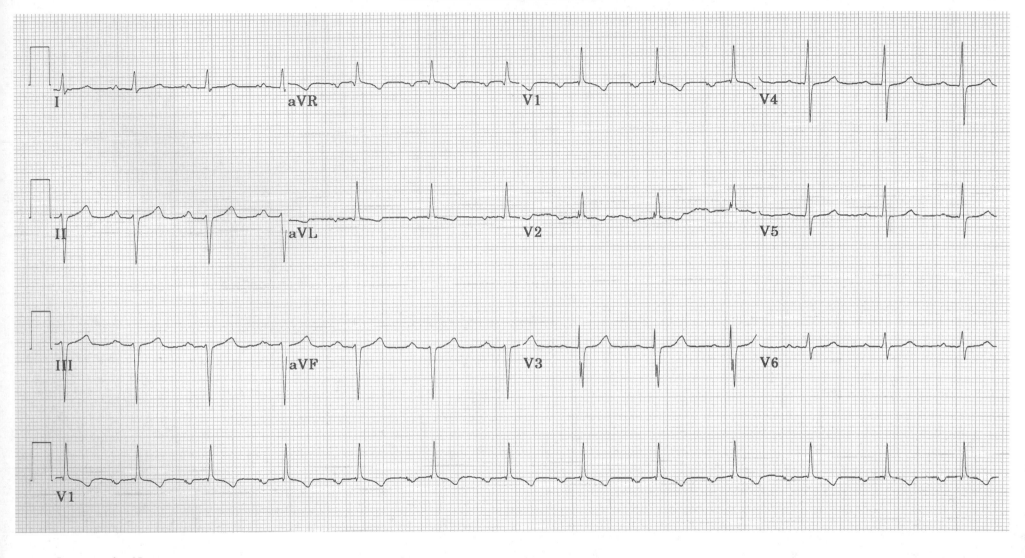

I aVR V1 V4

II aVL V2 V5

III aVF V3 V6

V1

Interpretation Notes: _____

_____

ECG 409 Thirty-four year old woman with a history of an atrioventricular canal and ostium primum atrial septal defect status post surgical repair who is readmitted for a cardiac evaluation. She is experiencing paroxysmal atrial dysrhythmias and is on no current medications.

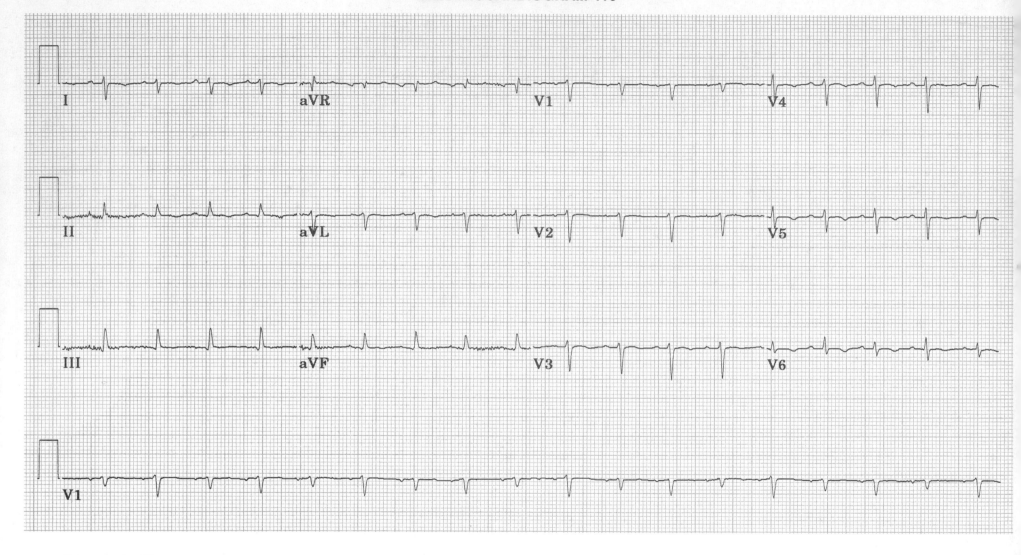

I   aVR   V1   V4

II   aVL   V2   V5

III   aVF   V3   V6

V1

Interpretation Notes: _____

_____

_____

ECG 410 Thirty-eight year old gentleman who presents with severe dyspnea of one week duration. An echocardiogram demonstrated a large pericardial effusion with evidence supporting cardiac tamponade. The patient underwent urgent surgical pericardial drainage.

ELECTROCARDIOGRAM 411

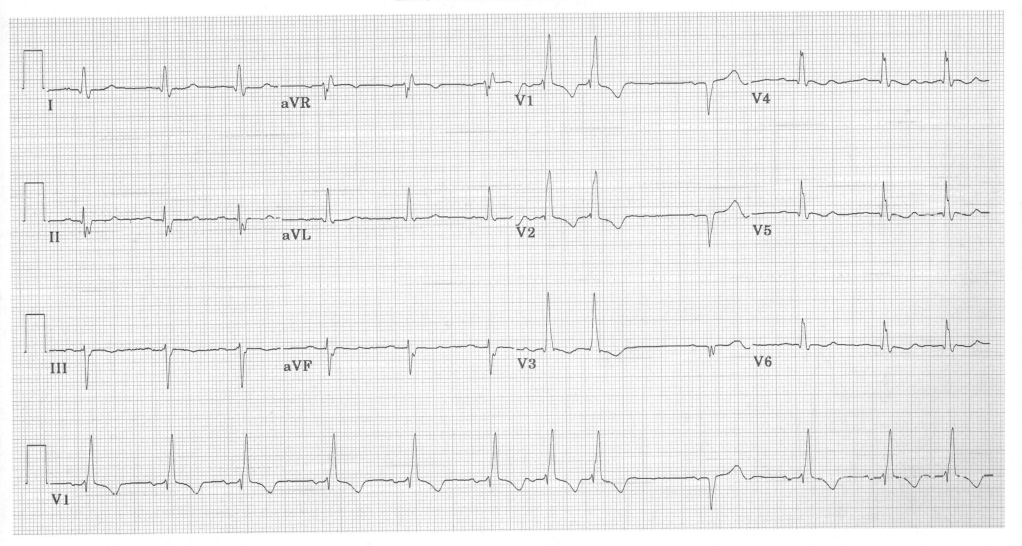

Interpretation Notes: _____

_____

ECG 411 Seventy-five year old gentleman with a prior anterior myocardial infarction who returns to the hospital with recent onset unstable angina pectoris. His medications at the time of this electrocardiogram included topical nitroglycerin, aspirin, atenolol, amlodipine, and intravenous heparin.

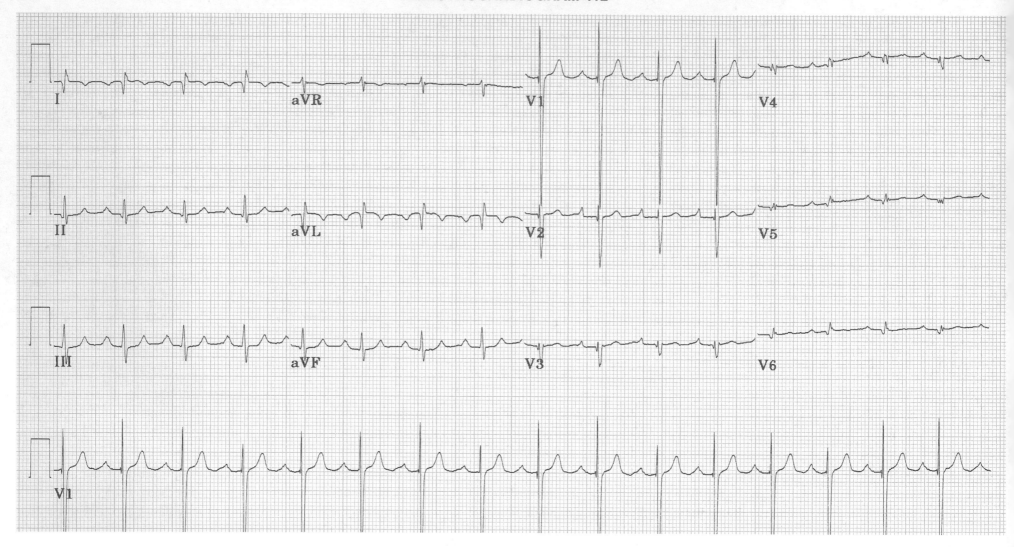

Interpretation Notes: _____

_____

ECG 412 Thirty year old woman with situs inversus, dextrocardia, and mild valvular pulmonic stenosis who returns for an outpatient cardiology follow-up evaluation.

ELECTROCARDIOGRAM 413

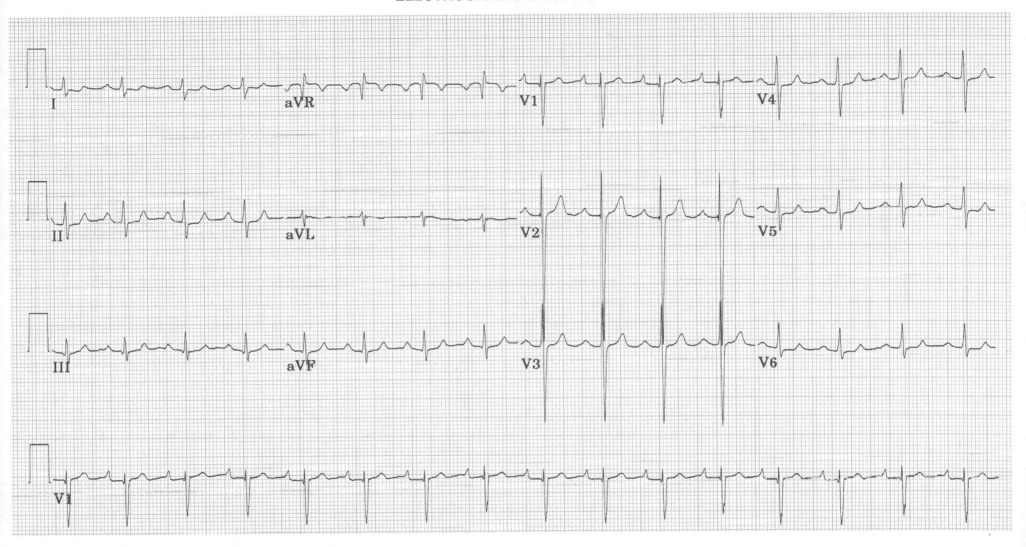

Interpretation Notes: _____

_____

ECG 413 Thirty year old woman with situs inversus, dextrocardia, and mild valvular pulmonic stenosis who returns for an outpatient cardiology evaluation.

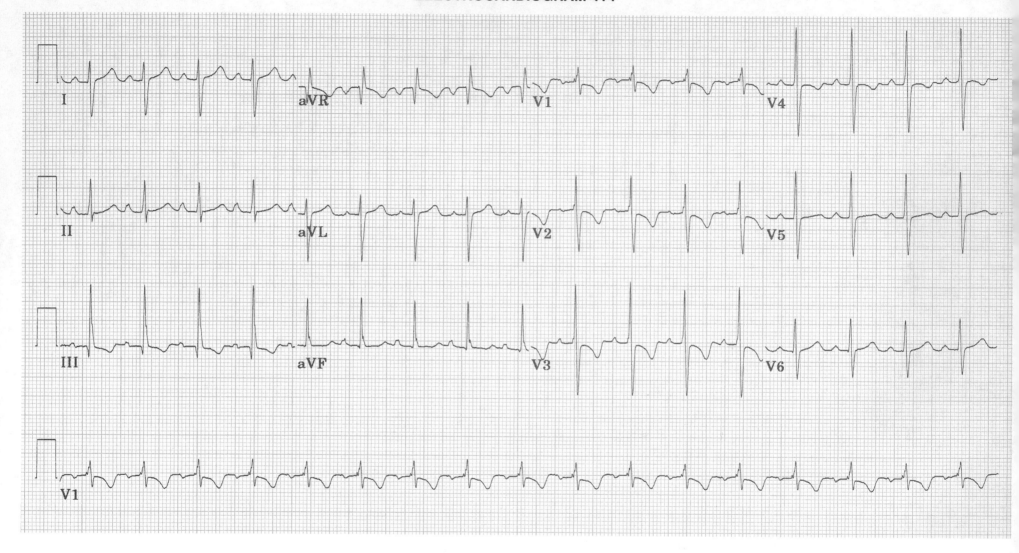

I aVR V1 V4

II aVL V2 V5

III aVF V3 V6

V1

Interpretation Notes: _____

_____

_____

ECG 414 Twenty year old woman who underwent a recent appendectomy. In the operating room she was difficult to oxygenate and upon further clinical questioning she noted a blue appearance with exertion. A follow-up cardiac evaluation demonstrated a secundum atrial septal defect and Eisenmenger's syndrome. The patient is currently on the lung transplant waiting list.

ELECTROCARDIOGRAM 415

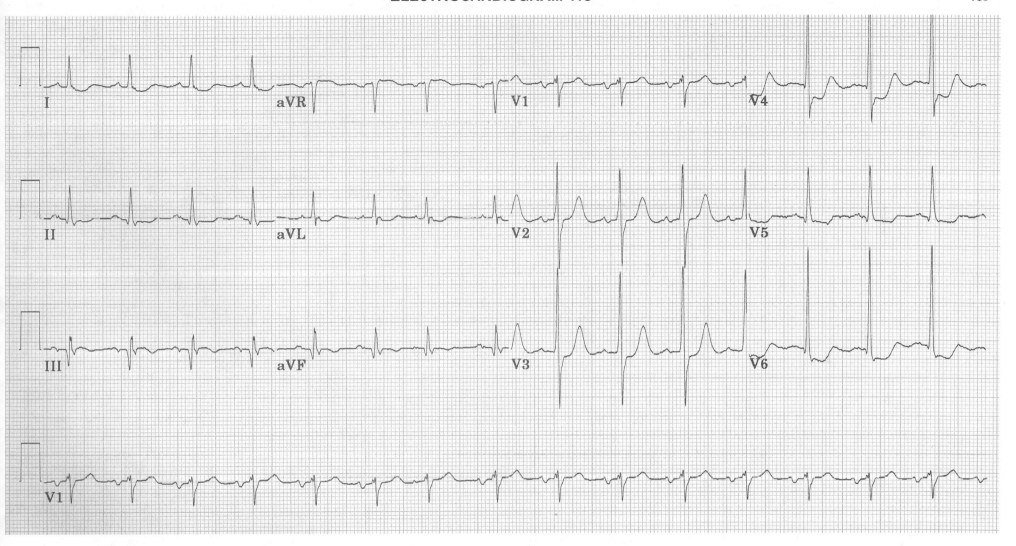

Interpretation Notes:

ECG 415 Seventy-seven year old woman admitted to the intensive care unit with an acute chest discomfort syndrome of cardiac origin. Serial cardiac enzymes confirmed the presence of acute myocardial injury and a non-Q wave myocardial infarction. A subsequent cardiac catheterization demonstrated severe three-vessel coronary artery disease and the patient was referred for successful coronary artery bypass graft surgery.

ELECTROCARDIOGRAM 416

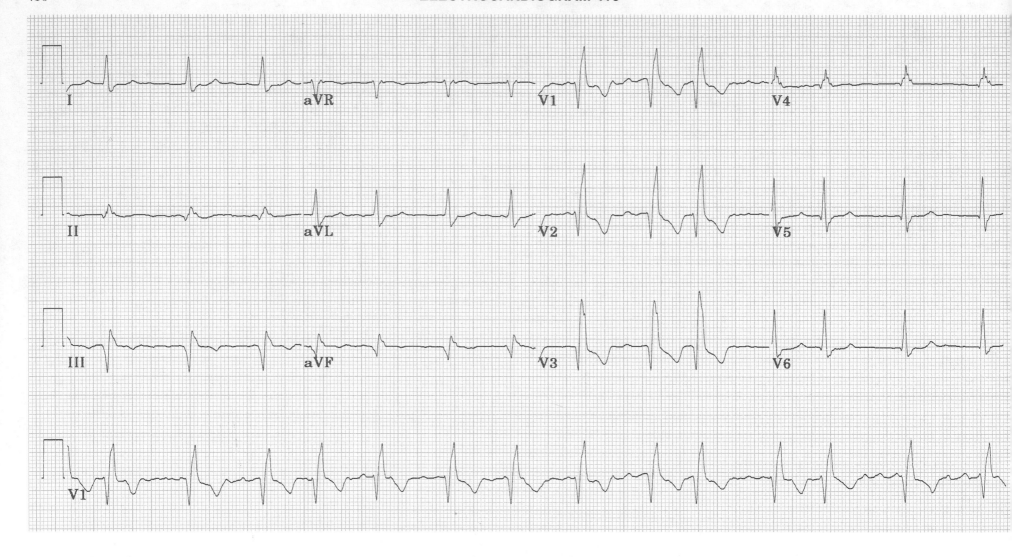

Interpretation Notes: _____

ECG 416 Seventy-nine year old woman with coronary artery disease who is recently status post coronary artery bypass graft surgery and aortic valve replacement. Her past medical history includes chronic atrial fibrillation and a transient ischemic attack. Her medications included enalapril, digoxin, hydralazine, furosemide, and potassium.

ELECTROCARDIOGRAM 417

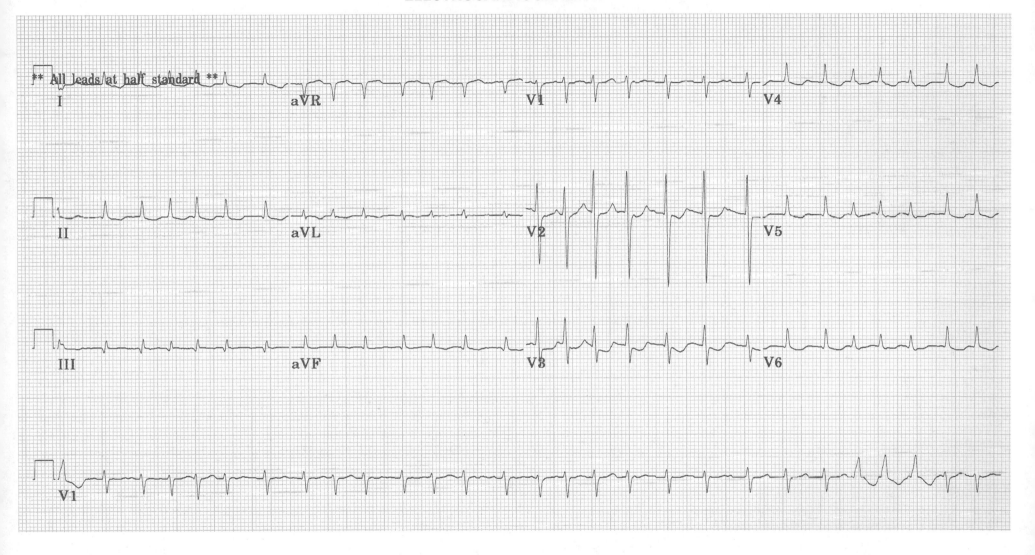

** All leads at half standard **

I   aVR   V1   V4

II   aVL   V2   V5

III   aVF   V3   V6

V1

Interpretation Notes: _____

_____

_____

ECG 417 Fifty-five year old gentleman with a history of hepatic cirrhosis accepted in hospital transfer for evaluation of increasing abdominal girth and suspected ascites. His medications included spironolactone, furosemide, potassium, and lactulose.

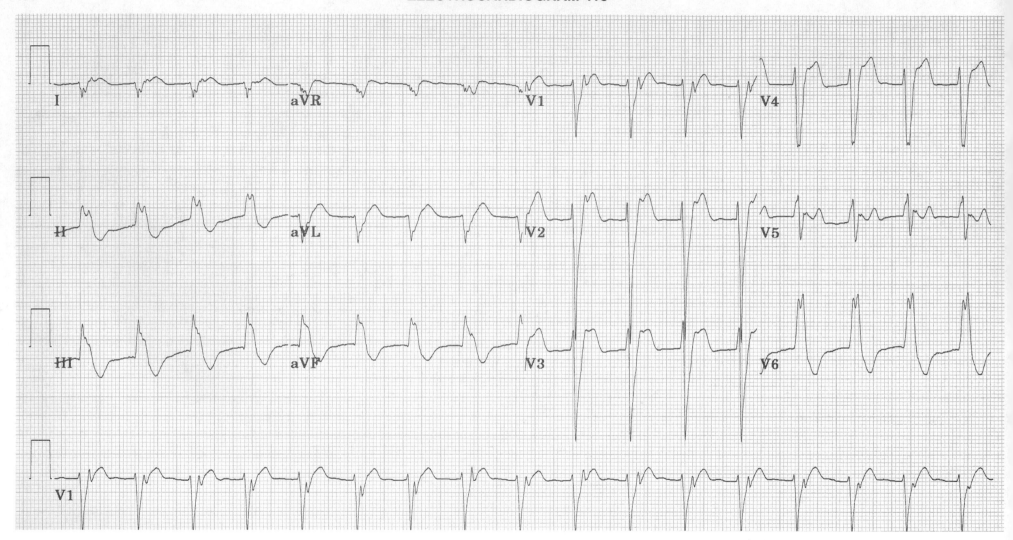

Interpretation Notes: _____

ECG 418 Forty-one year old woman with a history of a non-ischemic cardiomyopathy and severe left ventricular systolic dysfunction admitted for treatment of a congestive heart failure exacerbation. Medications at the time of this electrocardiogram included furosemide, metolazone, aspirin, digoxin, and captopril.

ELECTROCARDIOGRAM 419

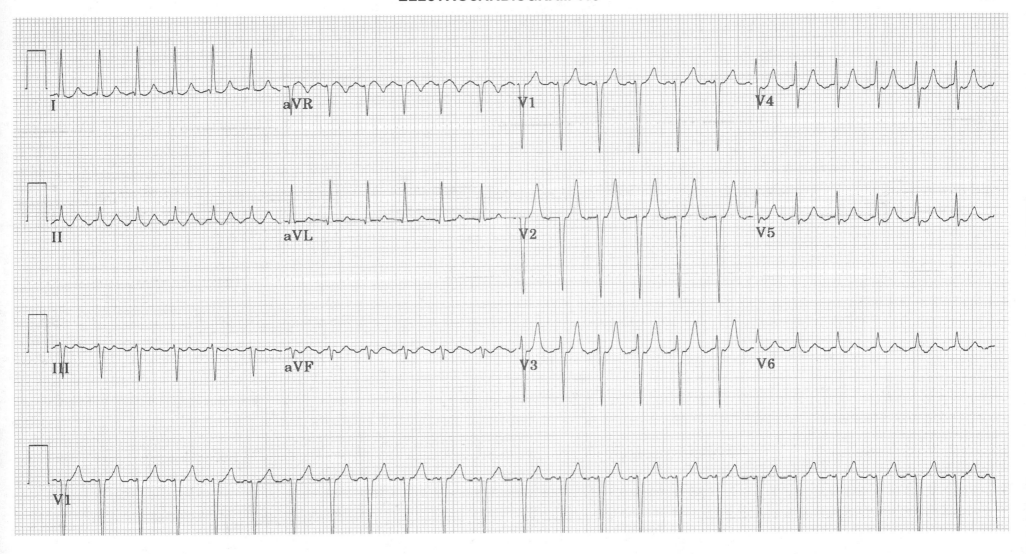

Interpretation Notes: _____

_____

ECG 419 Seventy-seven year old gentleman with a history of insulin requiring diabetes mellitus admitted to the hospital for evaluation of increasing abdominal girth and suspected hepatic cirrhosis. His medications included furosemide, spironolactone, and insulin.

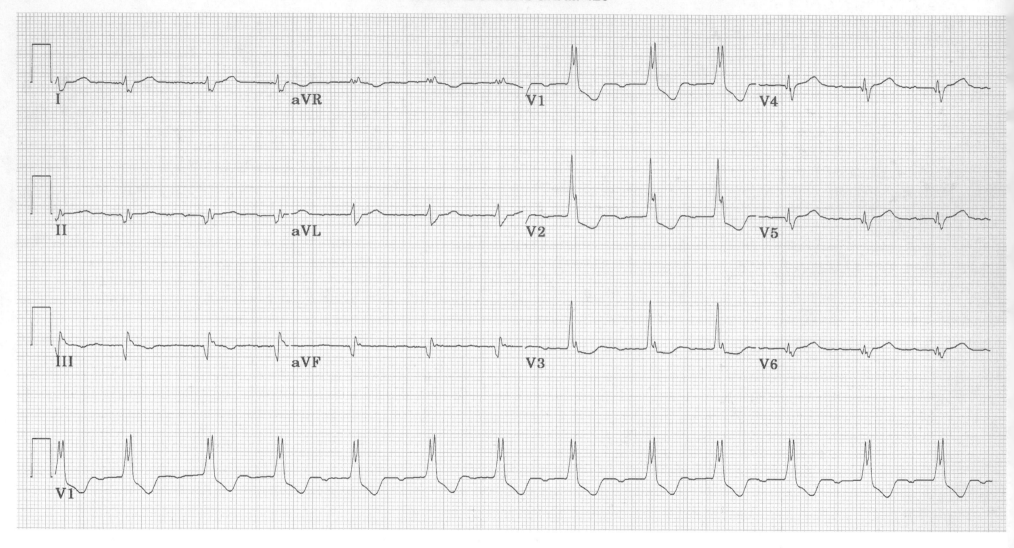

Interpretation Notes:

ECG 420 Seventy-nine year old gentleman status post coronary artery bypass graft surgery twice in the remote past, a prior myocardial infarction, and moderate left ventricular systolic dysfunction who re-presents to the hospital with recurrent angina pectoris. A subsequent cardiac catheterization demonstrated severe native coronary artery and graft vessel disease. This electrocardiogram was obtained prior to the patient undergoing his third open heart surgery procedure. Medications at the time of this electrocardiogram included aspirin, isosorbide mononitrate, and carvedilol.

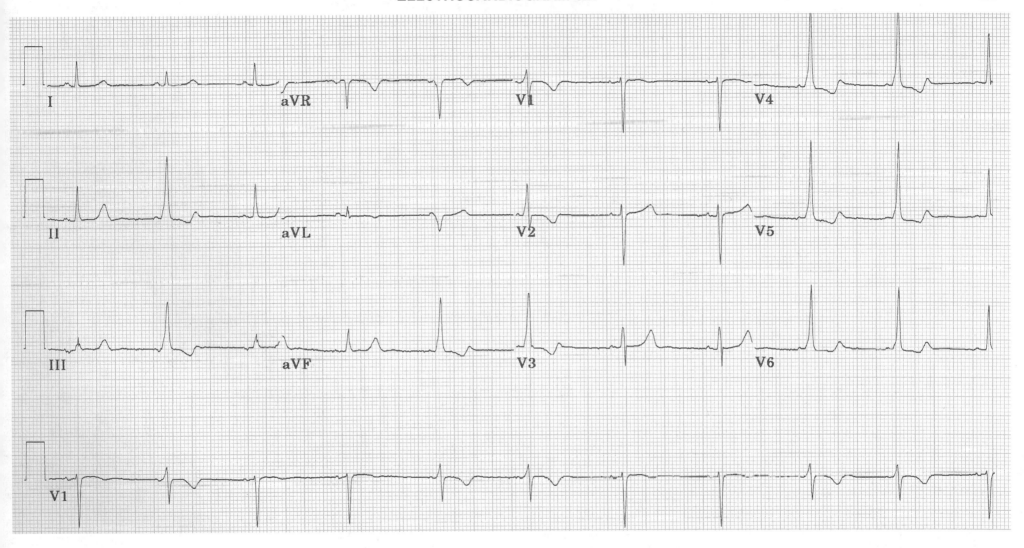

Interpretation Notes: _____

_____

ECG 421 Forty year old gentleman with infrequent palpitations whose routine electrocardiogram demonstrated the Wolff-Parkinson-White syndrome. He is referred by his local physician for further evaluation and possible treatment. Co-morbidities include hypertension. His medications included triamterene/hydrochlorothiazide and vitamins.

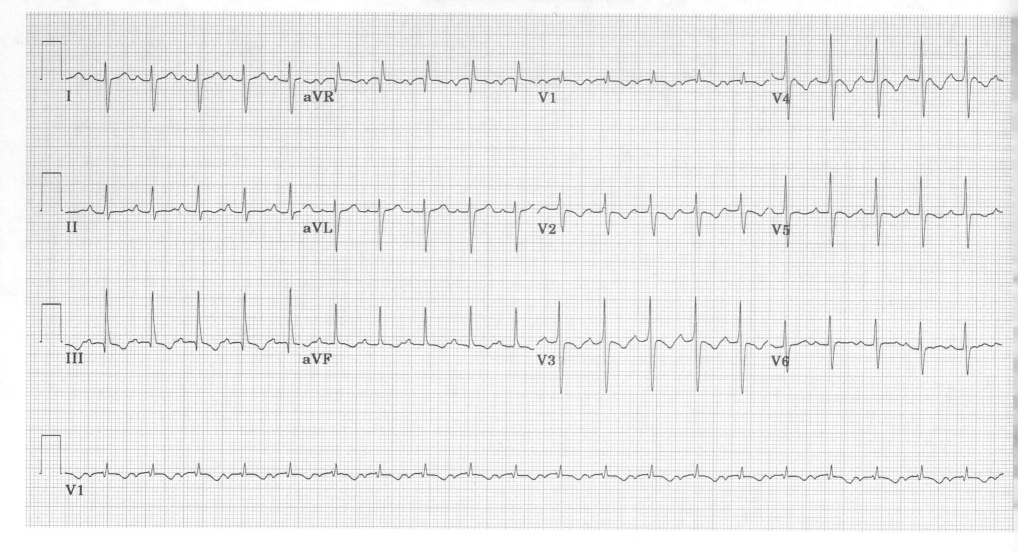

Interpretation Notes: _____

ECG 422 Twenty-two year old woman with primary pulmonary hypertension admitted for treatment of worsening right-sided congestive heart failure.

ELECTROCARDIOGRAM 423

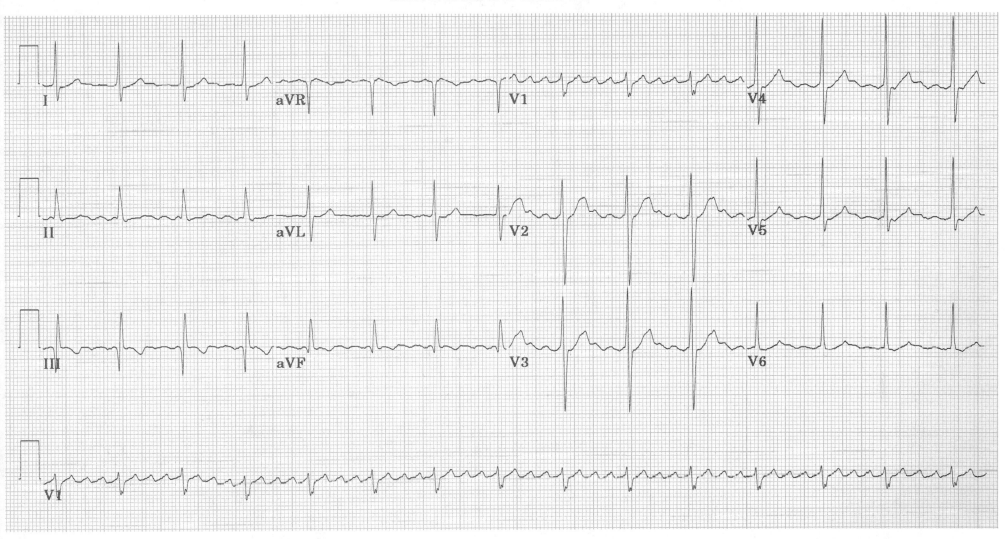

Interpretation Notes: _____

_____

ECG 423 Seventy-one year old gentleman with coronary artery disease status post coronary artery bypass graft surgery eight years prior to this electrocardiogram who is admitted for evaluation of recent syncope. A repeat cardiac catheterization demonstrated coronary artery disease progression. This patient underwent angioplasty of his right coronary artery and radiofrequency ablation of his atrial flutter.

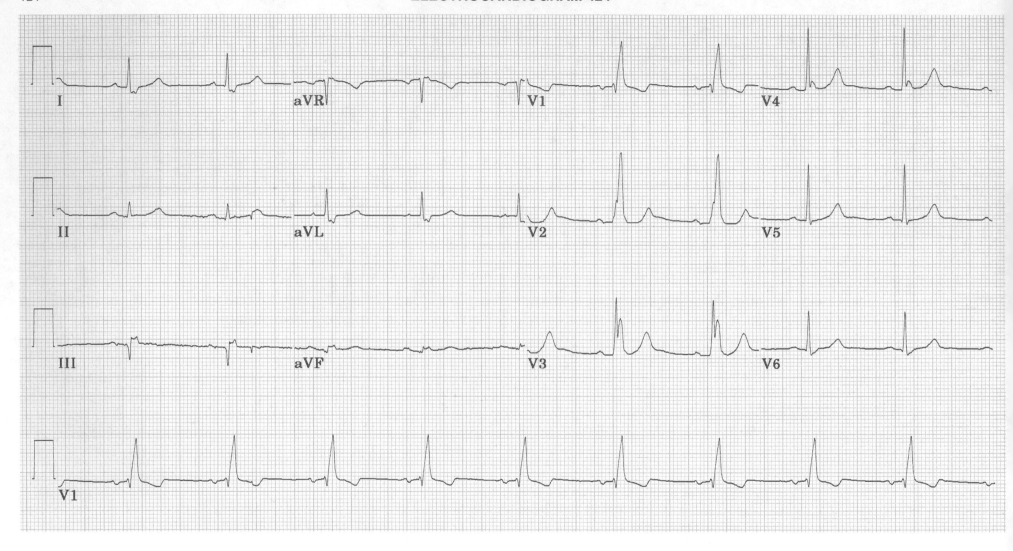

I aVR V1 V4

II aVL V2 V5

III aVF V3 V6

V1

Interpretation Notes: _____

ECG 424 Seventy-six year old gentleman with coronary artery disease status post remote coronary artery bypass surgery who now presents with acute onset chest discomfort. His past medical history includes hypertension, hyperlipidemia, and peptic ulcer disease. His medications included metoprolol, aspirin, ranitidine, and topical nitrates. A cardiac catheterization demonstrated advanced right coronary artery disease necessitating coronary artery stent placement.

ELECTROCARDIOGRAM 425

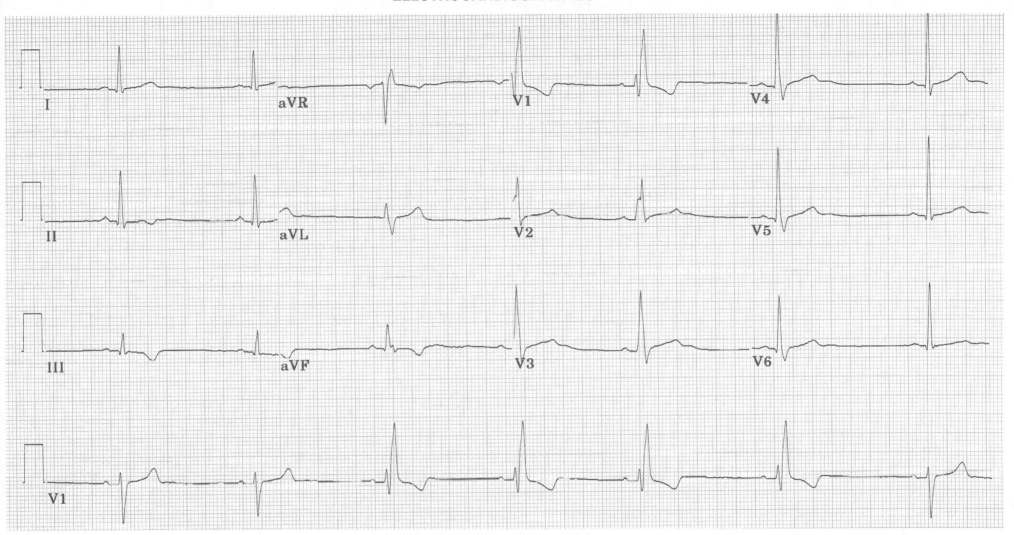

Interpretation Notes: _____

_____

ECG 425 Thirty-nine year old gentleman referred for a general physical examination. He has no known health problems with the exception of hyperlipidemia. He was on no medications.

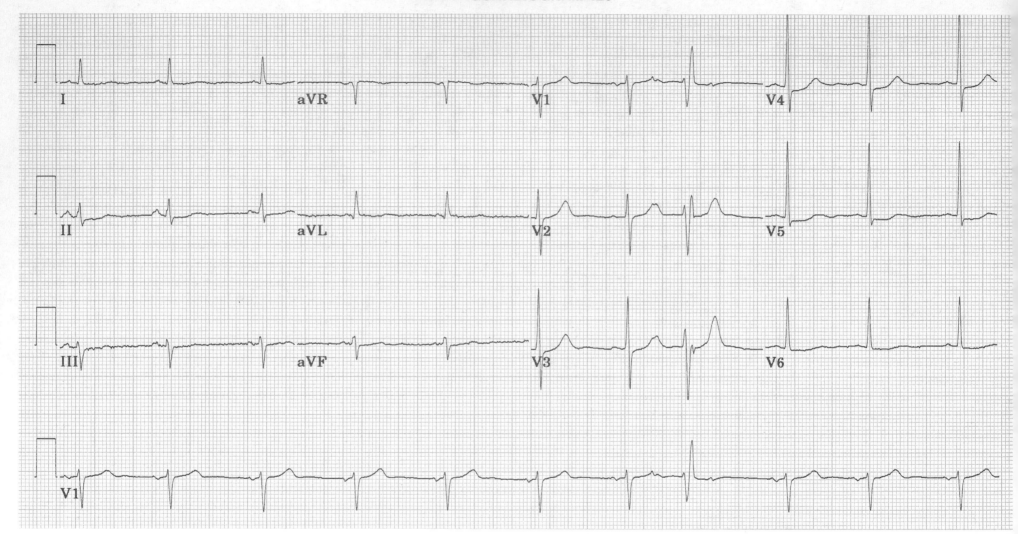

Interpretation Notes:_____

_____

_____

ECG 426 Seventy-five year old gentleman without a prior cardiac history self-referred for evaluation of chronic back pain.

ELECTROCARDIOGRAM 427

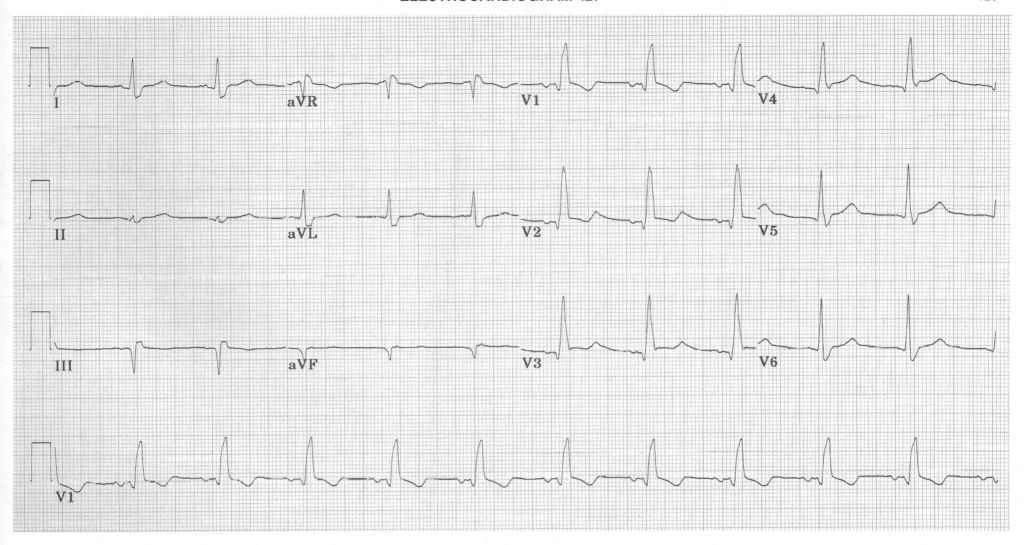

I aVR V1 V4

II aVL V2 V5

III aVF V3 V6

V1

Interpretation Notes: _____

_____

ECG 427 Sixty-eight year old gentleman with diffuse coronary artery obstructive disease and congestive heart failure who was found to have a significant amount of viable myocardium on a recent PET scan. He is now postoperative from coronary artery bypass graft surgery and a mitral valve repair.

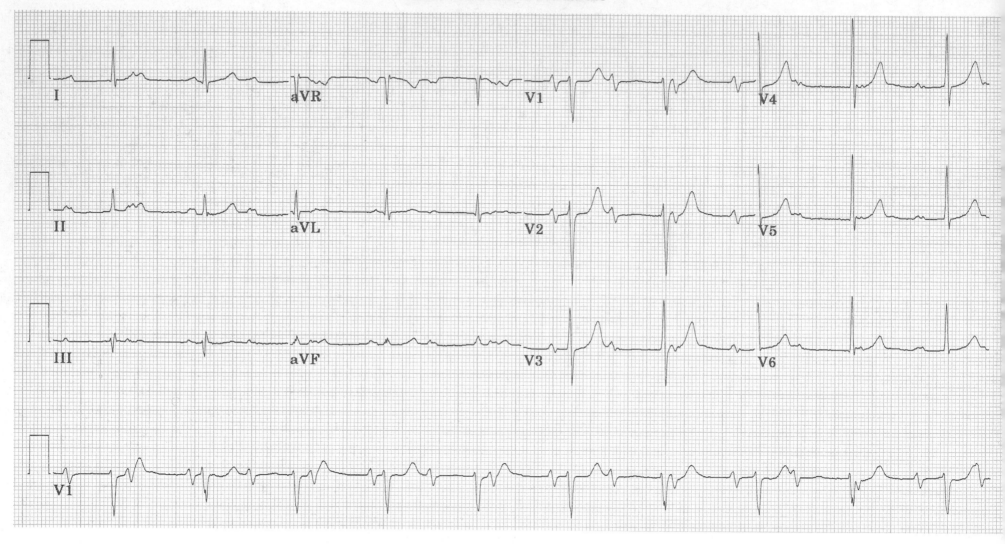

Interpretation Notes: _____

_____

ECG 428 Seventy-three year old gentleman with coronary artery disease who is status post four-vessel coronary artery bypass graft surgery two years prior to this electrocardiogram. He now returns for an outpatient cardiology follow-up evaluation. He has a history of a prior inferior myocardial infarction. Co-morbidities include non-insulin requiring diabetes mellitus. His medications included aspirin and vitamin E.

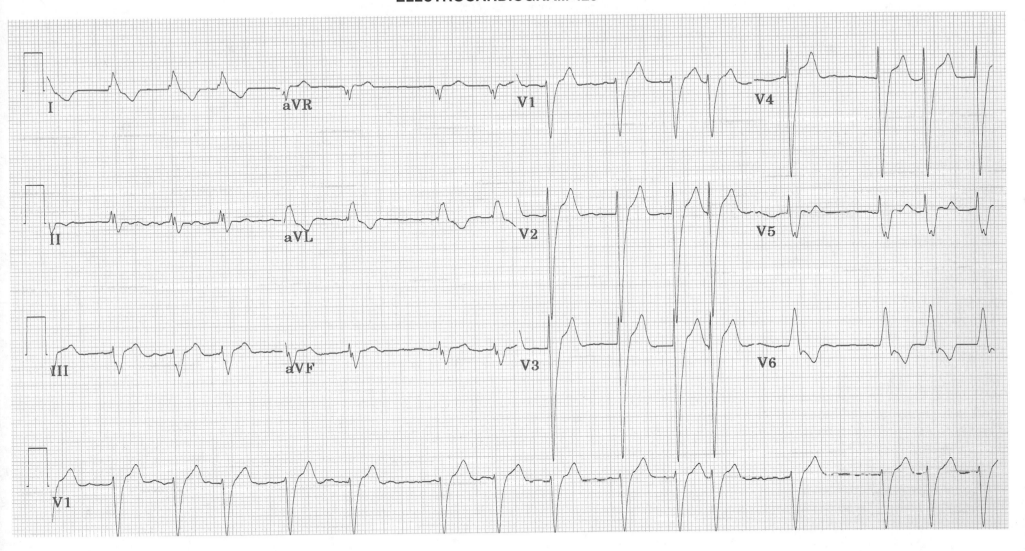

Interpretation Notes: _____

ECG 429 Forty-four year old man admitted to the hospital with worsening bilateral lower extremity edema. His past cardiac history includes aortic valve replacement secondary to severe aortic insufficiency and coronary artery bypass grafting two months prior to this electrocardiogram. He has moderately severe left ventricular systolic dysfunction and chronic atrial fibrillation. His medications at the time of this electrocardiogram included warfarin, digoxin, metoprolol, furosemide, lisinopril, and potassium.

ELECTROCARDIOGRAM 430

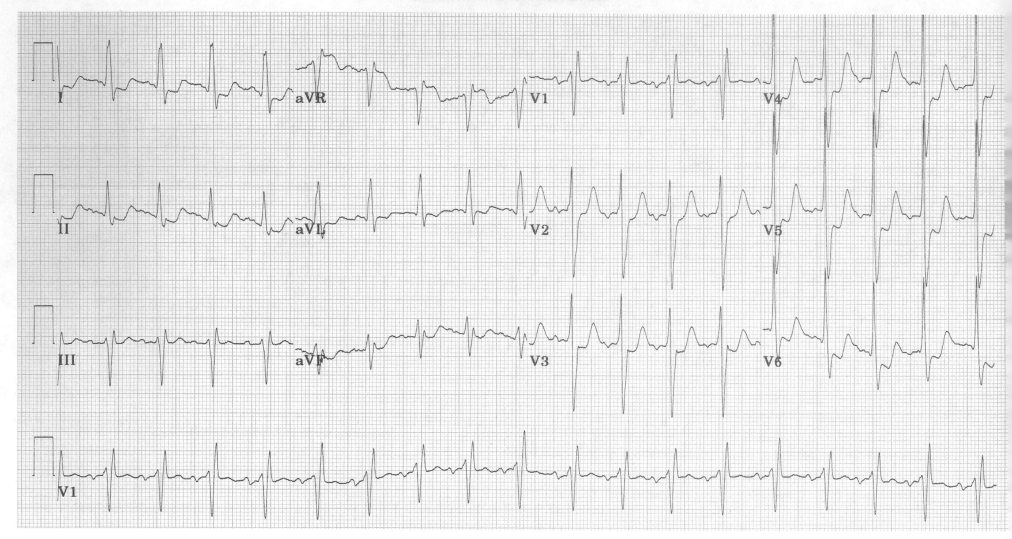

Interpretation Notes: _____

_____

ECG 430 Sixty-nine year old woman with a history of severe subaortic stenosis who presented to the hospital with a several day history of dyspnea consistent with congestive heart failure. A cardiac catheterization demonstrated a 100 mm Hg pressure gradient between the left ventricular outflow tract and the left ventricle. Her medications at the time of this electrocardiogram included diltiazem, furosemide, and doxazosin.

ELECTROCARDIOGRAM 431

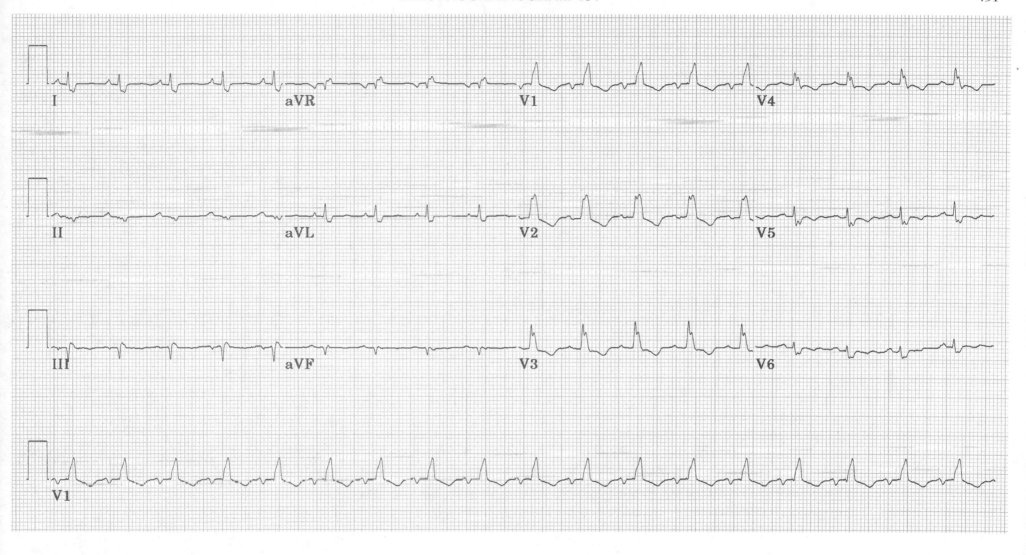

I   aVR   V1   V4

II   aVL   V2   V5

III   aVF   V3   V6

V1

Interpretation Notes: _____

_____

ECG 431 Sixty-three year old gentleman with constrictive pericarditis and coronary artery disease who is being seen preoperatively prior to planned pericardial stripping and coronary artery bypass graft surgery. His medications included lovastatin, aspirin, furosemide, and potassium.

432

ELECTROCARDIOGRAM 432

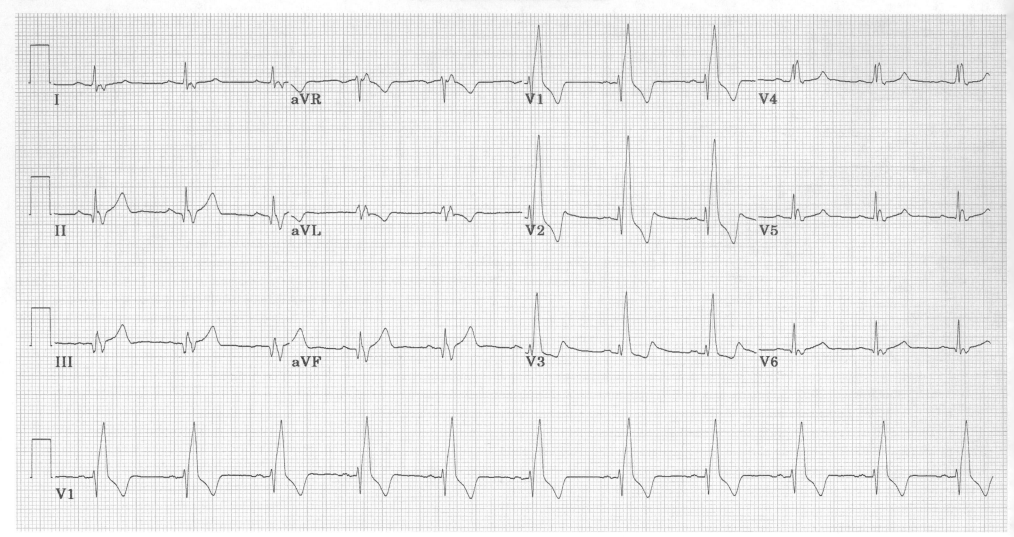

I   aVR   V1   V4

II   aVL   V2   V5

III   aVF   V3   V6

V1   V1

Interpretation Notes: _____

_____

ECG 432 Thirty year old gentleman with a history of Tetralogy of Fallot repaired at age seven who now returns for a follow-up evaluation. Co-morbidities include paroxysmal atrial flutter and paroxysmal atrial fibrillation. A recent echocardiogram demonstrated normal left ventricular systolic function and moderate right ventricular systolic dysfunction. His medications included atenolol, procainamide, and warfarin.

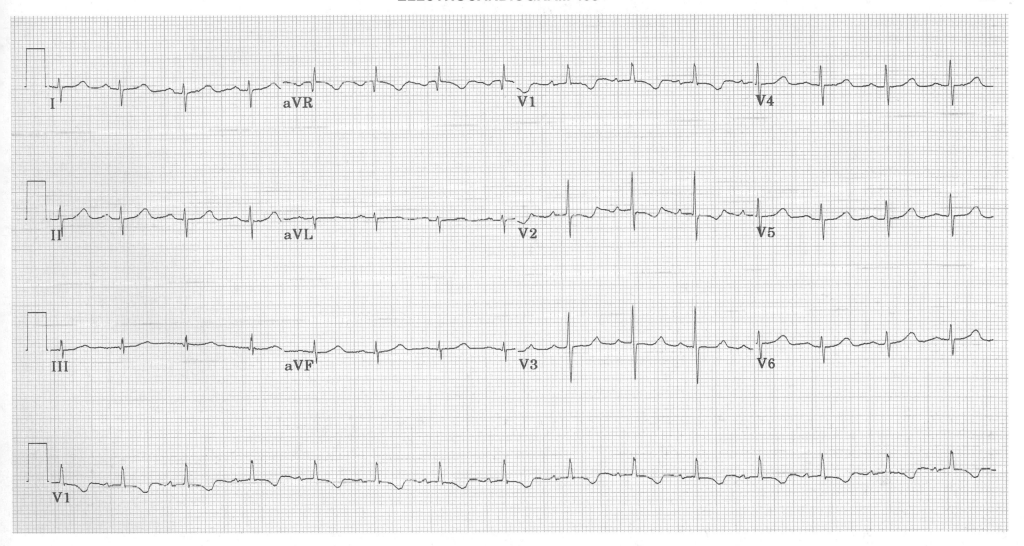

Interpretation Notes: _____

_____

ECG 433 Thirty year old woman with a history of primary pulmonary hypertension and a patent foramen ovale with a right-to-left interatrial shunt. Echocardiography demonstrated severe right ventricular systolic dysfunction. Her medications included intravenous epoprostenol, nebulized inhalers, and indapamide.

ELECTROCARDIOGRAM 434

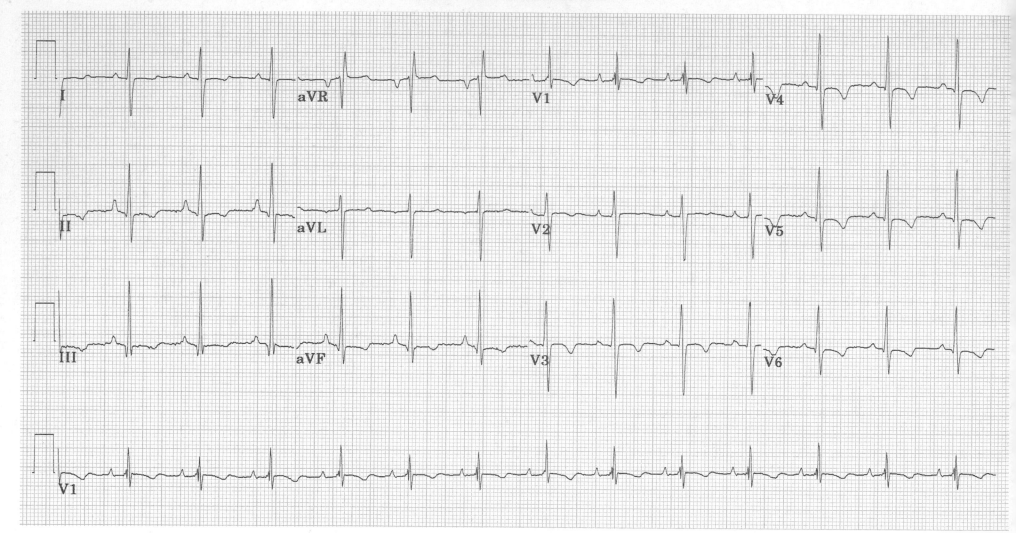

I aVR V1 V4

II aVL V2 V5

III aVF V3 V6

V1

Interpretation Notes: _____

_____

_____

ECG 434 Forty-eight year old gentleman with severe pulmonic stenosis who returns for an outpatient cardiac evaluation and consideration for cardiac surgery.

ELECTROCARDIOGRAM 435

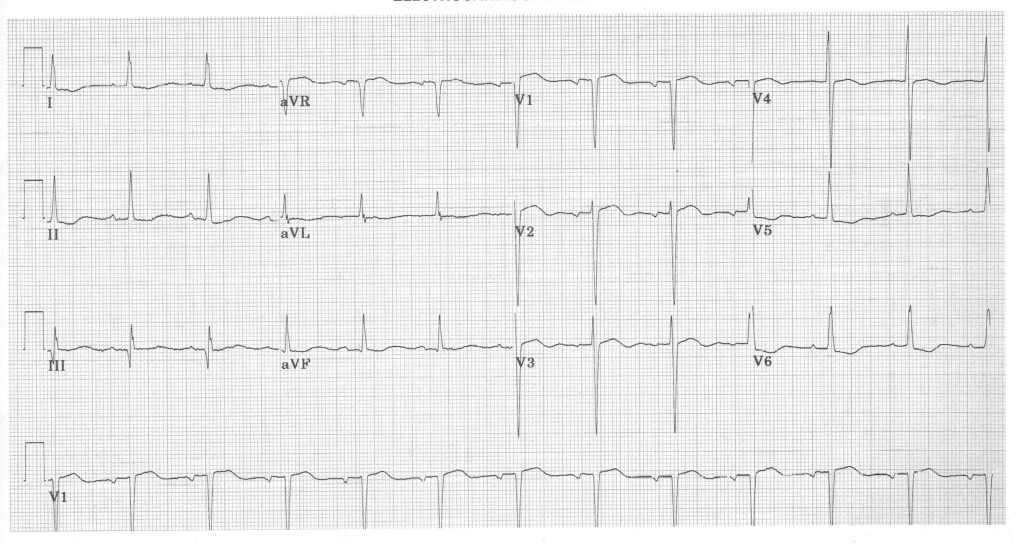

Interpretation Notes: _____

_____

ECG 435 Sixty-eight year old woman who presented to the hospital with angina pectoris in the setting of critical aortic stenosis. The patient underwent subsequent aortic valve replacement. Medications at the time of this electrocardiogram included digoxin, furosemide, potassium, and thyroxine.

ELECTROCARDIOGRAM 436

436

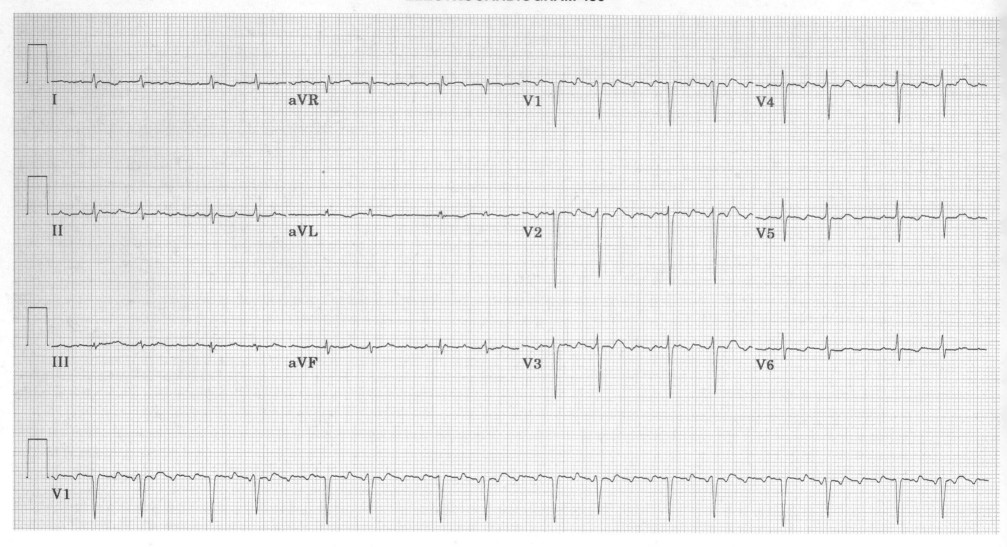

Interpretation Notes: _____

_____

_____

ECG 436 Sixty year old gentleman with two prior coronary artery bypass graft operations, constrictive pericarditis, and recurrent atrial arrhythmias who was scheduled for a near future radiofrequency ablation for persistent atrial flutter. His medications included nadolol, potassium, and furosemide.

ELECTROCARDIOGRAM 437

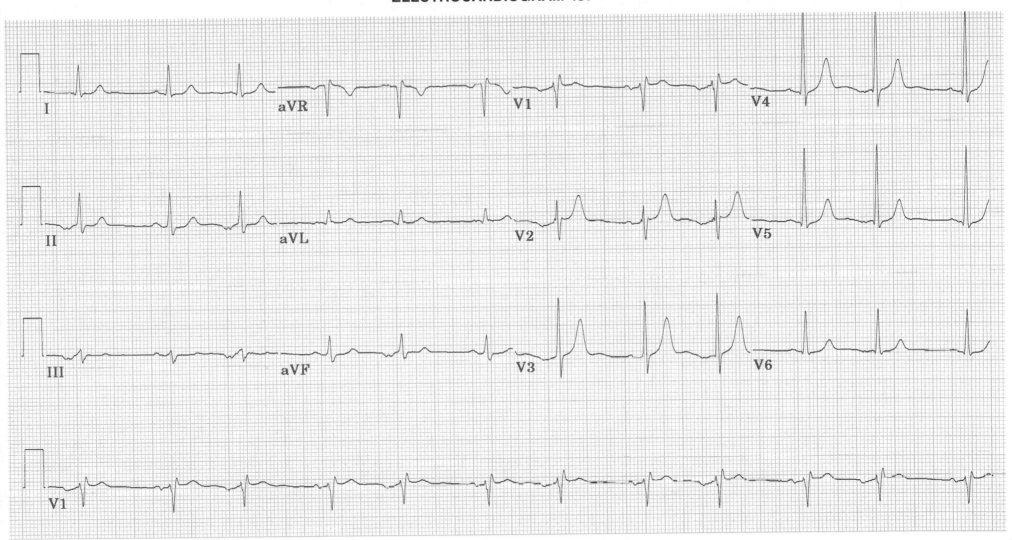

Interpretation Notes: _____

_____

_____

ECG 437 Sixty-six year old gentleman who is being seen in the preventive medicine department. He has no known health problems.

ELECTROCARDIOGRAM 438

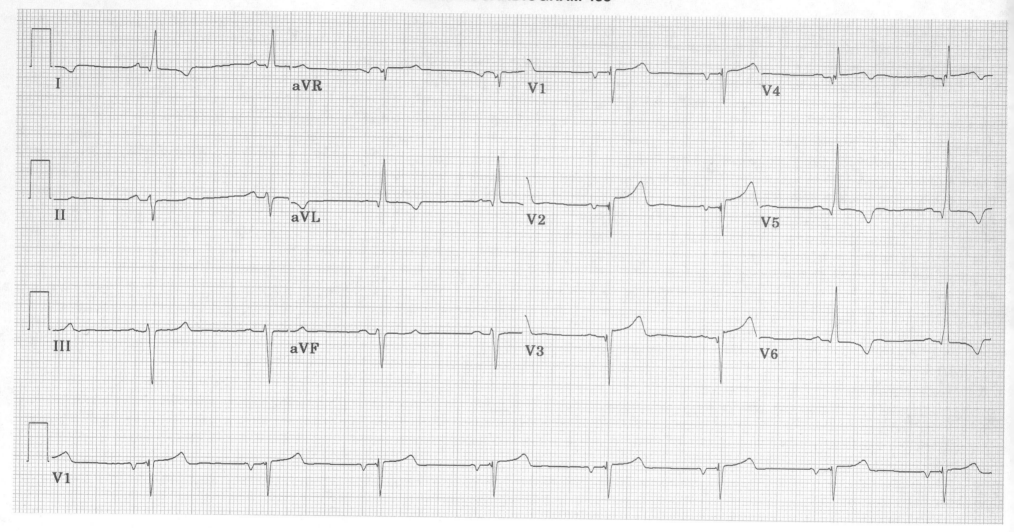

I	aVR	V1	V4
II	aVL	V2	V5
III	aVF	V3	V6
V1			

Interpretation Notes: _____

_____

ECG 438 Seventy-four year old gentleman status post a recent myocardial infarction referred for a second opinion. An echocardiogram demonstrated severe left ventricular systolic dysfunction involving the left anterior descending coronary artery territory. The ventricle was dilated but no aneurysm was seen. His medications included atenolol, enalapril, furosemide, aspirin, and warfarin.

ELECTROCARDIOGRAM 439

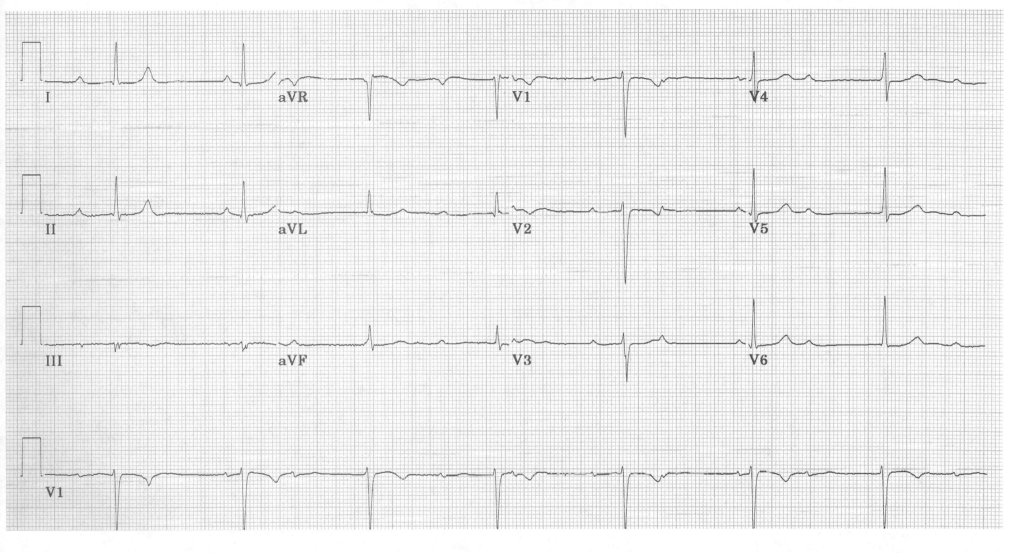

Interpretation Notes: _____

_____

_____

ECG 439 Twenty-nine year old woman thirty-seven weeks pregnant admitted to the hospital for close observation with pregnancy induced hypertension. She has known complete heart block without cardiovascular symptoms requiring no specific treatment or evaluation other than periodic holter monitoring.

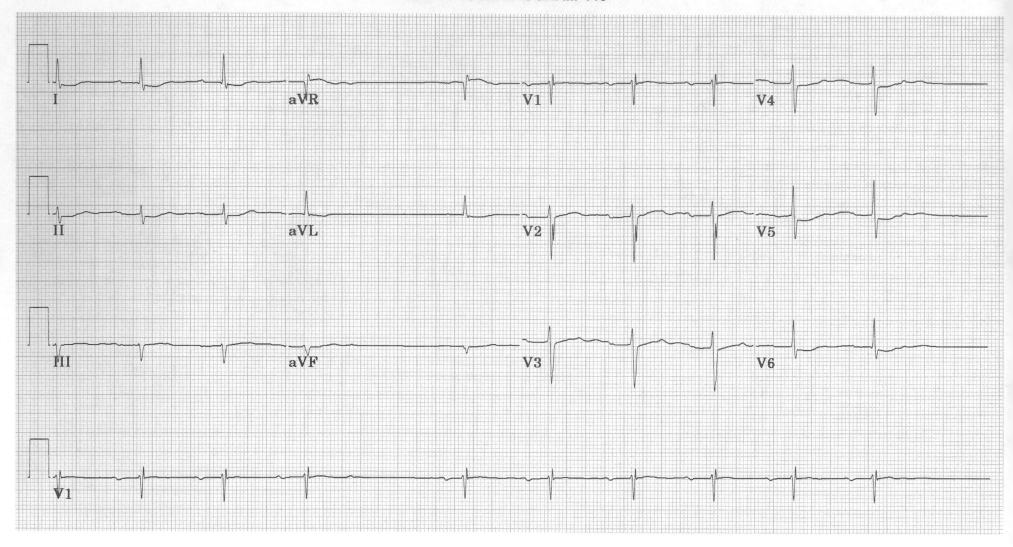

Interpretation Notes: _____

_____

_____

ECG 440 Sixty-six year old woman admitted to the hospital after a same day cardiac catheterization demonstrated severe three-vessel coronary artery obstructive disease. Her past history includes paroxysmal atrial fibrillation, rheumatic mitral stenosis, and esophageal spasm. Her medications included verapamil, digoxin, atorvastatin, ranitidine, and aspirin. Her serum potassium at the time of this electrocardiogram was 3.7 meq/L.

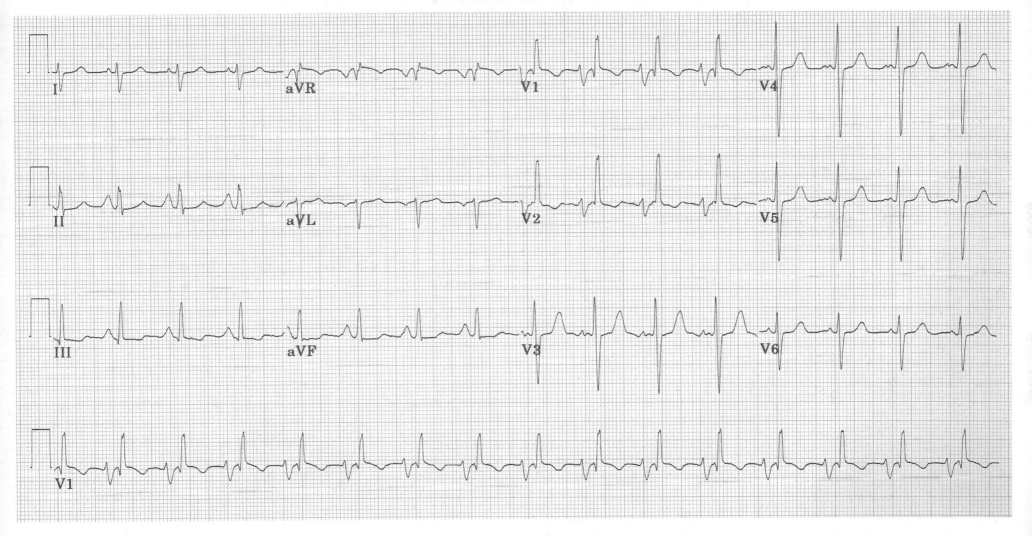

Interpretation Notes: _____

_____

ECG 441 Forty-eight year old gentleman with severe rheumatic mitral stenosis referred for mitral valve surgery. A recent echocardiogram demonstrated a dilated right ventricle with moderately severe right ventricular systolic dysfunction, severe tricuspid insufficiency, and severe pulmonary hypertension.

442

ELECTROCARDIOGRAM 442

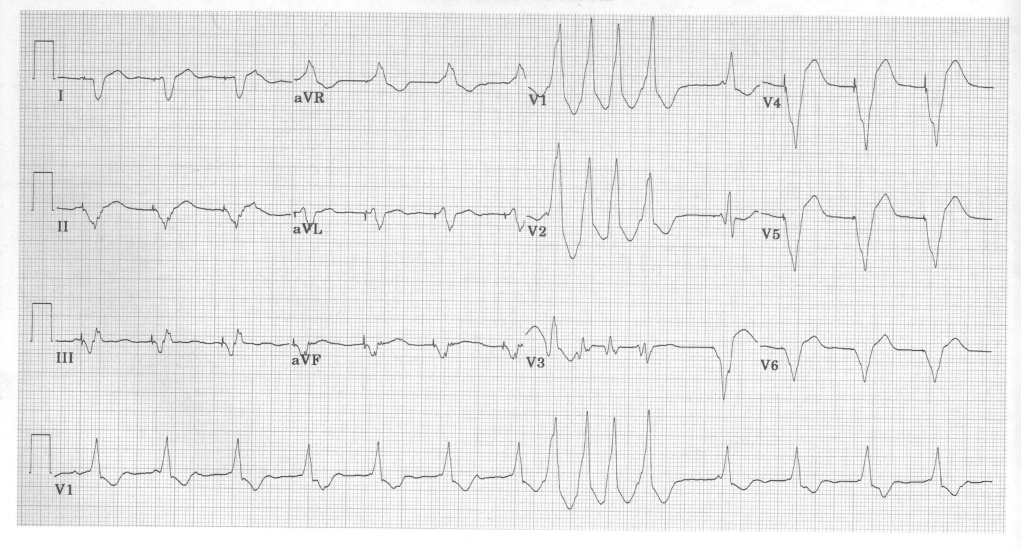

I aVR V1 V4

II aVL V2 V5

III aVF V3 V6

V1

Interpretation Notes: _____

ECG 442 Seventy-four year old woman with coronary artery disease and prior coronary artery bypass graft surgery who was urgently transferred from an outside hospital secondary to repeated implantable cardiac defibrillator discharges. The patient demonstrated drug refractory ventricular tachycardia and expired soon after hospital transfer.

ELECTROCARDIOGRAM 443

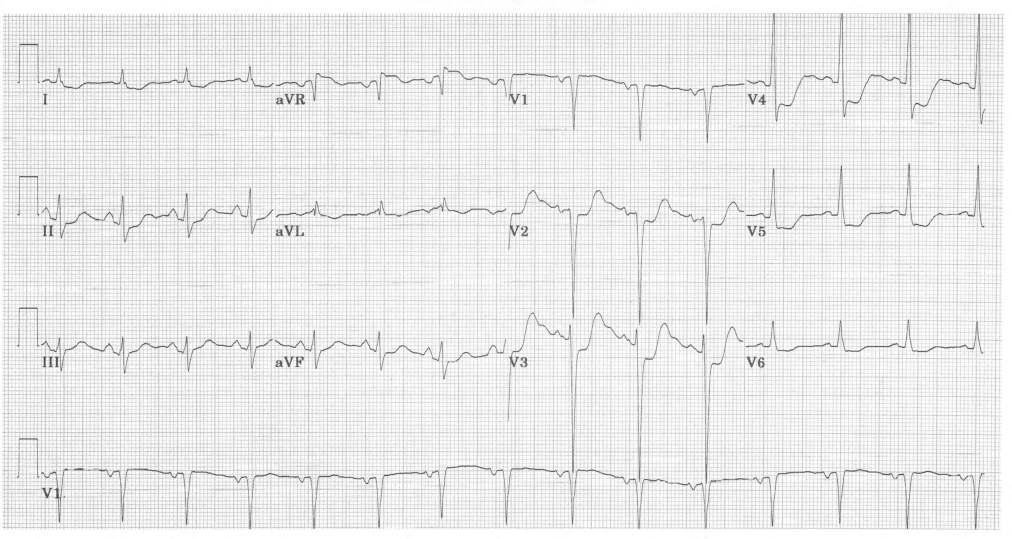

I aVR V1 V4

II aVL V2 V5

III aVF V3 V6

V1

Interpretation Notes: _____

_____

_____

ECG 443 Sixty-eight year old woman with coronary artery disease and prior coronary artery bypass graft surgery who re-presents to the outpatient clinic with a two week history of accelerating angina pectoris. Her medications included isosorbide dinitrate and quinidine. She was directly admitted to the hospital where a cardiac catheterization demonstrated severe multi-vessel coronary artery disease. The patient was referred for successful repeat coronary artery bypass graft surgery.

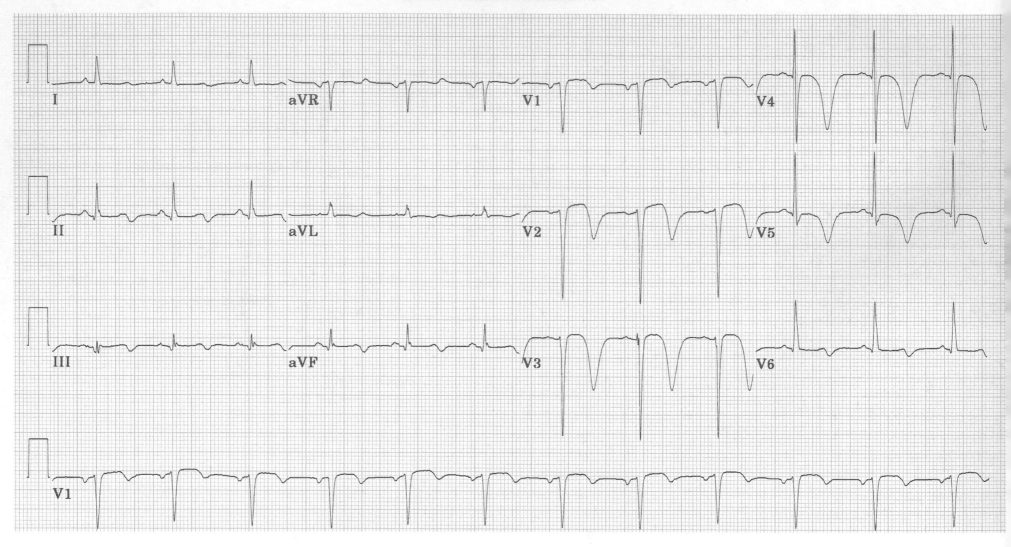

Interpretation Notes: _____

_____

_____

ECG 444 Fifty-one year old woman who presents acutely to the hospital with a chest discomfort syndrome. She underwent an urgent cardiac catheterization demonstrating a severe obstruction of the left anterior descending coronary artery. Percutaneous transluminal coronary angioplasty and stent placement was successfully performed. Serial cardiac enzymes were positive for acute myocardial injury.

ELECTROCARDIOGRAM 445

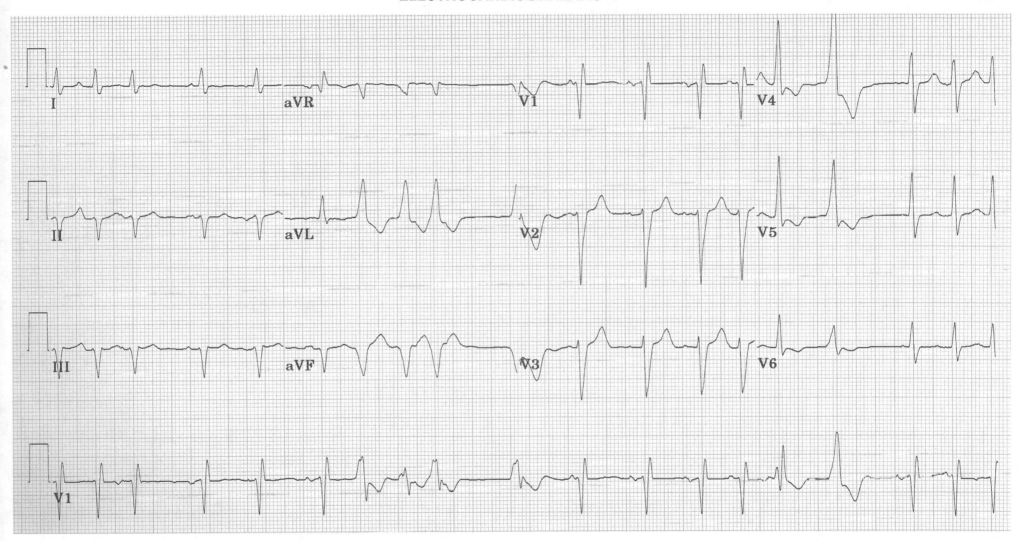

Interpretation Notes: _____

_____

ECG 445 Seventy-nine year old gentleman with severe aortic stenosis, chronic obstructive lung disease, and peripheral vascular disease admitted to the hospital with a congestive heart failure exacerbation. His medications included furosemide, digoxin, nebulized inhalers, and lisinopril.

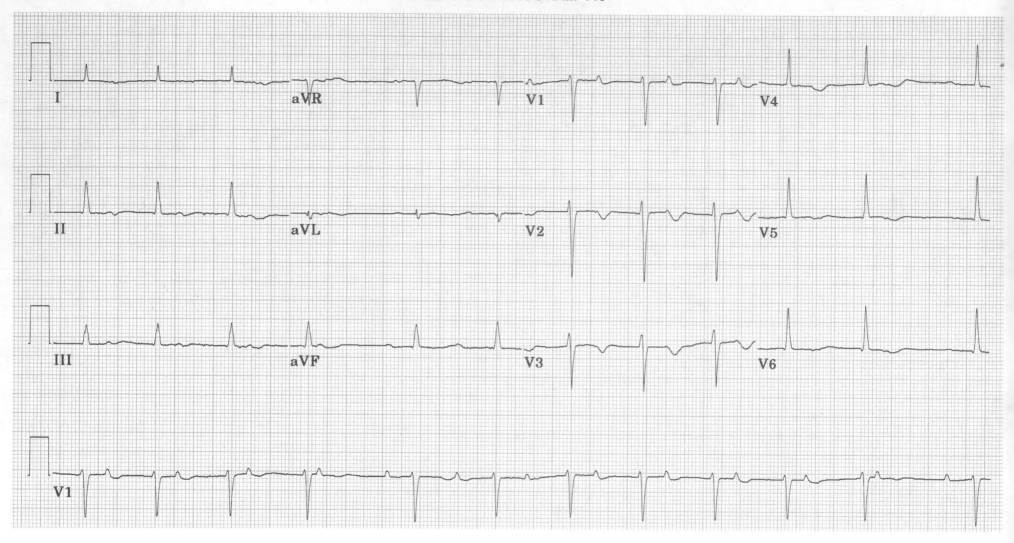

Interpretation Notes: _____

ECG 446 Seventy-three year old woman who is self-referred for cardiology follow-up in the presence of mild coronary artery disease. She remains active with a normal functional cardiac status. Her medications included gemfibrozil and quinidine.

ELECTROCARDIOGRAM 447

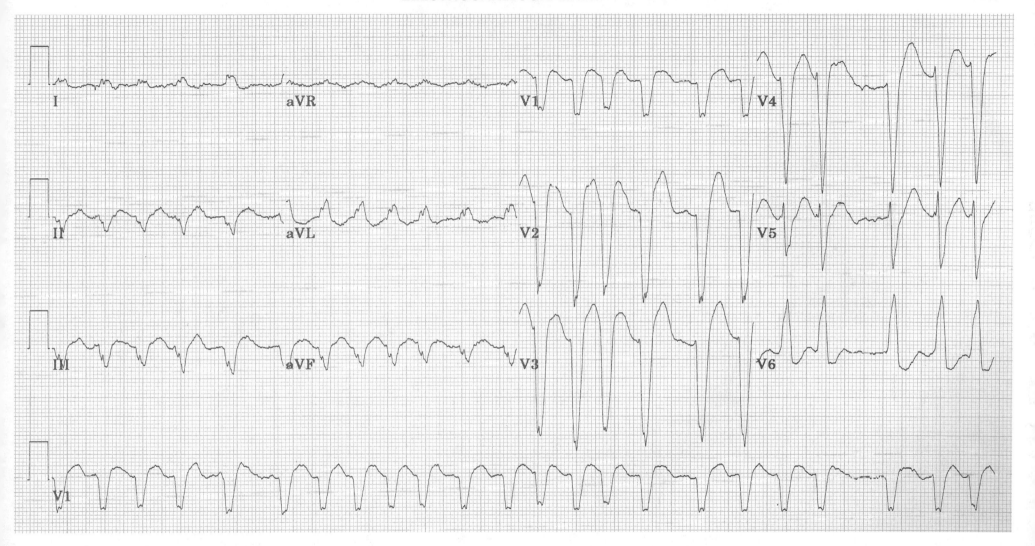

Interpretation Notes: _____

_____

ECG 447 Seventy-nine year old woman with a history of rectal carcinoma who is recently status post rectal surgery. Her past medical history includes a dilated cardiomy-opathy with severe global left ventricular systolic dysfunction, hypertension, and hypothyroidism.

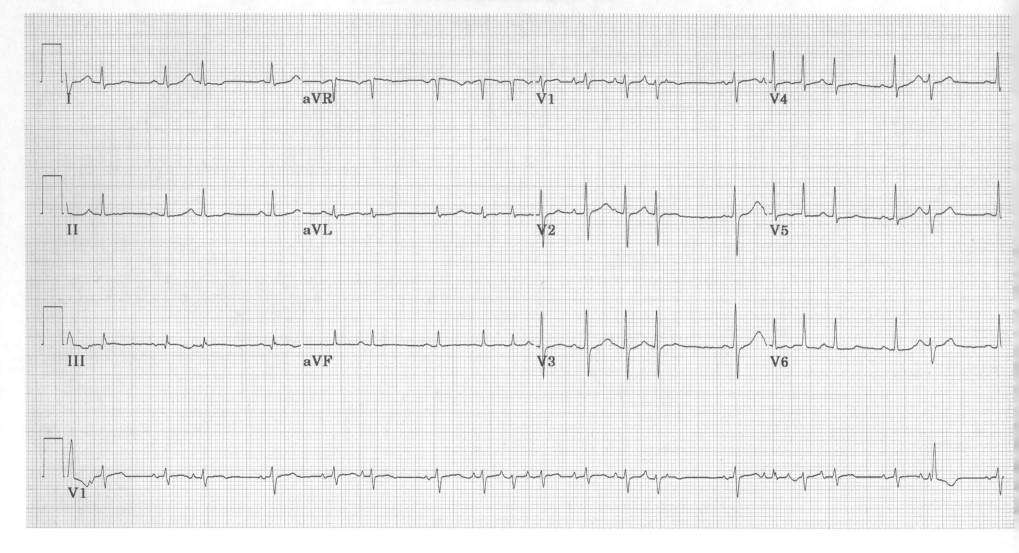

I   aVR   V1   V4

II   aVL   V2   V5

III   aVF   V3   V6

V1

Interpretation Notes: _____

ECG 448 Seventy-six year old woman with a history of endometrial carcinoma status post resection who is readmitted to the hospital with shortness of breath in the setting of lymphangitic pulmonary metastasis. She has had recurrent pleural effusions. Her past history includes paroxysmal atrial fibrillation. Her medications included aspirin, prednisone, atenolol, and hydrochlorothiazide.

ELECTROCARDIOGRAM 449

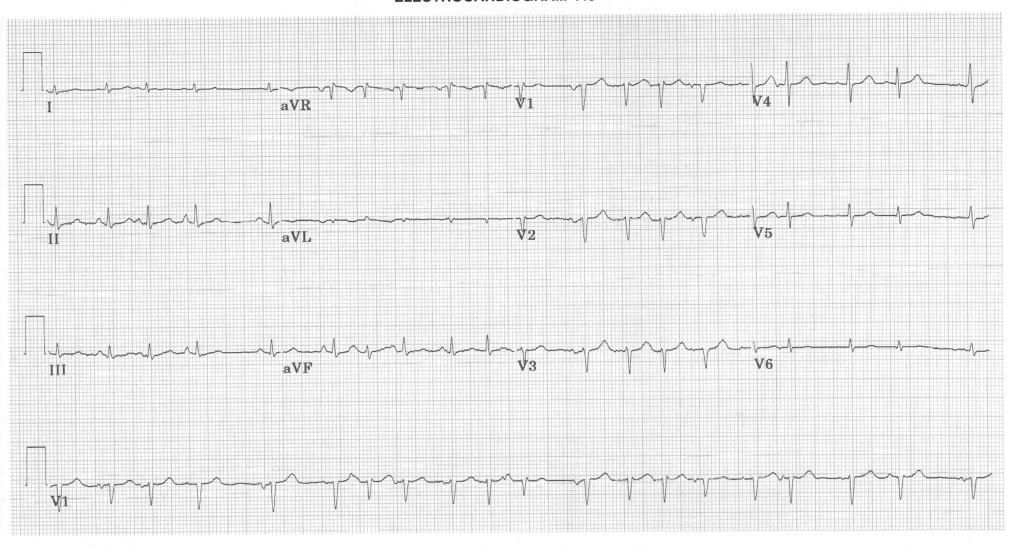

Interpretation Notes: _____

ECG 449 Seventy-two year old gentleman admitted to the hospital for further evaluation of an erythematous and bullous eruptive rash. His past medical history includes hypertension and chronic obstructive pulmonary disease for which he takes prednisone and numerous inhalers.

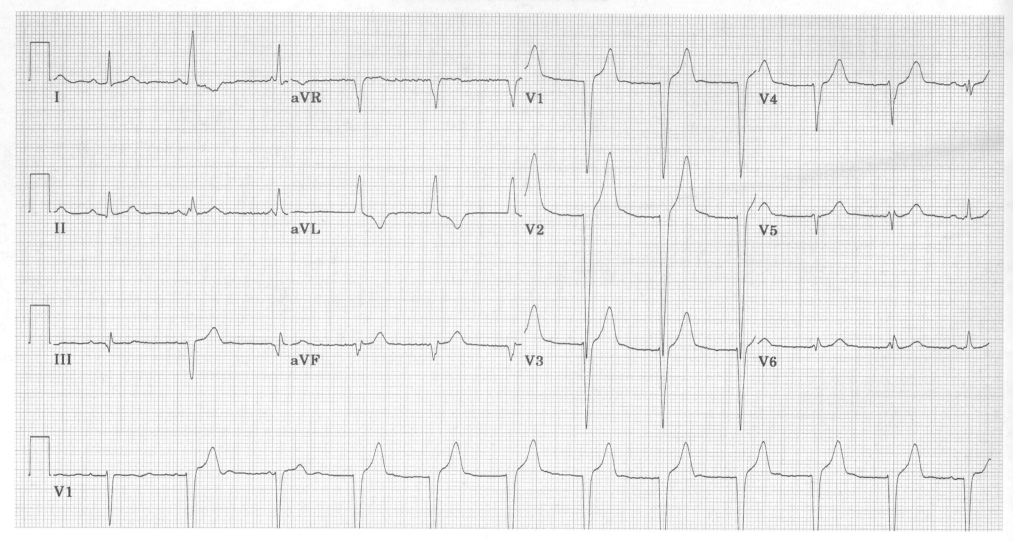

Interpretation Notes:_____

_____

ECG 450 Forty-seven year old woman who is admitted acutely to the hospital with mental status changes. A CT scan confirmed a subarachnoid hemorrhage and the patient subsequently underwent cerebral aneurysm clip placement.

ELECTROCARDIOGRAM 451

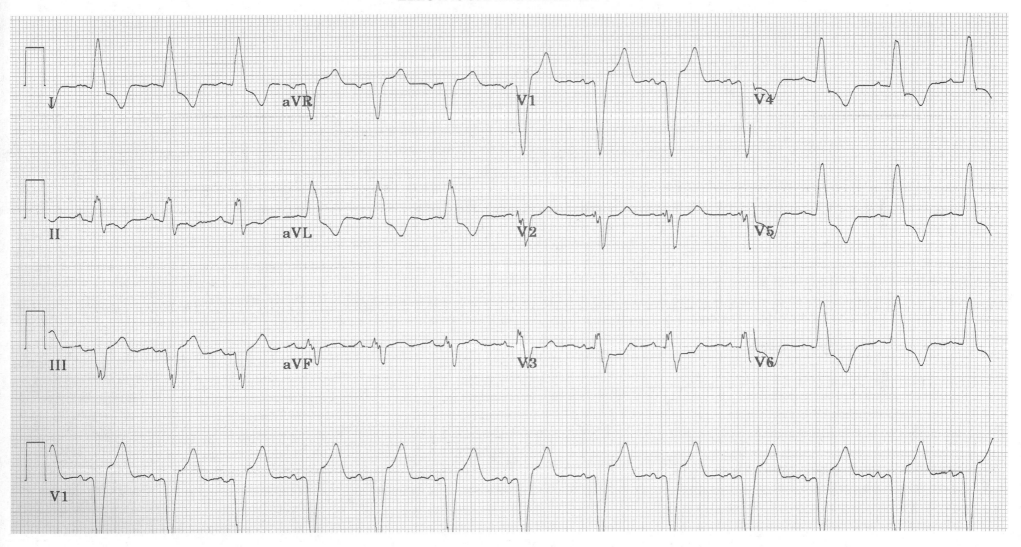

Interpretation Notes:_____

_____

_____

ECG 451 Seventy-two year old woman admitted acutely to the hospital for treatment of congestive heart failure. Her past cardiac history includes hypertrophic obstructive cardiomyopathy and paroxysmal atrial fibrillation. Her medications at the time of this electrocardiogram included sotalol and warfarin.

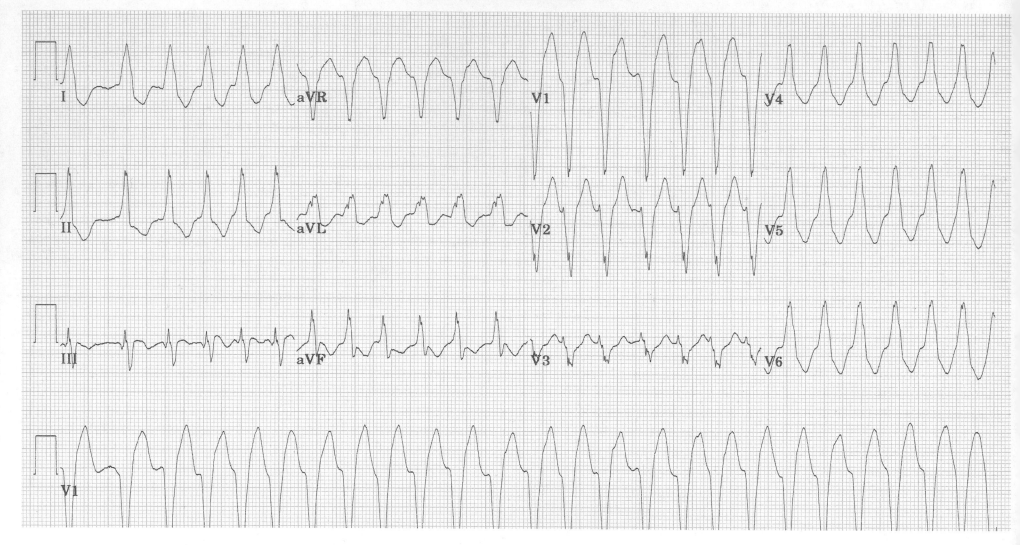

I aVR V1 V4

II aVL V2 V5

III aVF V3 V6

V1

Interpretation Notes: _____
_____
_____

ECG 452 Seventy-two year old woman admitted acutely to the hospital for treatment of paroxysmal atrial fibrillation. Her past cardiac history includes hypertrophic obstructive cardiomyopathy. Her medications at the time of this electrocardiogram included sotalol and warfarin.

ELECTROCARDIOGRAM 453

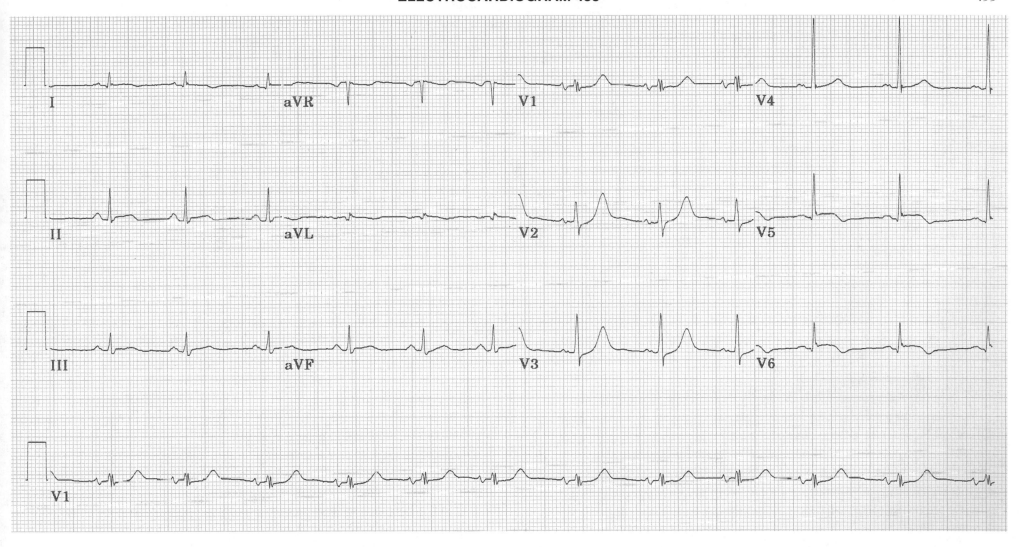

I aVR V1 V4

II aVL V2 V5

III aVF V3 V6

V1

Interpretation Notes:_____

_____

ECG 453 Sixty-seven year old woman accepted in hospital transfer after the sudden onset of acute chest discomfort and the accompanying electrocardiogram. A cardiac catheterization performed five days following this electrocardiogram demonstrated a severe proximal left circumflex coronary artery stenosis with an ulcerated plaque. This was successfully dilated by percutaneous transluminal coronary angioplasty.

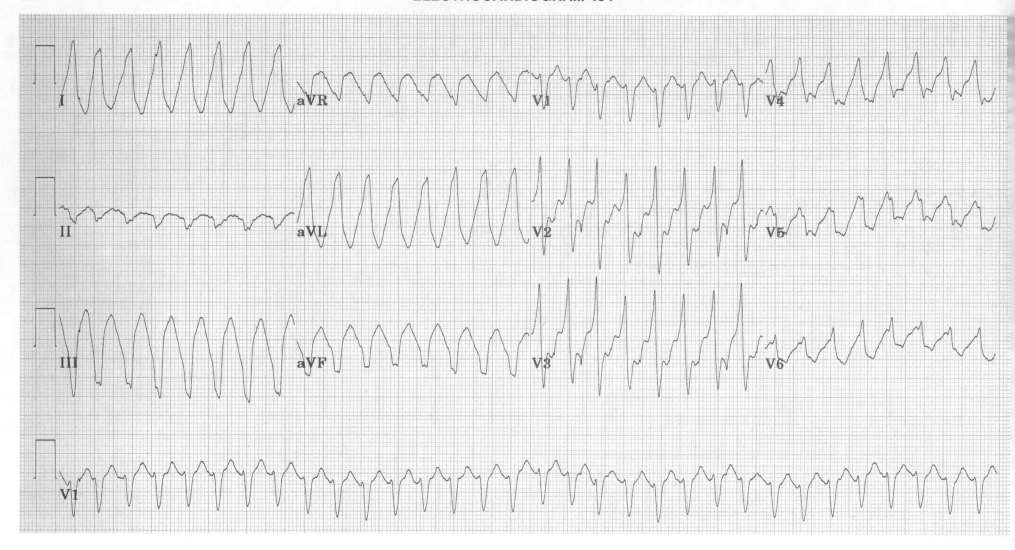

Interpretation Notes: _____

_____

_____

ECG 454 Eighty-two year old gentleman admitted to the hospital with acute pneumonia who was accepted in transfer to the coronary care unit for evaluation of suspected ventricular tachycardia. The patient has coronary artery disease status post coronary artery bypass graft surgery sixteen and three years prior to this electrocardiogram. Medications at the time of this electrocardiogram included amiodarone, atorvastatin, digoxin, topical nitroglycerin, and intravenous antibiotics.

ELECTROCARDIOGRAM 455

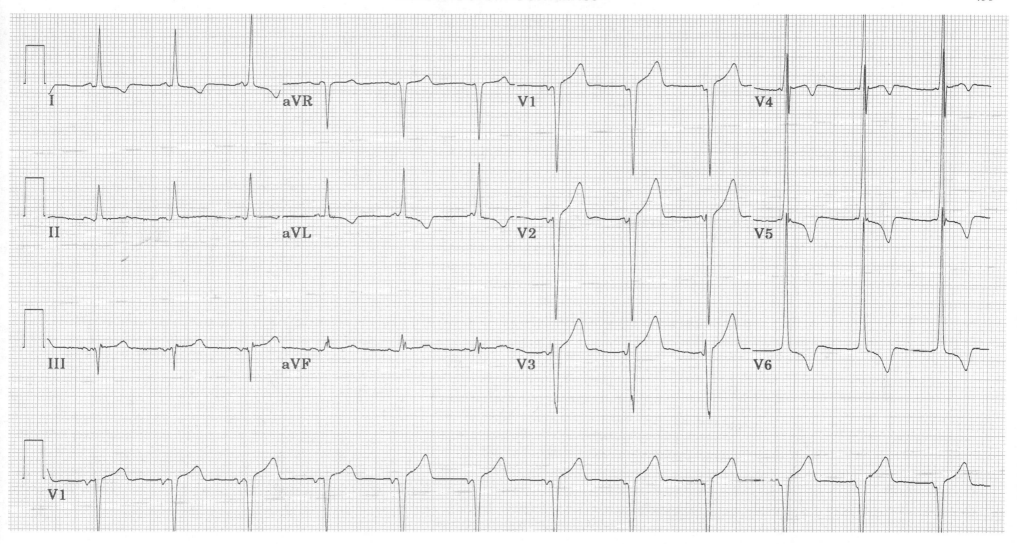

Interpretation Notes: _____

_____

ECG 455 Seventy-eight year old woman two days status post aortic valve replacement for severe aortic stenosis and multi-vessel coronary artery bypass grafting.

ELECTROCARDIOGRAM 456

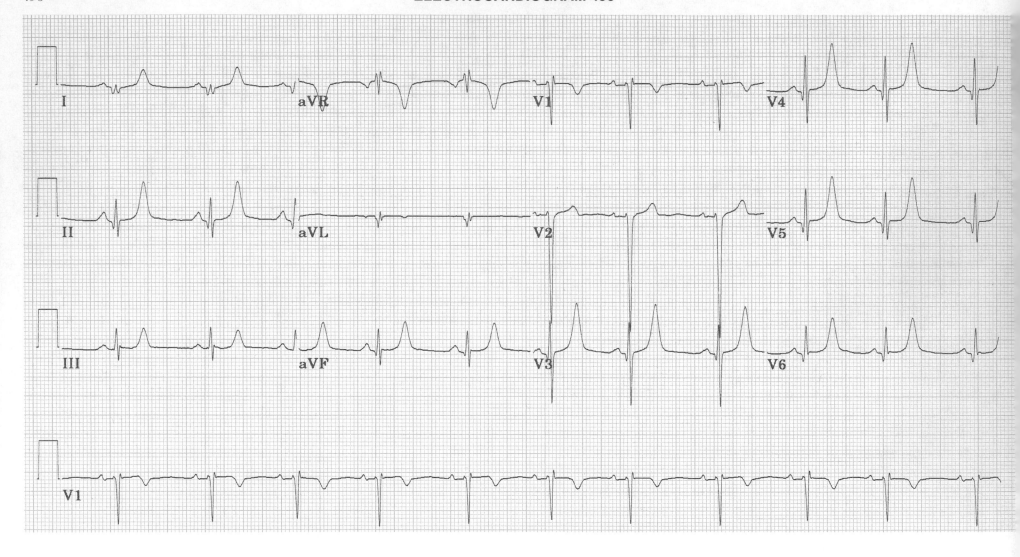

Interpretation Notes: _____

_____

_____

ECG 456 Thirty-one year old woman with hypertrophic obstructive cardiomyopathy who returns for a follow-up outpatient cardiac evaluation. She is currently without symptoms.

ELECTROCARDIOGRAM 457

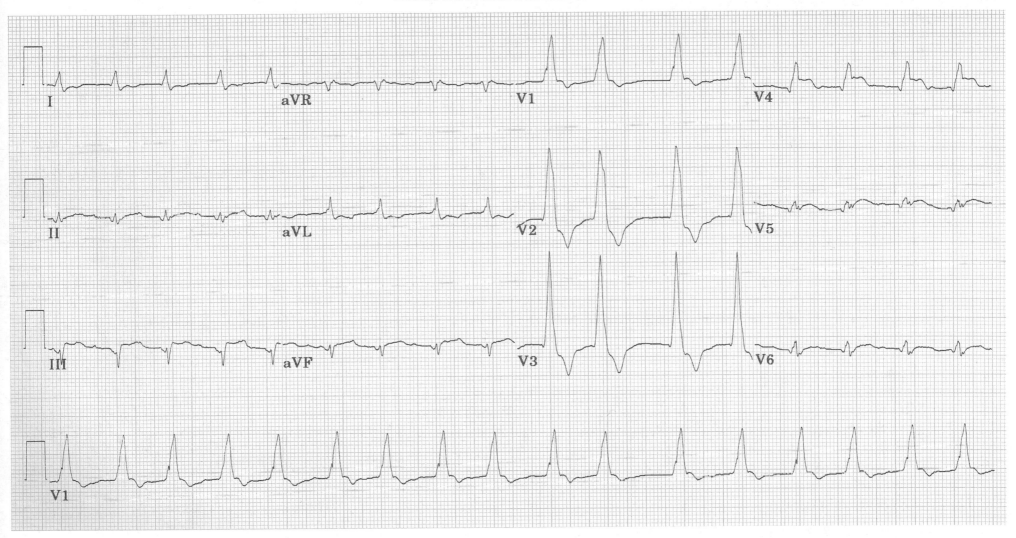

I   aVR   V1   V4

II   aVL   V2   V5

III   aVF   V3   V6

V1

Interpretation Notes: _____

_____

ECG 457 Eighty-four year old gentleman accepted in urgent hospital transfer after a cardiac arrest and successful resuscitation by paramedics. His past cardiac history includes severe three vessel coronary artery disease and mitral insufficiency. He is status post multi-vessel coronary artery bypass graft surgery and mitral valve replacement five years prior to this electrocardiogram. Medications at the time of this electrocardiogram included digoxin, furosemide, and aspirin.

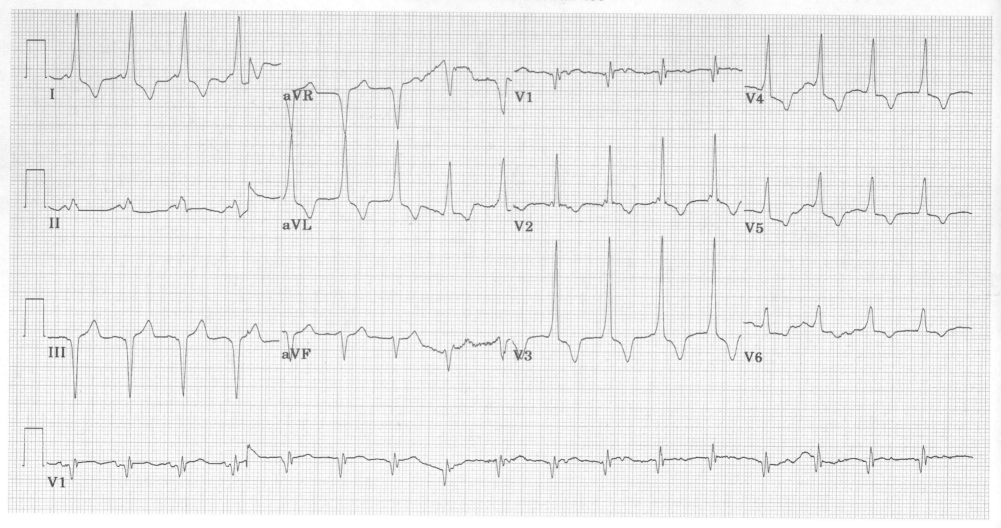

Interpretation Notes: _____

_____

_____

ECG 458 Sixty-one year old gentleman status post a prior myocardial infarction of unknown location who underwent coronary artery bypass graft surgery ten years before this electrocardiogram. He now re-presents to the outpatient cardiology clinic for evaluation of recent onset palpitations. A cardiac catheterization performed two years prior to this electrocardiogram demonstrated occlusions of several bypass grafts with normal left ventricular systolic function and mild inferior hypokinesis. Medications at the time of this tracing included lovastatin, nifedipine, isosorbide mononitrate, and aspirin.

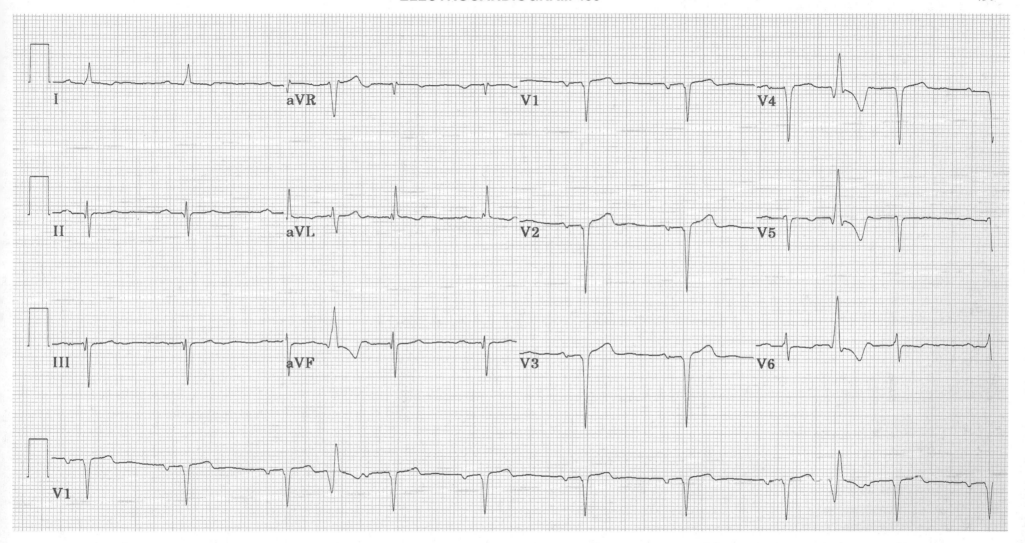

Interpretation Notes:_____

ECG 459 Fifty-three year old gentleman with diffuse coronary artery disease status post inferior and anterior myocardial infarctions fifteen years prior to this electrocardiogram who returns for routine cardiology follow-up. Subsequent to the myocardial infarctions the patient underwent ventricular aneurysmectomy. He continued with symptoms of stable angina pectoris in the setting of mild mitral insufficiency and moderate left ventricular systolic dysfunction. His medications included digoxin, furosemide, and captopril.

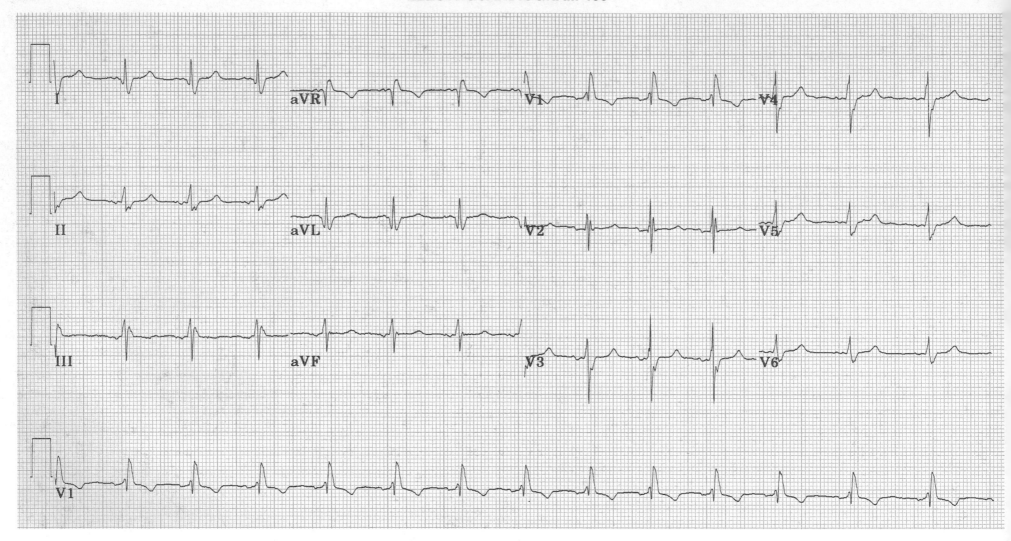

Interpretation Notes: _____

_____

ECG 460 Sixty-seven year old gentleman with a prior myocardial infarction who presents for cardiology follow-up. His medications included nifedipine and aspirin. A recent cardiac catheterization demonstrated akinesis of the anterior and anterolateral segments with significant left anterior descending coronary artery obstructive disease.

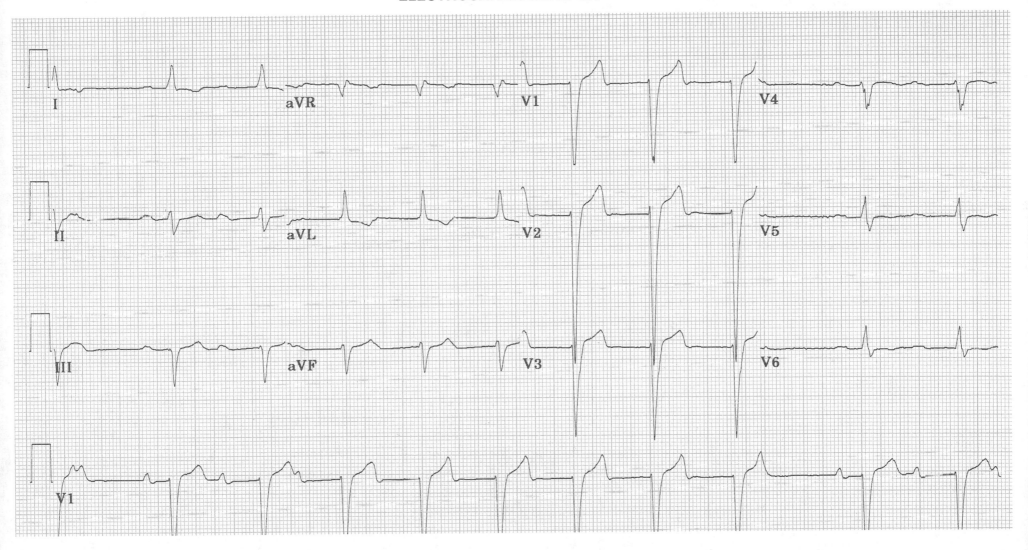

Interpretation Notes: _____

ECG 461 Seventy-three year old gentleman with coronary artery disease and severe ischemic left ventricular systolic dysfunction who returns for a follow-up evaluation of recurrent congestive heart failure. Co-morbidities include hypercholesterolemia, insulin requiring diabetes mellitus, hypertension, and peripheral vascular disease. Medications at the time of this electrocardiogram included thyroxine, metolazone, digoxin, furosemide, captopril, and procainamide.

462

ELECTROCARDIOGRAM 462

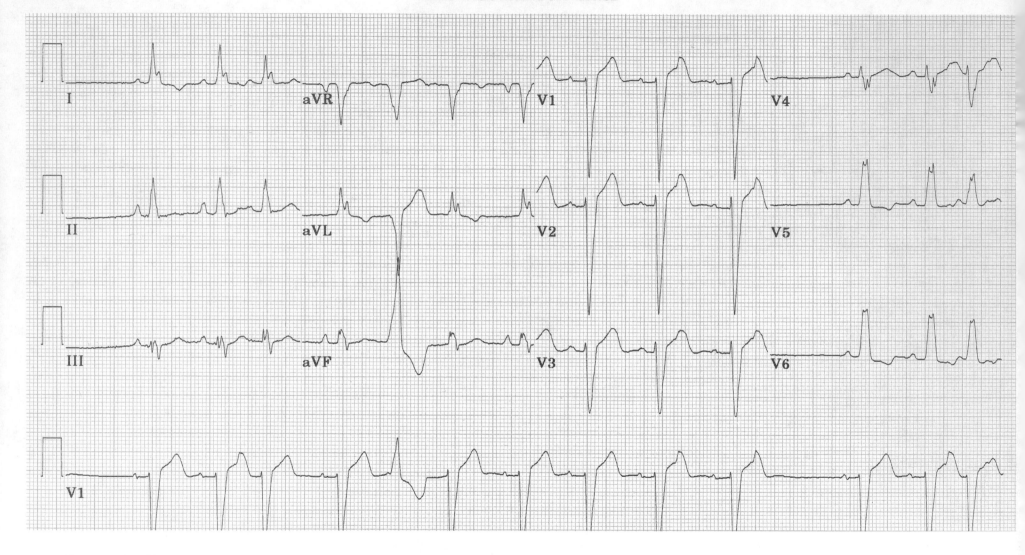

Interpretation Notes: _____

_____

_____

ECG 462 Forty-nine year old woman who presents acutely to the emergency room with shortness of breath and palpitations of two weeks duration. Her past medical history includes sleep apnea, rheumatoid arthritis, and Graves' disease. Her medications included thyroxine, clonidine, prednisone, and premarin.

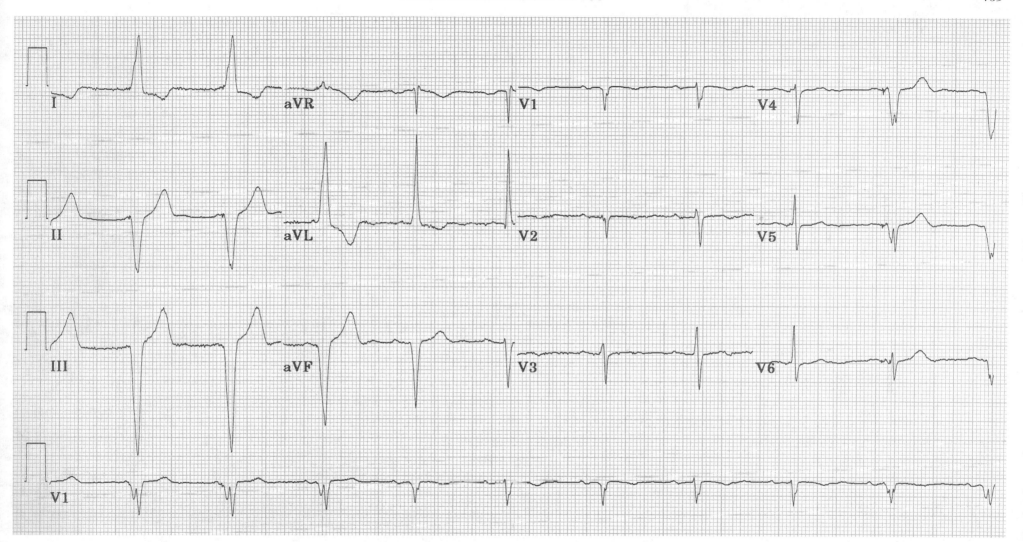

I aVR V1 V4

II aVL V2 V5

III aVF V3 V6

V1

Interpretation Notes: _____

_____

_____

ECG 463 Eighty-six year old woman with a recent cerebrovascular accident status post ventricular pacemaker placement secondary to recurrent atrial arrhythmias and the sick sinus syndrome.

464

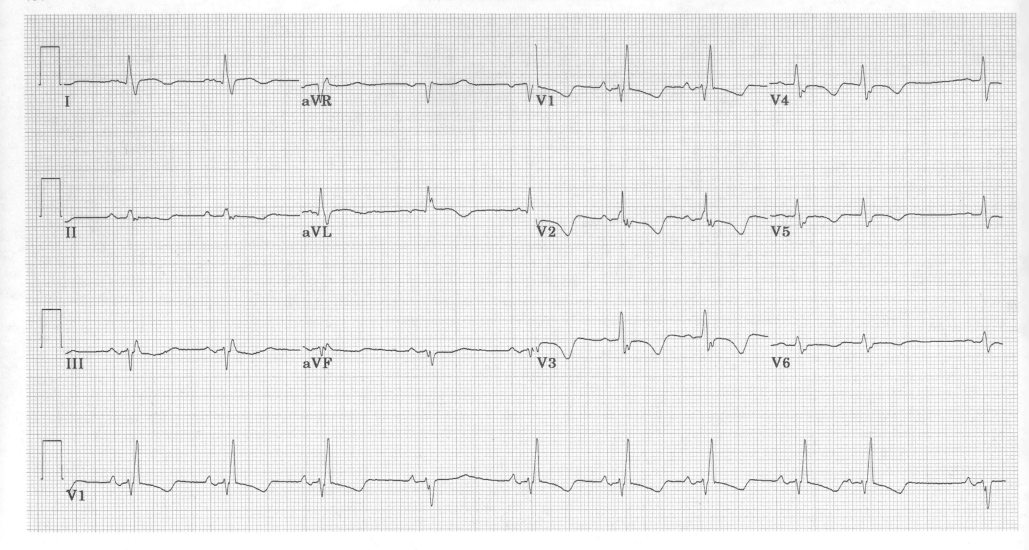

Interpretation Notes: _____

ECG 464 Eighty-one year old gentleman with a history of hypertensive heart disease and severe left ventricular hypertrophy who is admitted to the hospital for further evaluation of recurrent ventricular tachycardia and suspected congestive heart failure. His medications included amiodarone, furosemide, warfarin, and lisinopril.

ELECTROCARDIOGRAM 465

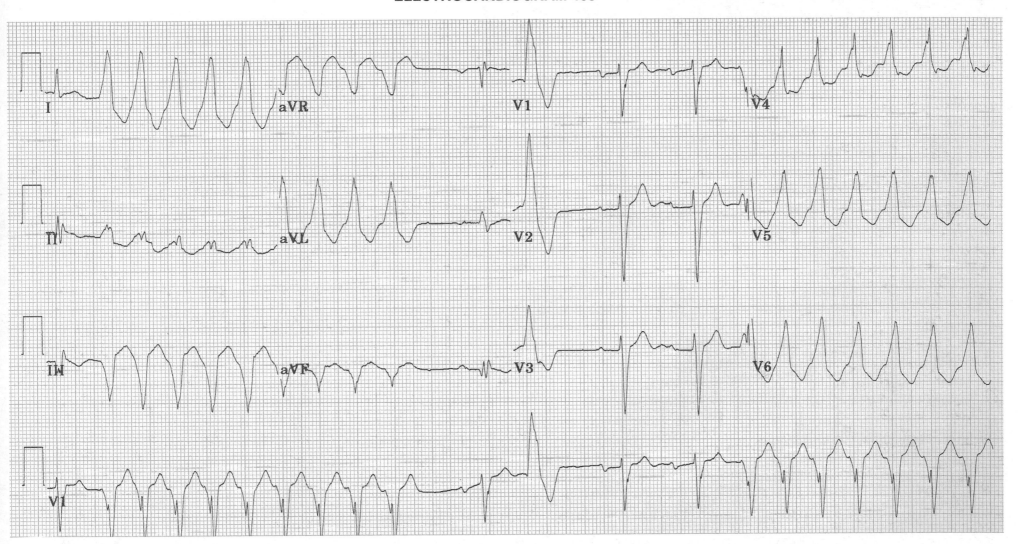

Interpretation Notes: _____

ECG 465 Seventy-four year old gentleman who is referred for a preoperative cardiac evaluation prior to planned knee replacement surgery. The patient has a pertinent past cardiac history including coronary artery bypass graft surgery one year prior to this electrocardiogram. A subsequent electrophysiology study demonstrated non-sustained ventricular tachycardia without inducible sustained cardiac dysrhythmias. Medications at the time of this electrocardiogram included potassium, digoxin, furosemide, simvastatin, captopril, and aspirin.

466

ELECTROCARDIOGRAM 466

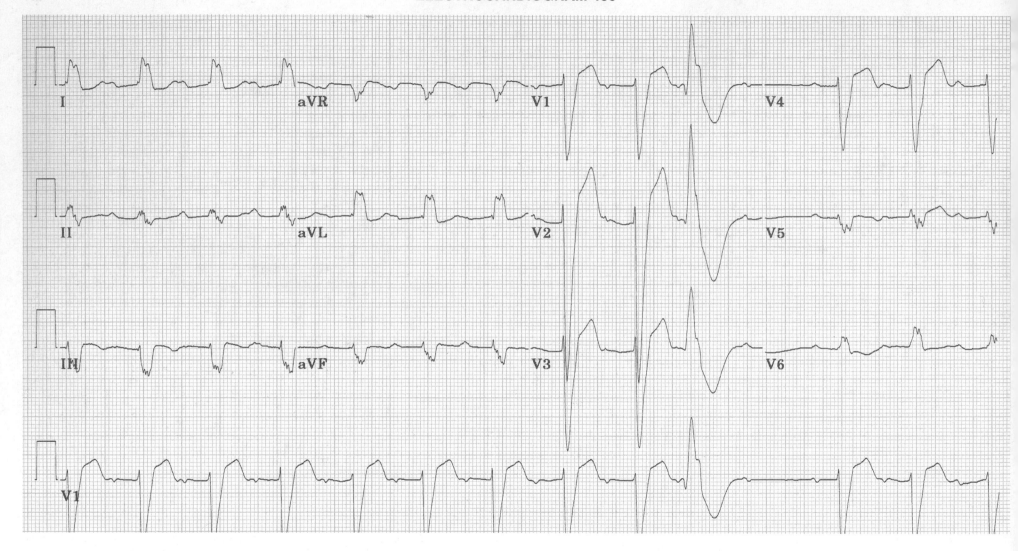

I aVR V1 V4

II aVL V2 V5

III aVF V3 V6

V1

Interpretation Notes:_____

_____

_____

ECG 466 Seventy-one year old gentleman with colon carcinoma status post resection who presents for follow-up cardiac evaluation in the outpatient clinic. An echocardiogram one year prior to this electrocardiogram demonstrated severe left ventricular systolic dysfunction felt secondary to chemotherapy toxicity. A co-morbidity includes paroxysmal atrial fibrillation. The patient's medications at the time of this electrocardiogram included digoxin, captopril, furosemide, and procainamide.

ELECTROCARDIOGRAM 467

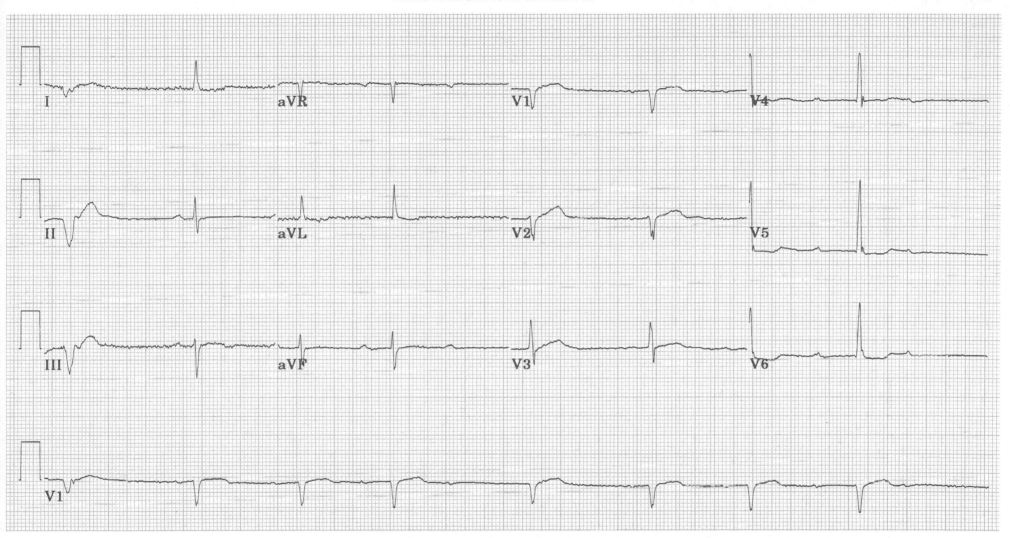

I aVR V1 V4

II aVL V2 V5

III aVF V3 V6

V1

Interpretation Notes: _____

_____

_____

ECG 467 Seventy-eight year old woman with non-insulin requiring diabetes mellitus, hypertension, and coronary artery disease admitted to the hospital for further evaluation and treatment of a venous stasis ulcer of the right foot. She has not undergone pacemaker implantation. She has a history of symptomatic premature atrial complexes for which she takes digoxin.

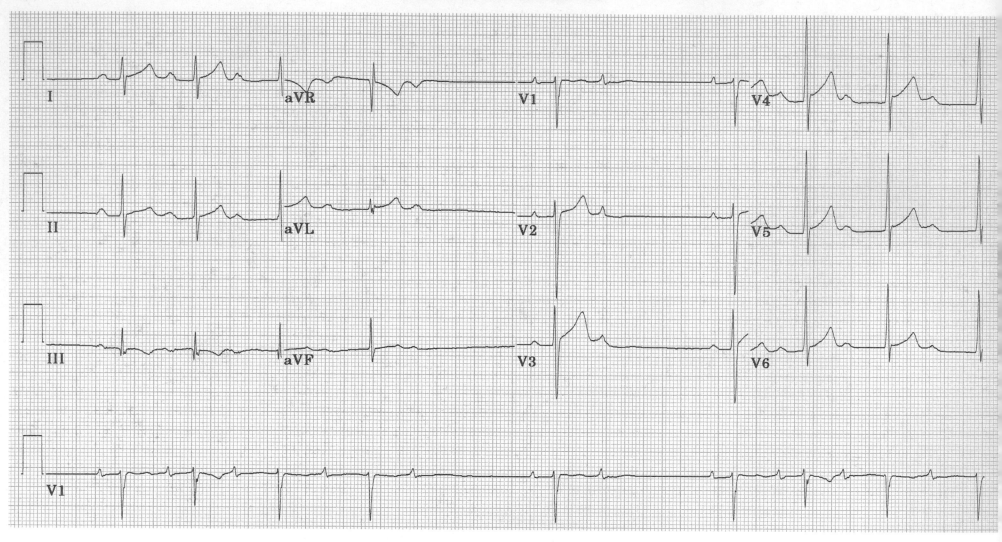

I aVR V1 V4

II aVL V2 V5

III aVF V3 V6

V1

Interpretation Notes: _____

_____

ECG 468 Twenty-four year old professional basketball player who is being evaluated for a pre-season physical examination. He has no known cardiac history.

ELECTROCARDIOGRAM 469

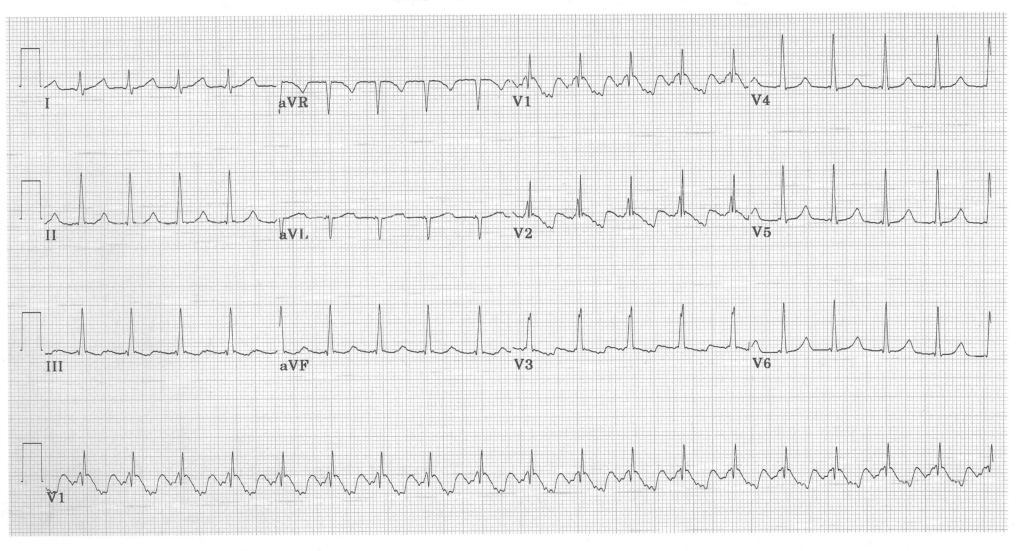

Interpretation Notes: _____
_____
_____

ECG 469 Thirty-six year old woman with rheumatic valvular heart disease and advanced mitral and tricuspid stenosis who underwent both mitral and tricuspid valve replacement two years prior to this electrocardiogram. The patient suffers from severe pulmonary hypertension and severe right ventricular systolic dysfunction.

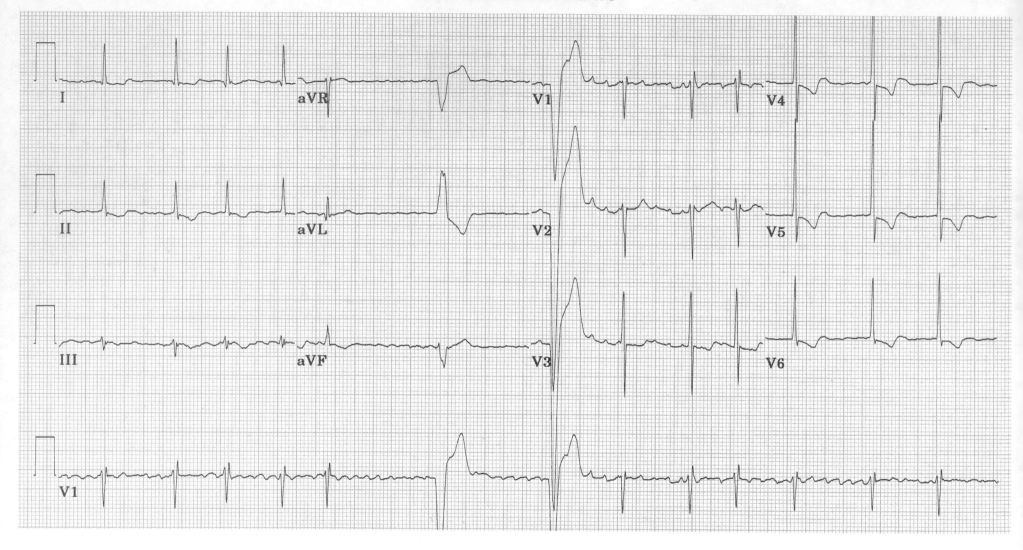

Interpretation Notes: _____

_____

ECG 470 Seventy-six year old gentleman with esophageal carcinoma status post esophagectomy who presents for outpatient follow-up. His past history includes coronary artery disease. He is status post coronary artery bypass graft surgery twelve years prior to this electrocardiogram. He also is known to suffer from chronic atrial fibrillation.

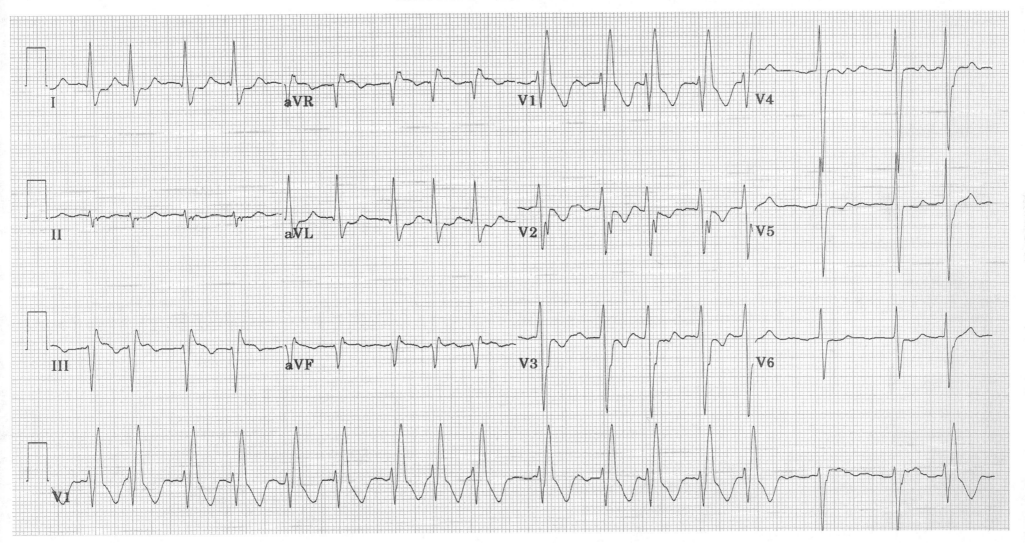

Interpretation Notes: _____

_____

ECG 471 Seventy-three year old woman with a history of aortic stenosis and hypertension who is readmitted to the hospital with shortness of breath secondary to rectal bleeding. A recent echocardiogram demonstrated normal left ventricular systolic function and severe aortic stenosis. Medications at the time of this electrocardiogram included iron, topical nitroglycerin, digoxin, diltiazem, and atenolol.

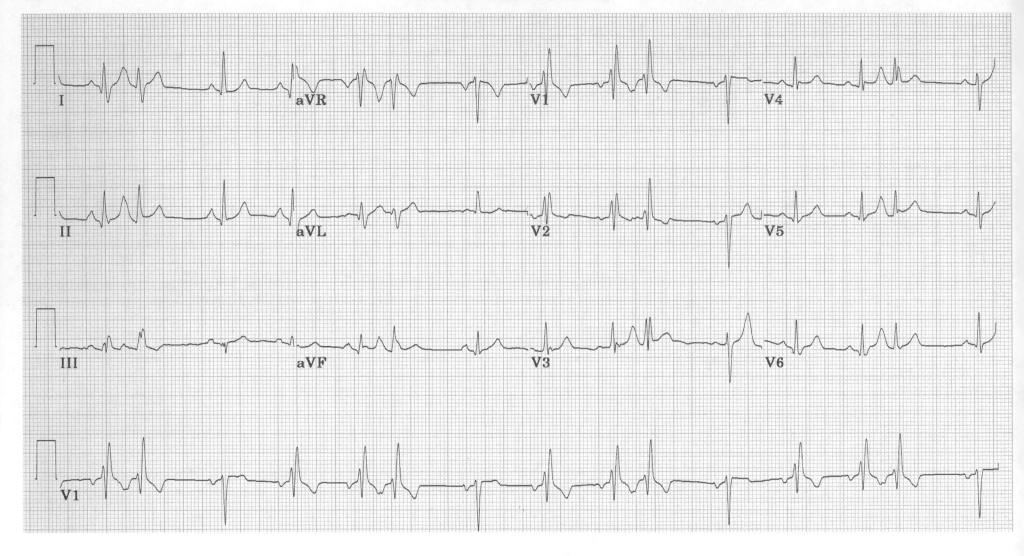

Interpretation Notes: _____

_____

ECG 472 Seventy-four year old woman with long-standing hypertension and hypertensive heart disease admitted from a nursing home for evaluation of a fever. Medications at the time of this electrocardiogram included diltiazem, aspirin, and levodopa.

ELECTROCARDIOGRAM 473

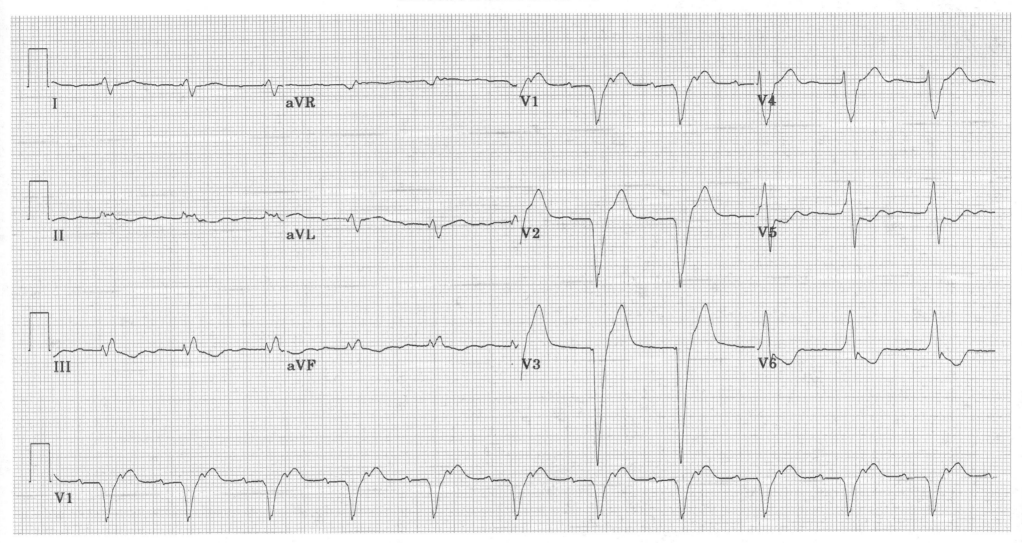

Interpretation Notes: _____

_____

ECG 473 Sixty year old gentleman status post aortic valve re-replacement who now presents to the hospital with a several day history of palpitations, associated dyspnea, and the above electrocardiogram.

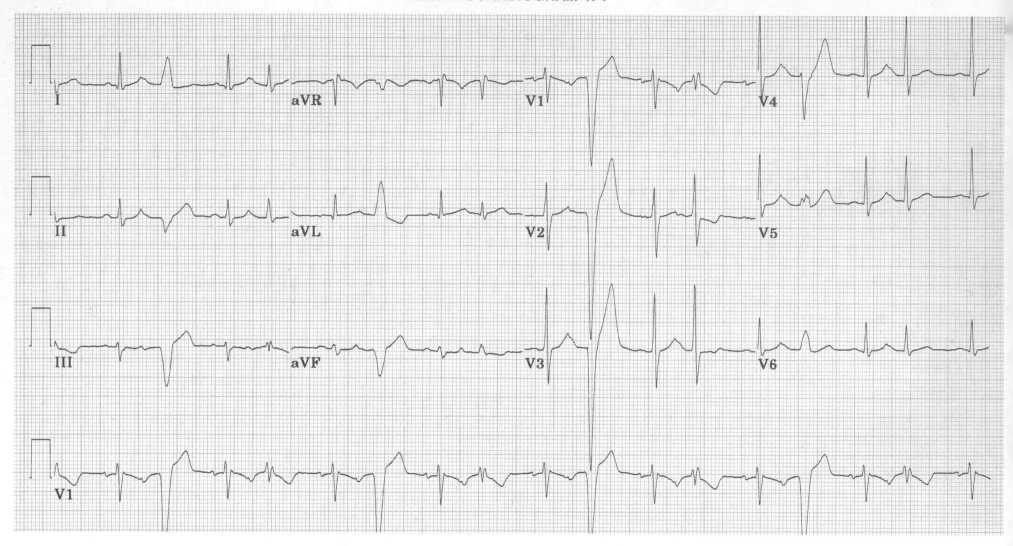

I   aVR   V1   V4

II   aVL   V2   V5

III   aVF   V3   V6

V1

Interpretation Notes: _____

_____

ECG 474 Fifty-eight year old gentleman with a history of esophageal carcinoma who is being seen in the arrhythmia outpatient clinic for evaluation of an abnormal holter monitor and suspected ventricular tachycardia. Medications at the time of this electrocardiogram included amiodarone and procainamide. In the outpatient clinic this electrocardiogram was interpreted as sinus tachycardia with atrial bigeminy and aberrant conduction. Both the amiodarone and procainamide were discontinued and a long-acting beta blocker was instituted.

ELECTROCARDIOGRAM 475

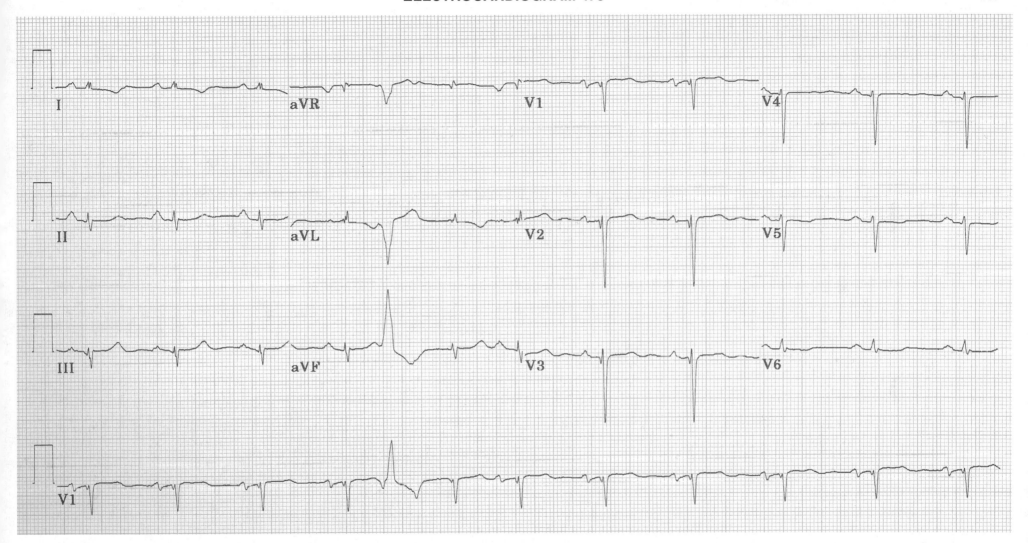

Interpretation Notes: _____

_____

ECG 475 Forty-seven year old gentleman with a history of an anterior myocardial infarction eight years prior to this electrocardiogram who re-presents with symptoms of angina pectoris. One year after his myocardial infarction he underwent multi-vessel coronary artery bypass graft surgery and left ventricular aneurysmectomy. Medications at the time of this electrocardiogram included metoprolol, aspirin, isosorbide dinitrate, and ticlodipine. A cardiac catheterization was obtained shortly after this electrocardiogram. This demonstrated compromise of the coronary arterial circulation to the native left circumflex coronary artery. The patient underwent successful percutaneous transluminal coronary angioplasty of a large left circumflex coronary artery branch vessel with symptom resolution.

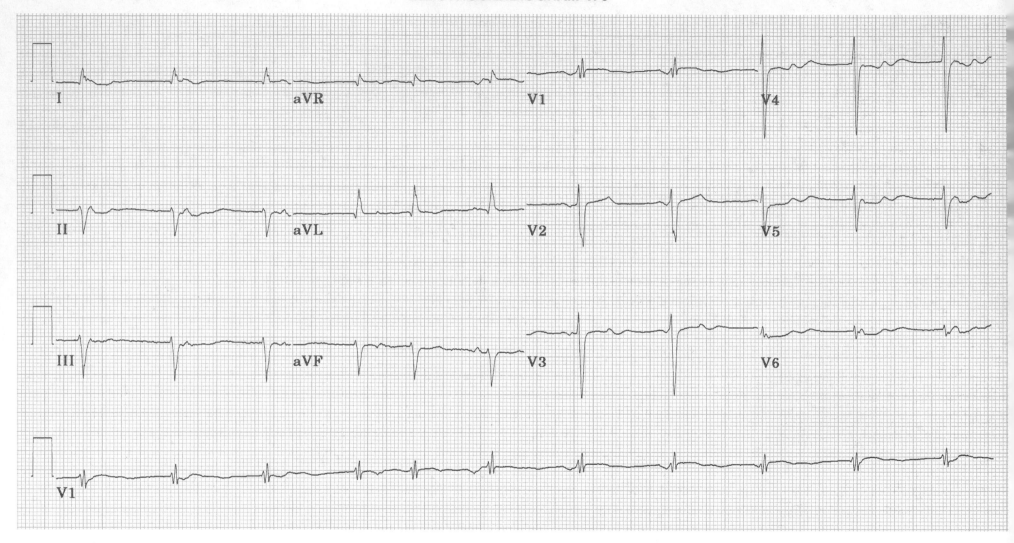

Interpretation Notes: _____

ECG 476 Thirty year old gentleman status post multiple prior cardiac surgeries in the setting of tricuspid valve atresia, a double outlet right ventricle, a large perimembranous ventricular septal defect, and an ostium primum atrial septal defect. The patient re-presents for evaluation of a perceived irregular heartbeat in the setting of known paroxysmal atrial arrhythmias.

ELECTROCARDIOGRAM 477

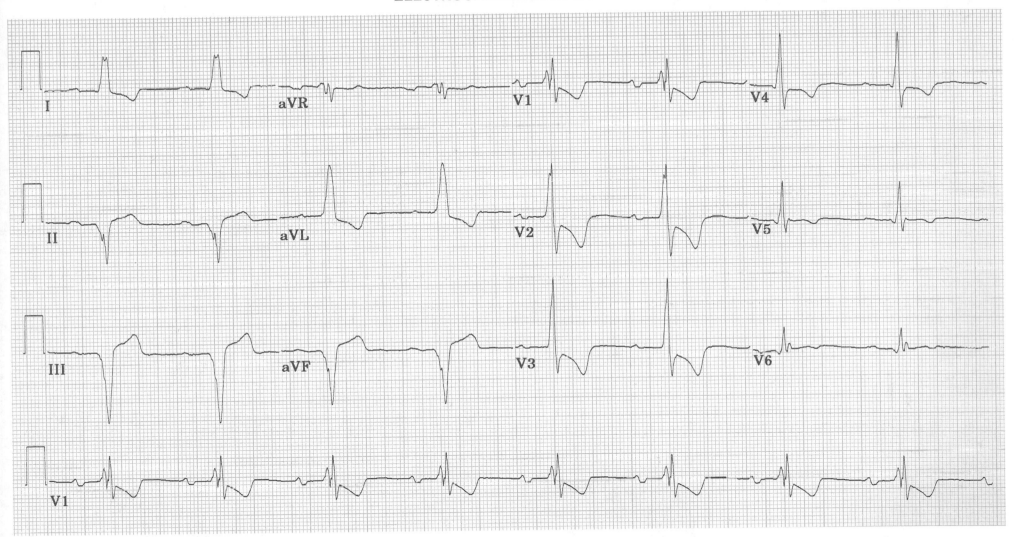

Interpretation Notes: _____

_____

ECG 477 Fifty-five year old gentleman with coronary artery disease and severe left ventricular systolic dysfunction status post coronary artery bypass surgery three years prior to this electrocardiogram. He is admitted to the hospital with a recurrent chest discomfort syndrome.

478

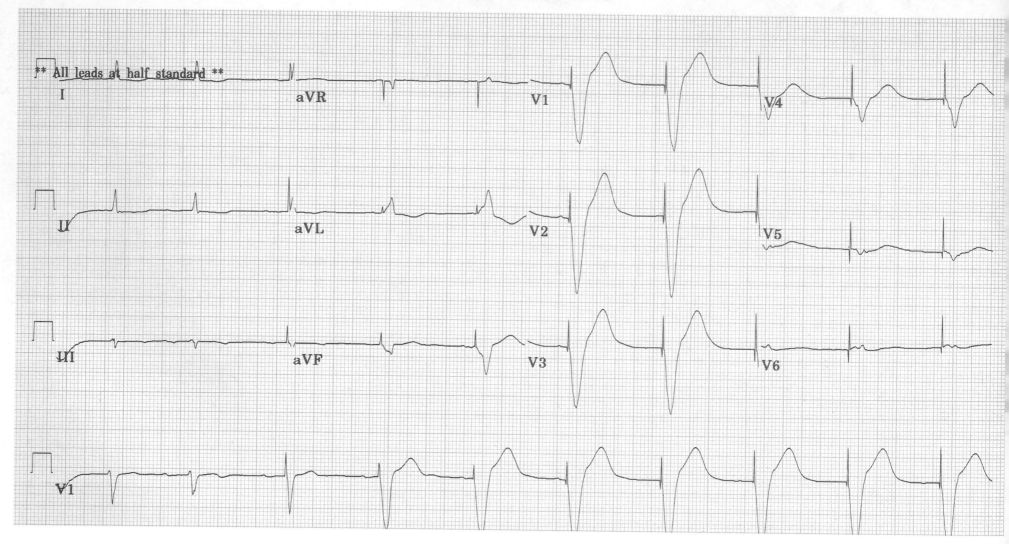

** All leads at half standard **

I   aVR   V1   V4

II   aVL   V2   V5

III   aVF   V3   V6

V1

Interpretation Notes: _____

_____

_____

ECG 478 Sixty-nine year old woman with advanced ischemic left ventricular systolic dysfunction status post multiple prior myocardial infarctions who presents for a routine outpatient cardiac follow-up evaluation. Other co-morbidities include complete heart block status post permanent pacemaker placement, congestive heart failure, and hypertension. Medications at the time of this electrocardiogram included amiodarone, enalapril, digoxin, and furosemide.

ELECTROCARDIOGRAM 479

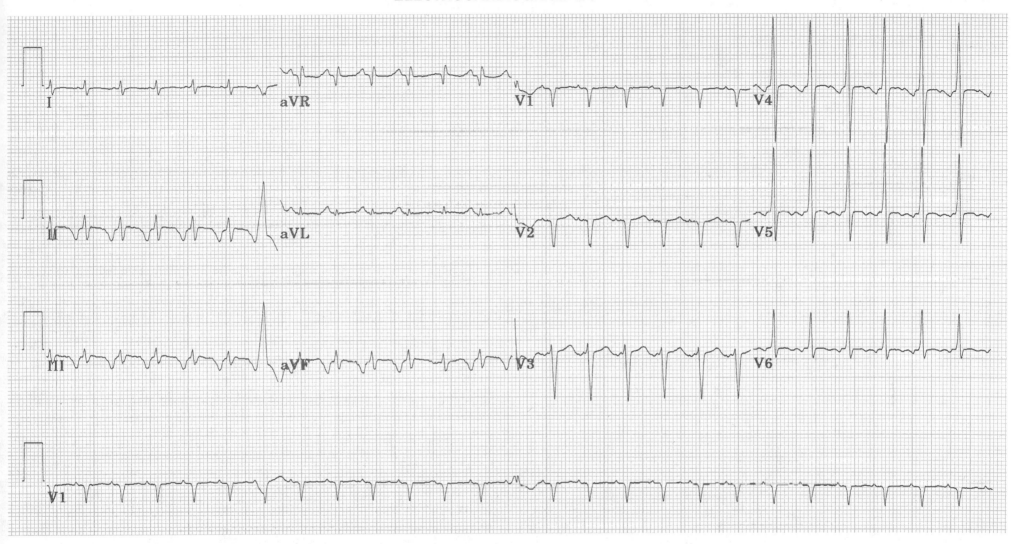

I aVR V1 V4

II aVL V2 V5

III aVF V3 V6

V1

Interpretation Notes: _____

_____

ECG 479 Seventy-six year old gentleman with ischemic heart disease status post two prior myocardial infarctions of uncertain location who returns for an outpatient evaluation. He has recently experienced a perceived rapid heartbeat. An echocardiogram demonstrated moderately severe regional left ventricular systolic dysfunction. Medications at the time of this electrocardiogram included enalapril, digoxin, and amiodarone. A co-morbidity included advanced chronic obstructive pulmonary disease.

ELECTROCARDIOGRAM 480

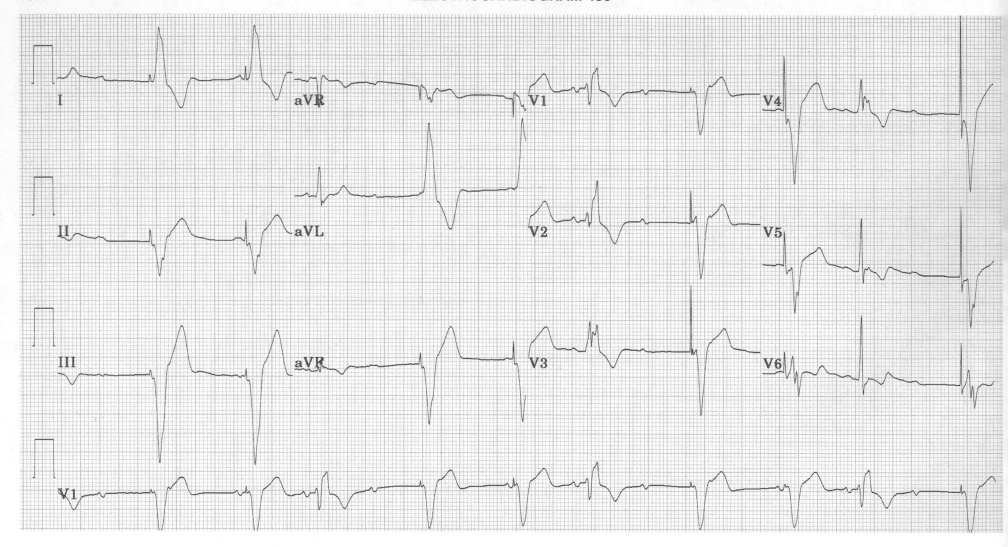

Interpretation Notes:_____

ECG 480 Fifty-three year old woman with bicuspid aortic valve stenosis status post aortic valve repair and ventricular pacemaker placement. The patient has a history of aortic coarctation and is status post coarctation repair twenty-seven years before this recent surgery.

ELECTROCARDIOGRAM 481

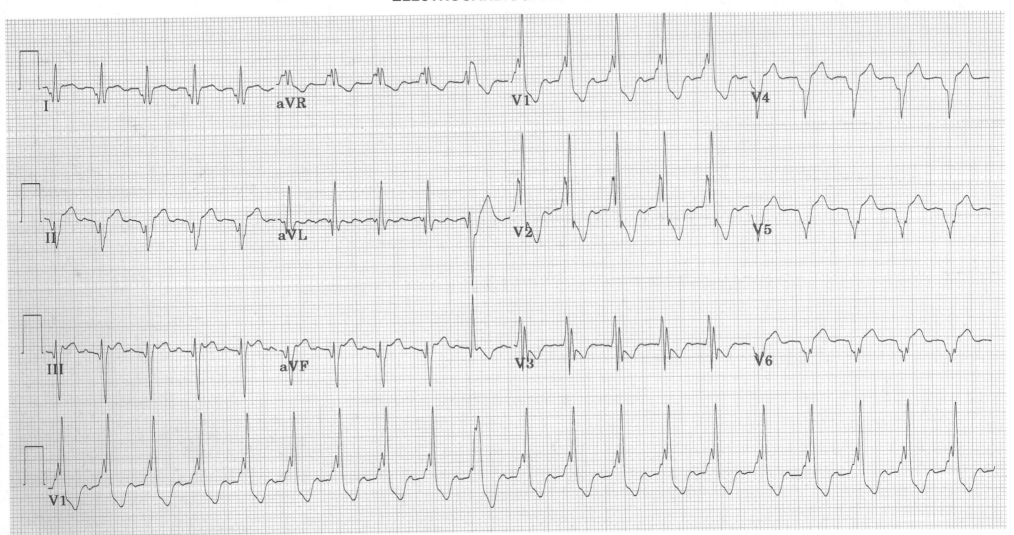

Interpretation Notes: _____

_____

ECG 481 Fifty-one year old gentleman admitted to the hospital acutely with a monoarticular arthritis. The patient subsequently developed bacteremia. He has coronary artery disease and an echocardiogram obtained at the time of this admission demonstrated inferolateral akinesis and moderately severe left ventricular systolic dysfunction. Co-morbid conditions include insulin requiring diabetes mellitus and renal insufficiency.

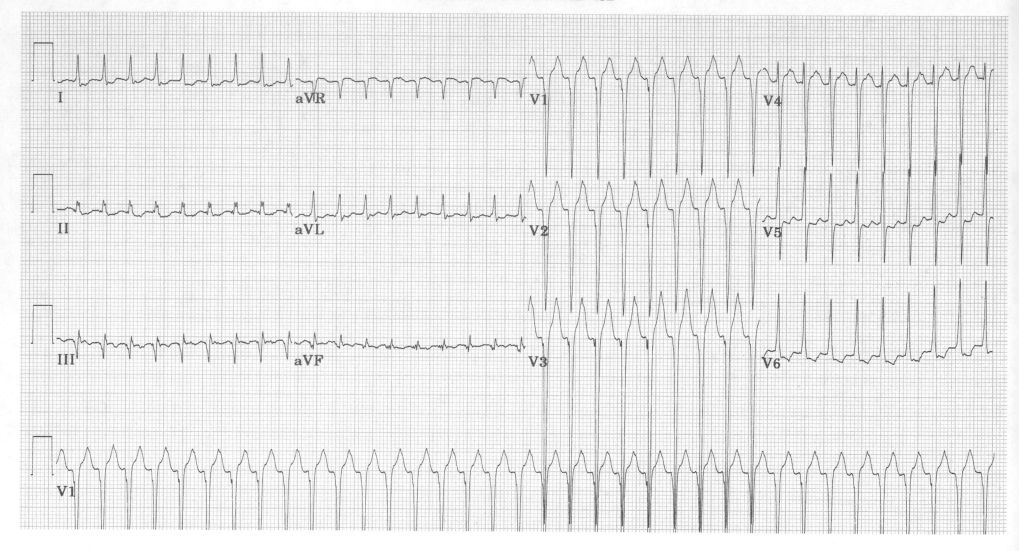

Interpretation Notes: _____

_____
_____

ECG 482 Forty-nine year old gentleman with metastatic lung cancer seen in cardiac consultation after the abrupt onset of palpitations and hypotension. His past cardiac history includes coronary artery disease and an inferior myocardial infarction twelve years prior to this electrocardiogram. He subsequently underwent three vessel coronary artery bypass graft surgery prior to the diagnosis of his malignancy.

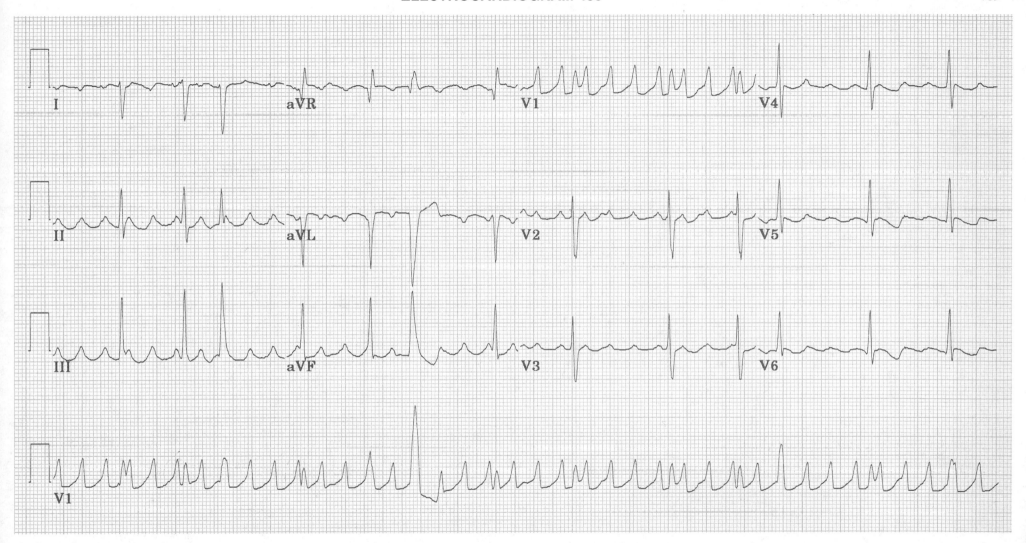

Interpretation Notes: _____

_____

ECG 483 Twenty-one year old woman who presents to the hospital with symptoms of right-sided congestive heart failure in the setting of an unrepaired atrial septal defect, a right-to-left interatrial shunt, and severe pulmonary hypertension compatible with Eisenmenger's syndrome. An echocardiogram demonstrated severe biventricular systolic dysfunction.

484

ELECTROCARDIOGRAM 484

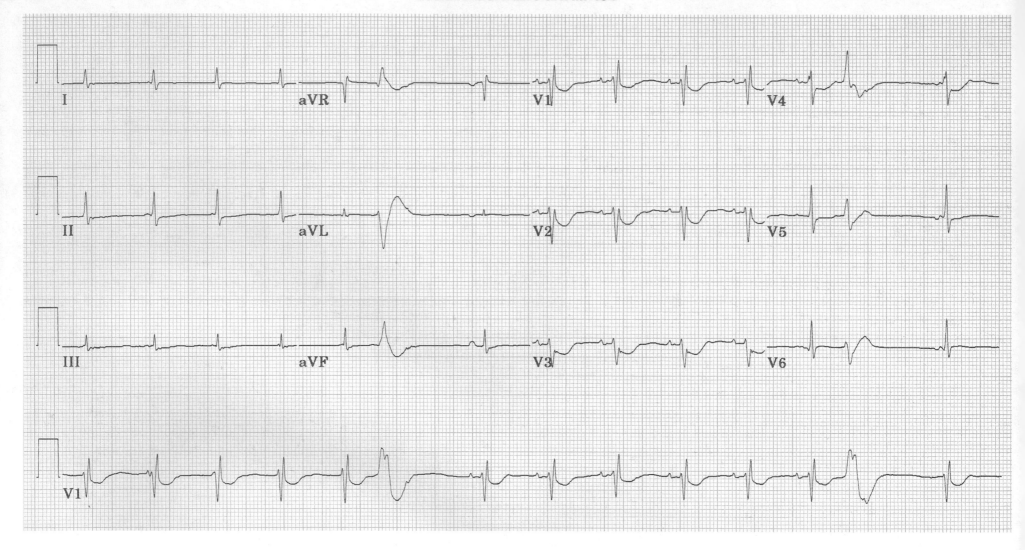

Interpretation Notes:

ECG 484 Seventy-eight year old woman with a recent posterior myocardial infarction and successful angioplasty to the left circumflex coronary artery who remains hospitalized secondary to paroxysmal sustained ventricular tachycardia. Medications at the time of this electrocardiogram included amiodarone, furosemide, intravenous nitroprusside, and aspirin.

ELECTROCARDIOGRAM 485

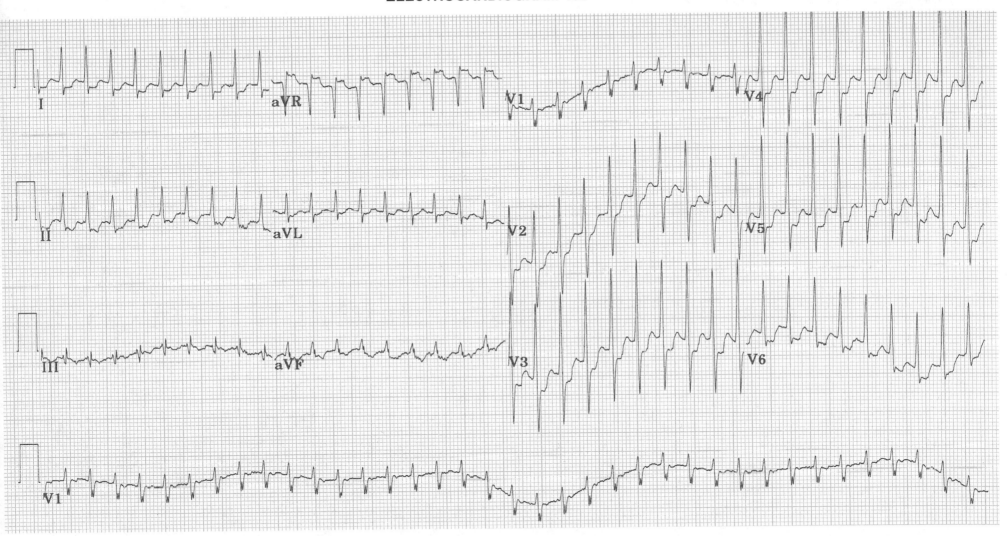

Interpretation Notes: _____

_____

ECG 485 Fifty-six year old woman admitted acutely to the hospital with a three day history of fever, chills, nausea, vomiting, and a productive cough of yellowish sputum. Her clinical presentation, exam, and chest x-ray were consistent with pneumonia. Co-morbid conditions included anemia, obesity, and chronic obstructive pulmonary disease. She also has a history of paroxysmal atrial fibrillation. Her medications at the time of this electrocardiogram included digoxin, metoprolol, and intravenous antibiotics.

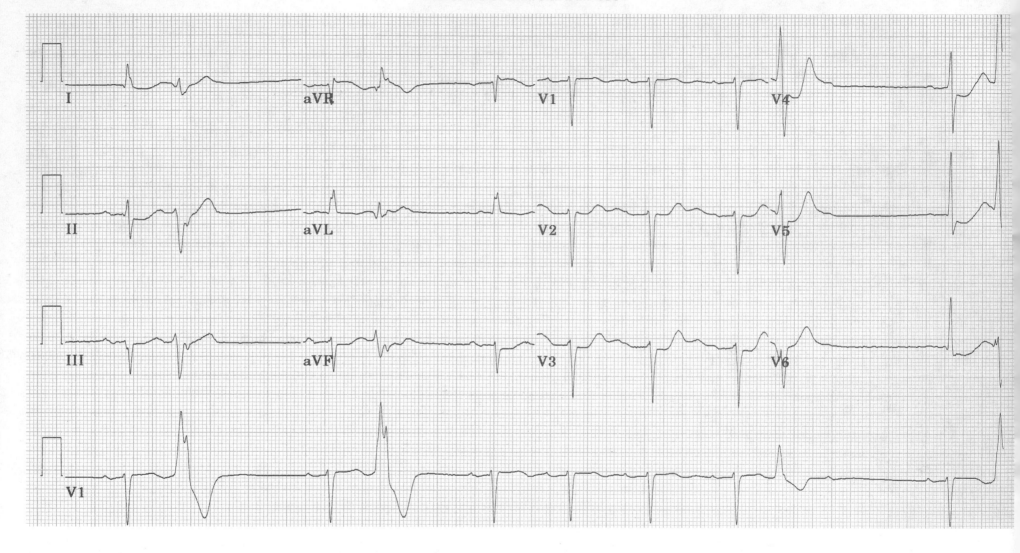

I   aVR   V1   V4

II   aVL   V2   V5

III   aVF   V3   V6

V1

Interpretation Notes:_____

_____

_____

ECG 486 Seventy-three year old gentleman with coronary artery disease and normal left ventricular systolic function who re-presents with symptoms of angina pectoris. Medications at the time of this electrocardiogram included topical nitroglycerin, diltiazem, lovastatin, triamterene/hydrochlorothiazide, and digoxin.

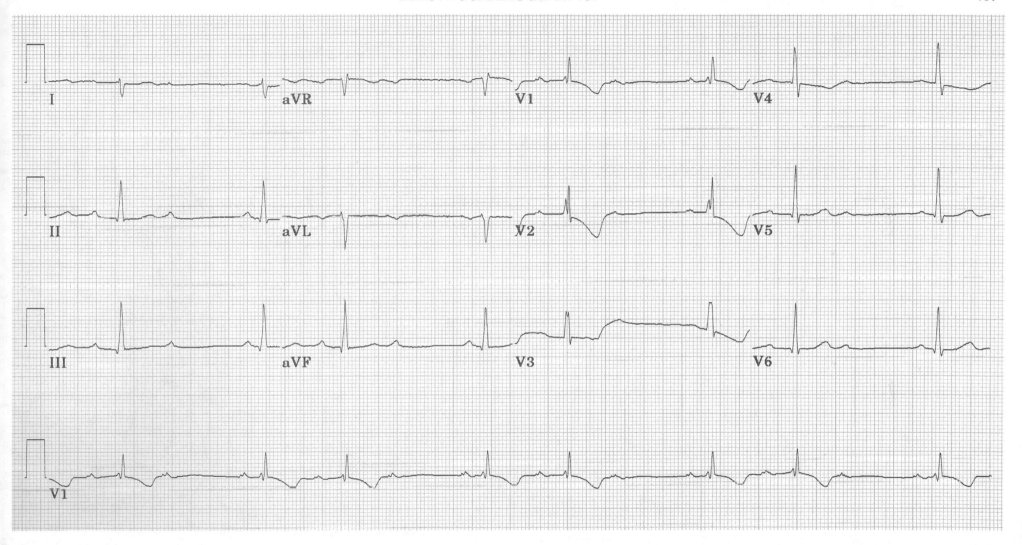

I	aVR	V1	V4
II	aVL	V2	V5
III	aVF	V3	V6
V1			

Interpretation Notes: _____

_____

_____

ECG 487 Thirty-six year old woman with rheumatic valvular heart disease including advanced mitral and tricuspid valve stenosis who underwent both mitral and tricuspid valve replacement two years prior to this electrocardiogram. The patient suffers from severe pulmonary hypertension and severe right ventricular systolic dysfunction.

488

ELECTROCARDIOGRAM 488

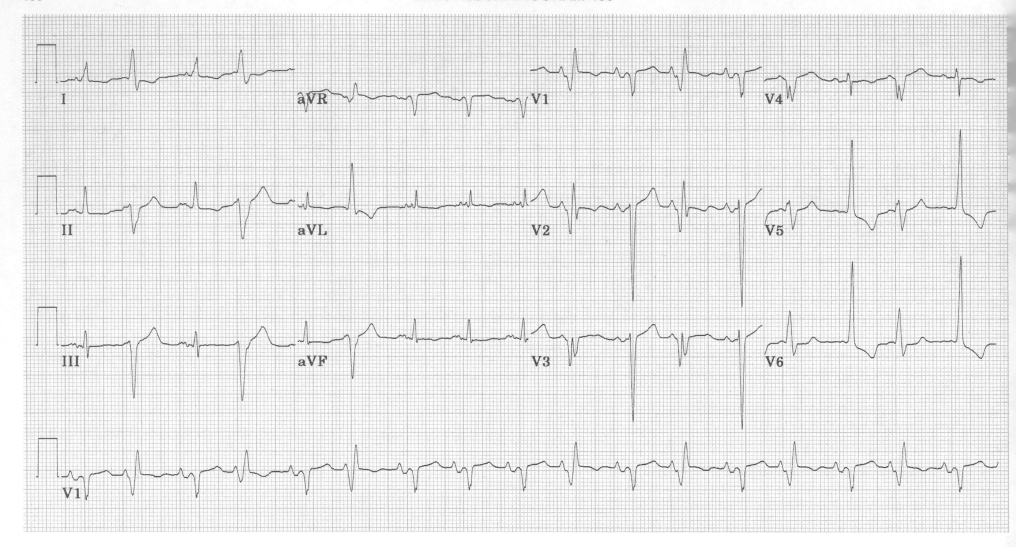

Interpretation Notes: _____

_____

ECG 488 Fifty-three year old gentleman who was accepted in hospital transfer for consideration of mitral valve reparative surgery. The patient suffers from severe mitral insufficiency. A recent cardiac catheterization demonstrated mild coronary artery disease with global moderately severe left ventricular systolic dysfunction and moderate pulmonary hypertension. Medications at the time of this electrocardiogram included captopril, aspirin, digoxin, furosemide, and potassium.

ELECTROCARDIOGRAM 489

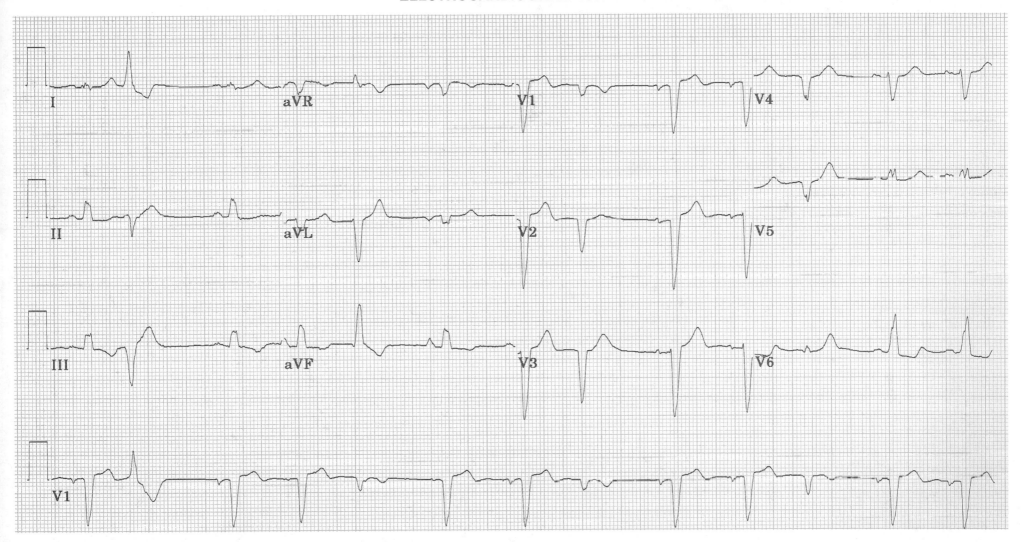

Interpretation Notes: _____

_____

_____

ECG 489 Seventy-two year old woman with prior inferior and anterior myocardial infarctions and resultant moderately severe depression of left ventricular systolic function who now presents for routine cardiology follow-up in the outpatient department. Co-morbidities include hypertension, non-sustained ventricular tachycardia, and peripheral vascular disease.

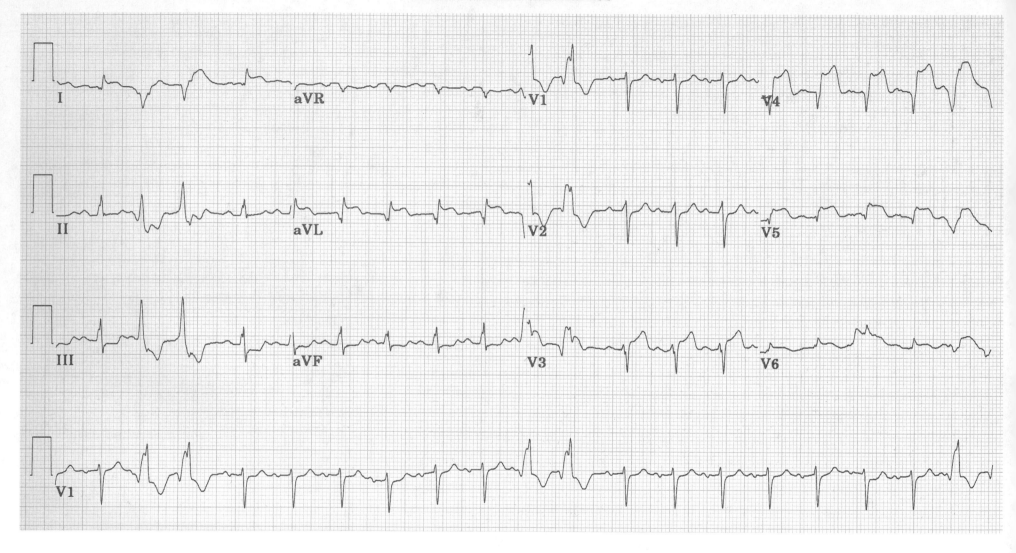

Interpretation Notes: _____

_____

_____

ECG 490 Fifty-five year old gentleman admitted to the hospital urgently with a recent onset chest discomfort syndrome felt consistent with an acute myocardial infarction. The patient underwent a cardiac catheterization demonstrating a subtotal occlusion of the left anterior descending coronary artery. Serial cardiac enzymes documented acute myocardial injury. His post myocardial infarction hospital course included recurrent ventricular tachycardia.

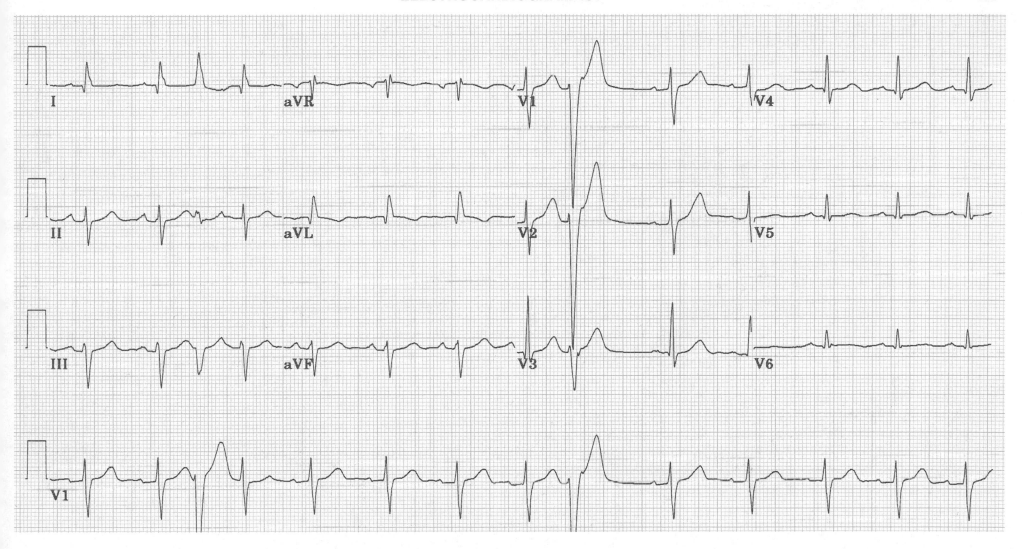

Interpretation Notes:_____

_____

ECG 491 Seventy-two year old gentleman with a history of a prior myocardial infarction of unknown location who presents for an outpatient cardiology follow-up examination. His medications at the time of this electrocardiogram included metoprolol, aspirin, and atorvastatin.

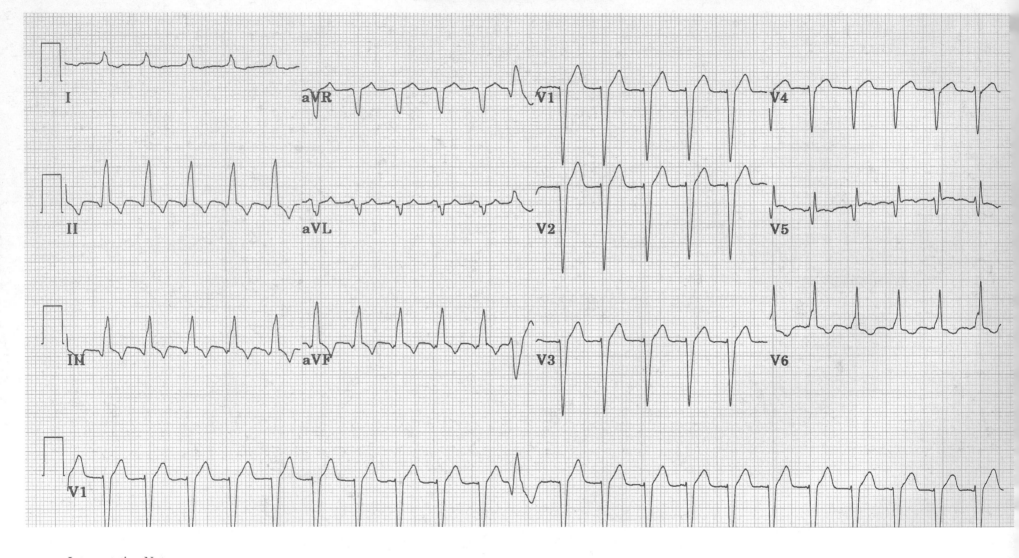

Interpretation Notes: _____

_____

ECG 492 Fifty-four year old gentleman with increasing symptoms of angina pectoris and dyspnea referred for coronary artery bypass graft surgery in the setting of multi-vessel coronary artery disease. Co-morbid conditions include chronic obstructive pulmonary disease and hyperlipidemia. Medications at the time of this electrocardiogram included verapamil and topical nitroglycerin.

ELECTROCARDIOGRAM 493

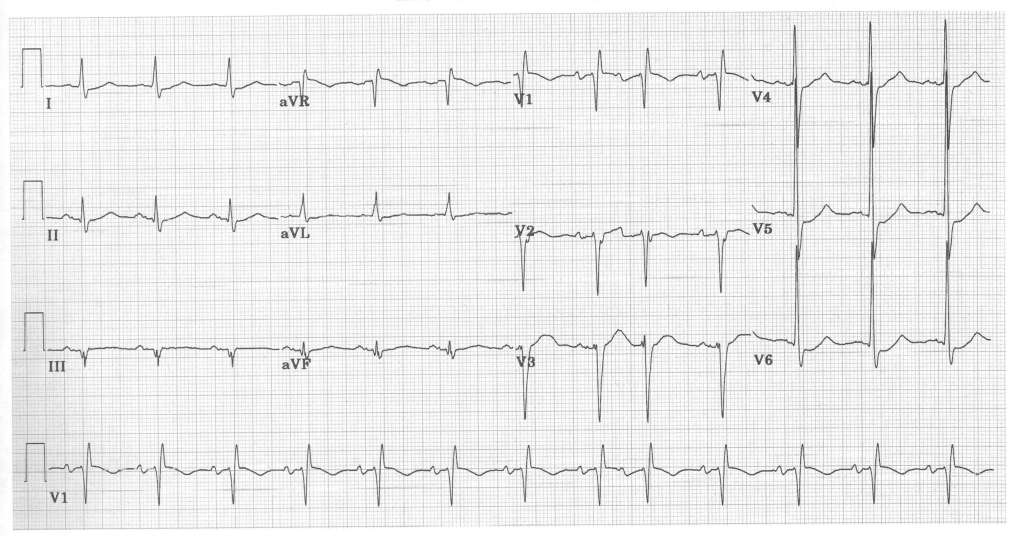

Interpretation Notes: _____

_____

ECG 493 Sixty-seven year old gentleman with a history of metastatic rectal carcinoma who returns for a routine cardiology follow-up examination. He has been diagnosed with paroxysmal atrial fibrillation. His medications included captopril, warfarin, and digoxin. He is currently asymptomatic from a cardiac standpoint.

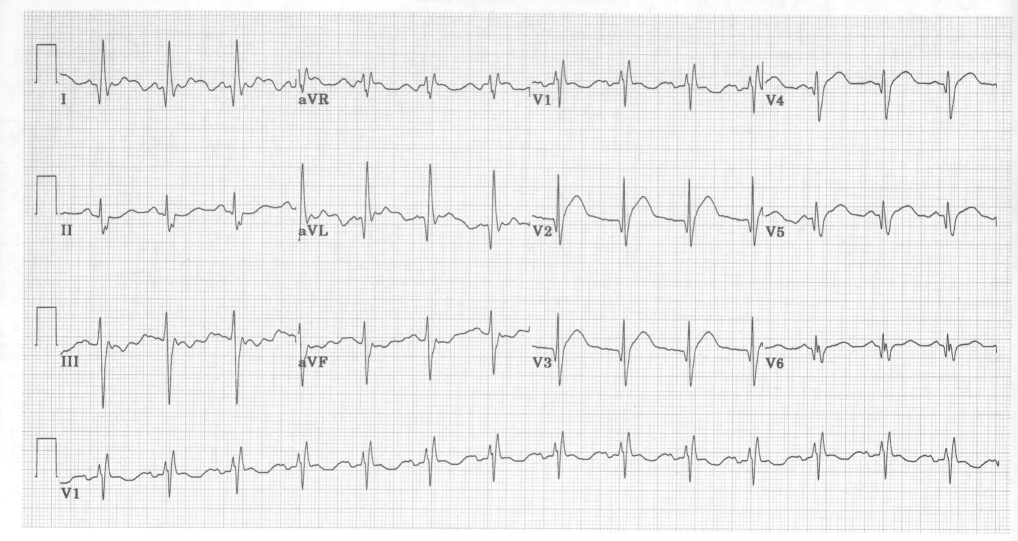

Interpretation Notes: _____

_____

_____

ECG 494 Seventy-one year old woman with an acute onset chest discomfort syndrome of two hours duration refractory to sublingual nitroglycerin. She presented to the hospital emergency room with the above electrocardiogram.

ELECTROCARDIOGRAM 495

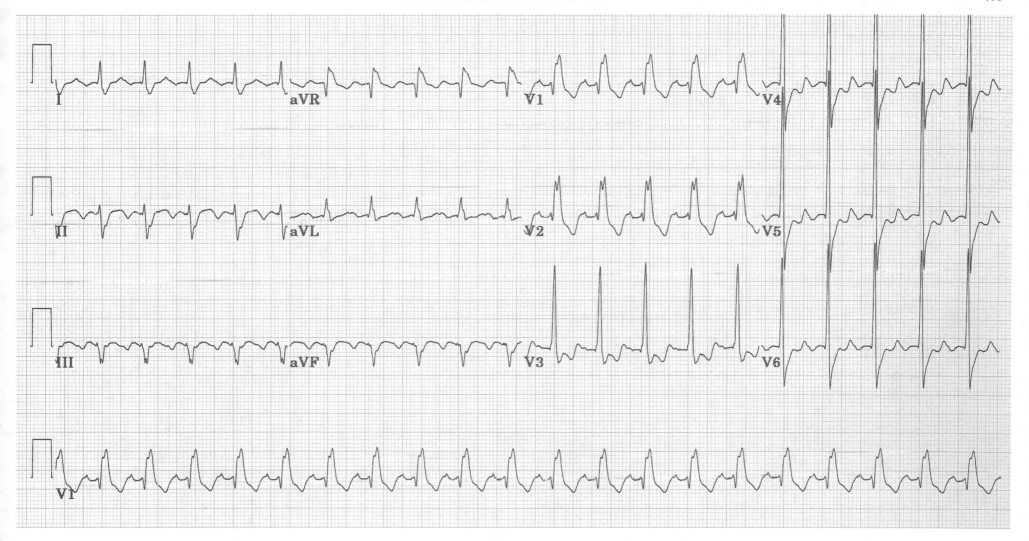

Interpretation Notes: _____

_____

ECG 495 Eighty-one year old woman with a history of severe aortic stenosis status post bioprosthetic aortic valve replacement and a prior inferior myocardial infarction who returns for outpatient cardiology follow-up. She has ongoing fatigue but no symptoms suggestive of arrhythmias. Her medications included enalapril, digoxin, and aspirin.

ELECTROCARDIOGRAM 496

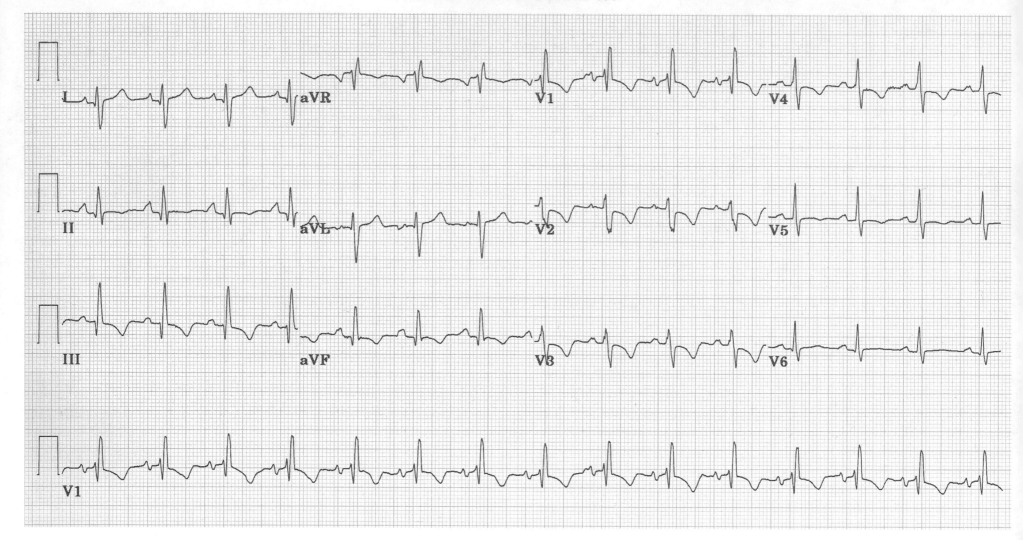

Interpretation Notes:_____

_____

_____

ECG 496 Fifty-seven year old woman with a history of adenocarcinoma of the rectum and a pulmonary embolism who presented to the hospital urgently secondary to severe shortness of breath and respiratory failure. Pulmonary angiography demonstrated evidence of remote and acute pulmonary emboli and severe pulmonary hypertension. The patient expired shortly after this electrocardiogram.

ELECTROCARDIOGRAM 497

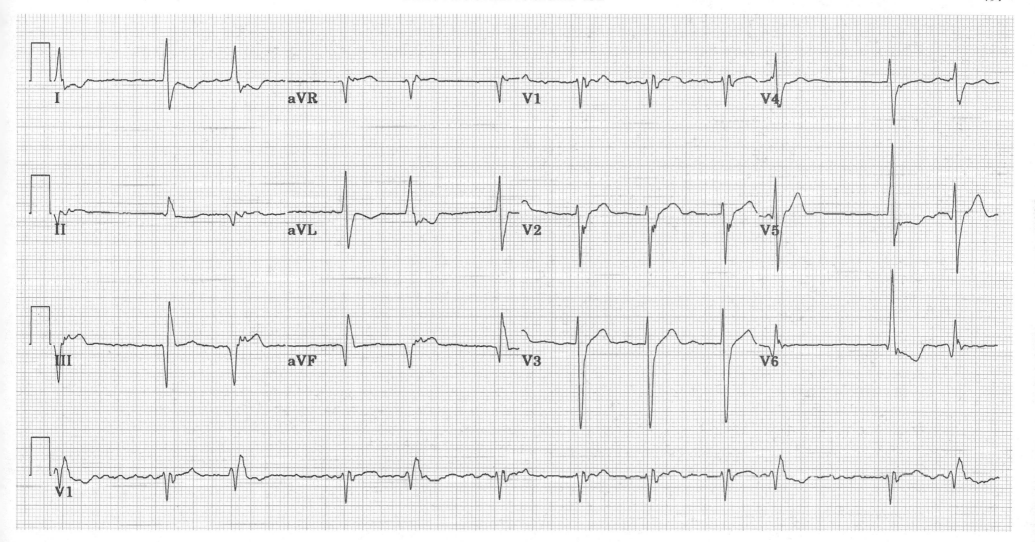

Interpretation Notes:_____

_____

_____

ECG 497 Sixty-three year old woman with a history of a remote myocardial infarction and coronary artery bypass graft surgery who returns for clinical evaluation in the setting of increasing dyspnea and progressive mitral stenosis. Her medications included bumetanide, lisinopril, potassium, and warfarin.

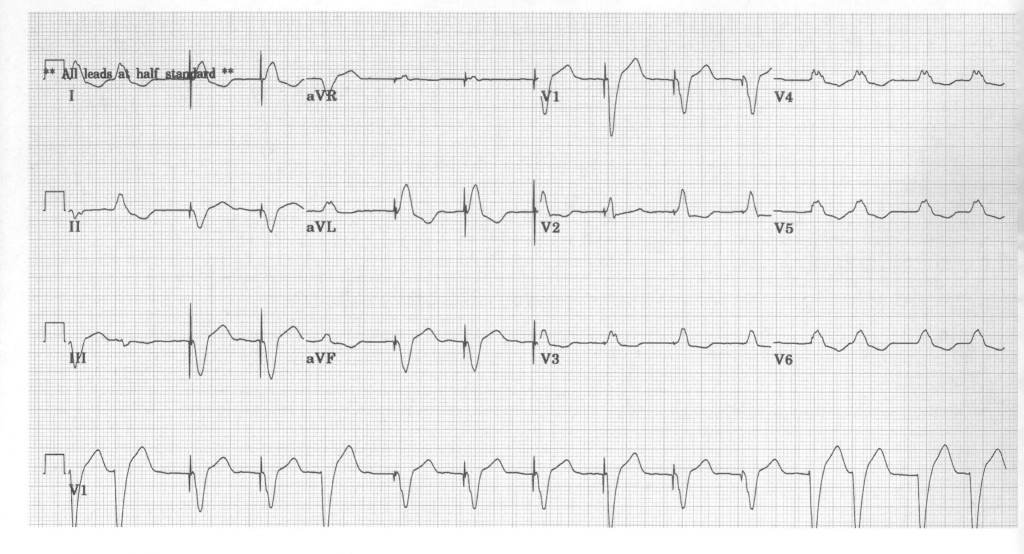

** All leads at half standard **

I   aVR   V1   V4

II   aVL   V2   V5

III   aVF   V3   V6

V1

Interpretation Notes: _____

_____

_____

ECG 498 Sixty-five year old gentleman with coronary artery disease status post remote coronary artery bypass graft surgery who was admitted acutely to the hospital with recurrent congestive heart failure. The patient has chronic atrial fibrillation and mitral insufficiency. He is status post permanent pacemaker placement for sick sinus syndrome. Medications at the time of this tracing included amiodarone, digoxin, isosorbide dinitrate, warfarin, and enalapril.

ELECTROCARDIOGRAM 499

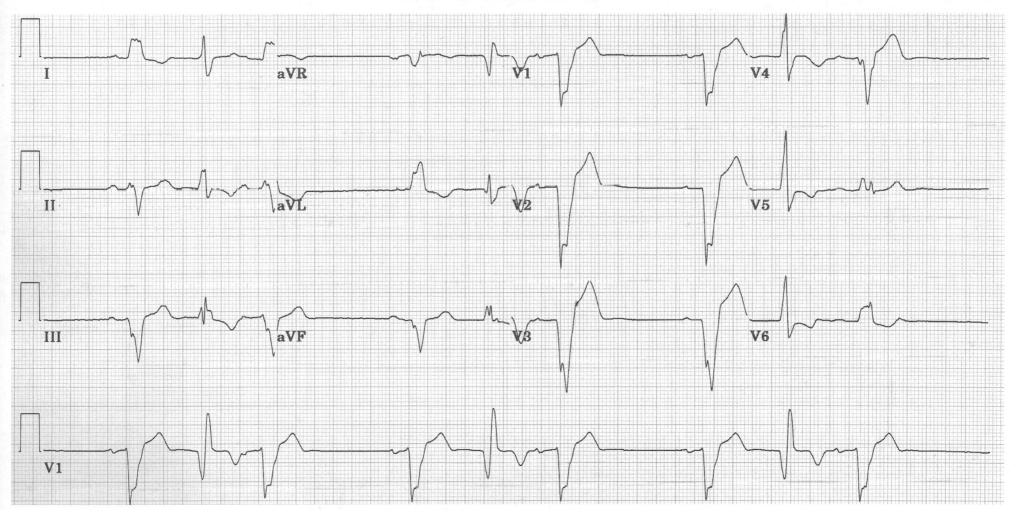

I aVR V1 V4

II aVL V2 V5

III aVF V3 V6

V1

Interpretation Notes: _____

_____

ECG 499 Fifty-five year old gentleman with an idiopathic dilated cardiomyopathy, congestive heart failure, and hypertension who returns for cardiology follow-up. His medications included warfarin, captopril, digoxin, furosemide, metoprolol, and sublingual nitroglycerin.

ELECTROCARDIOGRAM 500

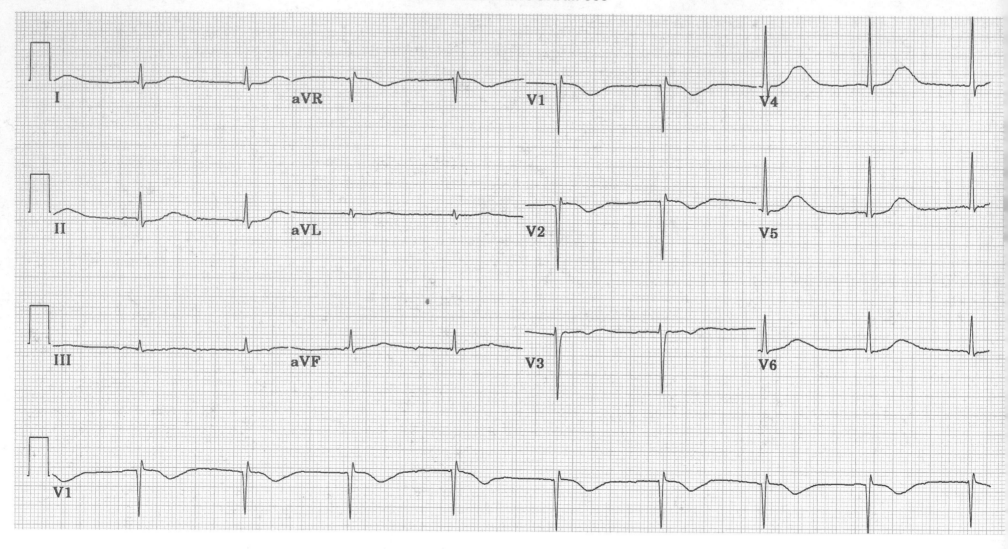

I aVR V1 V4

II aVL V2 V5

III aVF V3 V6

V1

Interpretation Notes: _____

_____

_____

ECG 500 Sixty-three year old gentleman status post a recent cardiac transplant in the setting of severe left ventricular systolic dysfunction and advanced ischemic cardiovascular disease who returns for a follow-up cardiac evaluation. Medications at the time of this electrocardiogram included digoxin, amiodarone, and captopril.

ELECTROCARDIOGRAM 501

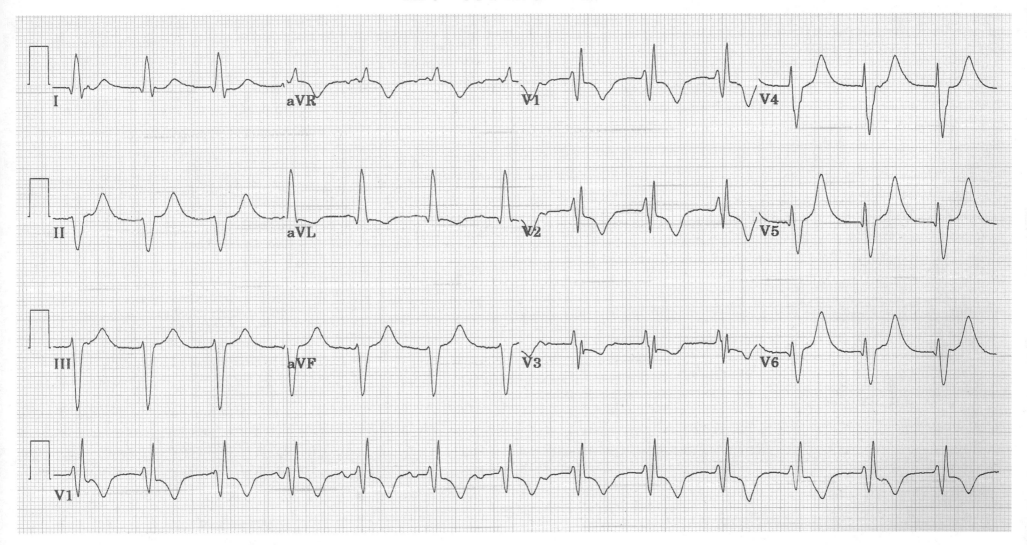

I aVR V1 V4

II aVL V2 V5

III aVF V3 V6

V1

Interpretation Notes:_____

ECG 501 Fifty-nine year old gentleman with a history of rheumatic heart disease status post aortic and mitral valve replacements six years prior to this electrocardiogram. He underwent a recent repeat mitral valve replacement in the setting of severe periprosthetic mitral regurgitation. The patient subsequently required a permanent pacemaker. Medications at the time of this electrocardiogram included enalapril and multi-vitamins.

ELECTROCARDIOGRAM 502

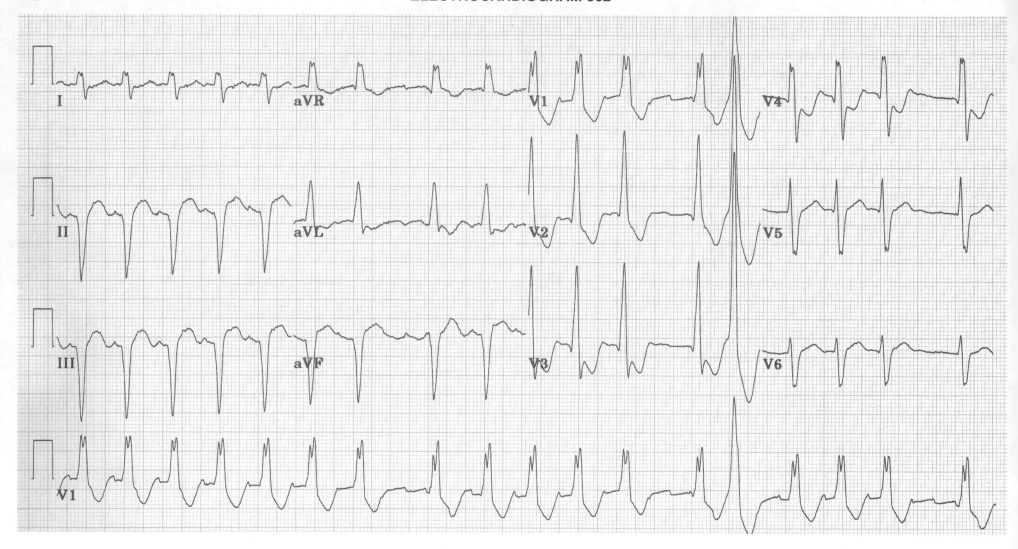

Interpretation Notes: _____

_____

ECG 502 Eighty-eight year old woman with a history of congestive heart failure of uncertain etiology who presents to the hospital acutely with shortness of breath and chest discomfort. Her medications at the time of this electrocardiogram included hydralazine, furosemide, and amiodarone.

ELECTROCARDIOGRAM 503

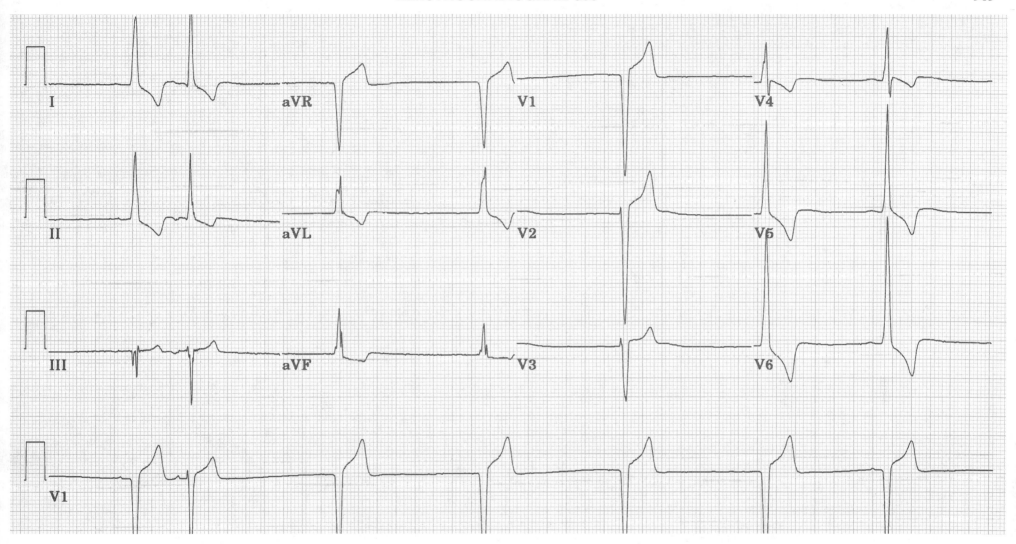

Interpretation Notes: _____

_____

ECG 503 Sixty-seven year old gentleman referred for a cardiac catheterization in the setting of hypertension and recent symptoms of profound exertional dyspnea. Medications at the time of this electrocardiogram included digoxin, nifedipine, and aspirin. An echocardiogram demonstrated left ventricular hypertrophy with normal left ventricular systolic function and severe aortic stenosis. The cardiac catheterization demonstrated normal coronary arteries. The patient was referred for successful aortic valve replacement.

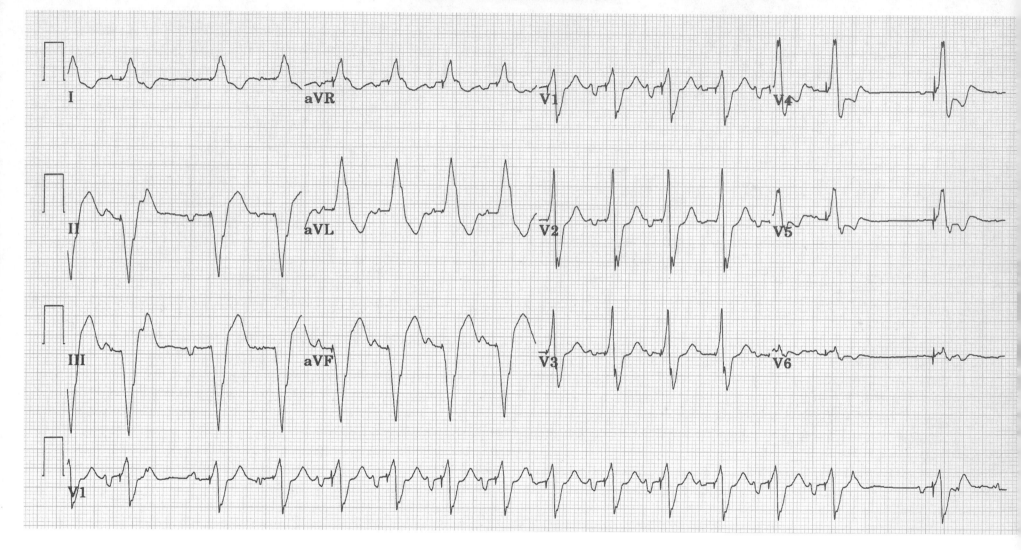

Interpretation Notes:

ECG 504 Sixty-eight year old gentleman status post repair of an ascending aortic dissection with aortic valve re-suspension and a single vessel coronary artery bypass graft procedure six years prior to this electrocardiogram who returns for a cardiology follow-up examination. He is experiencing progressive dyspnea and weakness. Medications at the time of this electrocardiogram included furosemide, potassium, and metolazone.

ELECTROCARDIOGRAM 505

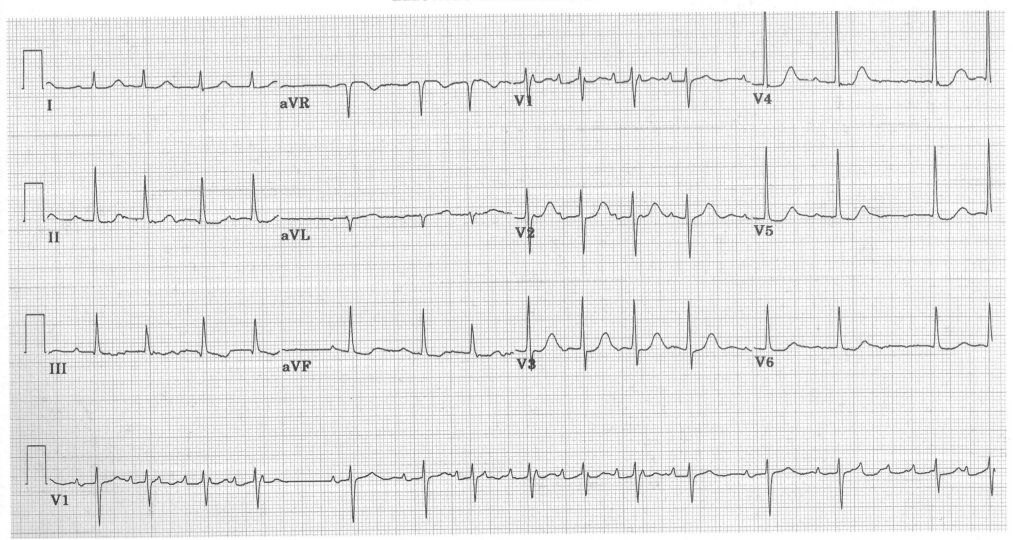

Interpretation Notes: _____

_____

_____

ECG 505 Seventy-one year old woman with long-standing hypertension and hypertensive heart disease documented on a recent echocardiogram. This patient was admitted to the hospital at the time of this electrocardiogram for antiarrhythmic therapy initiation in the setting of recurrent and drug refractory atrial arrhythmias.

506

ELECTROCARDIOGRAM 506

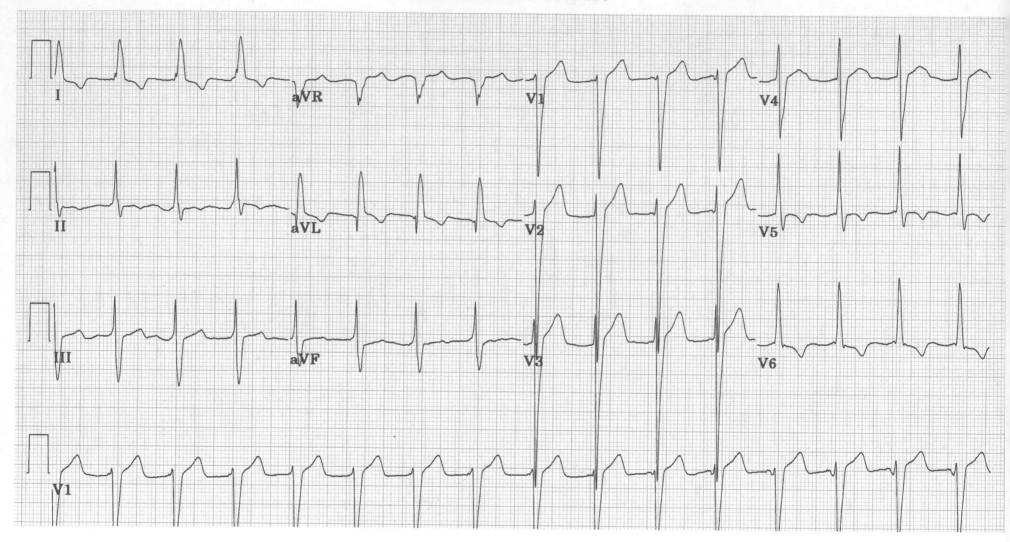

Interpretation Notes: _____

_____

_____

ECG 506 Thirty-five year old gentleman status post aortic valve replacement at age seventeen secondary to bacterial endocarditis now with recurrent aortic insufficiency. He is immediately postoperative aortic valve re-replacement.

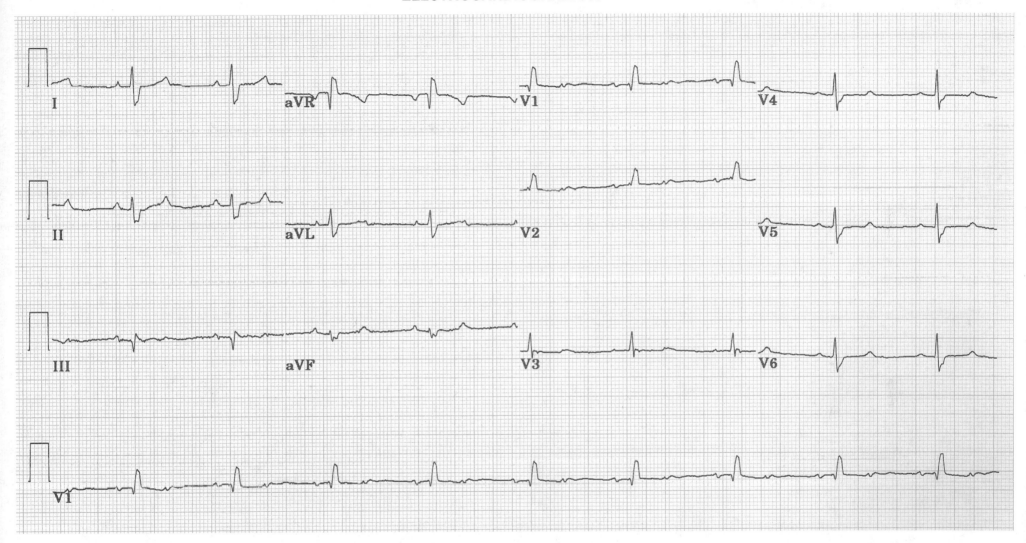

Interpretation Notes:

ECG 507 Seventy-five year old woman status post a remote mastectomy and radiation therapy admitted to the hospital with a three day history of increasing shortness of breath. An echocardiogram demonstrated moderate left ventricular systolic dysfunction of unknown etiology. The patient subsequently developed complete heart block and permanent pacemaker placement was required.

508

ELECTROCARDIOGRAM 508

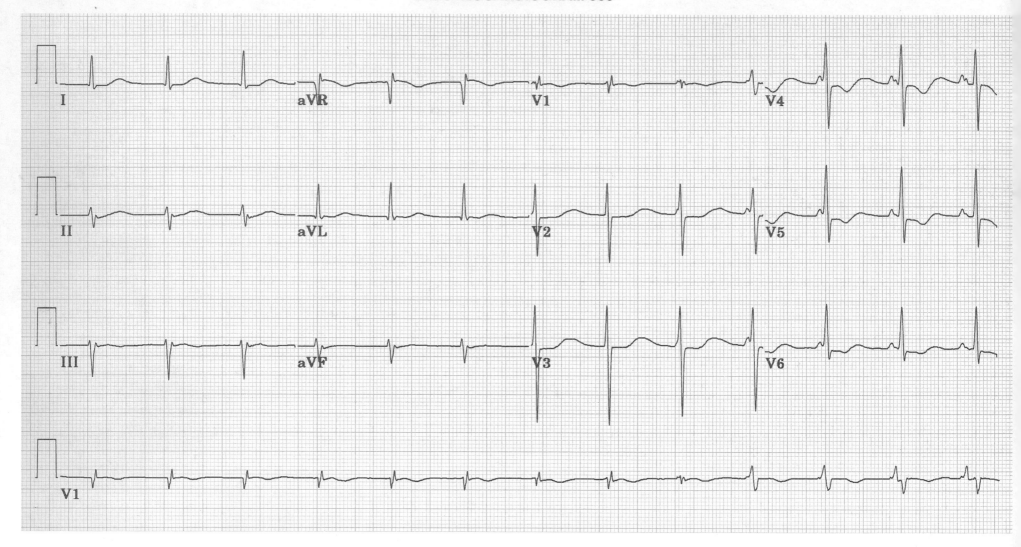

Interpretation Notes: _____

ECG 508 Sixty-seven year old woman with a history of chronic obstructive pulmonary disease, supraventricular tachycardia, and systemic hypertension admitted with a chronic obstructive pulmonary disease exacerbation. Her medications at the time of this electrocardiogram included phenobarbital, phenytoin, famotidine, methotrexate, colchicine, enalapril, and prednisone.

ELECTROCARDIOGRAM 509

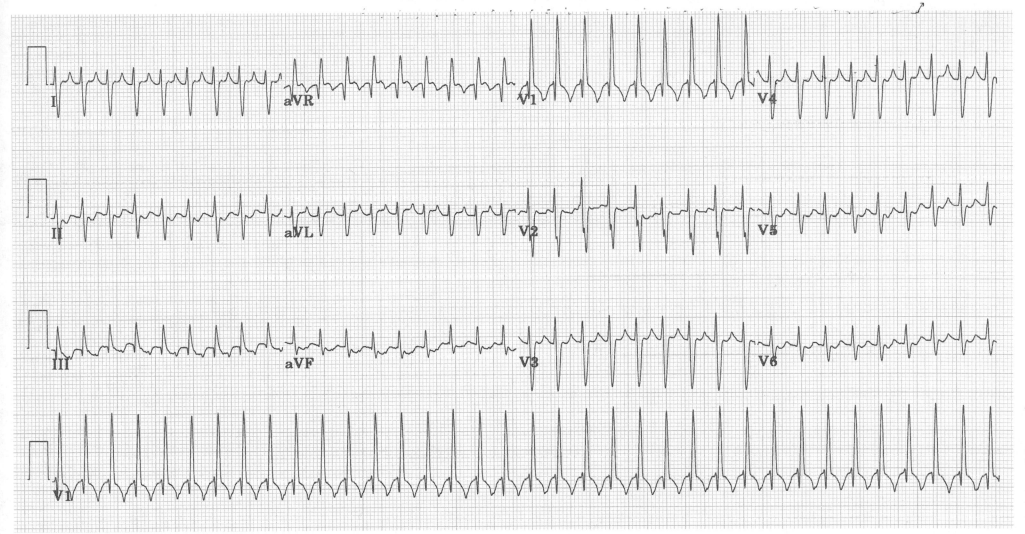

Interpretation Notes: _____

_____

ECG 509 Forty-one year old gentleman with a history of intravenous substance use, endocarditis, and prior mitral and tricuspid valve replacement who re-presents with symptoms and signs of congestive heart failure. He has also noted recent onset palpitations.

510

ELECTROCARDIOGRAM 510

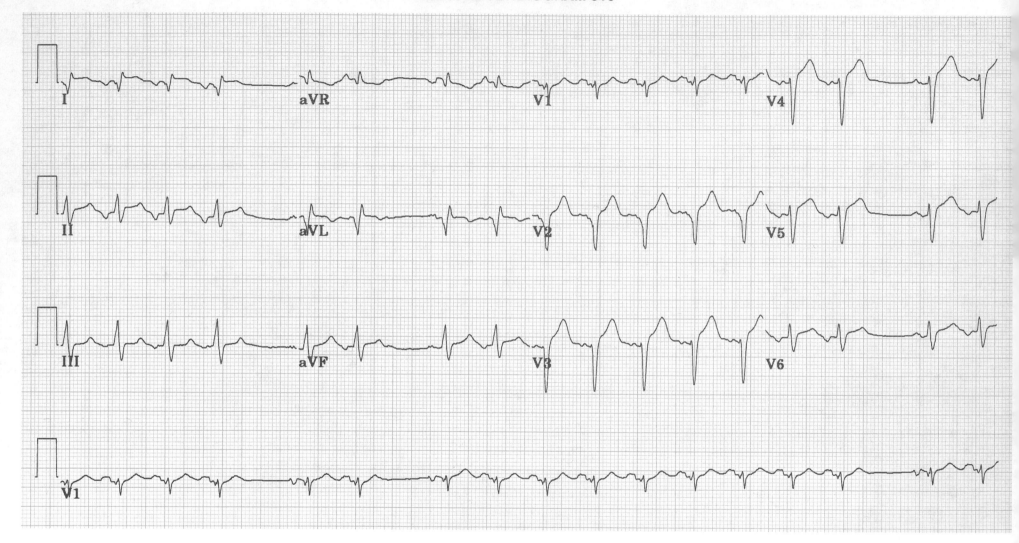

Interpretation Notes:_____

_____

_____

ECG 510 Fifty year old gentleman with coronary artery disease who presented acutely to the hospital with severe chest pressure. Serial cardiac enzyme analysis confirmed acute myocardial injury. The patient was subsequently referred for successful coronary artery bypass grafting. His medications at the time of this electrocardiogram included warfarin, enalapril, aspirin, digoxin, and furosemide.

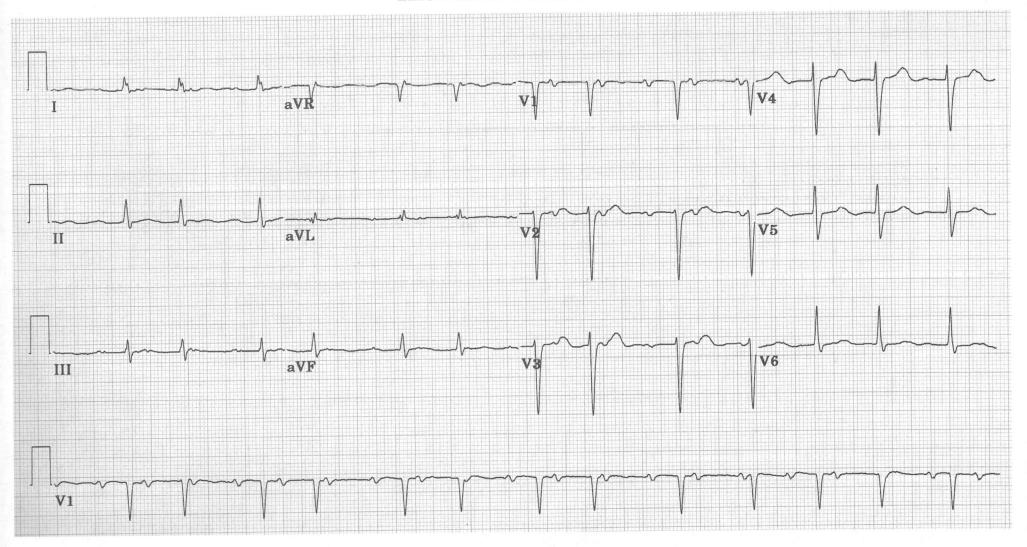

Interpretation Notes: _____

ECG 511 Seventy-two year old gentleman with multi-infarct dementia hospitalized for urosepsis. His past medical history includes hypertension, aspiration pneumonia, chronic obstructive pulmonary disease, and coronary artery disease. His medications included subcutaneous heparin and nebulized inhalers.

512

ELECTROCARDIOGRAM 512

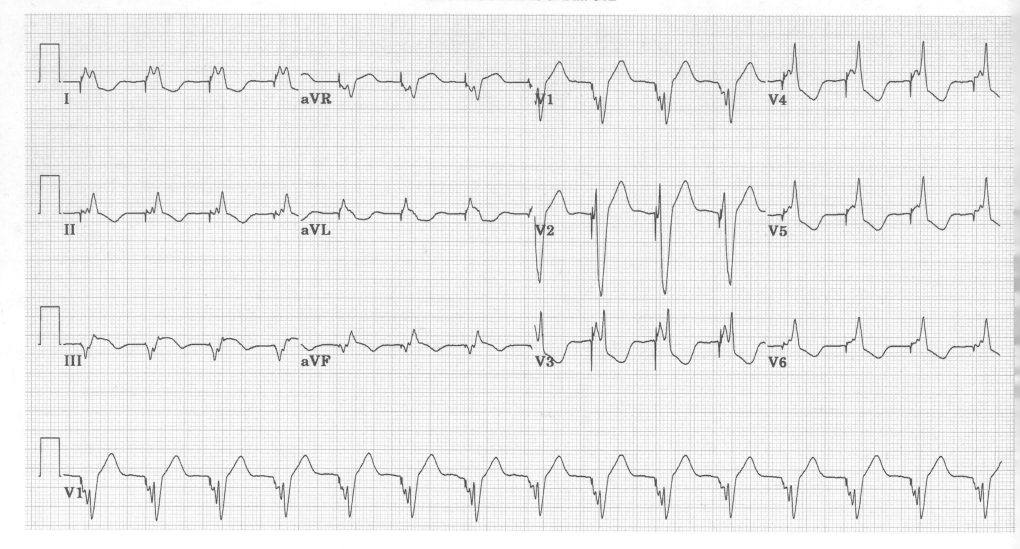

Interpretation Notes: _____

_____

ECG 512 Sixty-nine year old gentleman with an acute chest discomfort syndrome in the presence of a remote coronary artery bypass grafting procedure. Emergency cardiac catheterization was undertaken with a successful angioplasty and stent to the right coronary artery. This procedure was complicated by oliguric renal failure, pulmonary edema, and obtundation. The patient expired several days after the coronary intervention.

ELECTROCARDIOGRAM 513

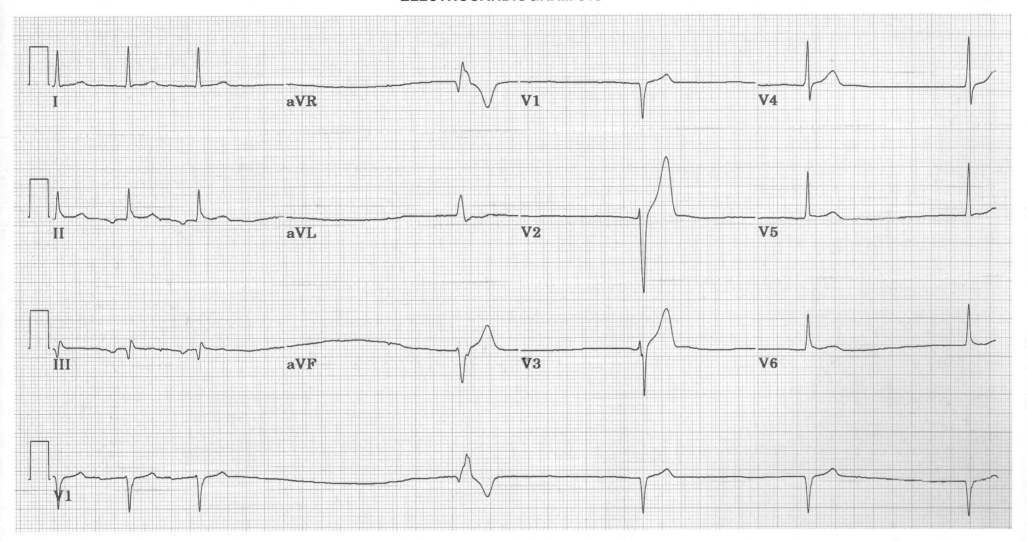

Interpretation Notes: _____

_____

ECG 513 Seventy year old gentleman who is status post recent mitral valve repair secondary to severe mitral valve prolapse and mitral insufficiency.

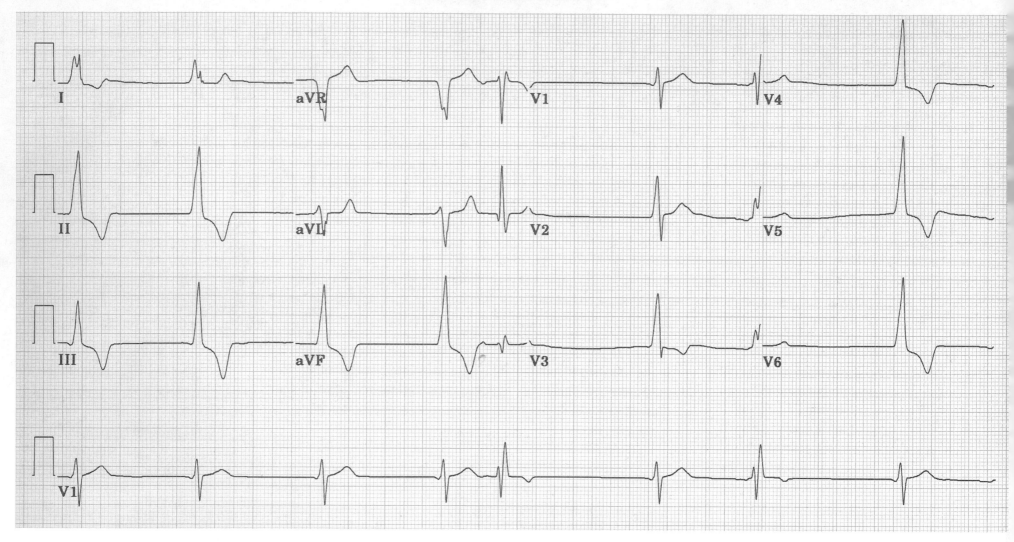

Interpretation Notes: _____

ECG 514 Sixty-two year old woman with coronary artery disease status post an inferoposterior myocardial infarction who now presents for elective mitral valve repair. She has severe ischemic mitral insufficiency. Her current symptoms are dyspnea upon exertion. Her medications at the time of this electrocardiogram included furosemide, atenolol, thyroxine, lisinopril, simvastatin, and aspirin.

ELECTROCARDIOGRAM 515

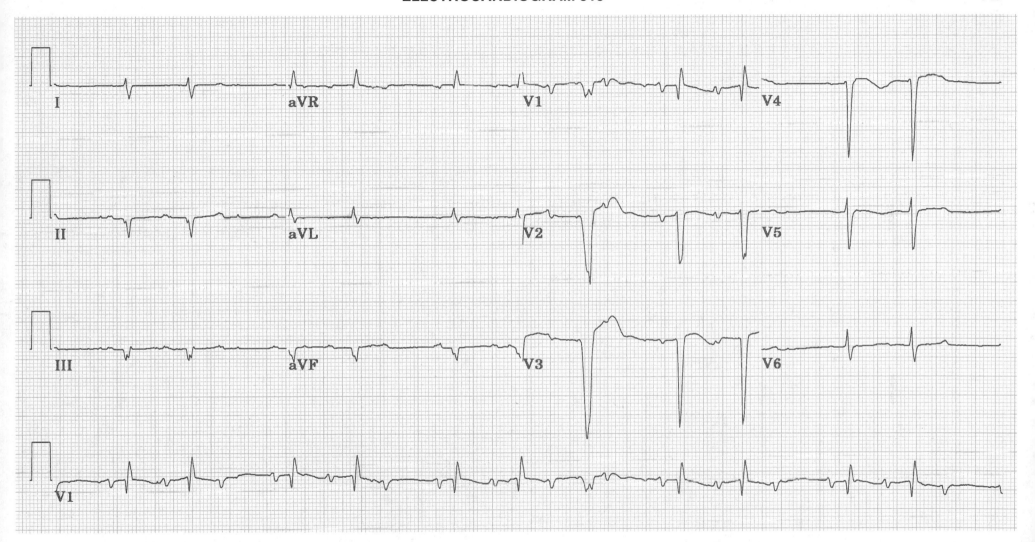

Interpretation Notes: _____

_____

ECG 515 Sixty-one year old gentleman status post cardiac transplantation with severe ischemic post transplantation vasculopathy. He has suffered both inferior and septal myocardial infarctions post transplantation. His medications at the time of this electrocardiogram included cyclosporine, prednisone, azathioprine, nifedipine, and famotidine.

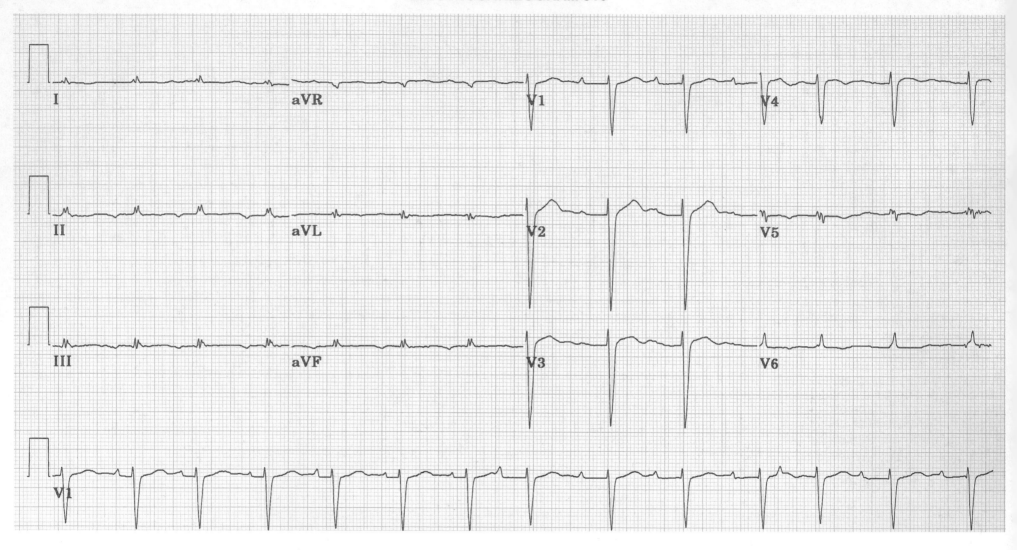

Interpretation Notes: _____

_____

_____

ECG 516 Sixty-five year old gentleman status post remote coronary artery bypass graft surgery and an inferior myocardial infarction with resultant severe left ventricular systolic dysfunction who is being seen as a cardiology outpatient. Co-morbid conditions include hypothyroidism, non-insulin requiring diabetes mellitus, and peripheral vascular disease. His medications included allopurinol, quinidine, bumetanide, captopril, warfarin, digoxin, and a multi-vitamin.

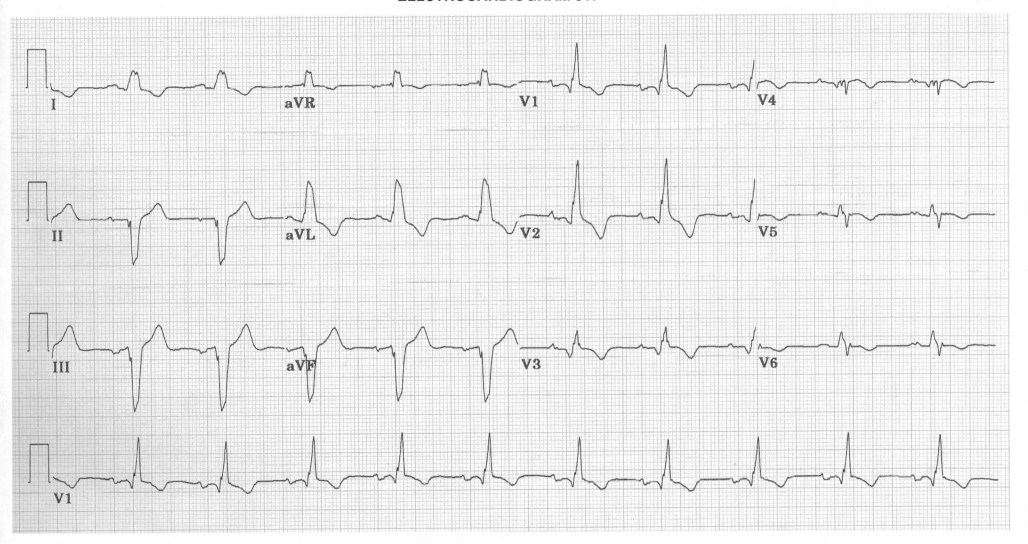

I aVR V1 V4

II aVL V2 V5

III aVF V3 V6

V1

Interpretation Notes:_____

ECG 517 Fifty-six year old gentleman with severe ischemic left ventricular systolic dysfunction admitted to the hospital for evaluation of near syncope. His echocardiogram demonstrated a left ventricular aneurysm. This patient underwent coronary artery bypass graft surgery three years prior to this electrocardiogram. Medications at the time of this tracing included captopril, aspirin, and digoxin.

ELECTROCARDIOGRAM 518

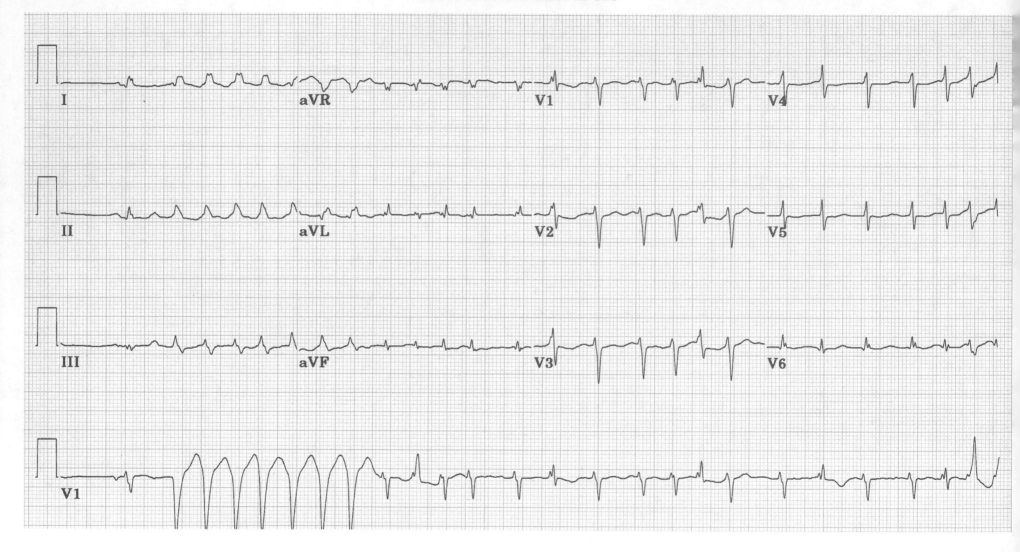

Interpretation Notes: _____

_____

ECG 518 Sixty-two year old gentleman with severe left ventricular systolic dysfunction who is four days status post coronary artery bypass graft surgery.

ELECTROCARDIOGRAM 519

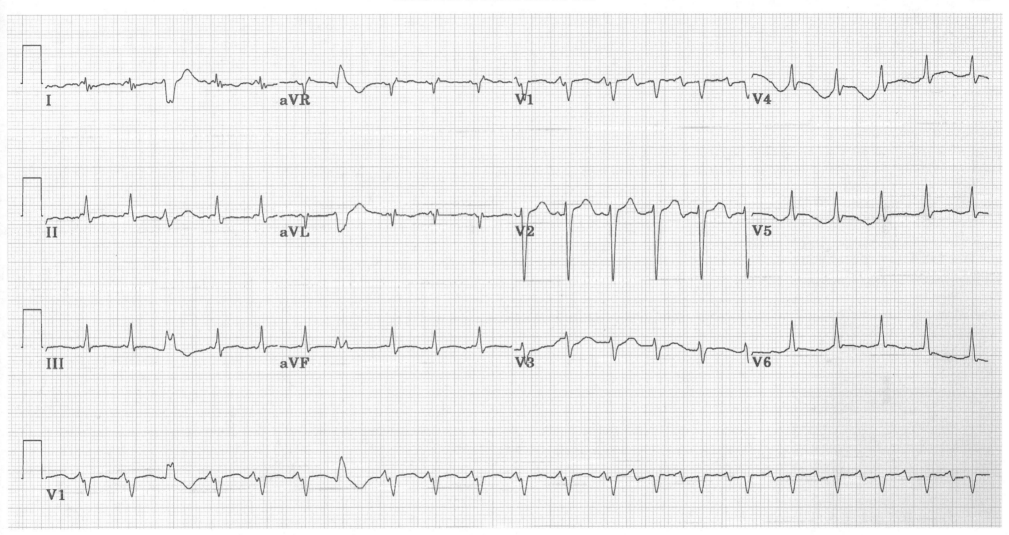

Interpretation Notes: _____

ECG 519 Seventy-two year old gentleman with multi-infarct dementia hospitalized for urosepsis. His past medical history includes hypertension, aspiration pneumonia, chronic obstructive pulmonary disease, and coronary artery disease. His medications included subcutaneous heparin and nebulized inhalers.

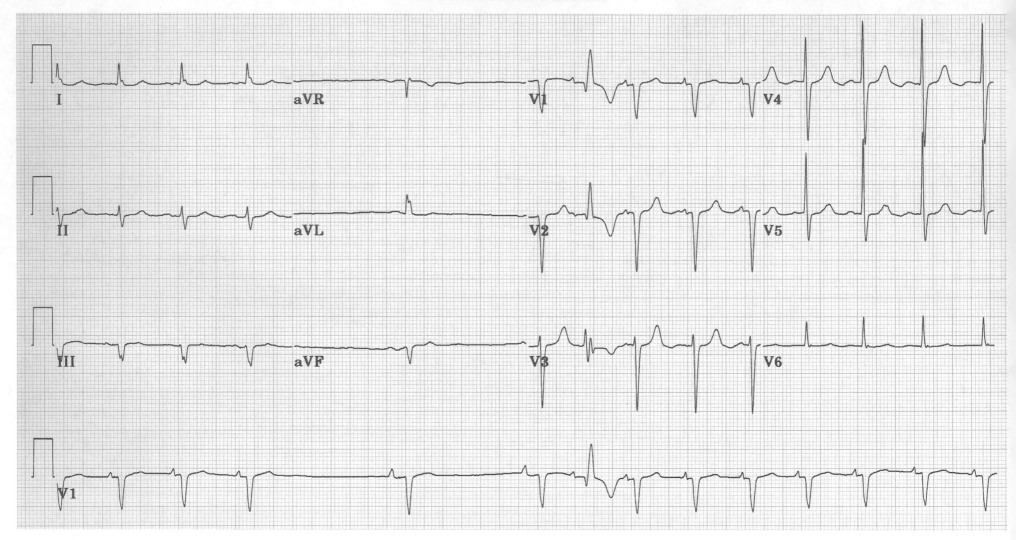

Interpretation Notes: _____

_____

_____

ECG 520 Seventy-six year old woman with paroxysmal ectopic atrial tachycardia who is being seen in the cardiology clinic after a recent elective electrical cardioversion. Her medications included digoxin, diltiazem, triamterene/ hydrochlorothiazide, and warfarin.

ELECTROCARDIOGRAM 521

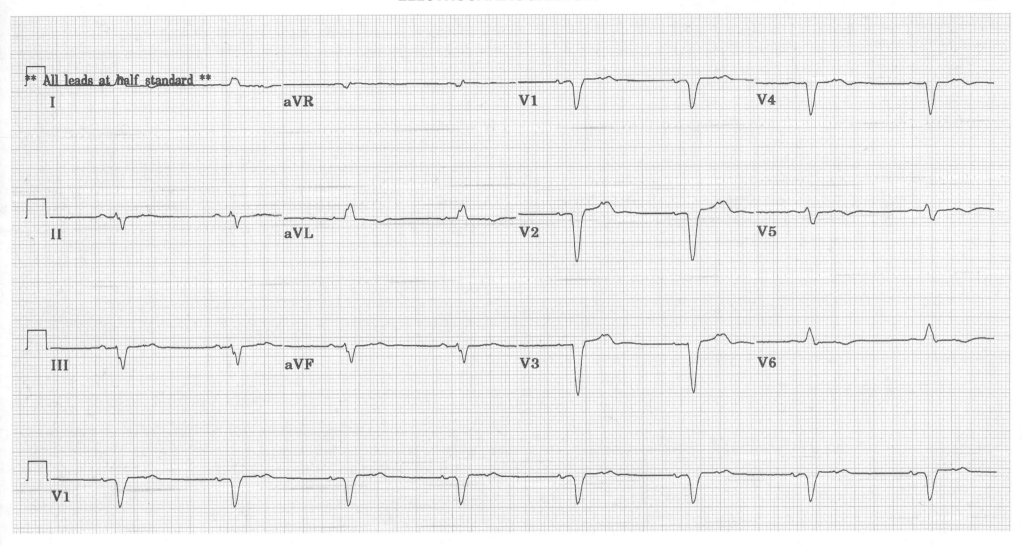

** All leads at half standard **

I   aVR   V1   V4

II   aVL   V2   V5

III   aVF   V3   V6

V1

Interpretation Notes: _____

_____

ECG 521 Ninety-two year old woman with an accelerating pattern of angina pectoris. A recent heart catheterization demonstrated normal coronary arteries and severe aortic stenosis.

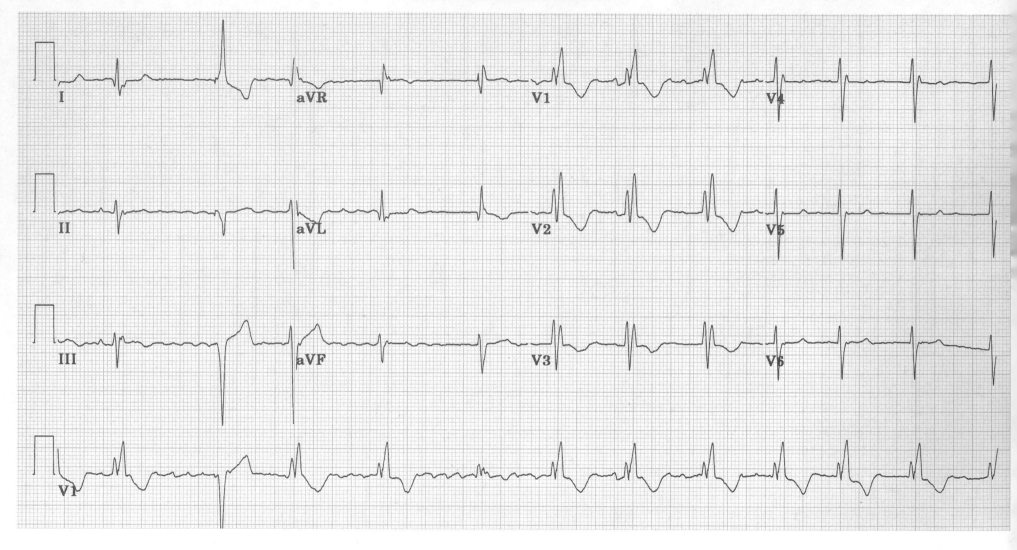

Interpretation Notes: _____

_____

ECG 522 Seventy-six year old gentleman who presents with fatigue and shortness of breath in the setting of severe aortic stenosis. The patient has a past history of rheumatic valvular heart disease undergoing a mechanical mitral valve replacement sixteen years prior to this electrocardiogram. He has also had a prior percutaneous coronary angioplasty to his left anterior descending coronary artery. A recent cardiac catheterization demonstrated normal left ventricular systolic function without evidence of a prior myocardial infarction. Medications at the time of this electrocardiogram included warfarin, furosemide, metoprolol, diltiazem, topical nitroglycerin, and aspirin.

ELECTROCARDIOGRAM 523

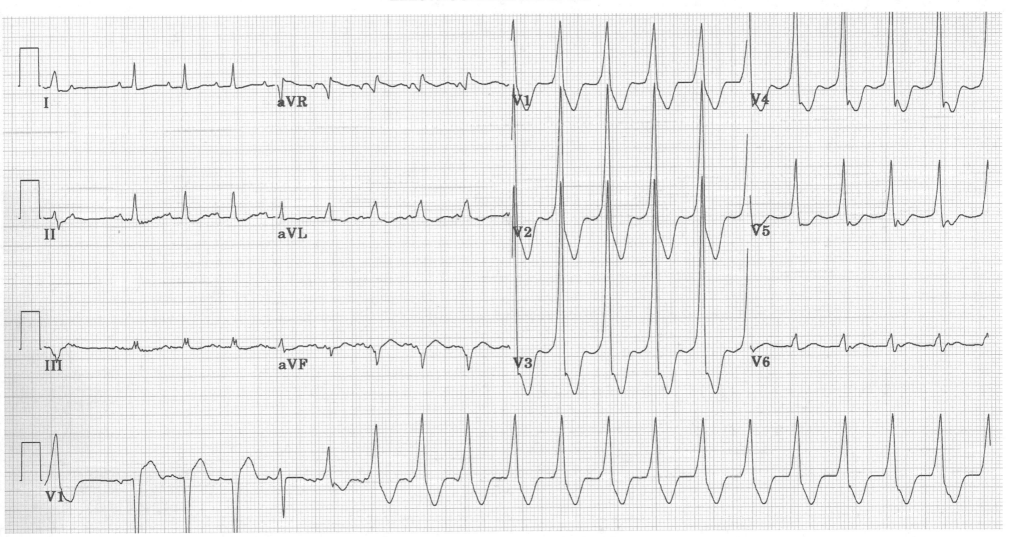

Interpretation Notes:_____

ECG 523 Sixty-six year old gentleman with metastatic prostate cancer and recent onset shortness of breath consistent with congestive heart failure. An echocardiogram demonstrated severe aortic stenosis. A cardiac catheterization demonstrated multi-vessel coronary artery disease. The patient underwent a palliative aortic valvuloplasty procedure which was deemed successful. Medications at the time of this electrocardiogram included enalapril, isosorbide dinitrate, nifedipine, furosemide, aspirin, insulin, quinidine, and digoxin.

524

ELECTROCARDIOGRAM 524

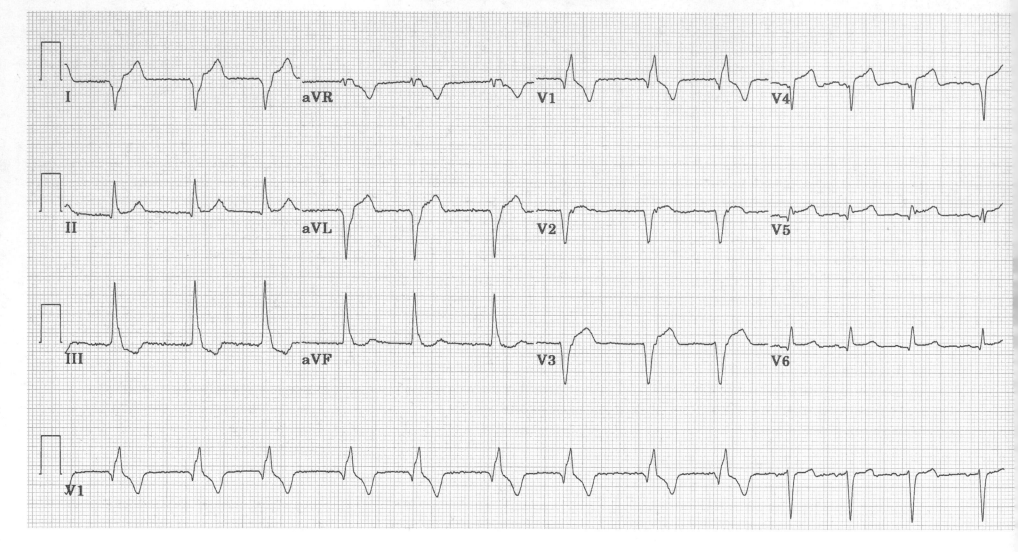

Interpretation Notes: _____

_____

ECG 524 Forty-one year old gentleman with a one hour history of acute chest discomfort who underwent urgent angioplasty and stent placement to his proximal left anterior descending coronary artery. The patient had an angioplasty to his right coronary artery six years prior to this electrocardiogram. He was on no medications at the time of this tracing.

ELECTROCARDIOGRAM 525

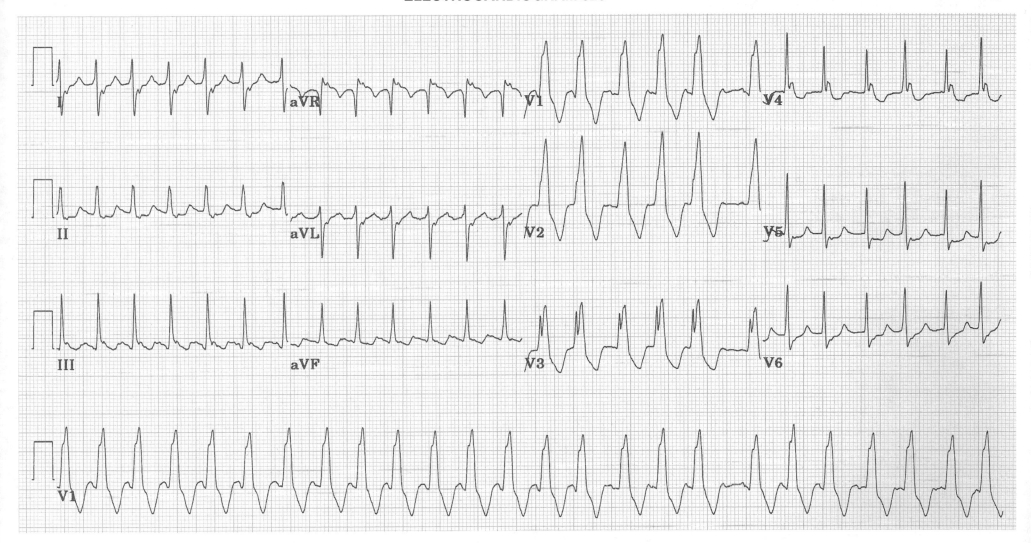

Interpretation Notes: _____

_____

ECG 525 Seventy-five year old woman referred for preoperative cardiac assessment in the setting of anticipated knee replacement. Her past history includes hypertension, long-standing diabetes mellitus, peripheral vascular disease, and hyperlipidemia. She is also status post remote coronary artery bypass graft surgery. Her medications included propafenone, potassium, furosemide, metoprolol, captopril, and warfarin.

526

ELECTROCARDIOGRAM 526

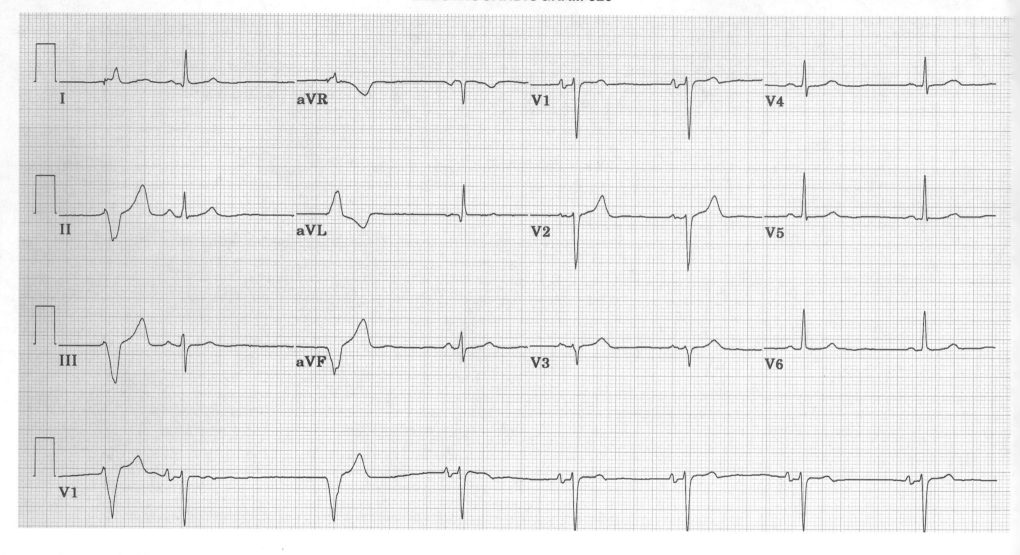

I aVR V1 V4

II aVL V2 V5

III aVF V3 V6

V1

Interpretation Notes: _____

_____

_____

ECG 526 Sixty-six year old gentleman with long-standing hypertension and dialysis requiring renal disease who is admitted to the hospital with facial herpes zoster. His past cardiac history includes a myocardial infarction ten years prior to this electrocardiogram followed by a percutaneous transluminal coronary angioplasty to both his left anterior descending and proximal ramus intermedius coronary arteries. A subsequent permanent pacemaker was placed for symptomatic bradycardia.

ELECTROCARDIOGRAM 527

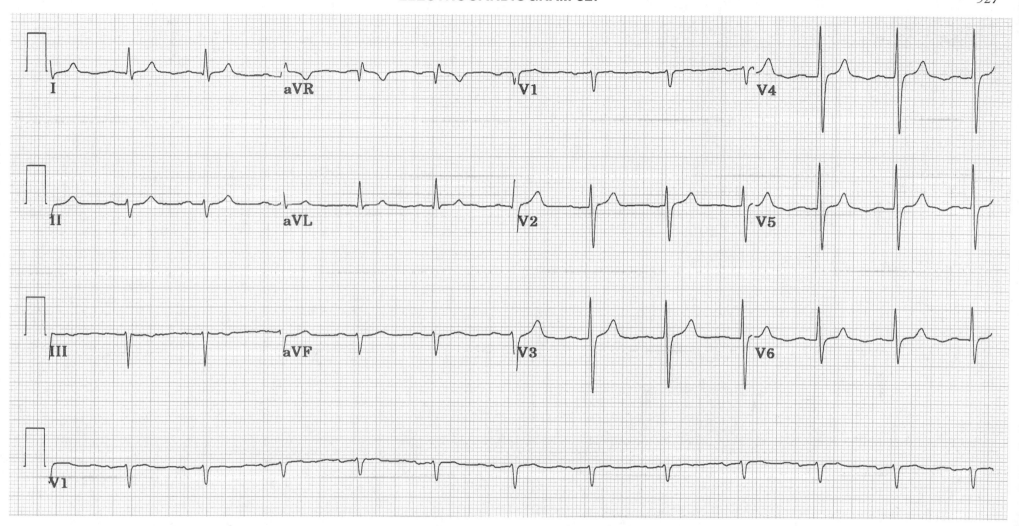

Interpretation Notes: _____

_____

_____

ECG 527 Sixty-two year old gentleman with recent symptoms of exertional dyspnea and a left shoulder ache. His past history included a heart catheterization six years previously documenting moderate coronary artery disease. Medical therapy was pursued for a short period. He was on no medications at the time of this electrocardiogram.

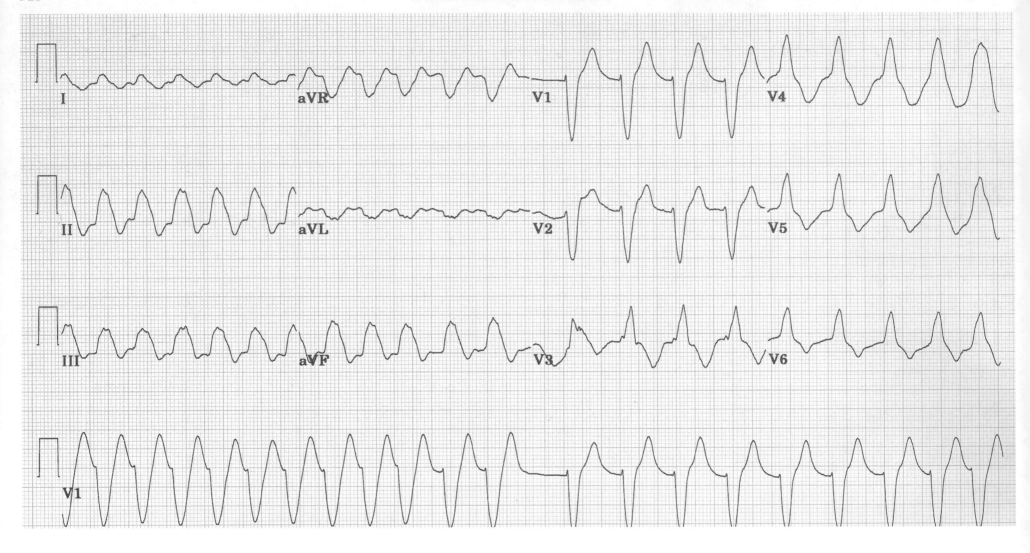

Interpretation Notes: _____

ECG 528 Sixty-seven year old woman with dialysis requiring renal failure who is recently postoperative exploratory laparotomy for an ischemic bowel. This patient became septic, hypotensive, and hyperkalemic. This electrocardiogram represents her terminal heart rhythm prior to expiring.

ELECTROCARDIOGRAM 529

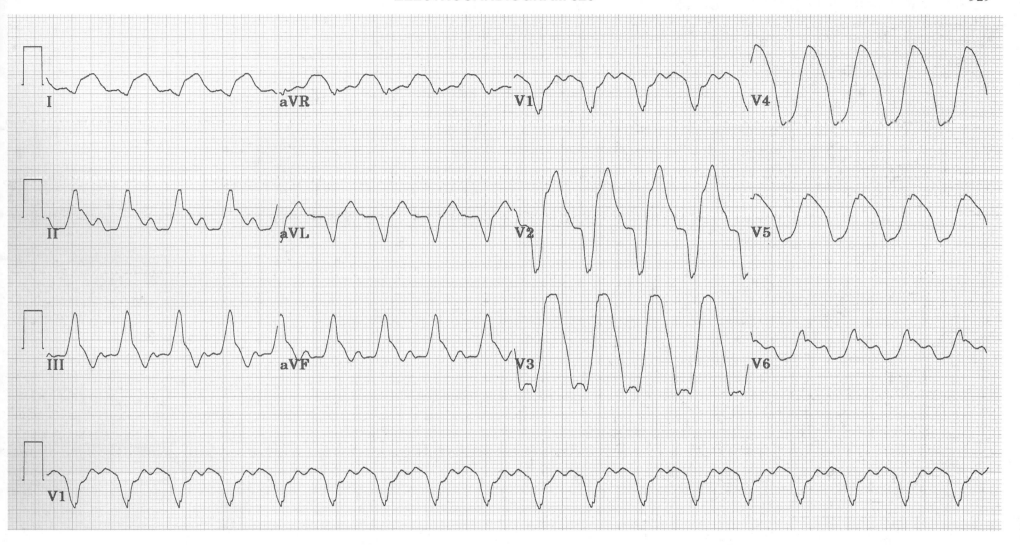

Interpretation Notes:_____

ECG 529 Sixty-seven year old woman with dialysis requiring renal failure who is recently postoperative exploratory laparotomy for an ischemic bowel. This patient became septic, hypotensive and hyperkalemic. This electrocardiogram represents her terminal heart rhythm prior to expiring.

ELECTROCARDIOGRAM 530

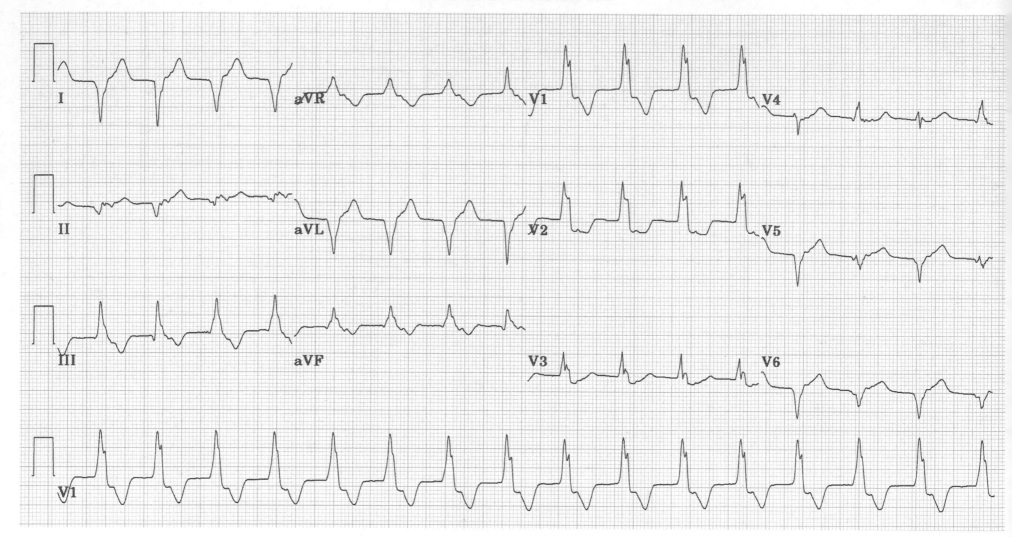

Interpretation Notes: _____

_____

_____

ECG 530 Seventy-five year old woman with a recent abnormal thallium stress test who is now referred for a cardiac catheterization. Her symptoms include dyspnea upon exertion. Her medications included digoxin, warfarin, isosorbide mononitrate, metoprolol, and lovastatin. This electrocardiogram was obtained shortly after an initially successful percutaneous transluminal coronary angioplasty to a left circumflex coronary artery branch. The procedure was complicated by abrupt vessel closure and acute myocardial injury.

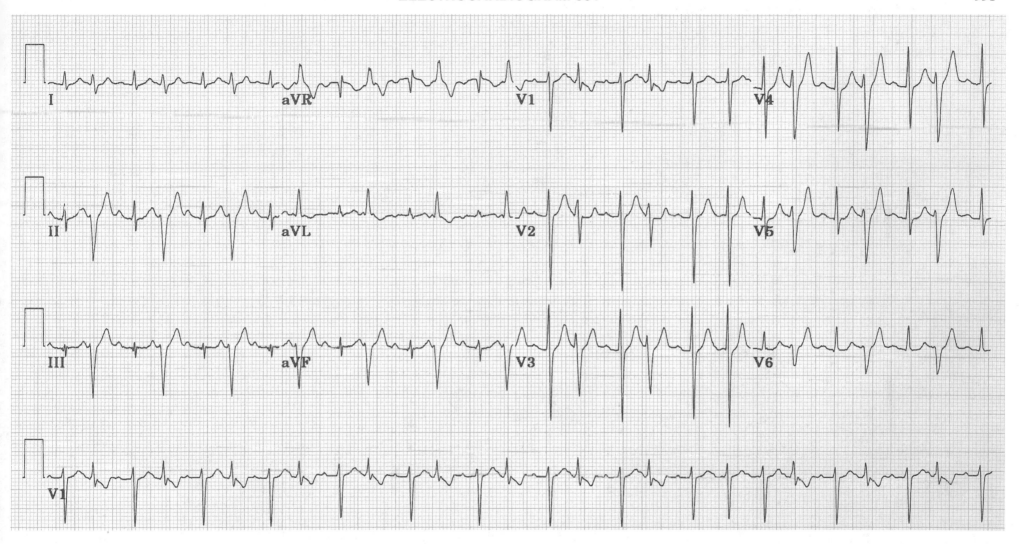

Interpretation Notes: _____

_____

ECG 531 Seventy-three year old gentleman with hyperthyroidism, hypertension, and no prior cardiac disease. This electrocardiogram was obtained as a preoperative evaluation prior to a thyroid nodule resection.

532

ELECTROCARDIOGRAM 532

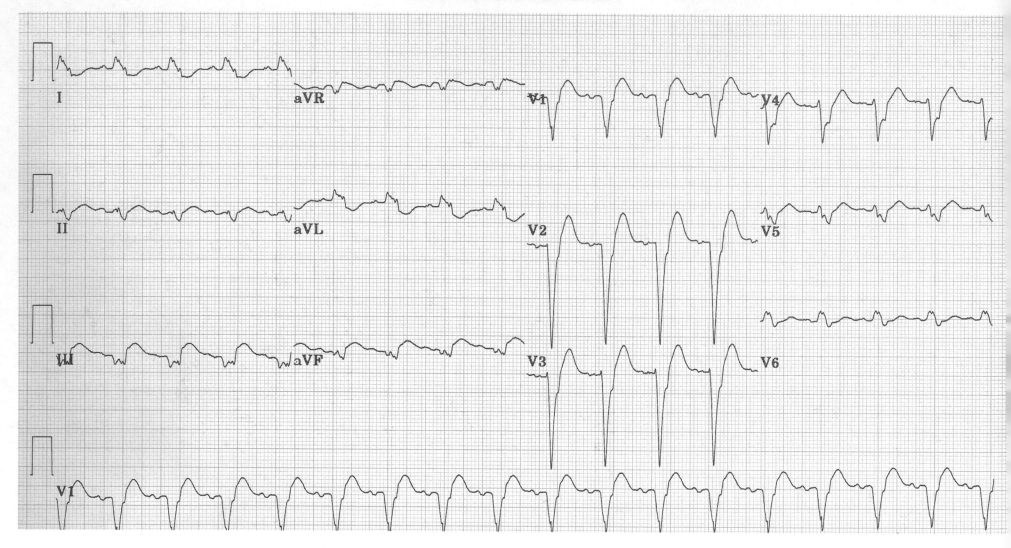

Interpretation Notes: _____

_____

_____

ECG 532 Fifty-six year old gentleman accepted in transfer from an outside hospital after suffering an acute inferior myocardial infarction. A cardiac catheterization demonstrated severe multi-vessel coronary artery disease. The patient was referred for coronary artery bypass surgery. Co-morbid conditions include insulin requiring diabetes mellitus, chronic renal insufficiency, hypertension, and anemia.

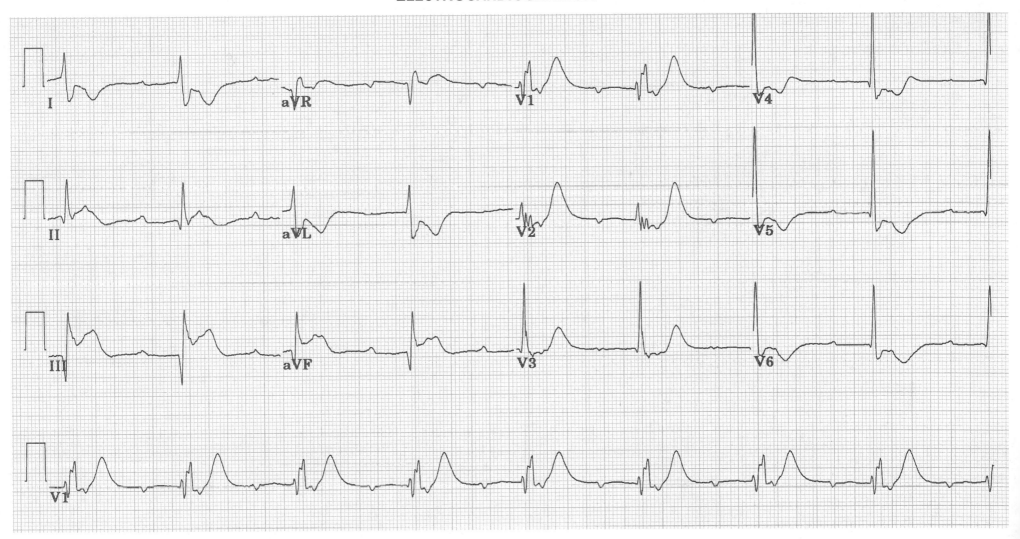

Interpretation Notes: _____

_____

ECG 533 Seventy year old gentleman with a chest discomfort syndrome who presented urgently to the hospital. His electrocardiogram demonstrated an acute inferior myocardial infarction. This patient subsequently developed advanced atrioventricular block with a prolonged HV interval detected during an electrophysiology study. A permanent pacemaker was placed. The patient underwent a cardiac catheterization and conservative medical management of his coronary artery disease.

ELECTROCARDIOGRAM 534

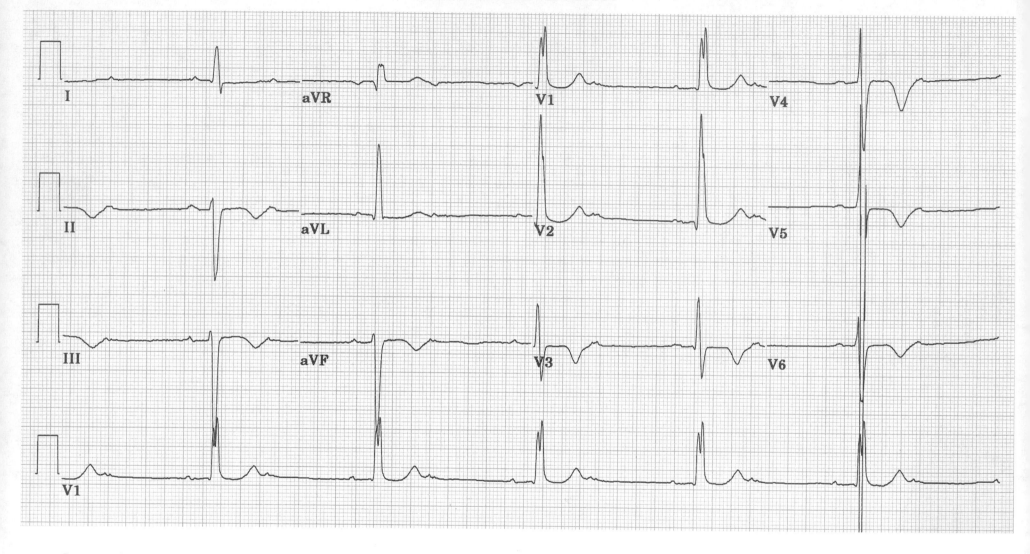

I   aVR   V1   V4

II   aVL   V2   V5

III   aVF   V3   V6

V1

Interpretation Notes: _____

_____

_____

ECG 534 Ninety-four year old woman admitted to the hospital with acute onset diarrhea and dehydration. She was noted to have lower extremity swelling with venous Doppler studies demonstrating an acute deep venous thrombosis. A subsequent ventilation perfusion scan was interpreted as high probability for an acute pulmonary embolism.

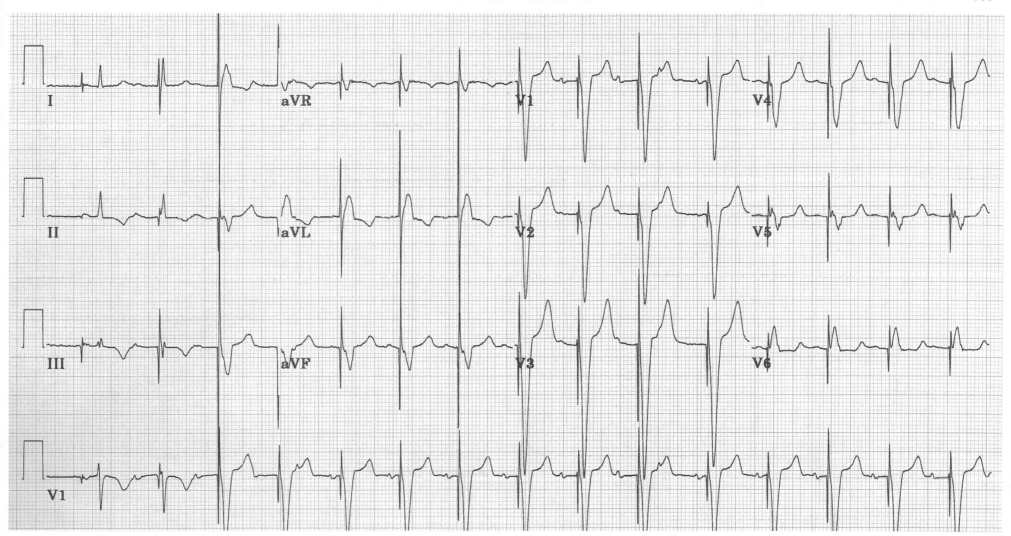

Interpretation Notes:_____

ECG 535 Seventy-two year old woman with advanced atrioventricular block necessitating prior permanent pacemaker placement who returns for a follow-up evaluation. Co-morbid conditions include coronary artery disease, hypertension, and hyperlipidemia. Medications at the time of this electrocardiogram included metoprolol, aspirin, and simvastatin.

ELECTROCARDIOGRAM 536

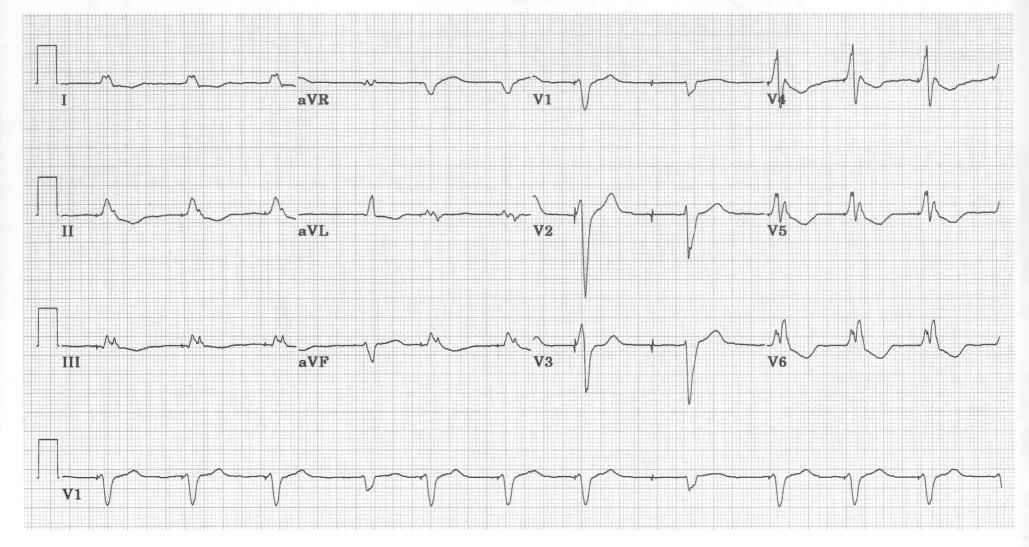

Interpretation Notes: _____

_____

ECG 536 Seventy-two year old gentleman with severe ischemic left ventricular systolic dysfunction, chronic atrial fibrillation, and advanced heart block admitted for pacemaker implantation. This electrocardiogram represents a routine tracing obtained after pacemaker placement. Interrogation of the pacemaker was abnormal and the patient underwent pacemaker lead repositioning.

ELECTROCARDIOGRAM 537

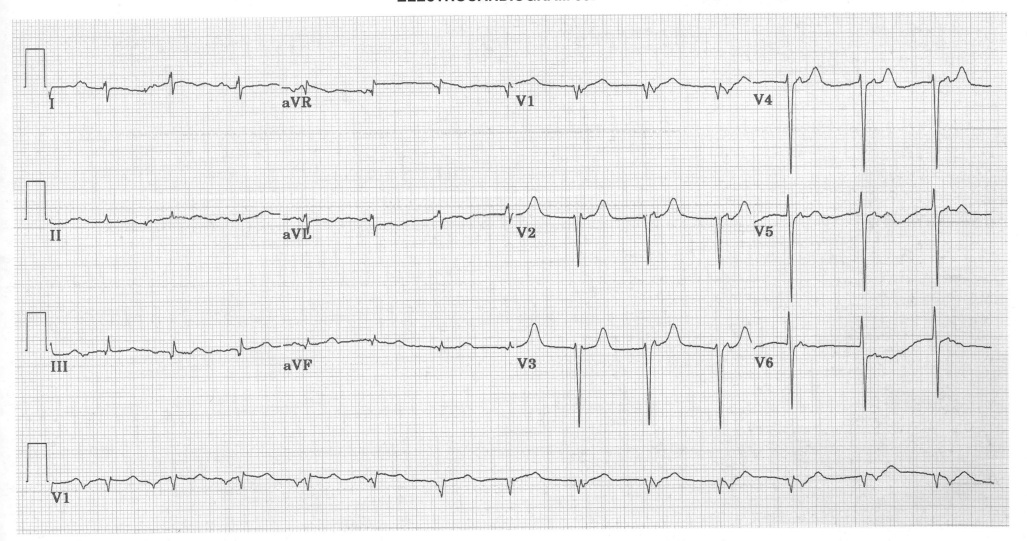

Interpretation Notes: _____

_____

ECG 537 Seventy-two year old gentleman with long-standing hypertension and hypertensive heart disease who presented to the hospital with increasing shortness of breath. These symptoms were most consistent with recent onset congestive heart failure.

538

ELECTROCARDIOGRAM 538

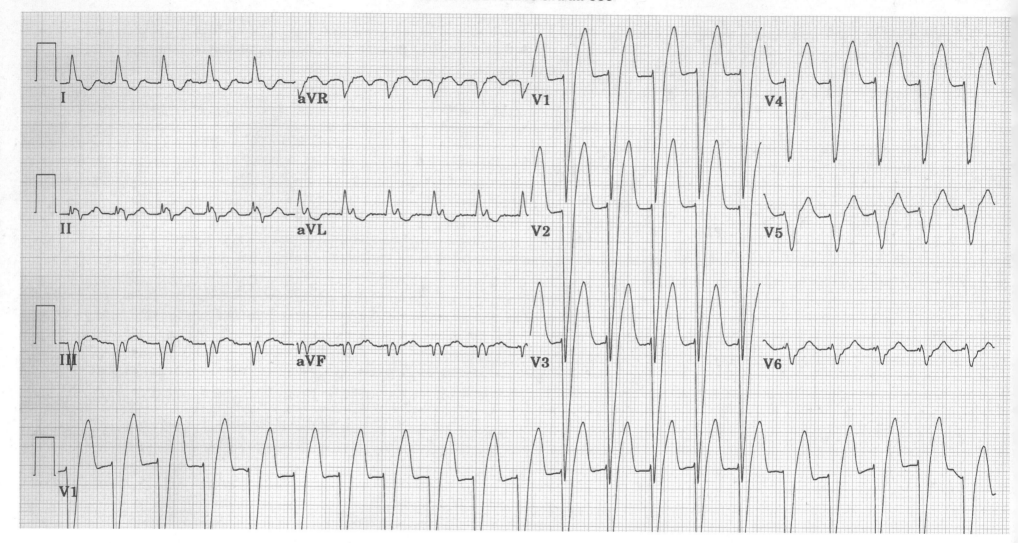

Interpretation Notes: _____

_____

ECG 538 Thirty-five year old gentleman with congenital heart disease including pulmonic stenosis and an atrial septal defect admitted for syncope. This electrocardiogram was obtained as part of his syncope evaluation.

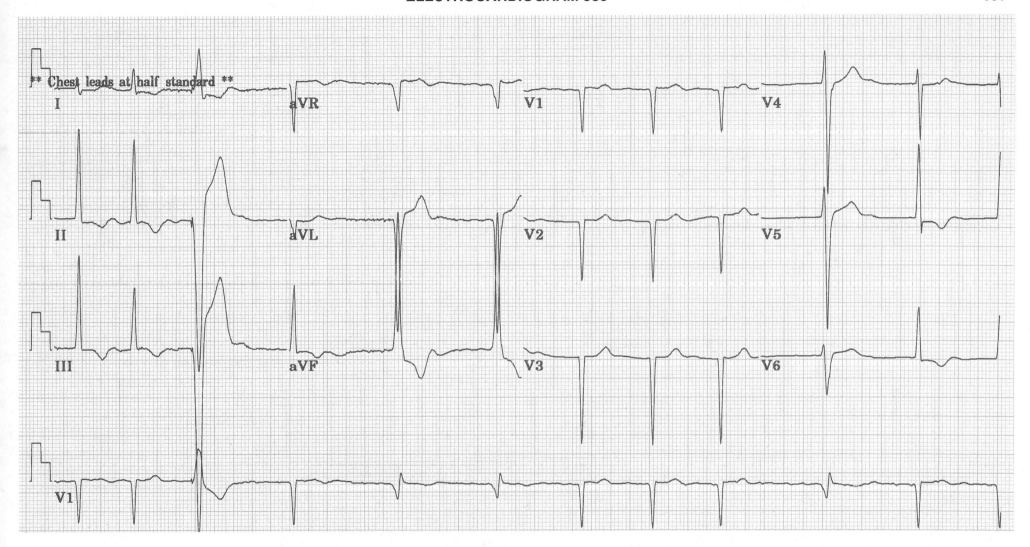

** Chest leads at half standard **

I aVR V1 V4
II aVL V2 V5
III aVF V3 V6
V1

Interpretation Notes: _____

ECG 539 Seventy-two year old gentleman admitted to the hospital with acute onset shortness of breath and pleuritic chest pain. His past medical history is significant for the myelodysplastic syndrome, permanent pacemaker placement, and squamous cell carcinoma of the head and neck.

540

ELECTROCARDIOGRAM 540

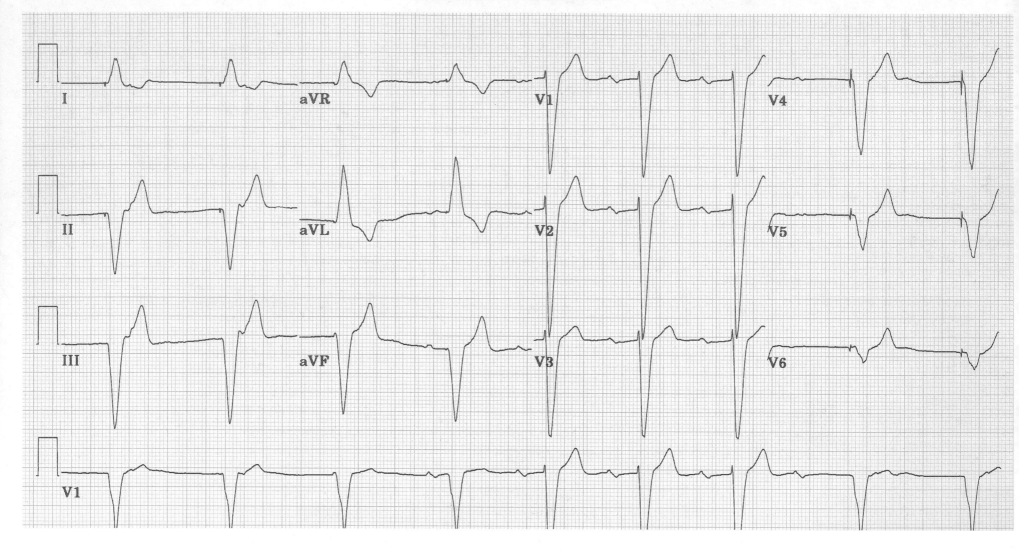

Interpretation Notes: _____

_____

ECG 540 Sixty-three year old gentleman with coronary artery disease and a prior myocardial infarction who presents for a routine pacemaker follow-up examination. He has a history of high degree atrioventricular block and is status post permanent pacemaker placement. Medications at the time of this electrocardiogram included nifedipine, hydrochlorothiazide, and aspirin.

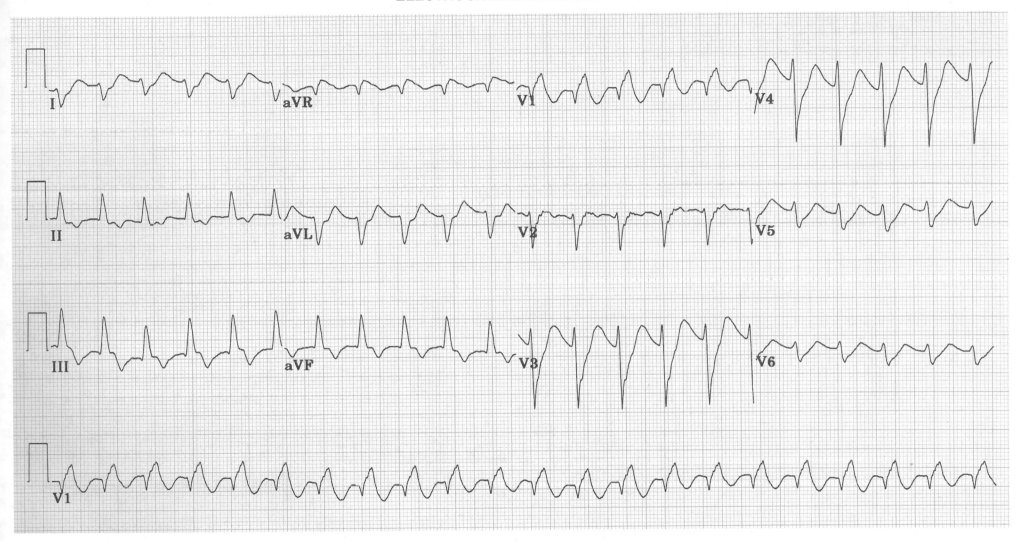

Interpretation Notes: _____

ECG 541 Eighteen year old gentleman with sepsis and multisystem organ failure in the setting of intractable seizures who expired shortly after this electrocardiogram. His serum potassium level was greater than 7.0 meq/L at the time of this electrocardiogram.

ELECTROCARDIOGRAM 542

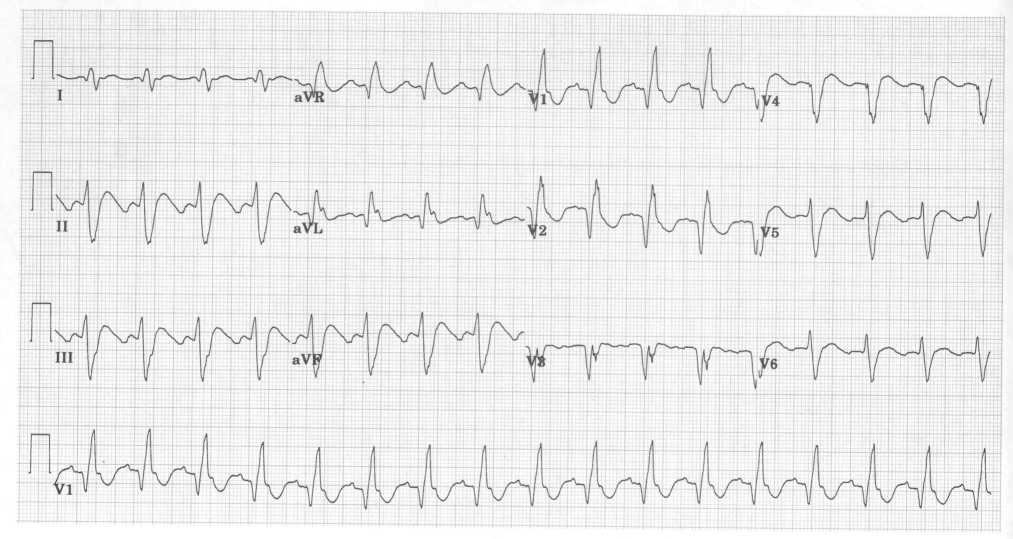

I aVR V1 V4

II aVL V2 V5

III aVF V3 V6

V1

Interpretation Notes: _____

_____

_____

ECG 542 Sixty-three year old gentleman status post a remote myocardial infarction of unknown location who re-presents with increasing symptoms of fatigue, shortness of breath, and lower extremity swelling. A recent echocardiogram demonstrated moderately severe left ventricular systolic dysfunction. Medications at the time of this tracing included amiodarone, quinidine, digoxin, aspirin, and furosemide.

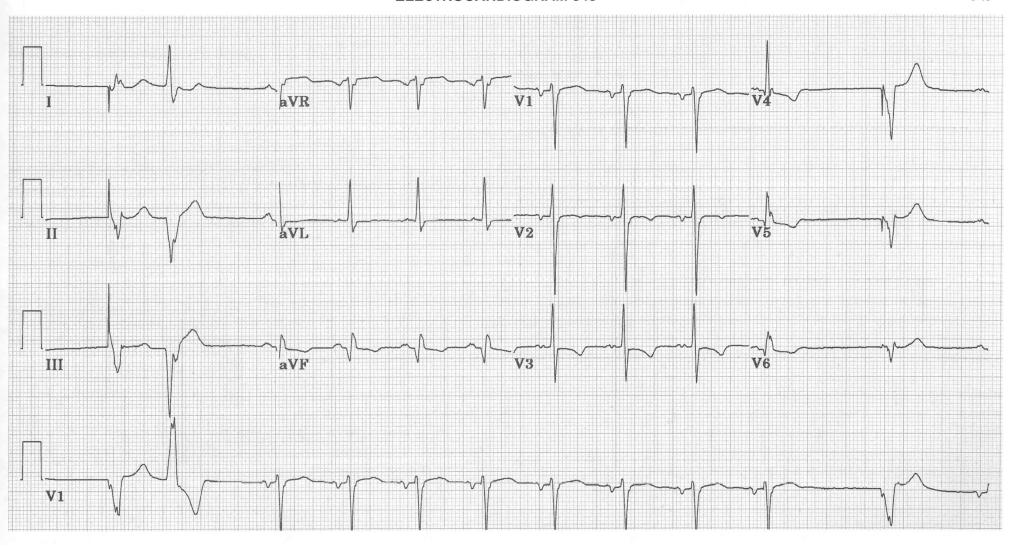

Interpretation Notes: _____
_____
_____

ECG 543 Seventy-two year old gentleman with severe coronary artery disease status post implantable cardiac defibrillator placement who is readmitted to the hospital with fevers and chills. Blood cultures returned positive for staphylococcus aureus.

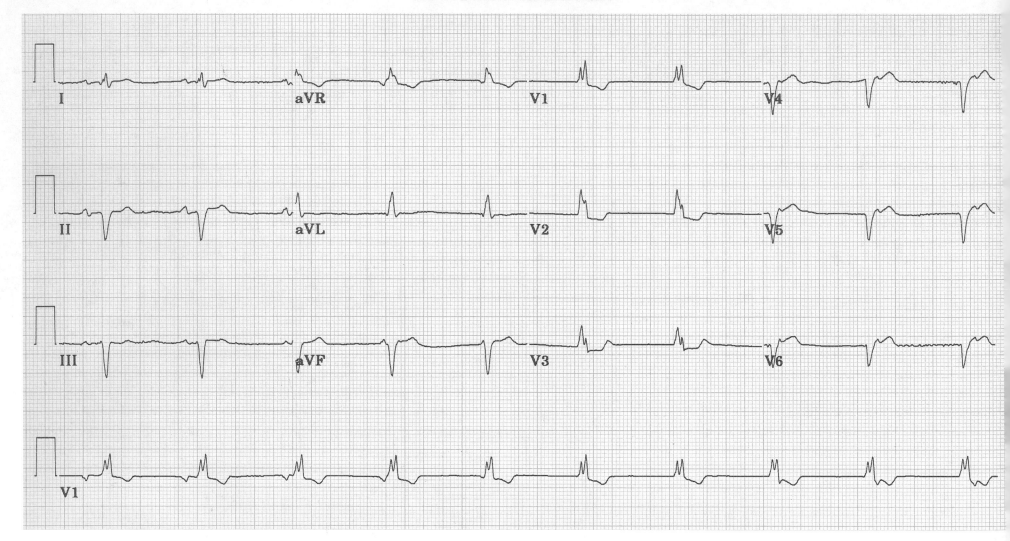

Interpretation Notes: _____

_____

ECG 544 Sixty-nine year old gentleman who re-presents for a second open heart surgery procedure in the setting of progressive angina, known coronary artery disease, moderate left ventricular systolic dysfunction, and severe mitral insufficiency. This tracing was obtained after a repeat coronary artery bypass grafting operation and mitral valve reparative surgery.

ELECTROCARDIOGRAM 545

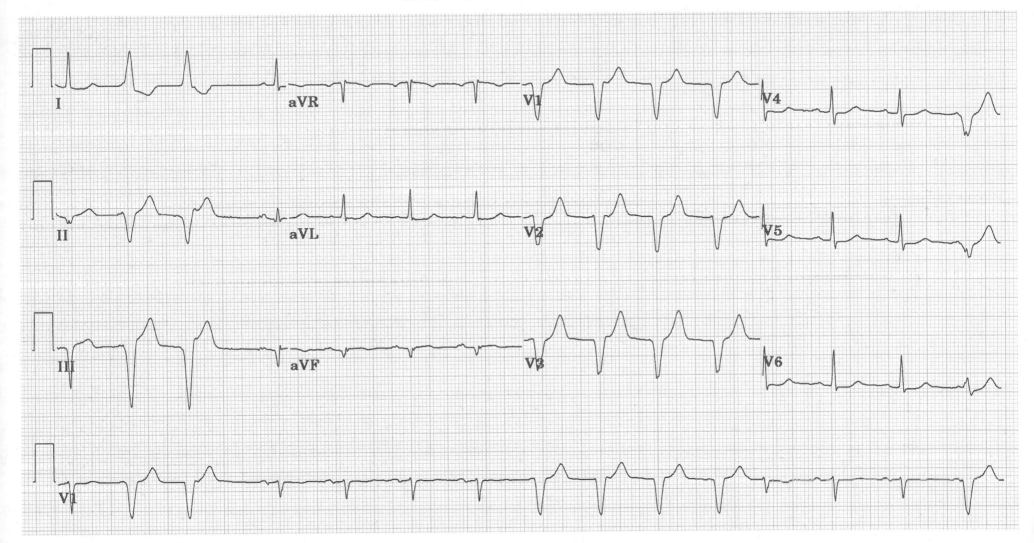

I aVR V1 V4

II aVL V2 V5

III aVF V3 V6

V1

Interpretation Notes: _____

_____

ECG 545 Sixty-one year old gentleman seen in cardiology outpatient follow-up after an acute inferior myocardial infarction three years prior to this electrocardiogram. This was followed by urgent right coronary artery percutaneous transluminal coronary angioplasty. He feels well with infrequent episodes of angina pectoris. His medications included metoprolol, aspirin, nicotinic acid, simvastatin, and vitamins.

ELECTROCARDIOGRAM 546

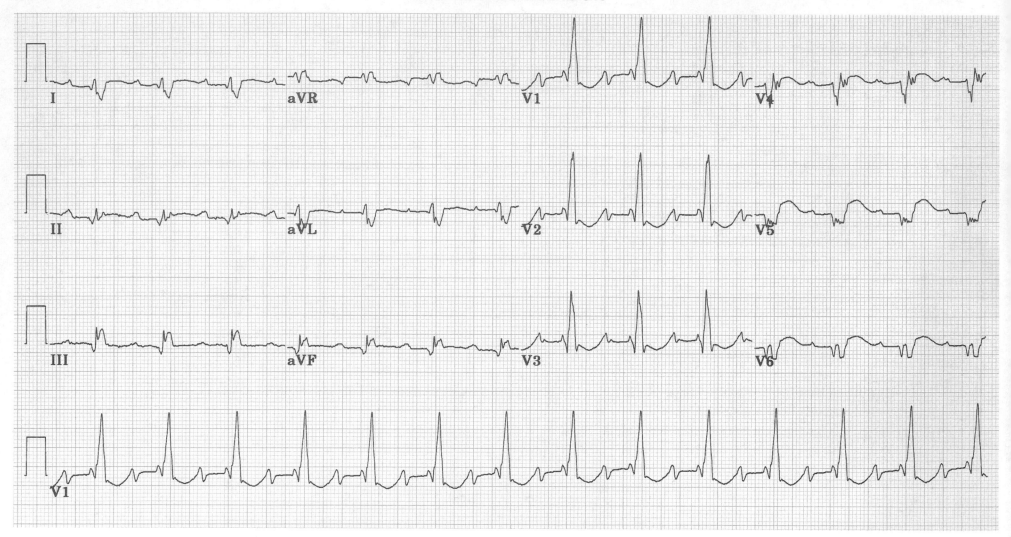

Interpretation Notes:_____

_____

ECG 546 Eighty-four year old woman transferred from an outside hospital and admitted to the Coronary Intensive Care Unit. She is status post a recent acute inferolateral myocardial infarction and experiencing post myocardial infarction angina pectoris. Her past medical history includes hypertension, peripheral vascular disease, and a cerebrovascular accident.

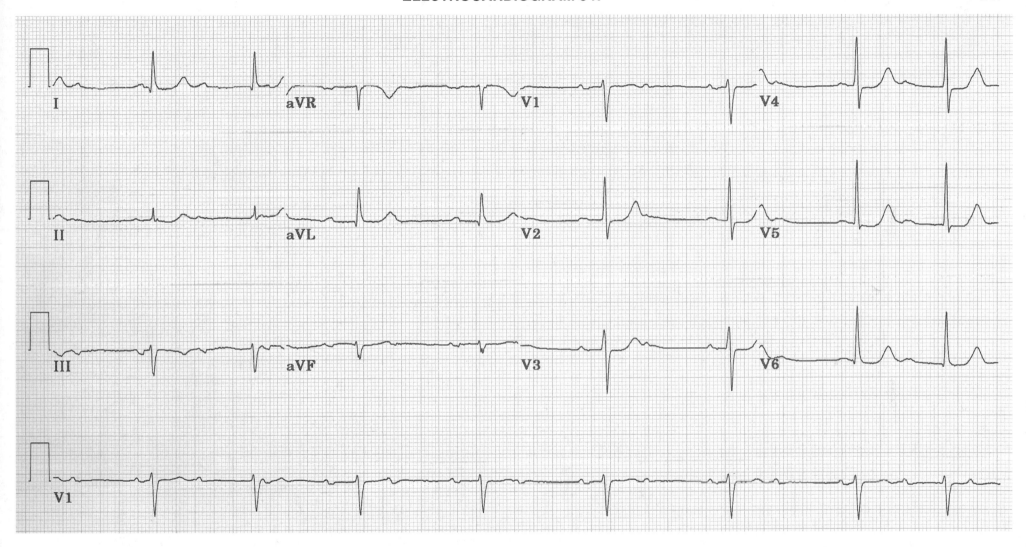

I aVR V1 V4
II aVL V2 V5
III aVF V3 V6
V1

Interpretation Notes: _____

_____

ECG 547 Seventy-five year old gentleman with long-standing hypertension who underwent electrocardiography on a routine basis during a preoperative urologic surgery evaluation. This demonstrated advanced atrioventricular block and a subsequent permanent pacemaker was placed.

548

ELECTROCARDIOGRAM 548

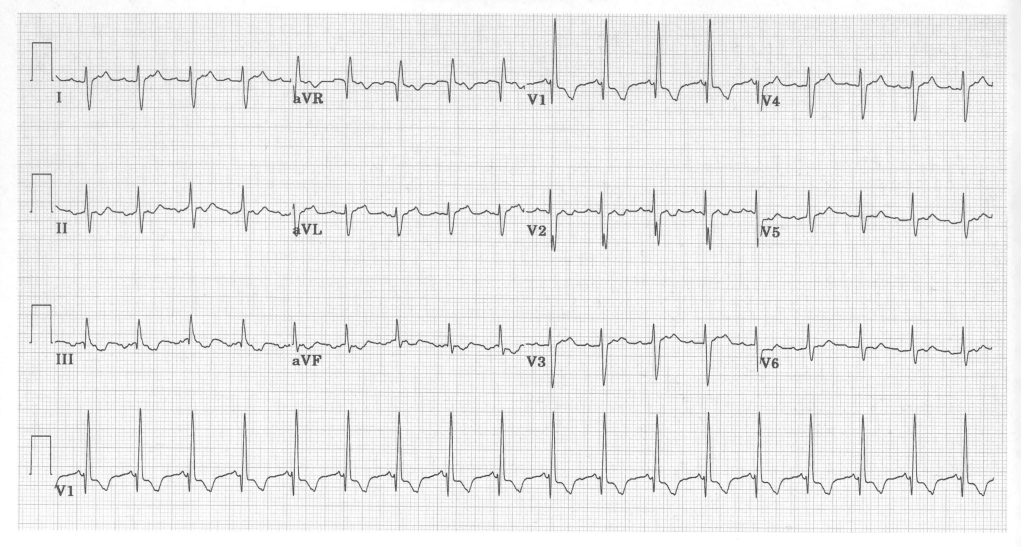

Interpretation Notes: _____

_____

ECG 548 Forty-one year old gentleman admitted to the hospital with alcohol intoxication and congestive heart failure. The patient is status post both mitral and tricuspid valve replacement secondary to endocarditis. His medications at the time of this electrocardiogram included furosemide, warfarin, atenolol, and topical nitroglycerin.

ELECTROCARDIOGRAM 549

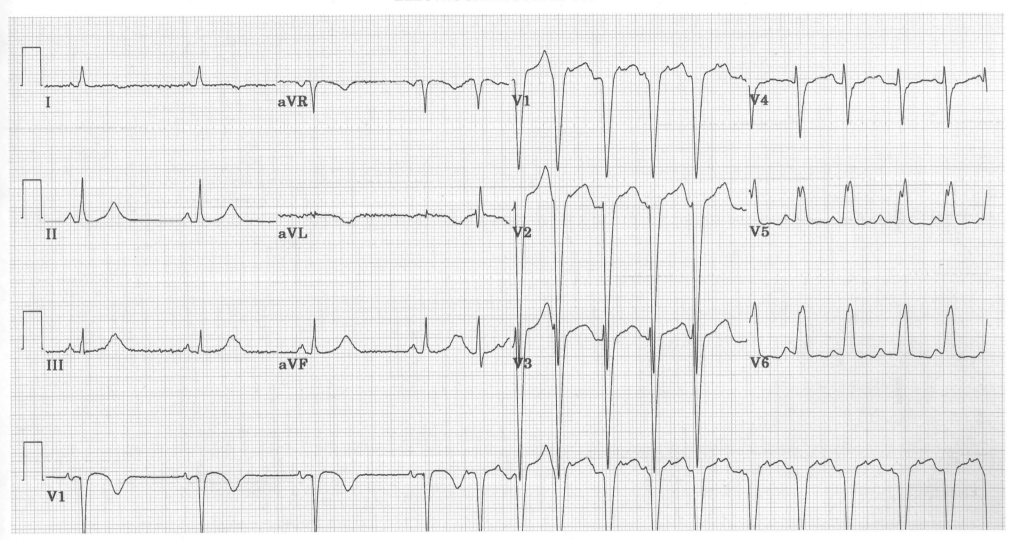

I	aVR	V1	V4
II	aVL	V2	V5
III	aVF	V3	V6

V1

Interpretation Notes: _____

_____

ECG 549 Sixty-three year old gentleman with paroxysmal atrial fibrillation, atrial tachycardia, and wide complex tachycardia in the setting of excessive alcohol use, hypertension, and hyperlipidemia.

ELECTROCARDIOGRAM 550

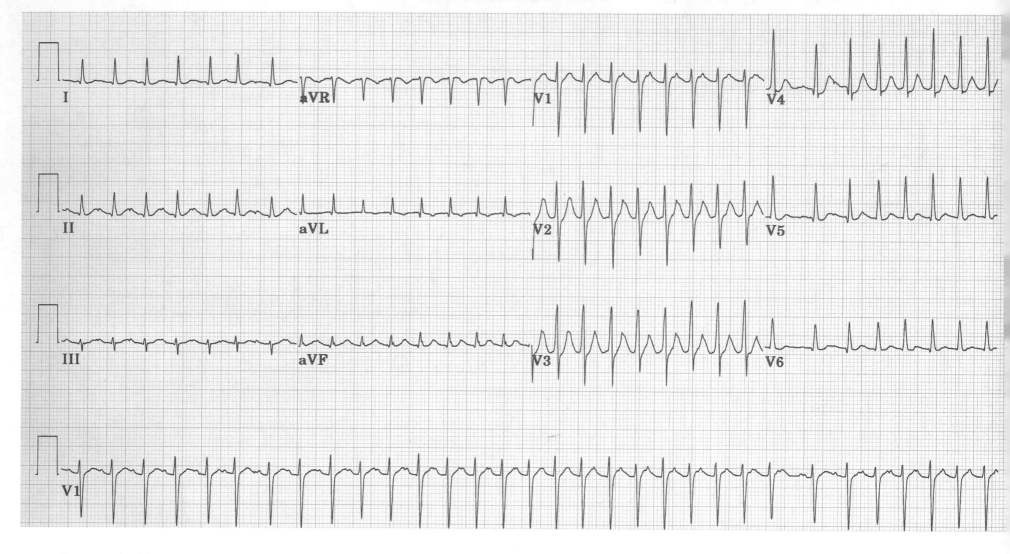

Interpretation Notes: _____

_____

ECG 550 Seventy-three year old gentleman who presented to the hospital with acute abdominal pain, fever, nausea, and vomiting. A computed tomography scan demonstrated diverticulitis and a contained abscess. This electrocardiogram was obtained postoperatively after a sigmoid colectomy and ileostomy was performed.

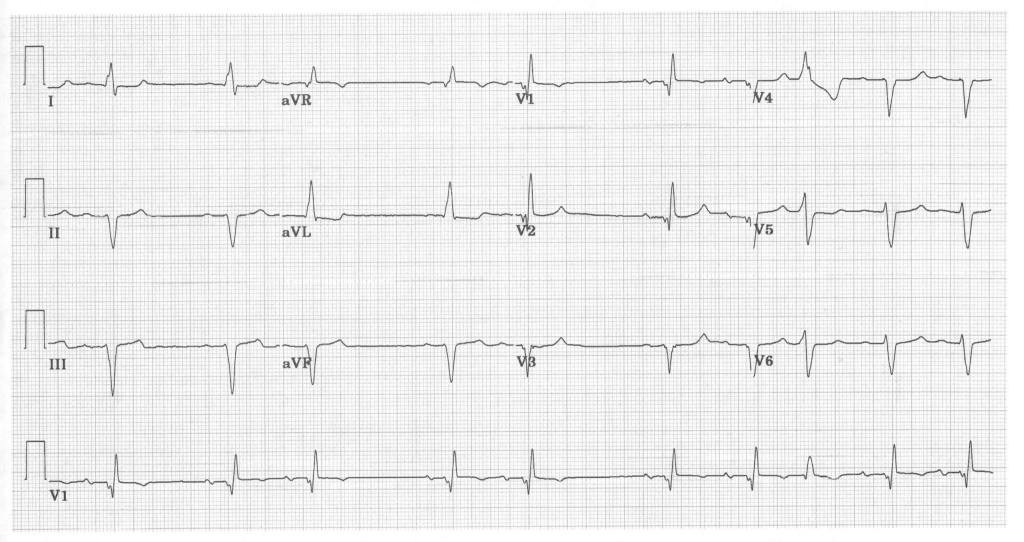

I aVR V1 V4

II aVL V2 V5

III aVF V3 V6

V1

Interpretation Notes: _____

ECG 551 Sixty-nine year old gentleman who presents to the hospital with symptoms of unstable angina. He is status post coronary artery bypass surgery, percutaneous transluminal coronary angioplasty, and stent placement to the left circumflex coronary artery. Co-morbidities include hypercholesterolemia. Medications included metoprolol, aspirin, and simvastatin.

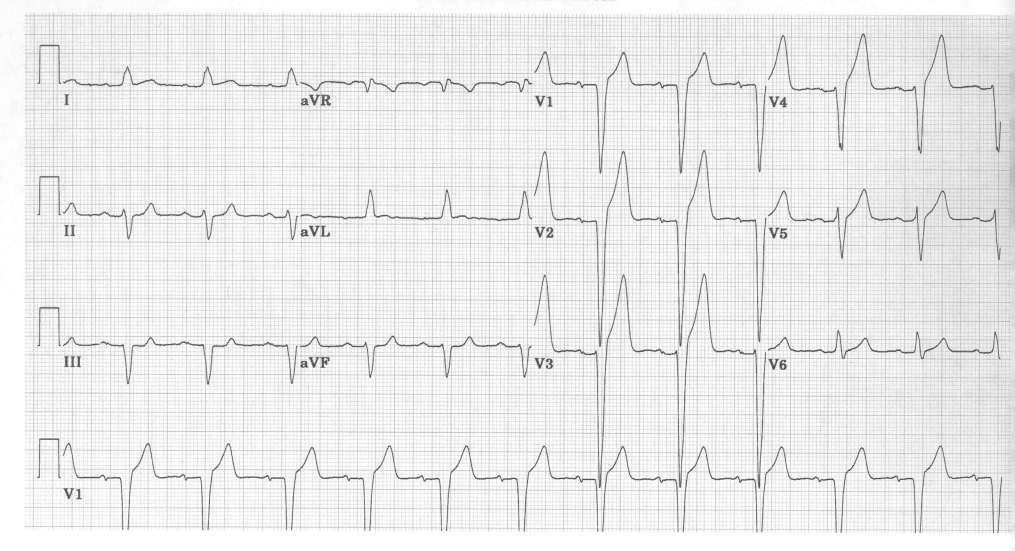

Interpretation Notes: _____

ECG 552 Eighty-two year old gentleman with recent syncope admitted to the hospital with an acute chest pain syndrome. An urgent cardiac catheterization demonstrated severe stenoses within the left anterior descending, first diagonal branch and right coronary arteries. Acute angioplasty was performed to the left anterior descending coronary artery stenosis.

ELECTROCARDIOGRAM 553

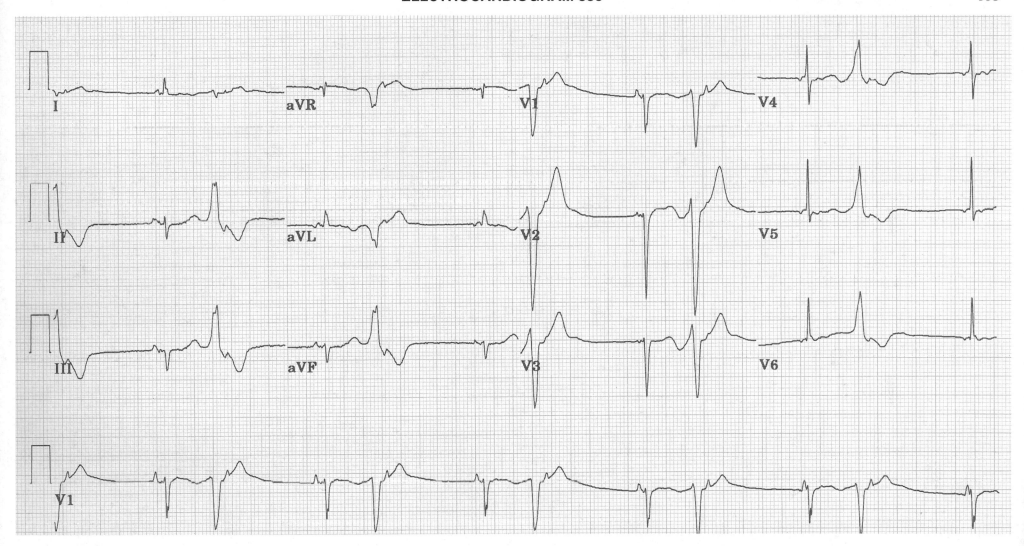

ECG 553 Seventy year old woman with a history of chronic renal insufficiency, a dilated cardiomyopathy, and deep venous thrombosis who presented to the hospital with a one week history of positional lightheadedness.

Interpretation Notes: _____
_____
_____

ELECTROCARDIOGRAM 554

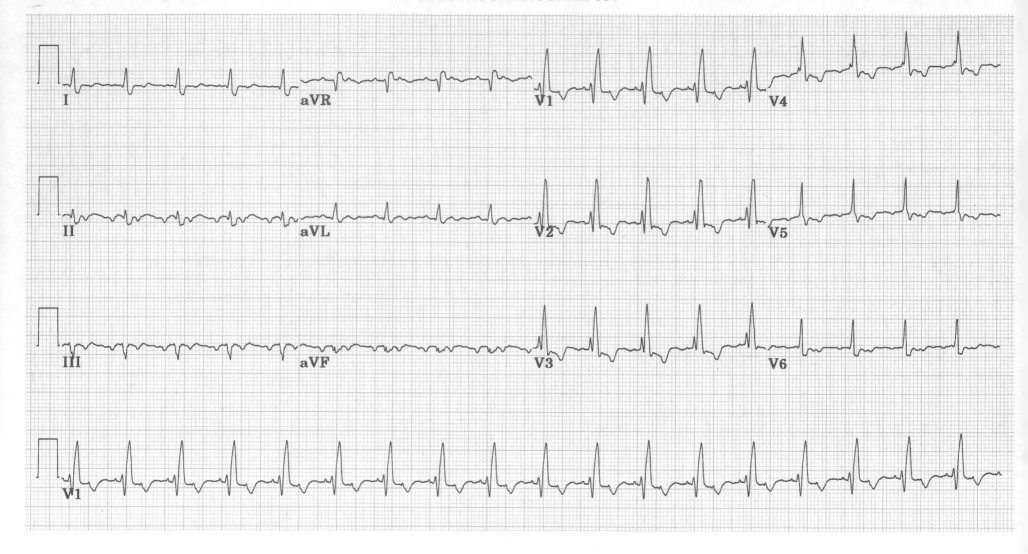

Interpretation Notes: _____

_____

ECG 554 Sixty-seven year old gentleman accepted in hospital transfer for further evaluation of recent onset shortness of breath. His past history includes long-term tobacco use. A chest x-ray suggested an acute pneumonia. An echocardiogram obtained during his hospitalization confirmed severe left ventricular systolic dysfunction. Medications at the time of this electrocardiogram included prednisone, theophylline, digoxin, and bumetanide.

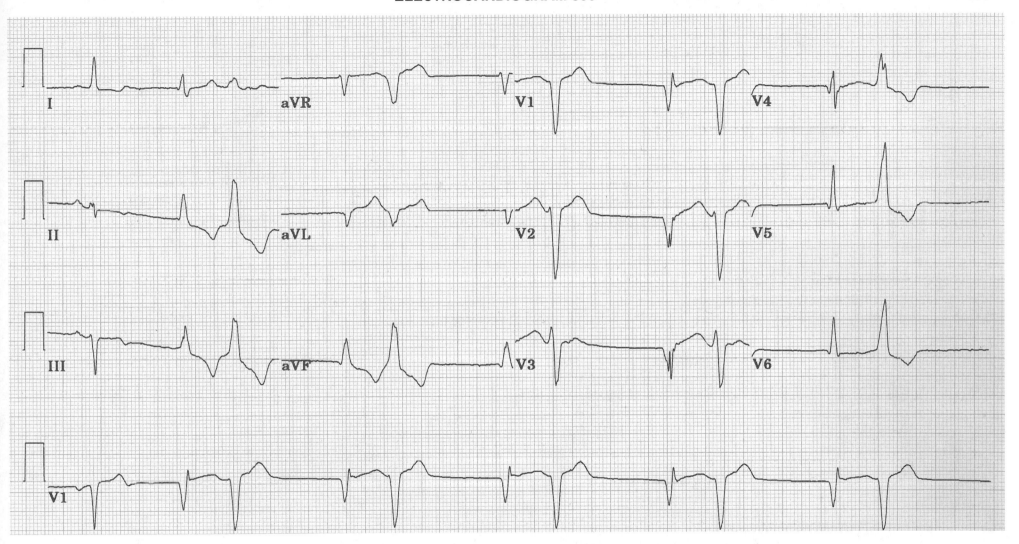

I aVR V1 V4

II aVL V2 V5

III aVF V3 V6

V1

Interpretation Notes: _____

_____

ECG 555 Seventy-seven year old gentleman with coronary artery disease, hypertension, and moderate left ventricular systolic dysfunction who developed acute substernal chest discomfort and diaphoresis after a transurethral resection of the prostate procedure earlier the same day. The patient has a history of a prior myocardial infarction in both the left anterior descending and right coronary artery distributions.

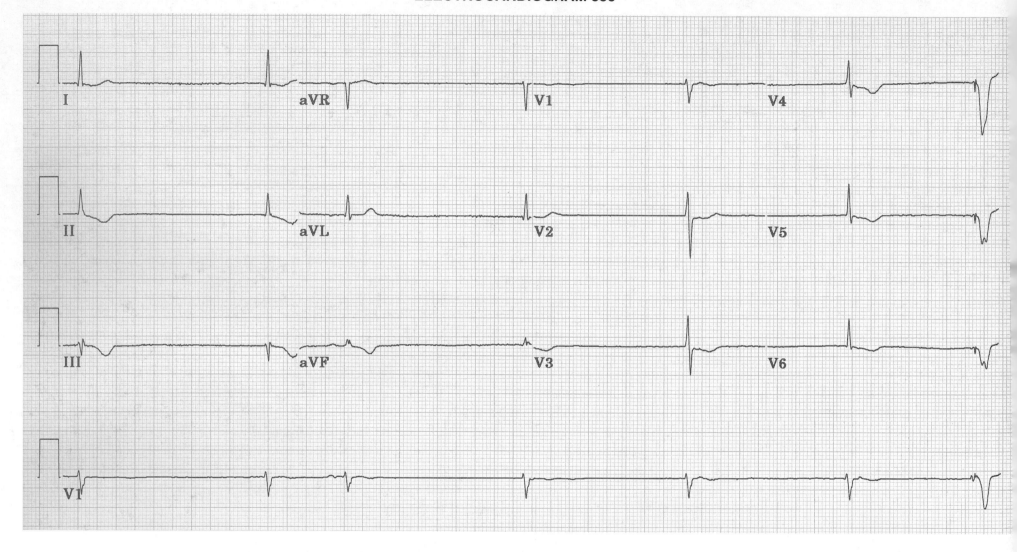

Interpretation Notes: _____

_____

ECG 556 Sixty-five year old woman status post recent mitral valve and tricuspid valve repair in the setting of severe coronary artery obstructive disease and prior coronary artery bypass graft surgery.

ELECTROCARDIOGRAM 557

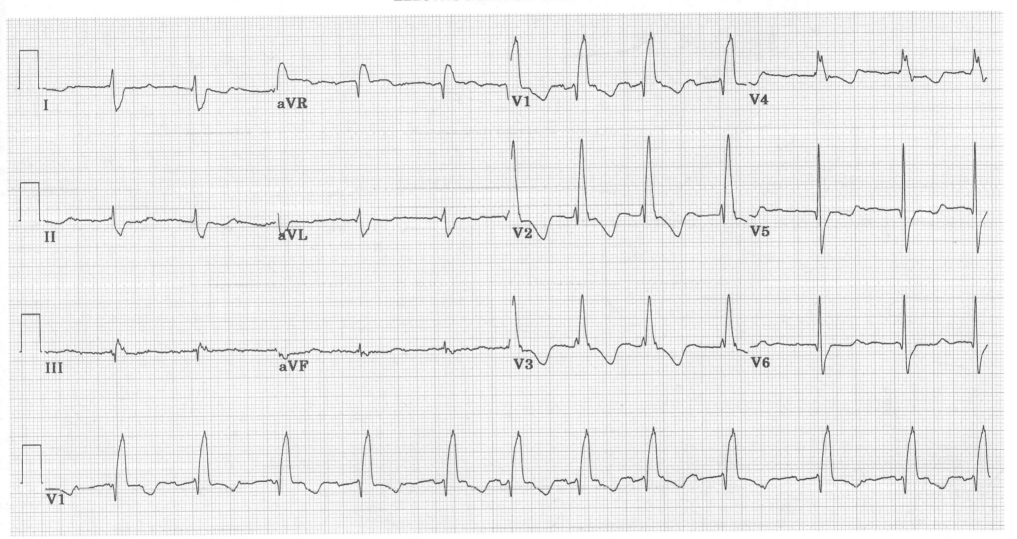

Interpretation Notes: _____

_____

ECG 557 Forty-two year old woman with Tetralogy of Fallot who is status post surgical repair. An echocardiogram demonstrated a dilated right ventricle with moderate dysfunction, severe left and right atrial enlargement, moderate mitral insufficiency, and moderately severe tricuspid insufficiency. A left ventricular to right atrial shunt was also identified.

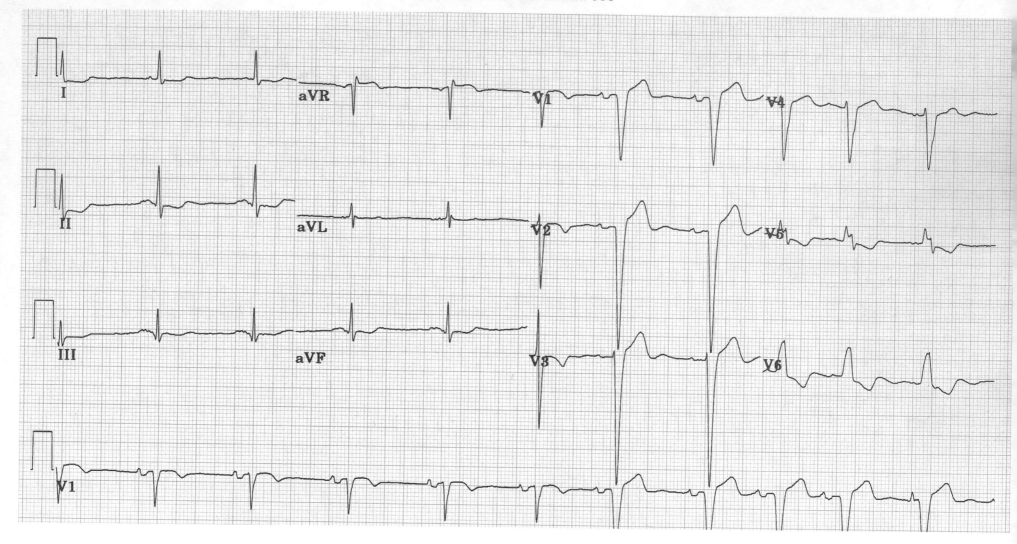

Interpretation Notes: _____

_____

ECG 558 Eighty-two year old woman with a history of coronary artery bypass graft surgery six years prior to this electrocardiogram who returns for a cardiac evaluation. She is experiencing rapid and irregular heart beating. She also has a history of paroxysmal atrial flutter. Her medications included sotalol, potassium, and aspirin.

ELECTROCARDIOGRAM 559

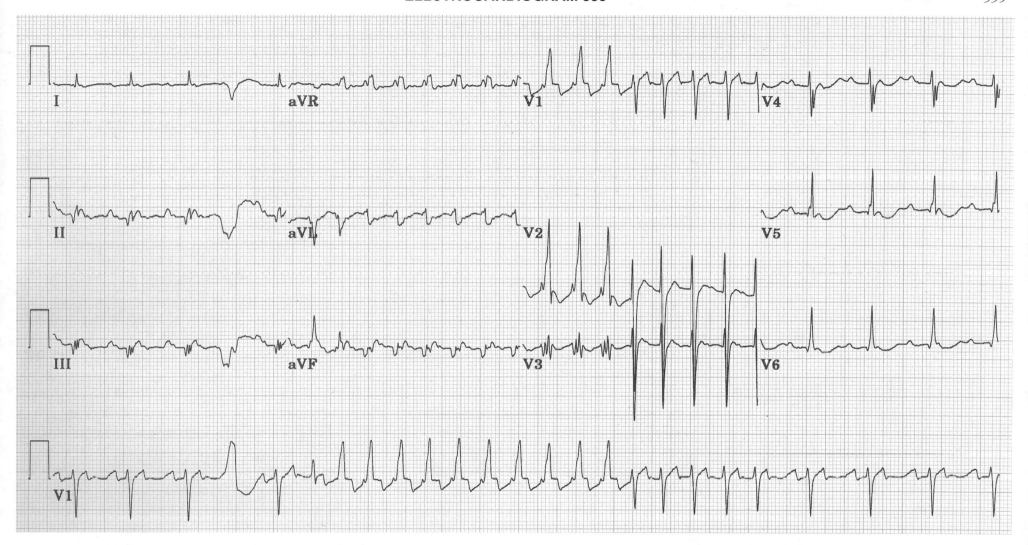

Interpretation Notes: _____

_____

ECG 559 Forty-eight year old gentleman who presents acutely to the hospital with a several week history of worsening shortness of breath. An echocardiogram demonstrated severe left ventricular systolic dysfunction, moderately severe right ventricular systolic dysfunction and severe mitral insufficiency. Medications at the time of this electrocardiogram included intravenous dobutamine, intravenous milrinone, lisinopril, furosemide, and warfarin.

560

ELECTROCARDIOGRAM 560

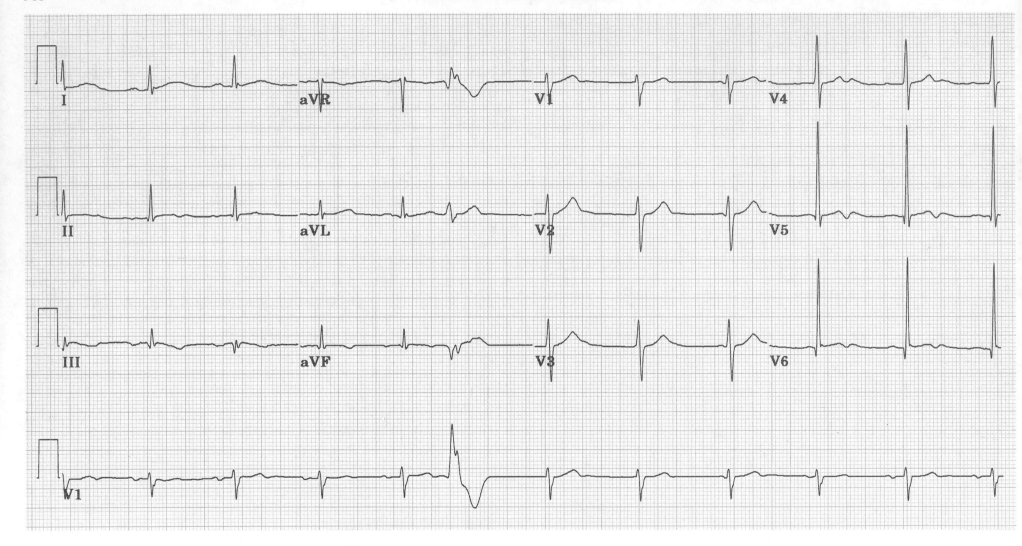

Interpretation Notes:_____

ECG 560 Fifty-six year old gentleman with severe mitral insufficiency secondary to mitral valve prolapse who is immediately postoperative mitral valve cardiac surgical repair.

ELECTROCARDIOGRAM 561

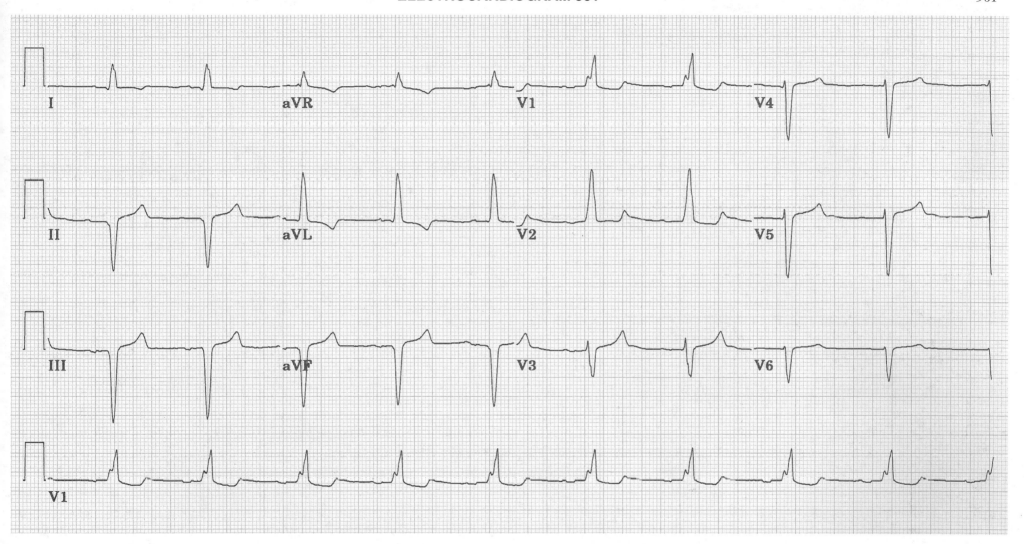

I aVR V1 V4

II aVL V2 V5

III aVF V3 V6

V1

Interpretation Notes: _____

_____

ECG 561 Seventy-five year old gentleman status post prior coronary artery bypass graft surgery and an inferior myocardial infarction who is immediately status post repeat coronary artery bypass graft surgery. The patient also underwent an aortic valve and ascending aorta replacement. His past medical history includes hypertension and hyperlipidemia. Medications at the time of this tracing included amlodipine, sotalol, and aspirin.

562

ELECTROCARDIOGRAM 562

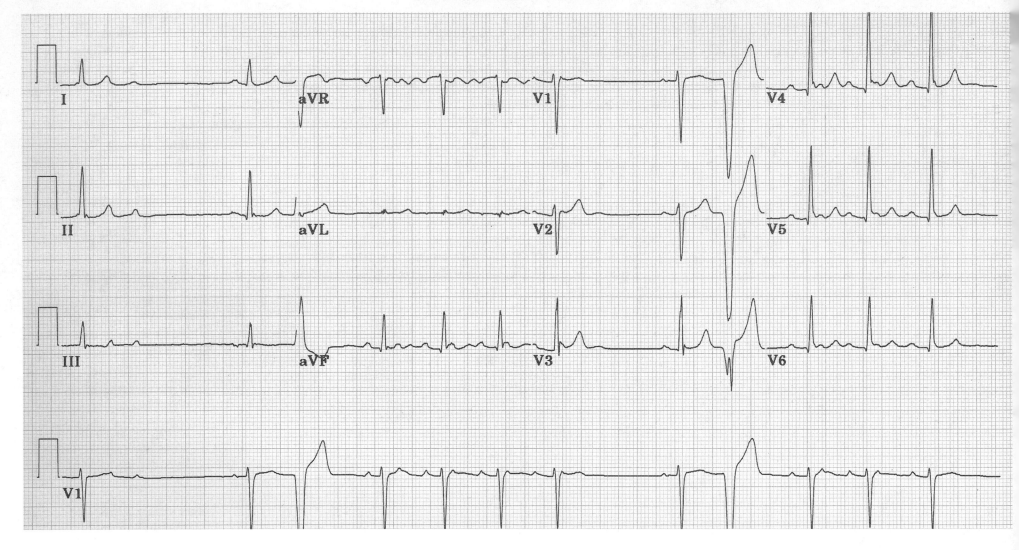

Interpretation Notes:_____

_____

_____

ECG 562 Fifty-four year old gentleman who is being seen in the outpatient department for evaluation of recurrent atrial arrhythmias. His medications included thyroxine, digoxin, and a multi-vitamin.

ELECTROCARDIOGRAM 563

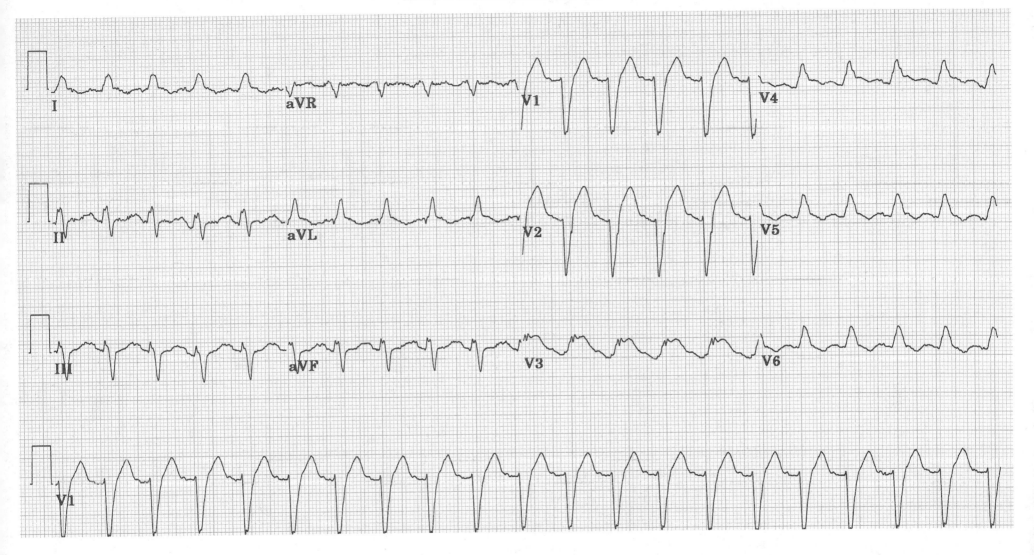

Interpretation Notes: _____

ECG 563 Sixty-four year old gentleman with an anterior myocardial infarction and percutaneous transluminal coronary angioplasty of the left anterior descending coronary artery two months prior to this electrocardiogram who was emergently admitted to the hospital after suffering a cardiopulmonary arrest. The patient suffered from anoxic encephalopathy and expired soon thereafter.

564

ELECTROCARDIOGRAM 564

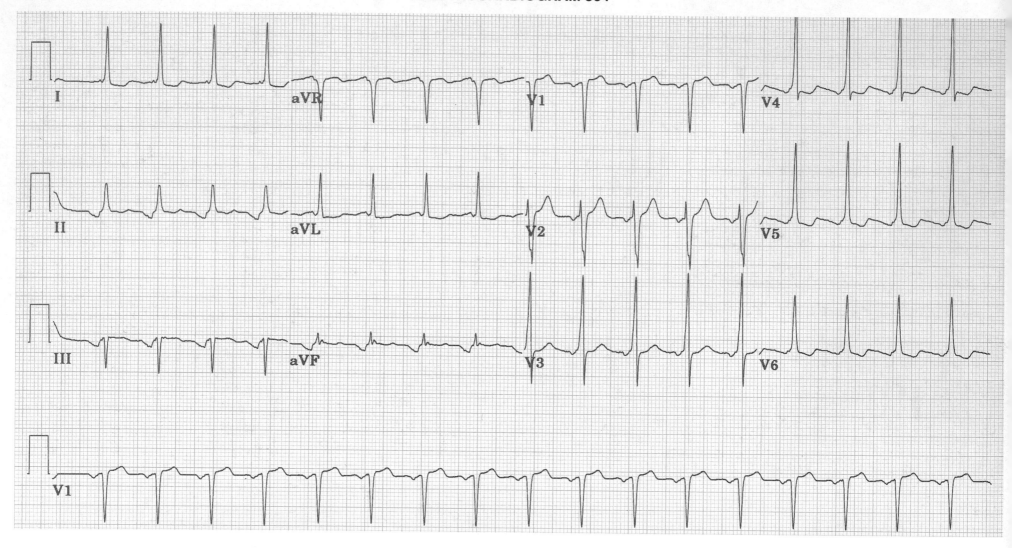

Interpretation Notes: _____

_____

_____

ECG 564 Seventy-seven year old gentleman self-referred for a cardiac evaluation in the setting of increasing exertional chest discomfort over the past two months. A subsequent cardiac catheterization demonstrated multi-vessel coronary artery disease. He was referred for successful coronary artery bypass graft surgery. His medications at the time of this electrocardiogram included procainamide, carvedilol, lisinopril, and intravenous heparin.

ELECTROCARDIOGRAM 565

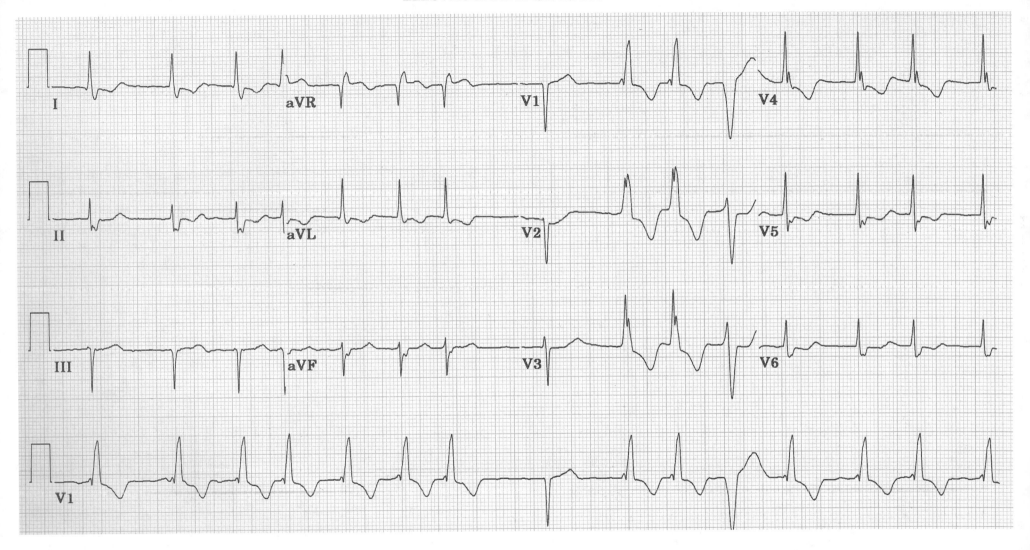

Interpretation Notes:

ECG 565 Seventy-four year old woman status post St. Jude aortic valve replacement secondary to bacterial endocarditis who re-presents to the hospital with symptoms consistent with unstable angina. Her past history includes coronary artery disease and remote coronary artery bypass graft surgery, atrial fibrillation, and peripheral vascular disease. Medications at the time of this electrocardiogram included metoprolol, aspirin, digoxin, and warfarin.

566

ELECTROCARDIOGRAM 566

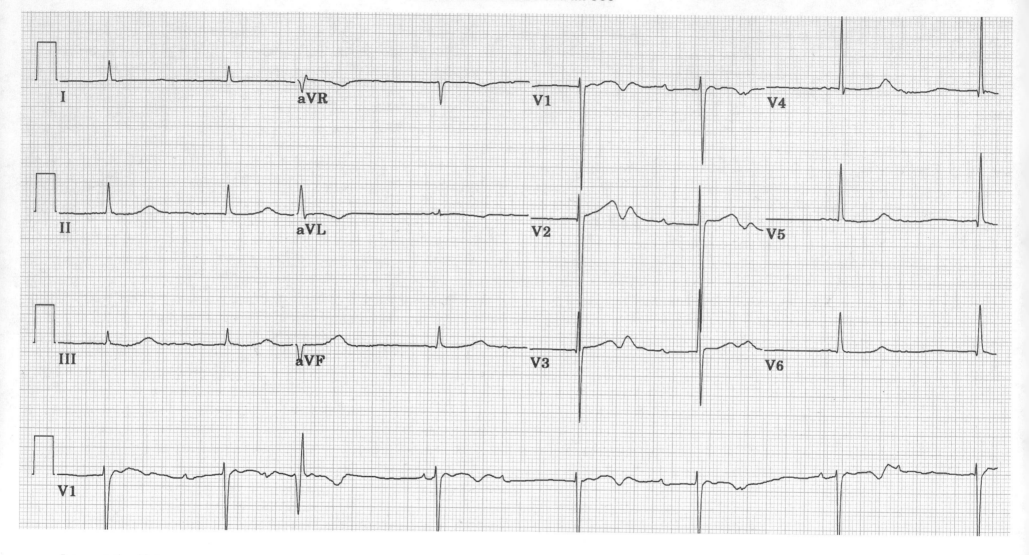

I aVR V1 V4

II aVL V2 V5

III aVF V3 V6

V1

Interpretation Notes:_____

_____

_____

ECG 566 Eighty-four year old gentleman with coronary artery disease status post coronary artery bypass graft surgery ten years prior to this electrocardiogram who presents to the hospital with recent onset exertional shortness of breath. His presentation was consistent with congestive heart failure. His medications at the time of this electrocardiogram included isosorbide mononitrate, doxazosin, nadolol, and felodipine.

ELECTROCARDIOGRAM 567

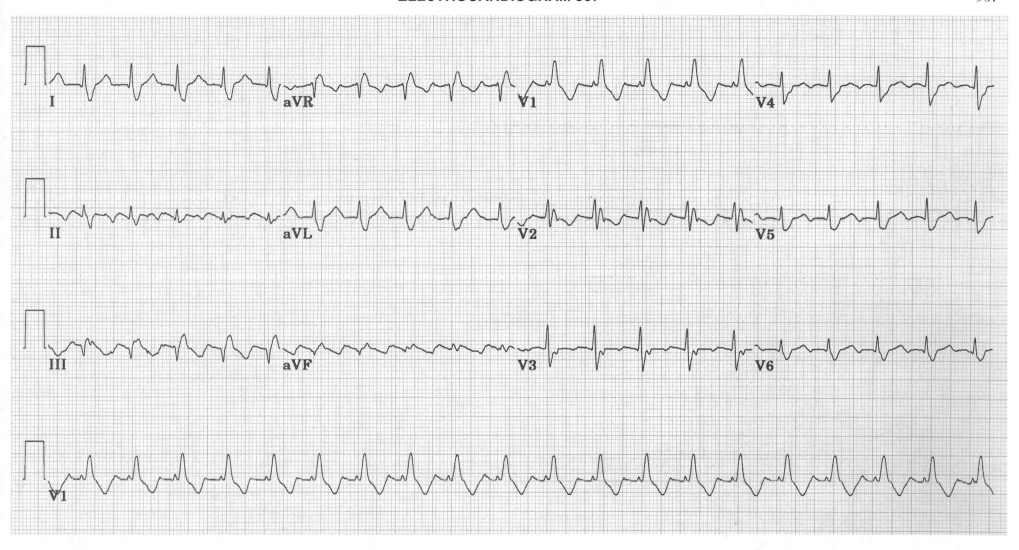

Interpretation Notes: _____

_____

_____

ECG 567 Sixty-one year old gentleman with episodic palpitations in the presence of hypertension. This electrocardiogram was obtained during a symptomatic episode of cardiac palpitations. His medication at the time of this electrocardiogram included hydrochlorothiazide.

568

ELECTROCARDIOGRAM 568

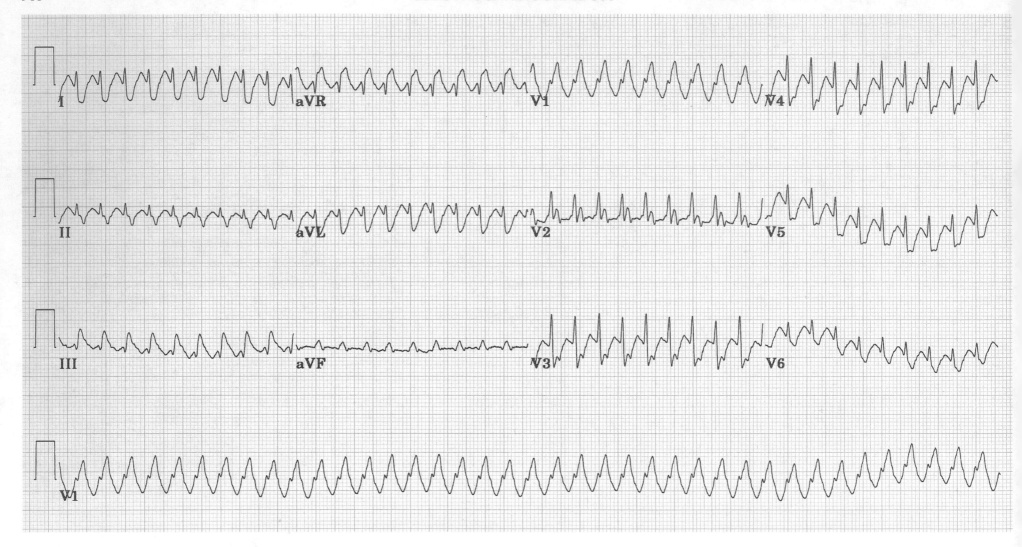

Interpretation Notes: _____

_____

_____

ECG 568 Sixty-one year old gentleman with symptoms of episodic palpitations and hypertension. This electrocardiogram was obtained during a symptomatic episode of cardiac palpitations. His medications at the time of this electrocardiogram included hydrochlorothiazide.

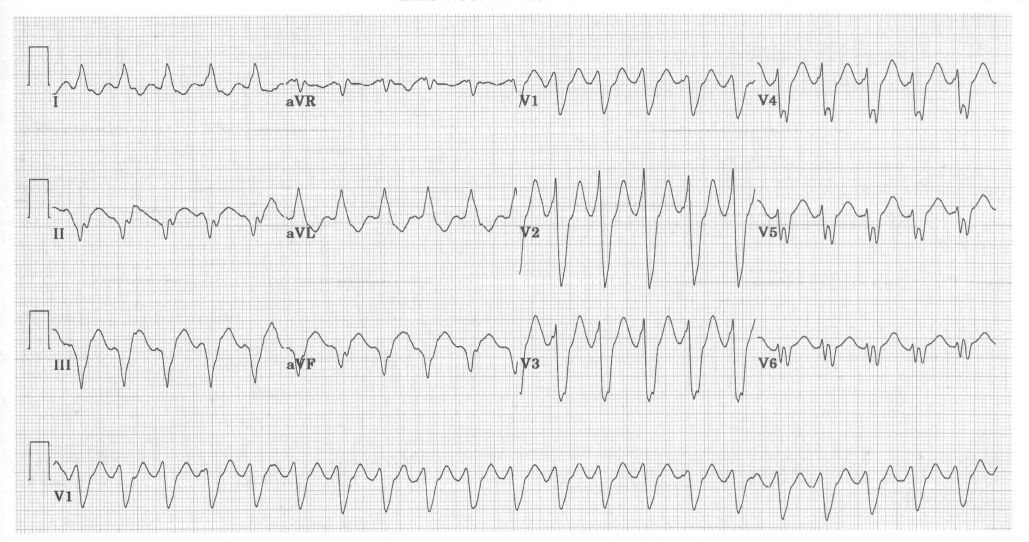

Interpretation Notes: _____

ECG 569 Fifty-three year old gentleman with a remote myocardial infarction admitted urgently to the hospital after a syncopal episode. The patient has a history of paroxysmal ventricular tachycardia and is status post implantable cardiac defibrillator placement. His medications at the time of this electrocardiogram included captopril, amiodarone, digoxin, nadolol, isosorbide dinitrate, and furosemide.

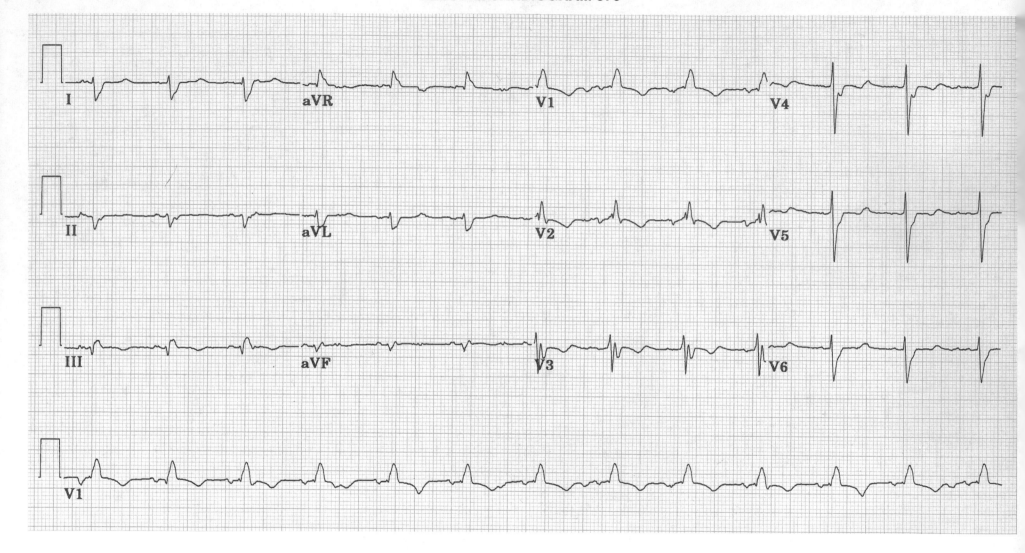

Interpretation Notes: _____

_____

_____

ECG 570 Forty-one year old gentleman status post a recent cardiac transplantation who re-presents for symptomatic management of severe right-sided congestive heart failure. His medications included thyroxine, prednisone, immunosuppressive agents, bumetanide, and nebulized inhalers.

ELECTROCARDIOGRAM 571

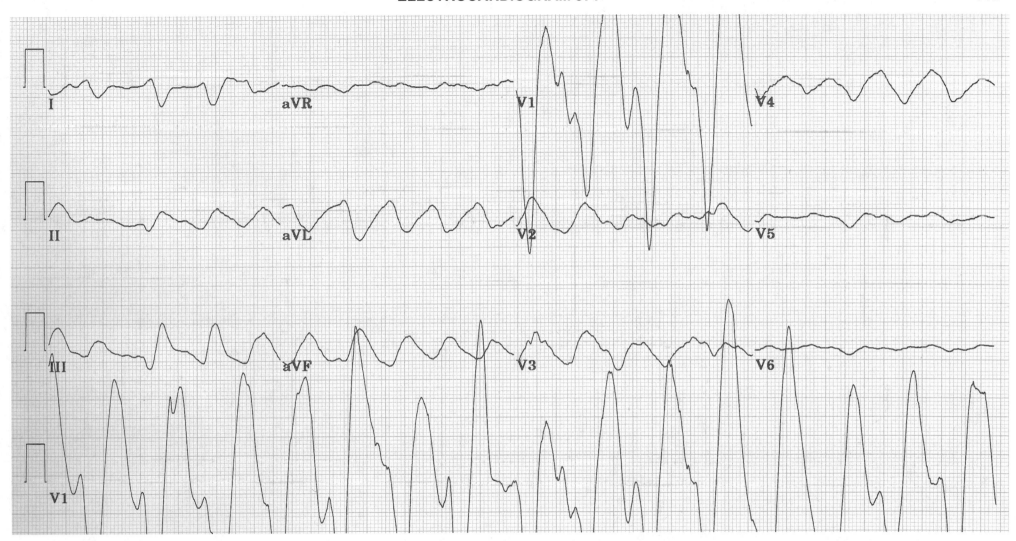

Interpretation Notes: _____

_____

ECG 571 Sixty-two year old woman with severe peripheral vascular disease who underwent a recent emergency aorto-bifemoral bypass graft. This was complicated by acute renal failure and progressive clinical deterioration. This electrocardiogram was obtained during an unsuccessful resuscitation.

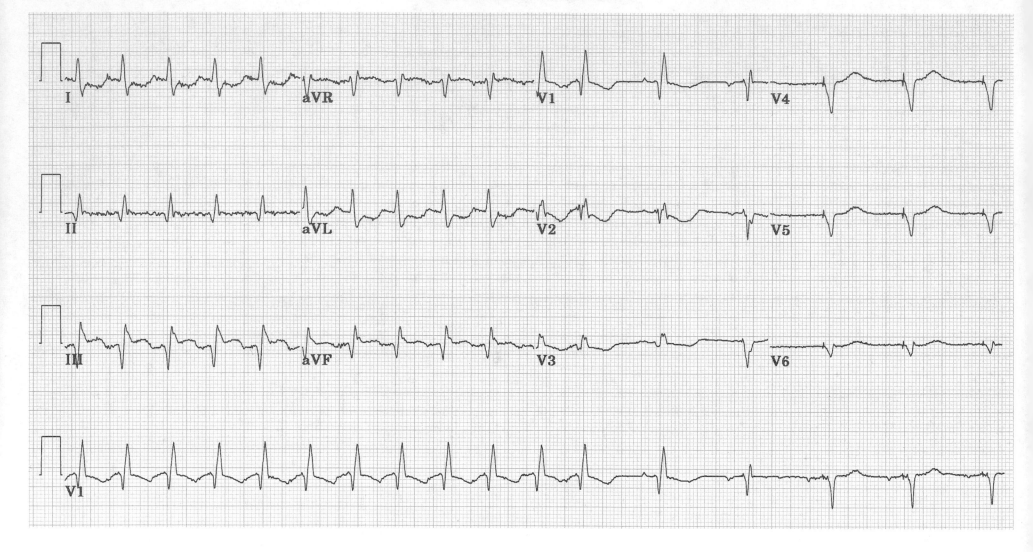

Interpretation Notes:

ECG 572 Sixty-nine year old woman with coronary artery disease and severe left ventricular systolic dysfunction who presents with symptoms and signs of acute myocardial injury. Her medications at the time of this electrocardiogram included carvedilol, amiodarone, enalapril, isosorbide mononitrate, and furosemide.

ELECTROCARDIOGRAM 573

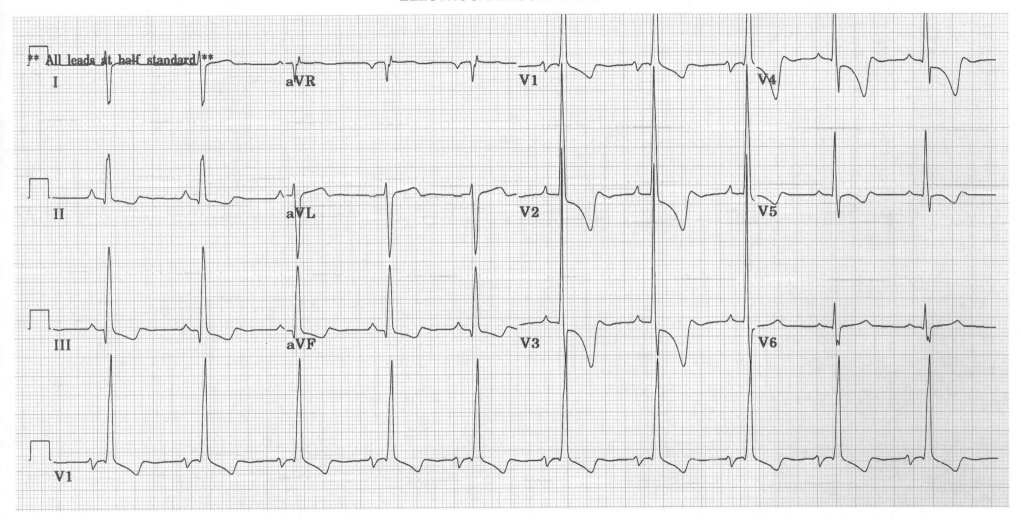

** All leads at half standard **

I   aVR   V1   V4

II   aVL   V2   V5

III   aVF   V3   V6

V1

Interpretation Notes: _____

_____

ECG 573 Fourteen year old gentleman being seen in the pediatric outpatient clinic in the setting of critical pulmonary stenosis, severe right ventricular hypertrophy and New York Heart Association functional class IV symptoms. An echocardiogram confirmed the presence of severe pulmonic stenosis, a moderate sized atrial septal defect with right-to-left interatrial flow, and severe pulmonary hypertension.

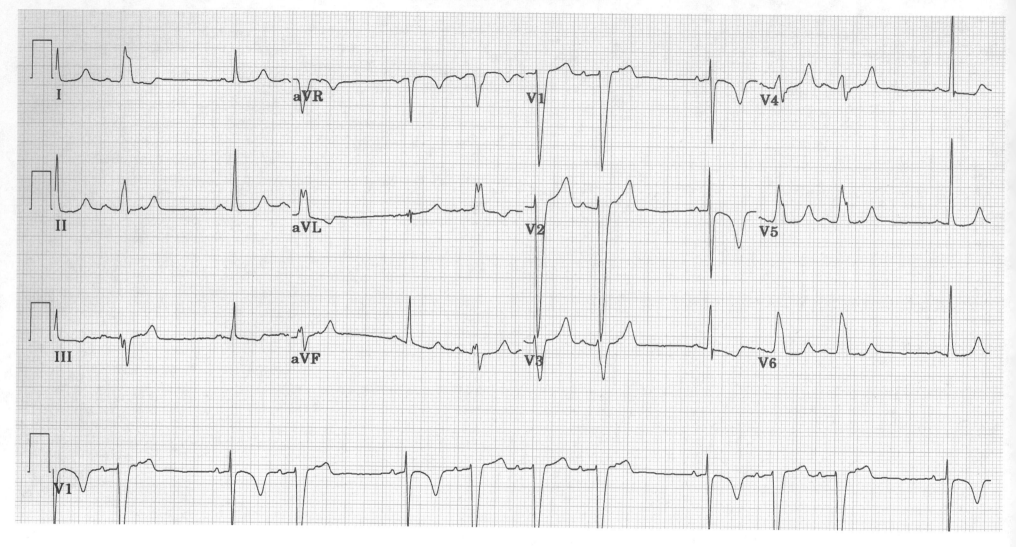

Interpretation Notes: _____

_____

_____

ECG 574 Seventy-two year old woman with a history of multi-vessel coronary artery disease status post recent coronary artery bypass graft surgery. This tracing was obtained in the hospital several days postoperatively. She also has a history of paroxysmal atrial fibrillation and supraventricular cardiac dysrhythmias. Medications at the time of this electrocardiogram included furosemide, diltiazem, aspirin, lovastatin, and sotalol.

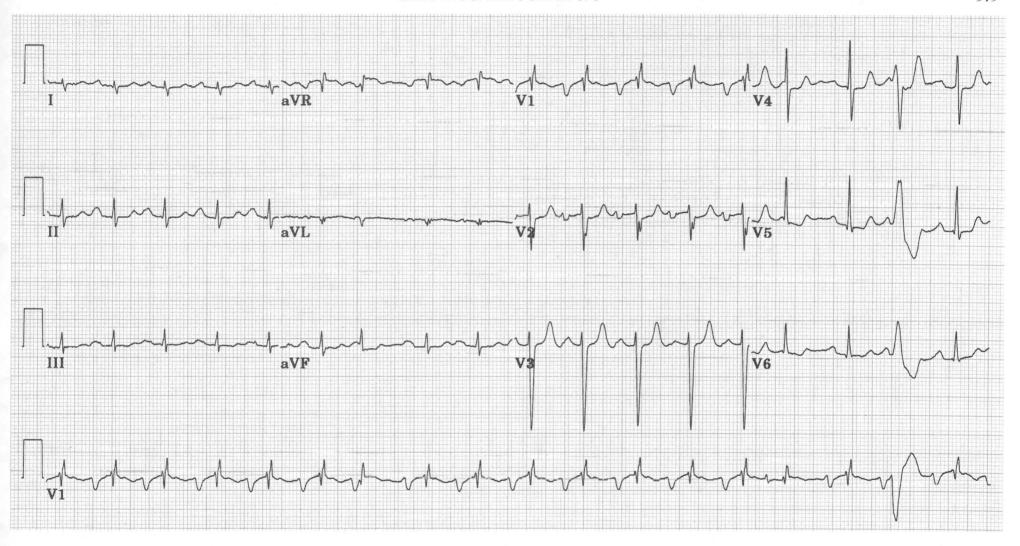

I aVR V1 V4

II aVL V2 V5

III aVF V3 V6

V1

Interpretation Notes: _____

_____

ECG 575 Sixty-four year old woman admitted with recurrent congestive heart failure. A recent echocardiogram demonstrated severe left and right atrial enlargement, severe mitral stenosis, severe dilatation and dysfunction of the right ventricle, severe tricuspid regurgitation, and pulmonary hypertension.

576

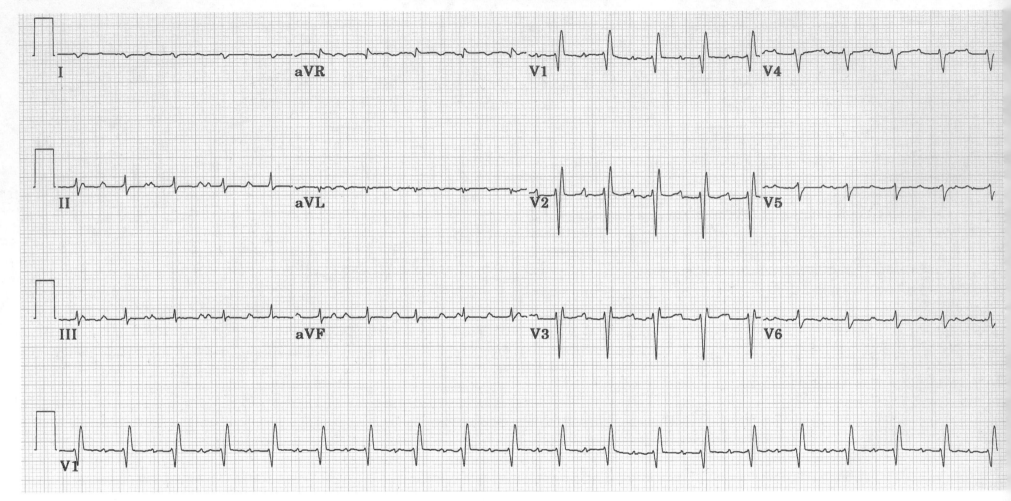

I aVR V1 V4

II aVL V2 V5

III aVF V3 V6

V1

Interpretation Notes: _____

_____

ECG 576 Fifty-seven year old gentleman status post cardiac transplantation four years prior to this electrocardiogram now with severe biventricular dysfunction secondary to cardiac transplant rejection. His medications included aspirin, warfarin, azathioprine, and lisinopril.

ELECTROCARDIOGRAM 577

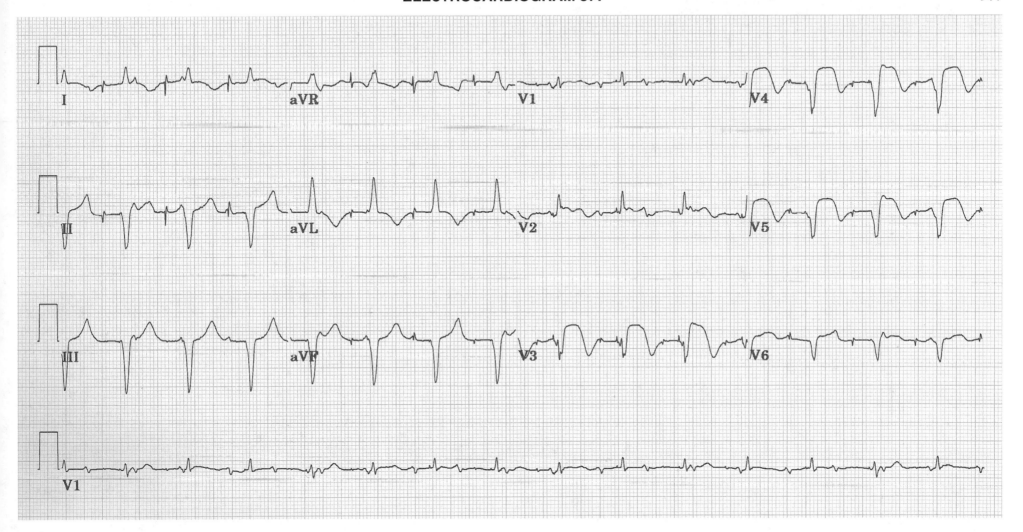

Interpretation Notes: _____

_____

_____

ECG 577 Eighty-five year old woman who presented to the hospital with respiratory distress. A temporary atrioventricular pacemaker and intra-aortic balloon pump were placed and the patient was taken urgently to the cardiac catheterization laboratory. An attempt at urgent angioplasty of a totally occluded left anterior descending coronary artery was unsuccessful. The patient expired a short time later.

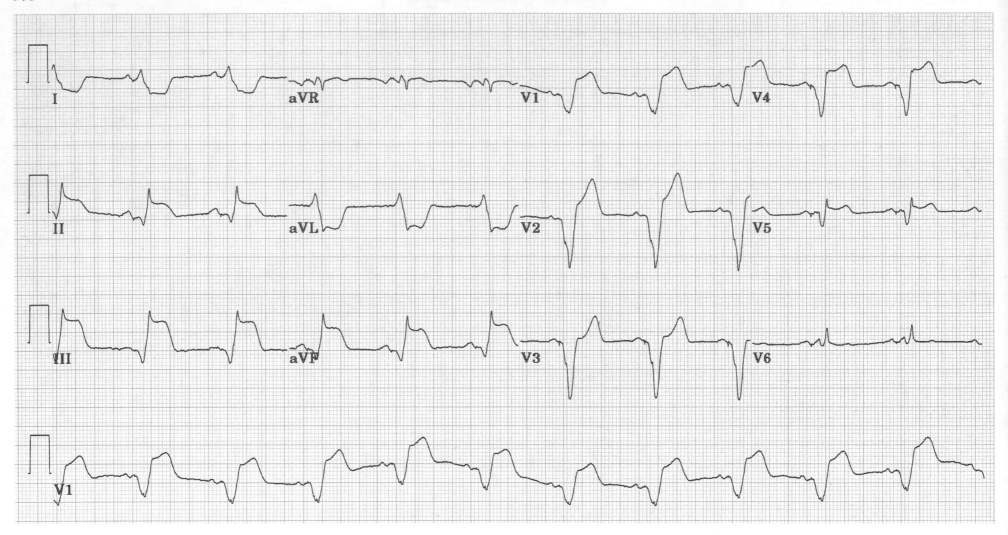

Interpretation Notes: _____

_____

_____

ECG 578 Fifty year old woman undergoing percutaneous alcohol ablation for hypertrophic obstructive cardiomyopathy who was directly admitted to the hospital with an acute chest discomfort syndrome. A subsequent echocardiogram demonstrated inferior akinesis with moderate right ventricular systolic dysfunction.

ELECTROCARDIOGRAM 579

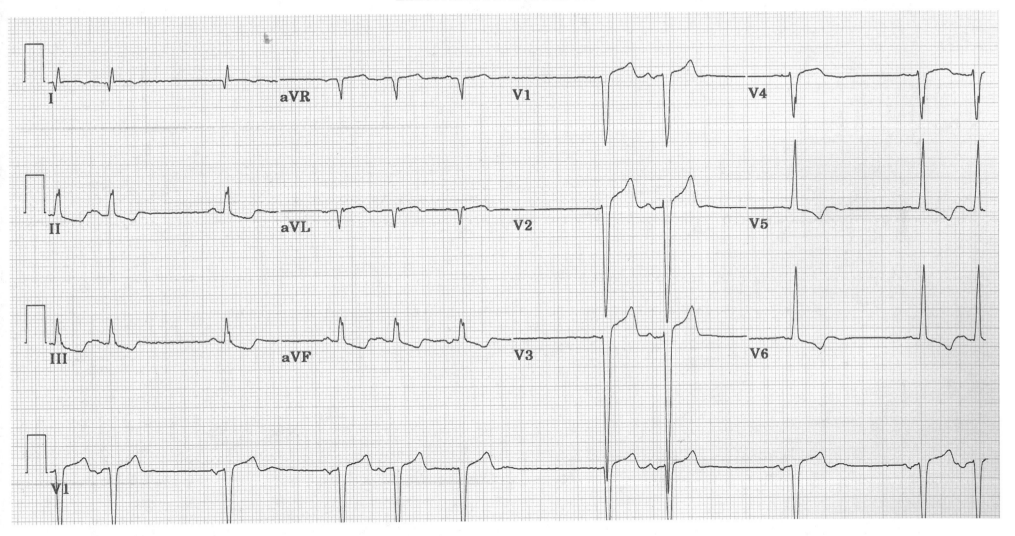

Interpretation Notes: _____

ECG 579 Seventy-seven year old gentleman with coronary artery disease who presents to the hospital with signs and symptoms of an acute cerebrovascular accident. A recent echocardiogram demonstrated severe regional left ventricular systolic dysfunction with an estimated left ventricular ejection fraction of 20%. His medications at the time of this electrocardiogram included lisinopril, digoxin, aspirin, furosemide, and potassium.

ELECTROCARDIOGRAM 580

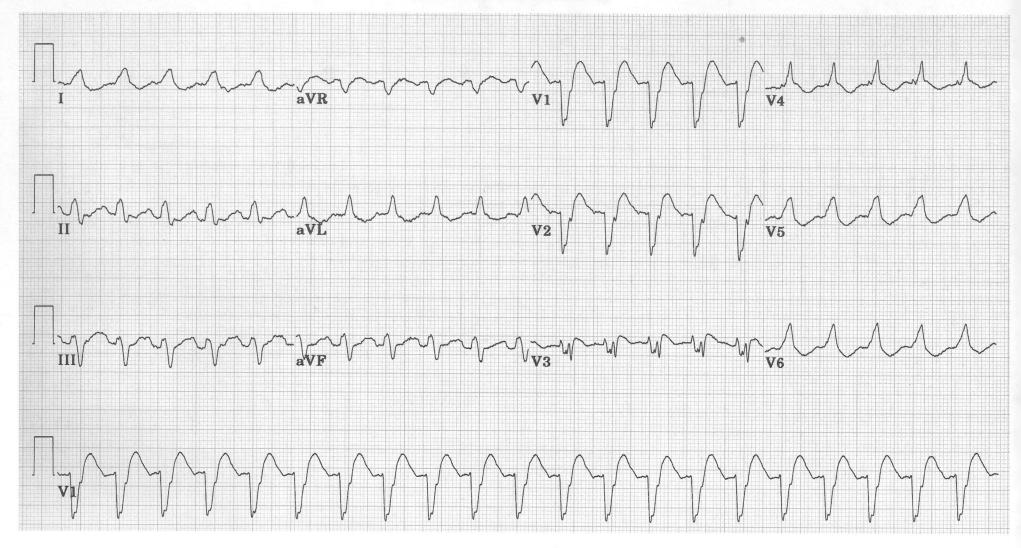

I   aVR   V1   V4

II   aVL   V2   V5

III   aVF   V3   V6

V1

Interpretation Notes:_____

_____

ECG 580 Sixty-four year old gentleman with a history of an anterior myocardial infarction and percutaneous transluminal coronary angioplasty of the left anterior descending coronary artery two months before this electrocardiogram who was emergently admitted to the hospital after suffering a cardiopulmonary arrest at home. The patient suffered from anoxic encephalopathy and expired soon thereafter.

ELECTROCARDIOGRAM 581

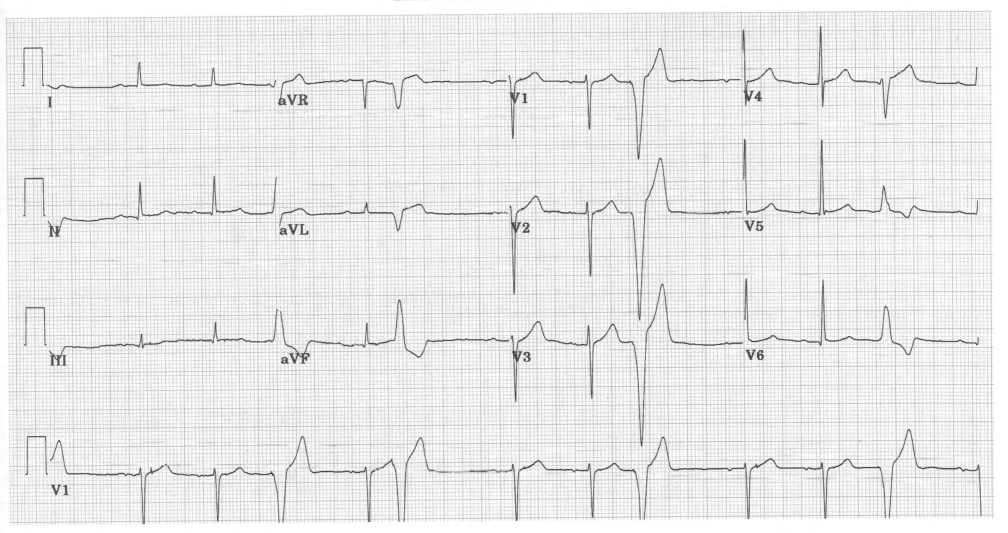

Interpretation Notes:_____

_____

ECG 581 Fifty-four year old gentleman with severe mitral insufficiency secondary to mitral valve prolapse referred for mitral valve reparative surgery. He overall feels well. He is on no current medications.

582

ELECTROCARDIOGRAM 582

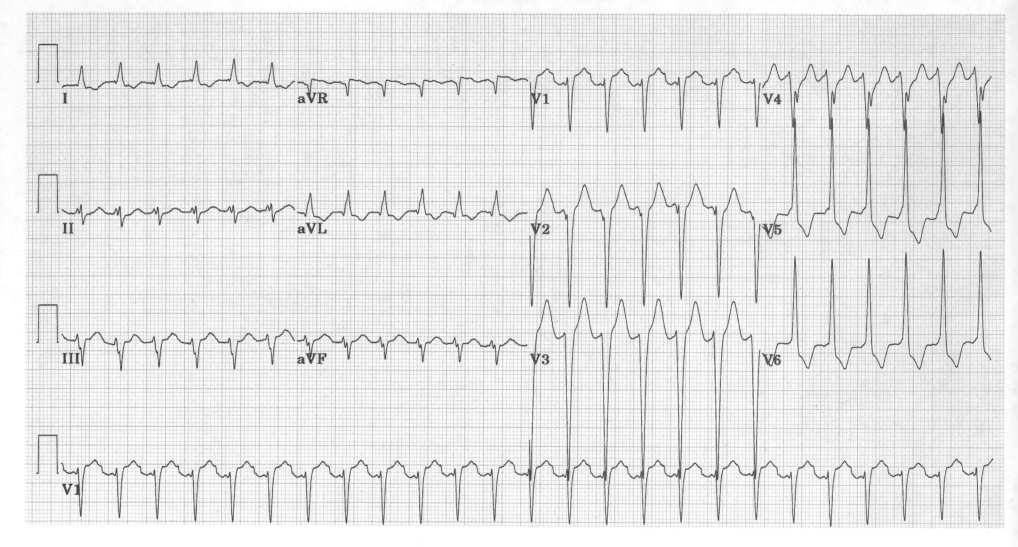

Interpretation Notes: _____

_____

_____

ECG 582 Fifty-two year old woman with severe aortic insufficiency who presents acutely to the hospital with symptoms of profound shortness of breath. Her physical exam and chest x-ray confirmed pulmonary edema. The patient was medically stabilized and referred for aortic valve replacement surgery.

ELECTROCARDIOGRAM 583

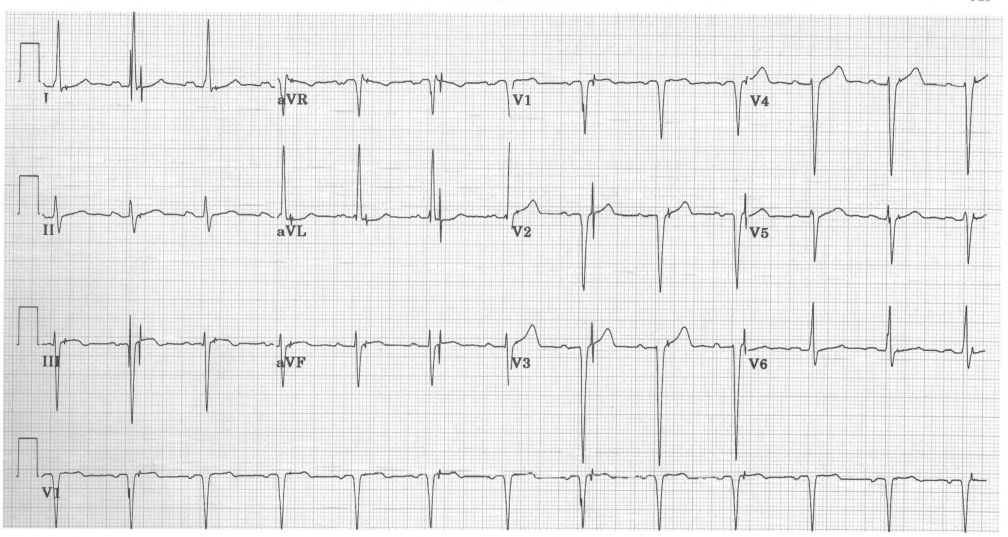

Interpretation Notes: _____

_____

_____

ECG 583 Fifty-one year old woman with long-standing rheumatic heart disease readmitted with pulmonary edema. An echocardiogram demonstrated severe prosthetic valve aortic stenosis and aortic insufficiency. This tracing was obtained shortly after aortic valve re-replacement.

584

ELECTROCARDIOGRAM 584

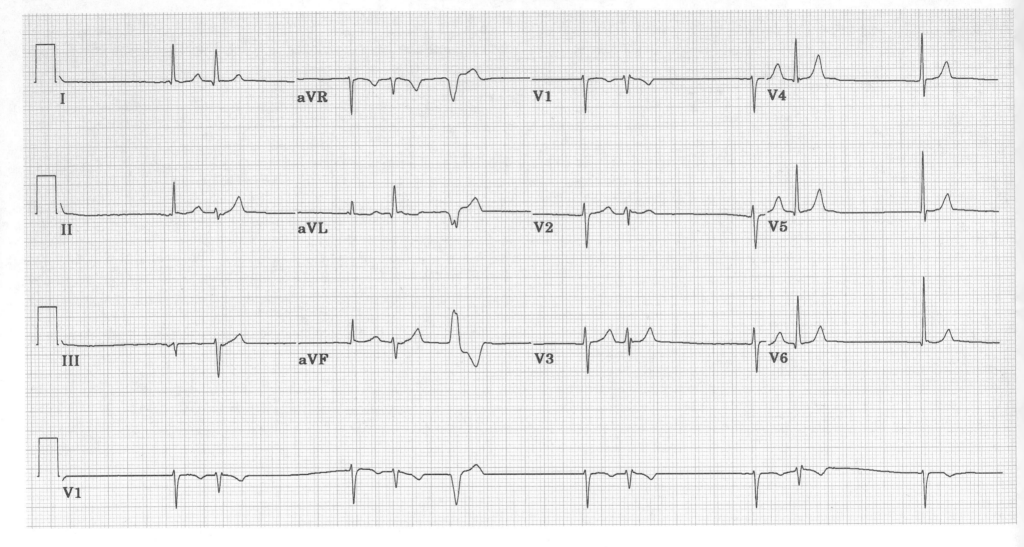

Interpretation Notes: _____

ECG 584 Fifty-nine year old woman who recently underwent mitral valve re-replacement secondary to severe perivalvular mitral regurgitation. Her past medical history includes hypertension, paroxysmal atrial fibrillation, and osteoarthritis.

ELECTROCARDIOGRAM 585

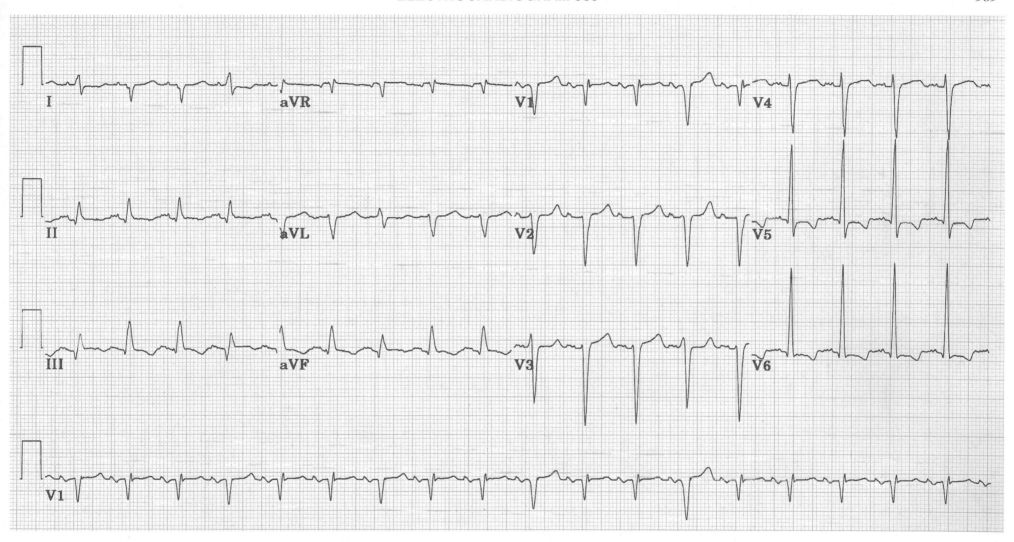

Interpretation Notes:_____

_____

ECG 585 Fifty-four year old gentleman with a history of an inferior myocardial infarction and left ventricular aneurysm formation who re-presents for evaluation of new onset congestive heart failure. A recent echocardiogram demonstrated moderately severe mitral insufficiency and moderate regional left ventricular systolic dysfunction.

ELECTROCARDIOGRAM 586

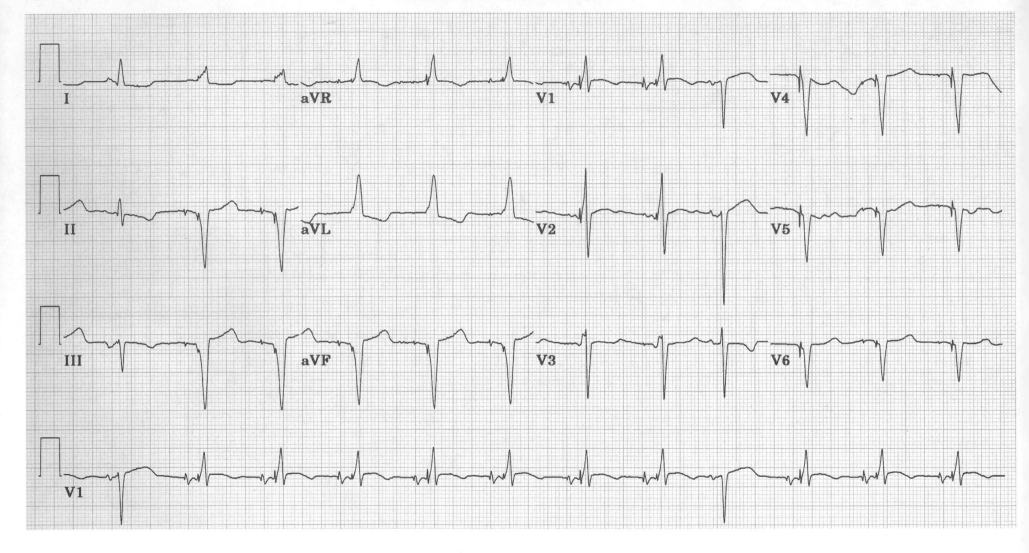

Interpretation Notes:_____

_____

_____

ECG 586 Seventy-three year old woman with severe mitral insufficiency secondary to bileaflet mitral valve prolapse recently postoperative mitral valve surgical repair. She has a history of sick sinus syndrome and underwent permanent pacemaker placement several years prior to this electrocardiogram.

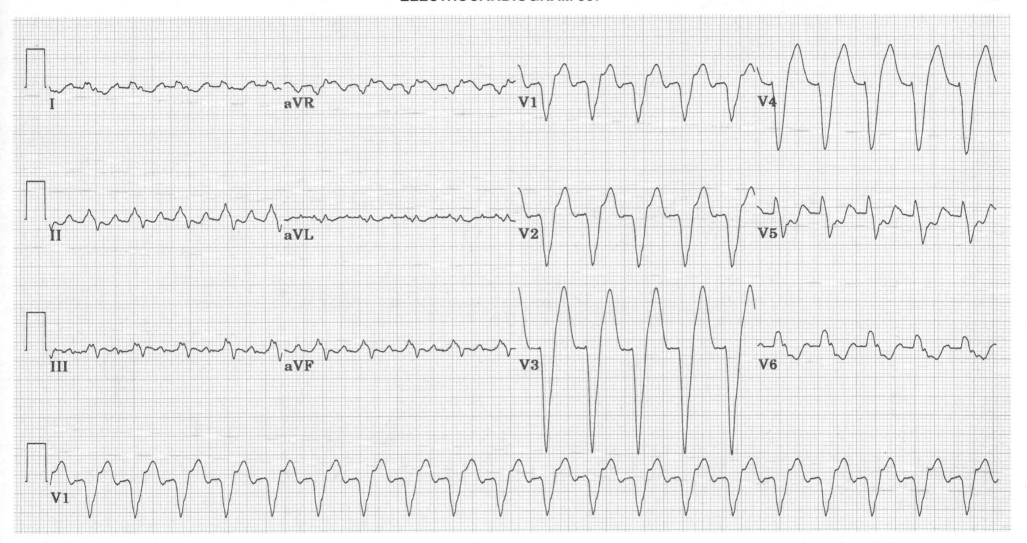

Interpretation Notes: _____

ECG 587 Eighty-three year old gentleman with coronary artery disease status post aortic valve replacement who is admitted for further evaluation of recurrent atrial and ventricular dysrhythmias. His past medical history includes non-insulin requiring diabetes mellitus, pulmonary fibrosis, and paroxysmal atrial fibrillation.

588

ELECTROCARDIOGRAM 588

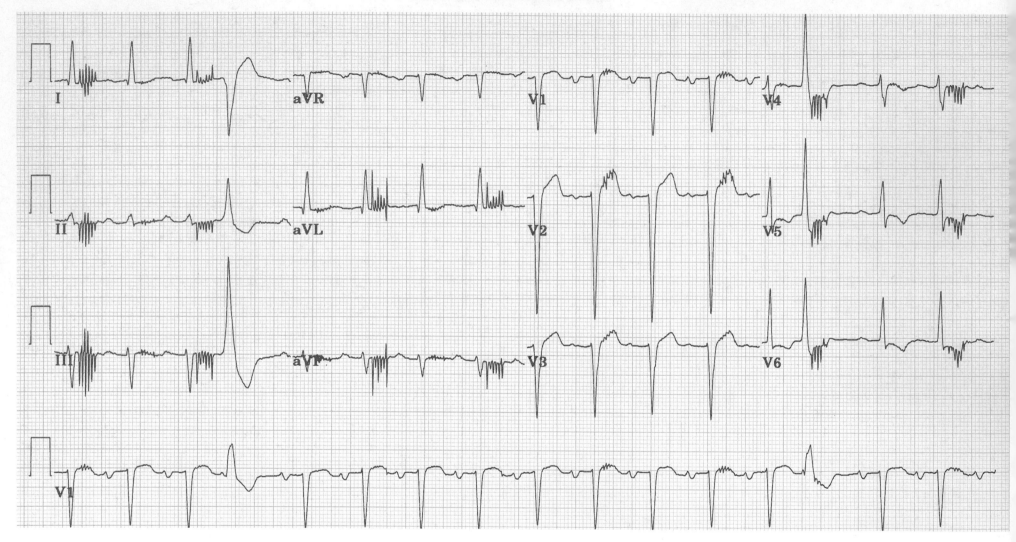

Interpretation Notes: _____

_____

_____

ECG 588 Fifty-nine year old woman who underwent the cardiomyoplasty procedure three years prior to this electrocardiogram who returns to the outpatient congestive heart failure clinic. Her medications at the time of this electrocardiogram included furosemide, digoxin, captopril, and potassium.

ELECTROCARDIOGRAM 589

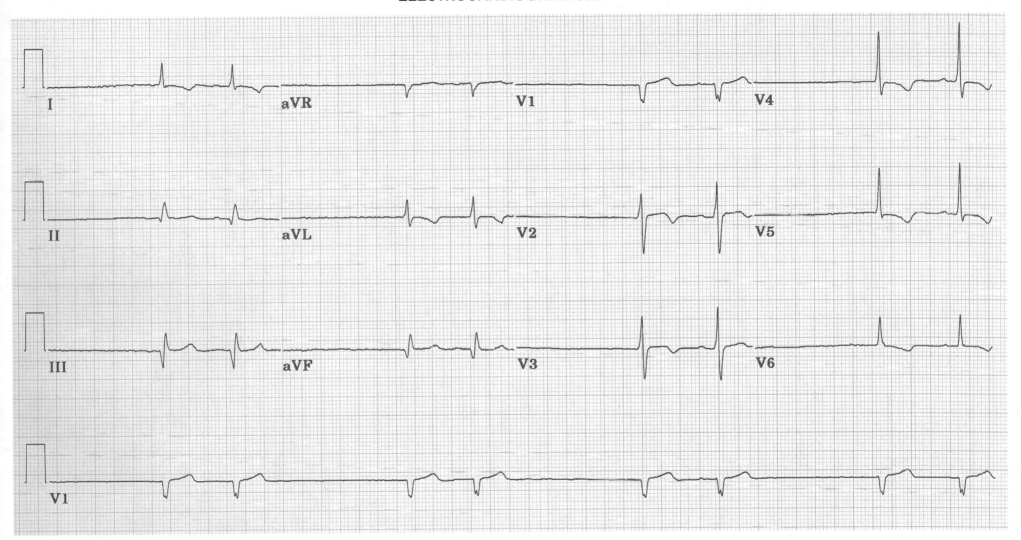

I   aVR   V1   V4

II   aVL   V2   V5

III   aVF   V3   V6

V1

Interpretation Notes:_____

_____

ECG 589 Sixty-nine year old gentleman with symptoms of progressive congestive heart failure who is recently postoperative coronary artery bypass graft surgery. Medications at the time of this electrocardiogram included amiodarone, digoxin, enalapril, aspirin, and simvastatin. A recent echocardiogram demonstrated a left ventricular ejection fraction of approximately 15% to 20%.

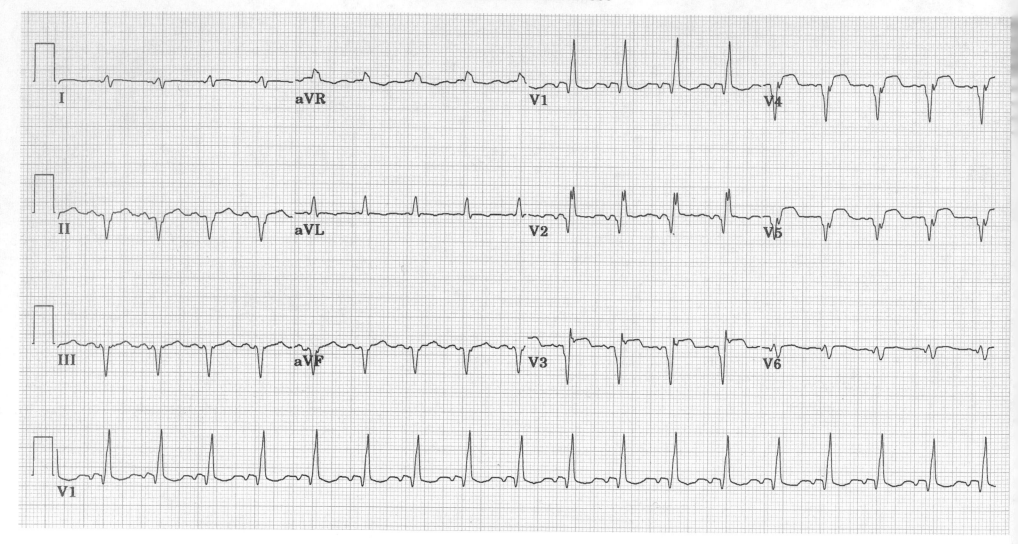

Interpretation Notes: _____

_____

_____

ECG 590 Sixty-four year old gentleman with severe coronary artery disease, a prior anterior myocardial infarction, and left ventricular aneurysm formation who is admitted for evaluation and treatment of new-onset congestive heart failure. At the time of this electrocardiogram an acute myocardial infarction was excluded. The patient subsequently underwent successful cardiac transplantation surgery.

ELECTROCARDIOGRAM 591

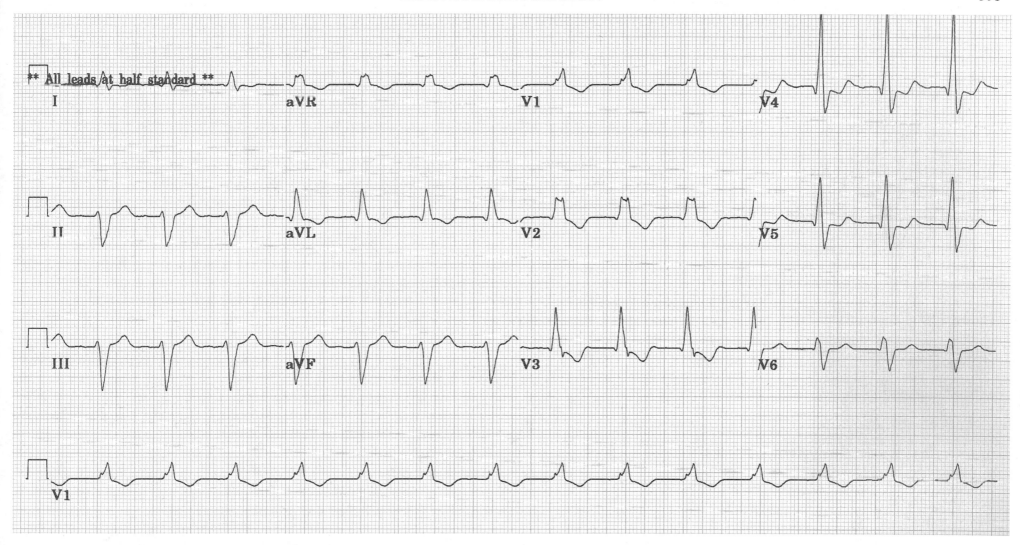

** All leads at half standard **

I aVR V1 V4

II aVL V2 V5

III aVF V3 V6

V1

Interpretation Notes: _____

_____

_____

ECG 591 Fifty-four year old gentleman with a recent episode of chest discomfort referred for coronary artery bypass graft surgery. A cardiac catheterization demonstrated severe coronary artery disease and normal left ventricular systolic function without evidence of a prior myocardial infarction. Co-morbid medical conditions include severe peripheral vascular disease and a prior cerebrovascular accident. The patient also has suffered from a staphylococcus aureus bacteremia and probable endocarditis.

592

ELECTROCARDIOGRAM 592

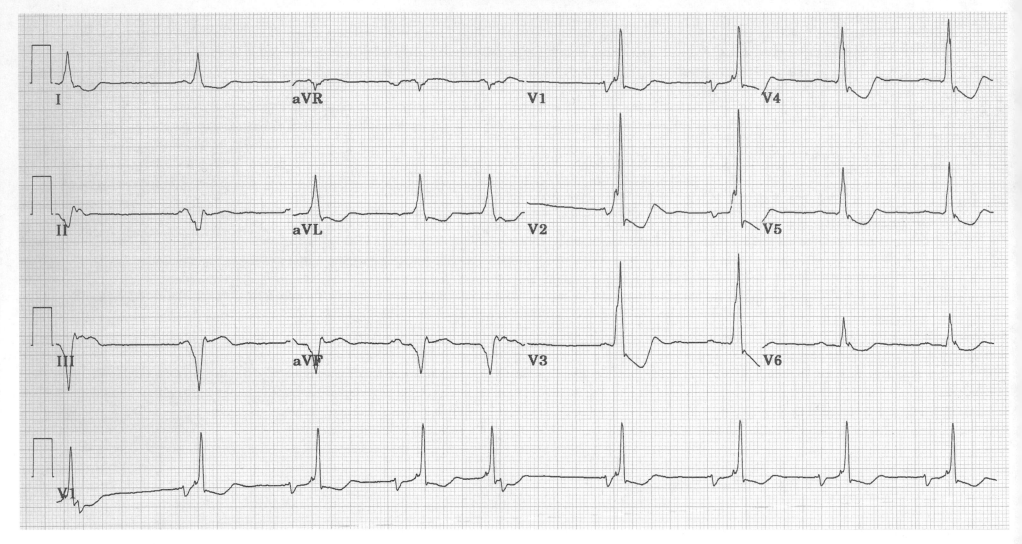

Interpretation Notes: _____

ECG 592 Sixty-eight year old gentleman with severe left ventricular systolic dysfunction secondary to ischemic heart disease who re-presented to the hospital with signs and symptoms of congestive heart failure. His medications at the time of this electrocardiogram included amiodarone, digoxin, fosinopril, aspirin, furosemide, and potassium.

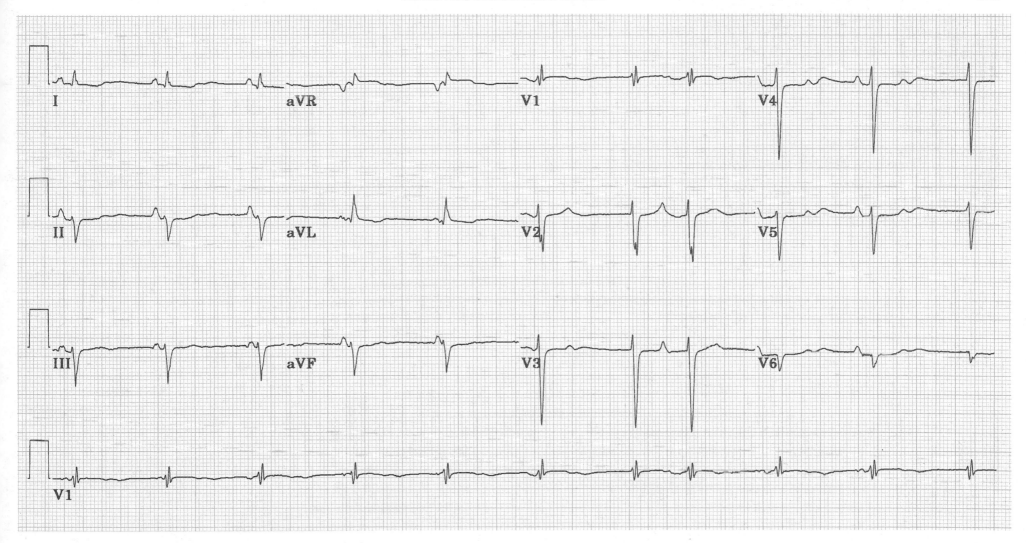

Interpretation Notes: _____

_____

ECG 593 Thirty year old gentleman status post multiple prior cardiac surgeries for tricuspid valve atresia, a double outlet right ventricle, a large perimembranous ventricular septal defect, and an ostium primum atrial septal defect. The patient re-presents for evaluation of a perceived irregular heartbeat.

ELECTROCARDIOGRAM 594

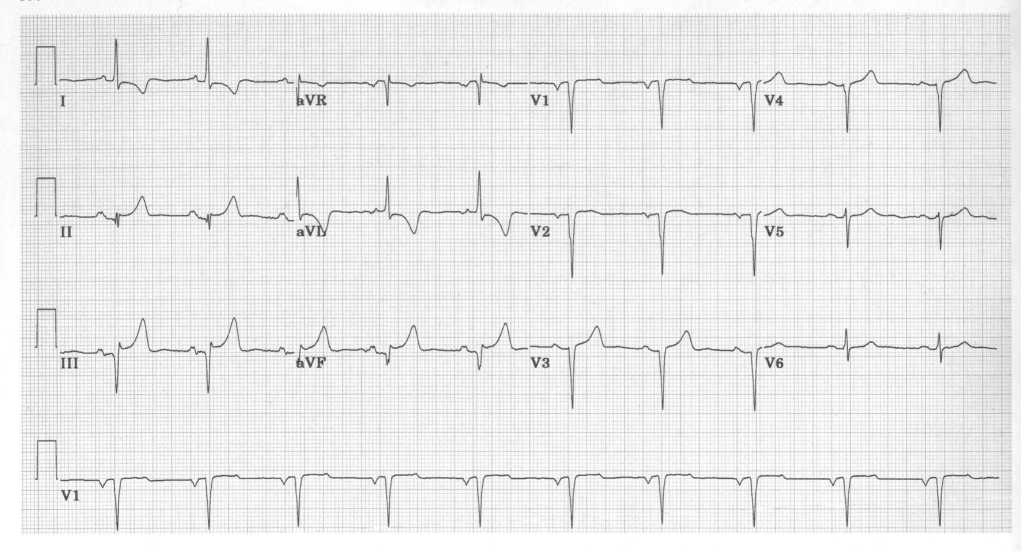

I aVR V1 V4

II aVL V2 V5

III aVF V3 V6

V1

Interpretation Notes: _____

_____

_____

ECG 594 Fifty-two year old woman who presents to the hospital emergency room with a recent onset accelerating pattern of chest discomfort. Dobutamine echocardiography demonstrated no inducible myocardial ischemia and moderately severe concentric left ventricular hypertrophy. In the absence of a hypertension history these findings supported hypertrophic obstructive cardiomyopathy.

ELECTROCARDIOGRAM 595

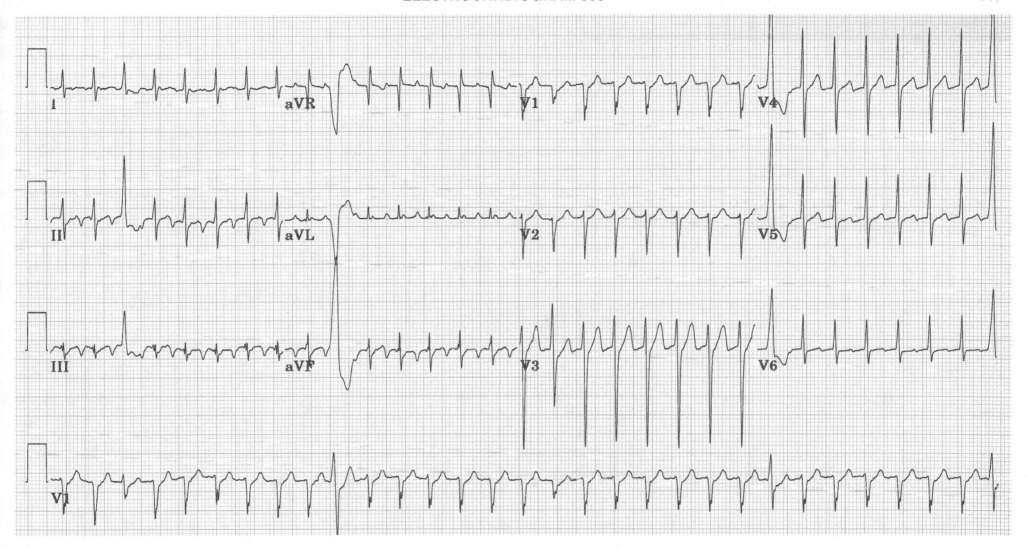

Interpretation Notes: _____

_____

_____

ECG 595 Seventy-two year old gentleman with recently diagnosed myasthenia gravis admitted for rehabilitation. His past medical history includes diabetes mellitus, chronic obstructive pulmonary disease, recurrent atrial fibrillation, and coronary artery disease.

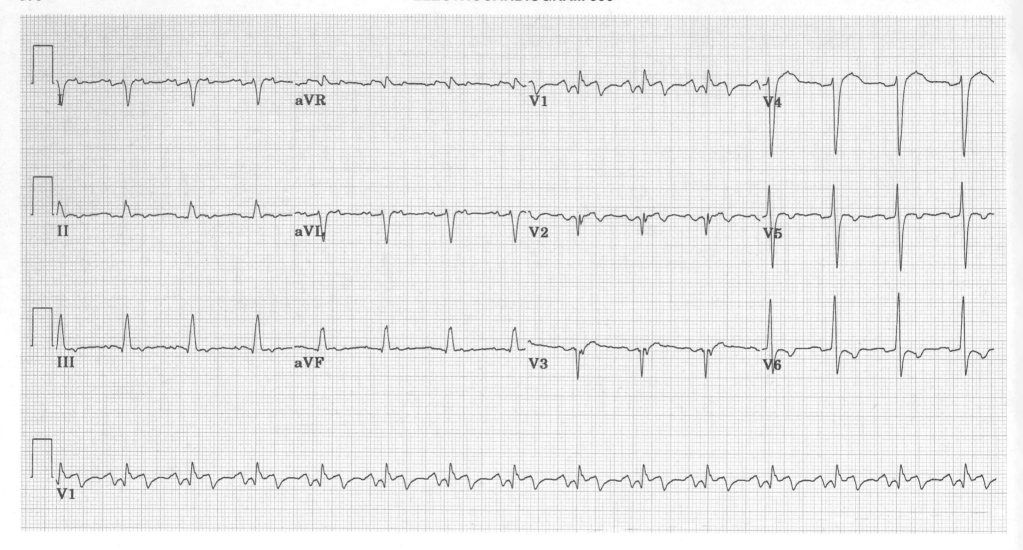

Interpretation Notes: _____

_____

_____

ECG 596 Thirty-five year old gentleman with a non-ischemic dilated cardiomyopathy and a recent history of syncope scheduled for implantable cardiac defibrillator placement. An electrophysiology study demonstrated inducible sustained monomorphic ventricular tachycardia. His medications included amiodarone, digoxin, lisinopril, furosemide, and potassium.

ELECTROCARDIOGRAM 597

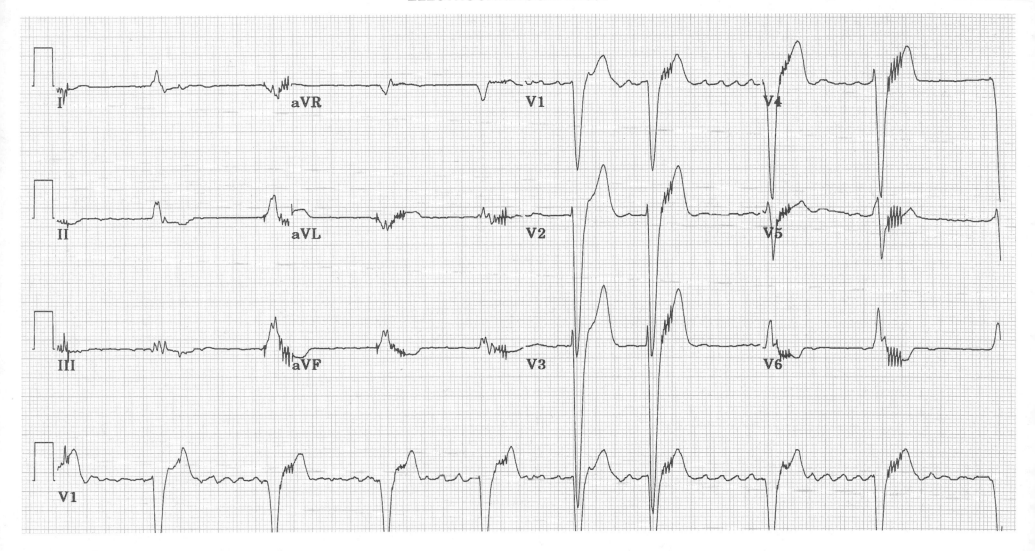

Interpretation Notes: _____

ECG 597 Sixty-four year old gentleman status post a ventricular cardiomyoplasty procedure one year prior to this electrocardiogram secondary to a non-ischemic dilated cardiomyopathy who returns for an outpatient cardiac follow-up examination. Co-morbidities include chronic atrial fibrillation, non-insulin requiring diabetes mellitus, and hypertension. His medications included captopril, digoxin, metoprolol, furosemide, potassium, and warfarin.

598

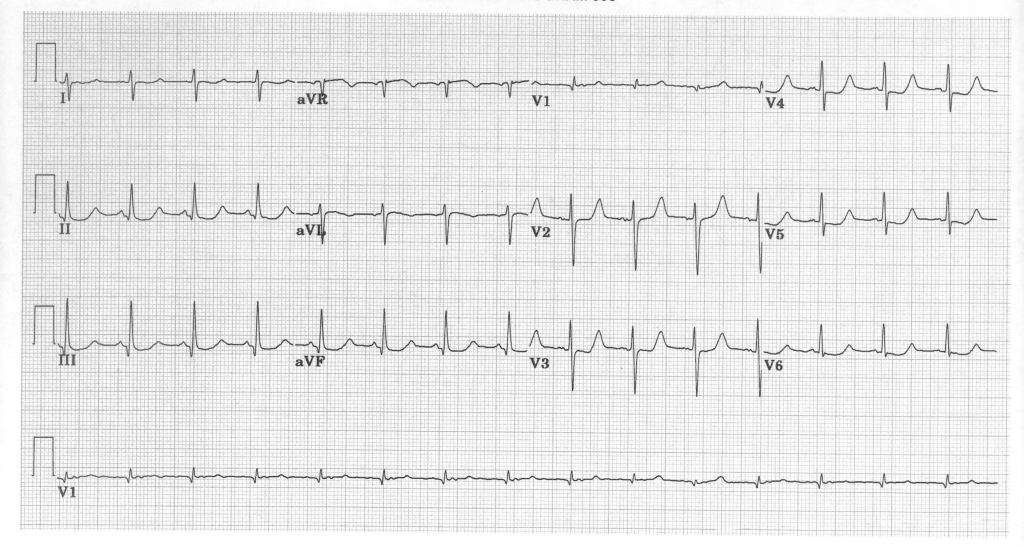

Interpretation Notes:_____

_____

_____

ECG 598 Forty-five year old woman with bicuspid aortic valve stenosis and insufficiency referred for aortic valve replacement. Her medications at the time of this electrocardiogram included thyroxine.

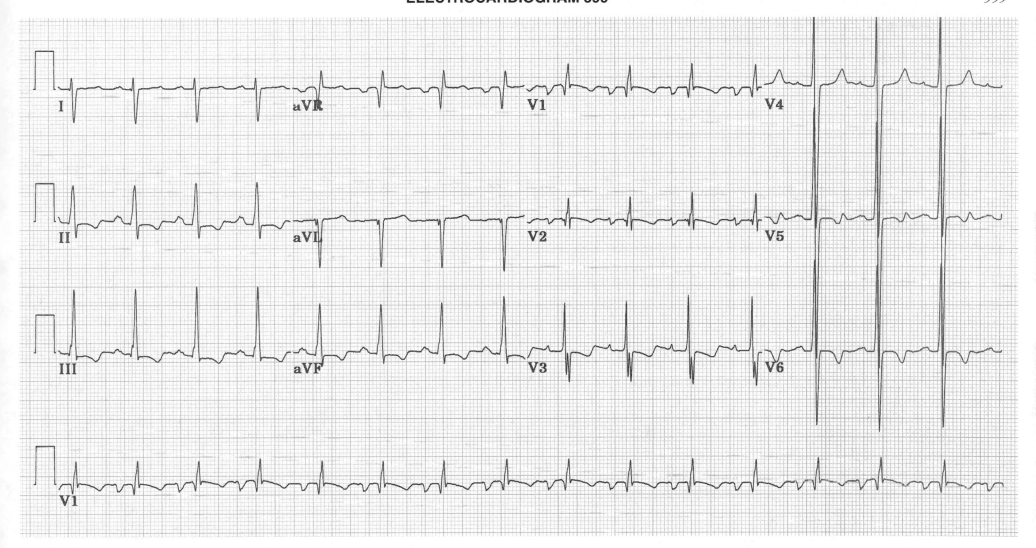

Interpretation Notes: _____

ECG 599 Thirty-five year old woman with primary pulmonary hypertension admitted to the hospital with increasing shortness of breath. An echocardiogram performed at the time of this hospitalization demonstrated a dilated right ventricle with severe right ventricular systolic dysfunction and right ventricular hypertrophy, a small left ventricle with mildly reduced systolic function, and an atrial septal defect with prominent right-to-left interatrial shunting. Medications at the time of this electrocardiogram included nifedipine, furosemide, and warfarin.

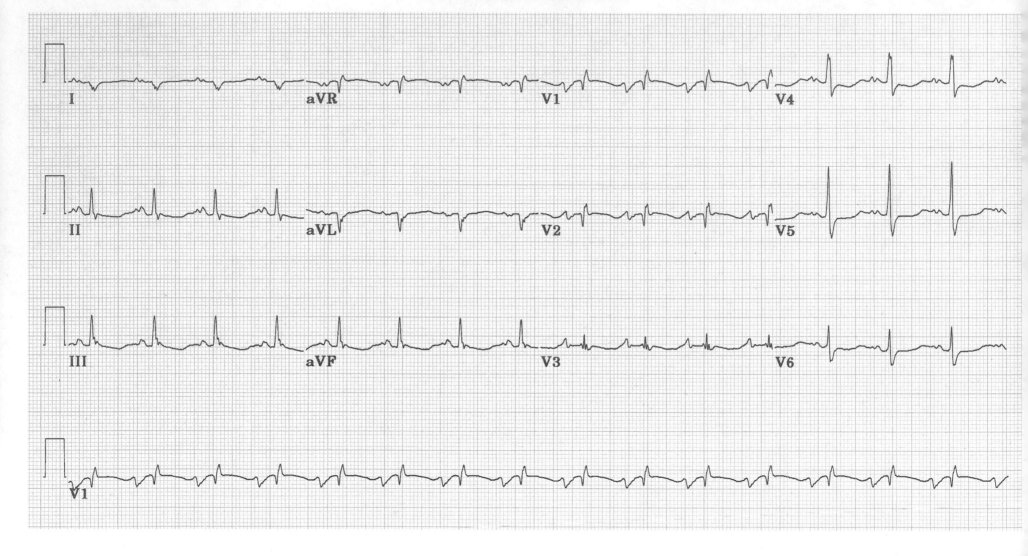

I	aVR	V1	V4
II	aVL	V2	V5
III	aVF	V3	V6

V1

Interpretation Notes: _____

_____

_____

ECG 600 Sixty-four year old woman with Ebstein's anomaly who returns for a cardiology outpatient follow-up evaluation. Her medications included amiodarone, captopril, potassium, digoxin, and furosemide. A past cardiac catheterization demonstrated a proximal left circumflex coronary artery occlusion.

ELECTROCARDIOGRAM 601

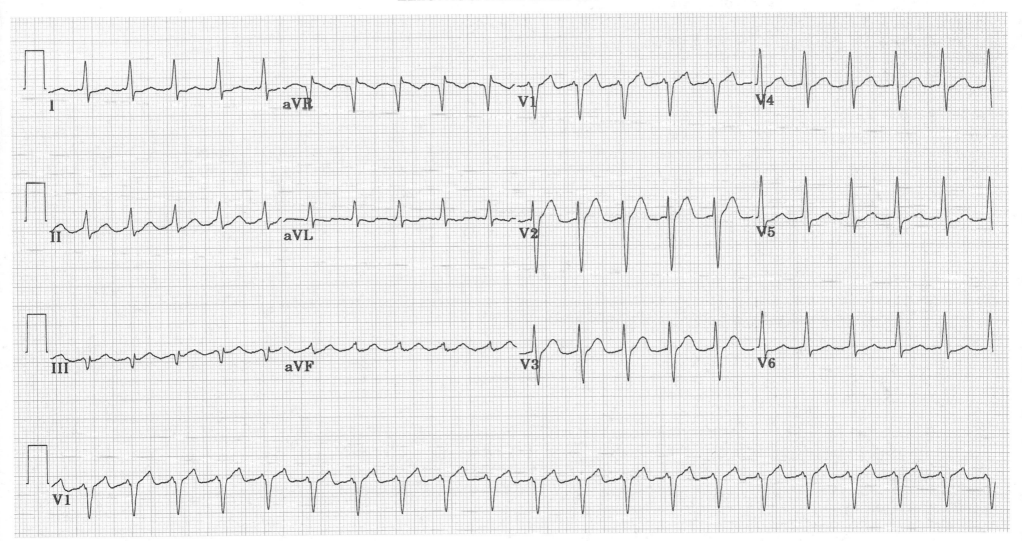

Interpretation Notes: _____

_____

ECG 601 Forty-eight year old gentleman with recurrent palpitations referred for radiofrequency catheter ablation.

ELECTROCARDIOGRAM 602

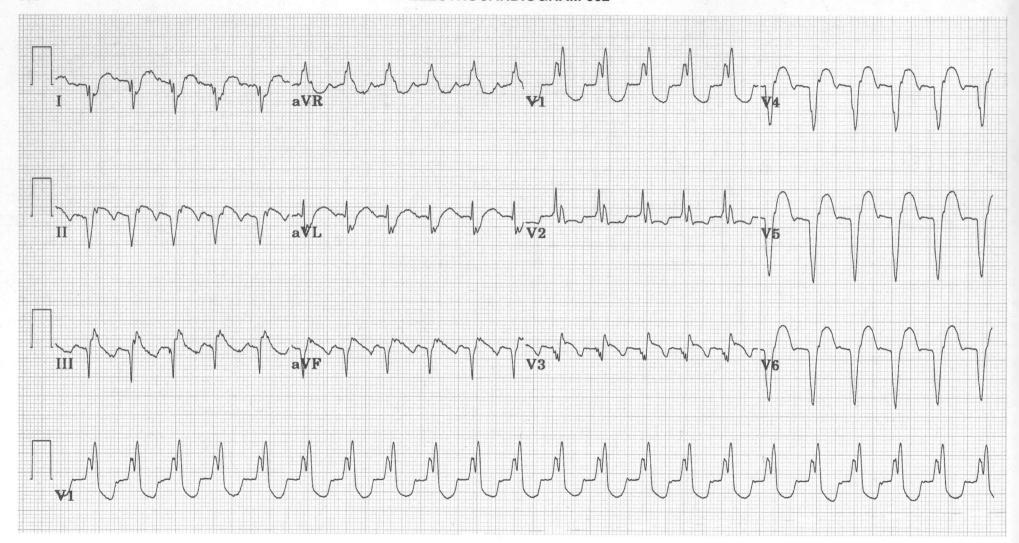

Interpretation Notes: _____

_____

_____

ECG 602 Sixty-seven year old gentleman transferred from an outside hospital after a recent anterior myocardial infarction. The myocardial infarction was complicated by anterolateral papillary muscle rupture. The patient subsequently underwent a left ventricular assist device implantation followed by coronary artery bypass grafting and mitral valve replacement.

ELECTROCARDIOGRAM 603

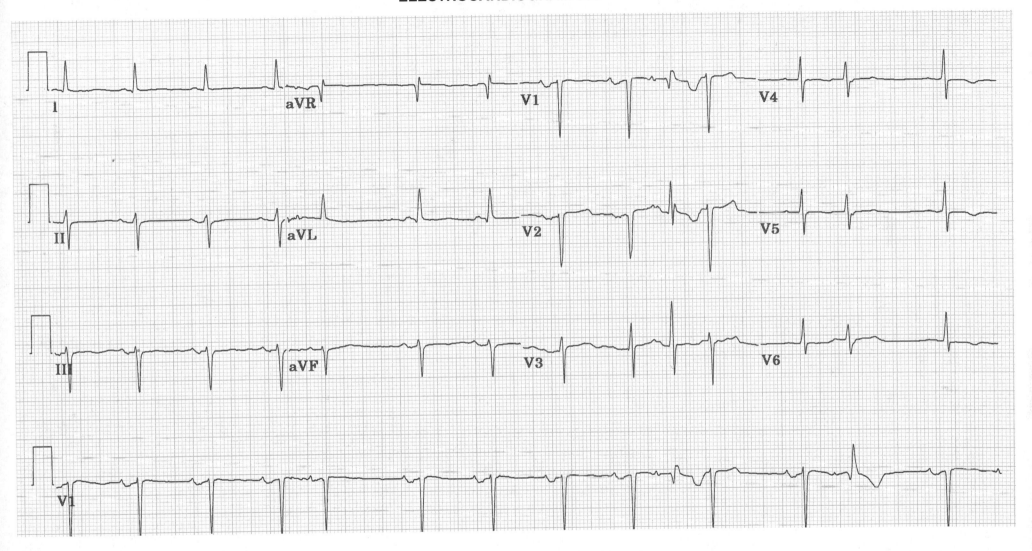

Interpretation Notes: _____

ECG 603 Seventy-seven year old woman who is being seen in the preoperative anesthesia department prior to planned eye surgery. She has a history of hypertension and non-insulin requiring diabetes mellitus. Her medications included amlodipine, potassium, and theophylline.

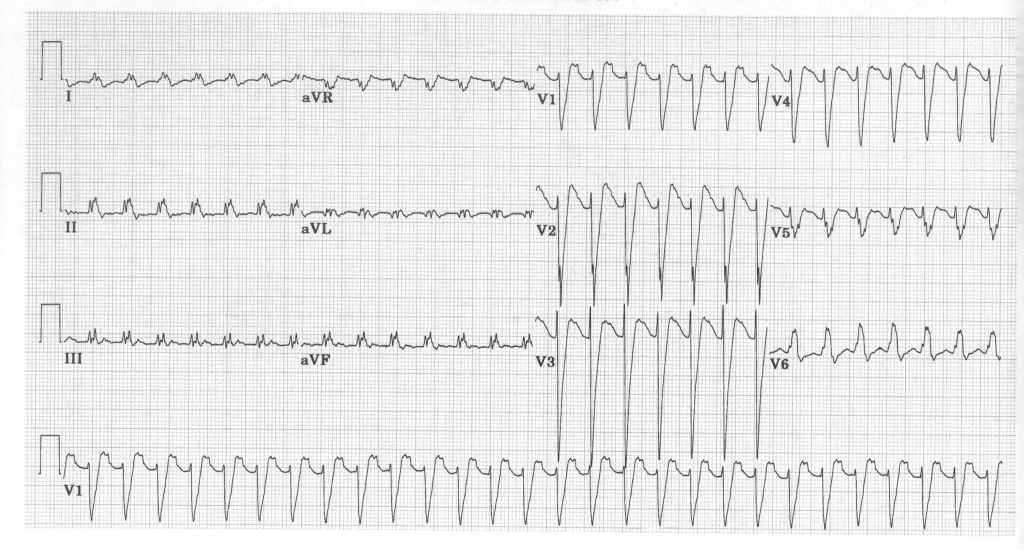

I aVR V1 V4

II aVL V2 V5

III aVF V3 V6

V1

Interpretation Notes: _____

_____

ECG 604 Forty-seven year old woman accepted in hospital transfer for evaluation of advanced congestive heart failure. Her past medical history includes chronic renal insufficiency and Hodgkin's lymphoma. Her medications included intravenous milrinone, thyroxine, digoxin, estrogen, and metolazone.

ELECTROCARDIOGRAM 605

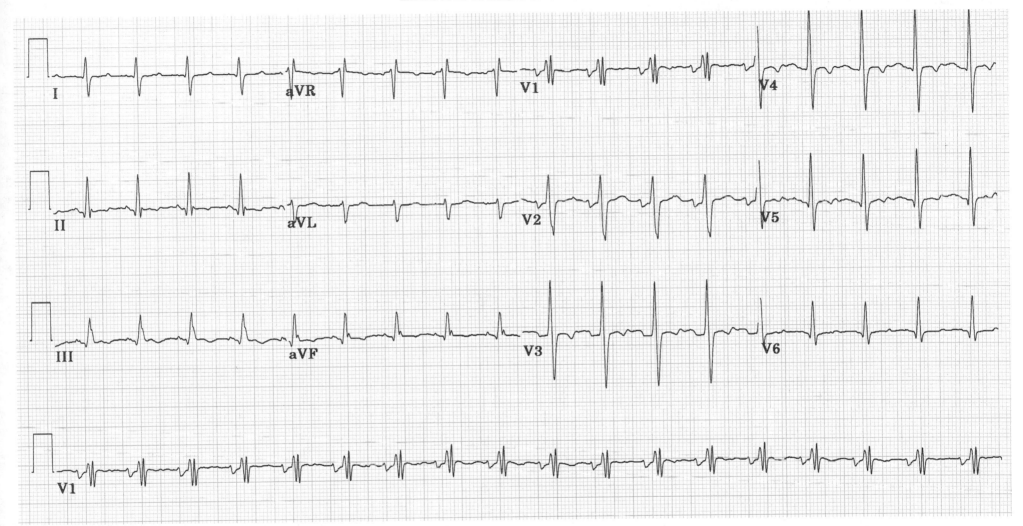

Interpretation Notes: _____

ECG 605 Forty-eight year old gentleman with severe ischemic left ventricular systolic dysfunction status post orthotopic cardiac transplantation. This electrocardiogram represents a post cardiac transplantation tracing in the presence of cardiac transplant vasculopathy.

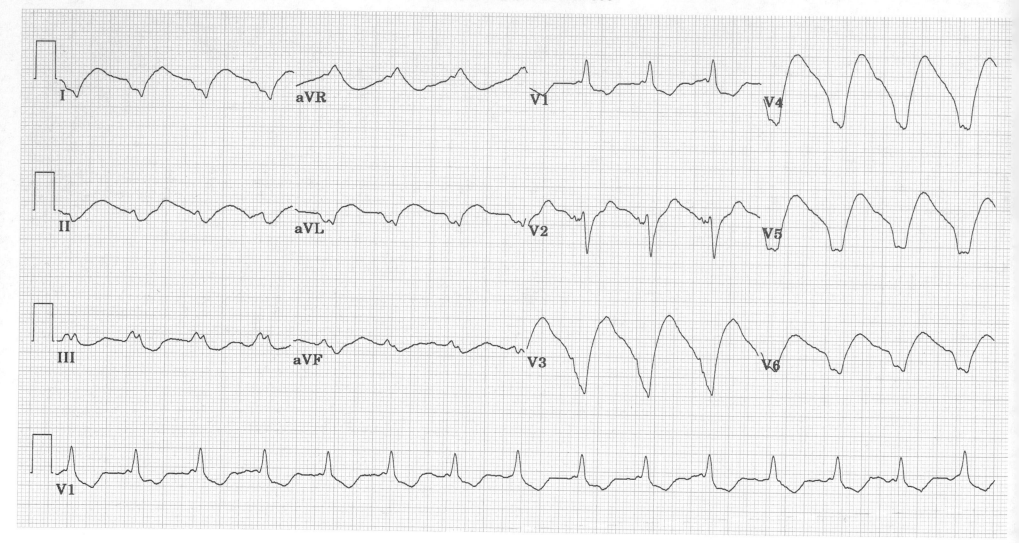

I   aVR   V1   V4

II   aVL   V2   V5

III   aVF   V3   V6

V1

Interpretation Notes: _____

_____

_____

ECG 606 Sixty-two year old gentleman with severe left ventricular systolic dysfunction and ischemic heart disease who presented to the hospital with intractable congestive heart failure. He was placed on a left ventricular assist device and was awaiting cardiac transplantation.

ELECTROCARDIOGRAM 607

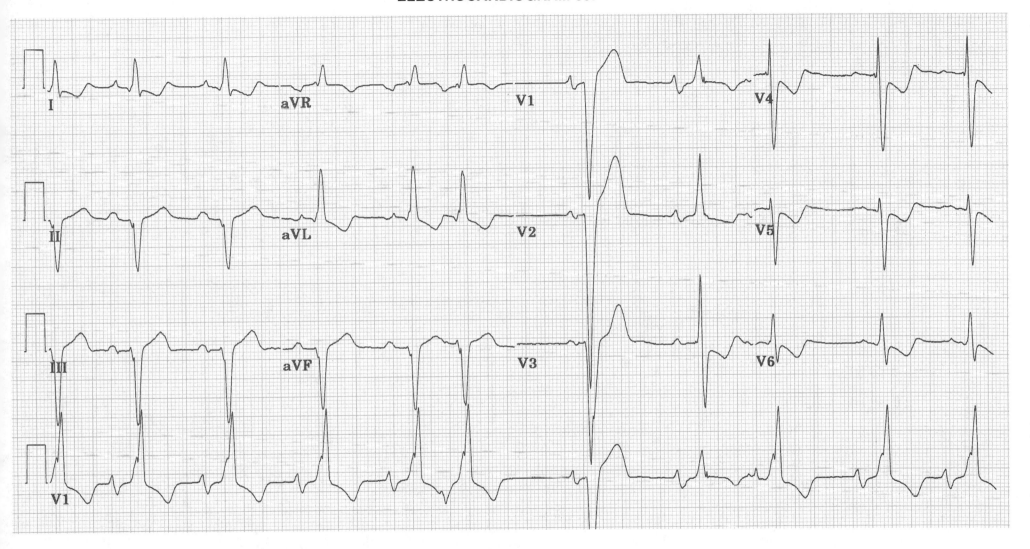

Interpretation Notes: _____

ECG 607 Thirty-four year old gentleman who presented to the hospital with near syncope. He has hypertrophic obstructive cardiomyopathy and moderately severe mitral insufficiency. He had undergone a recent cardiac catheterization demonstrating normal coronary arteries.

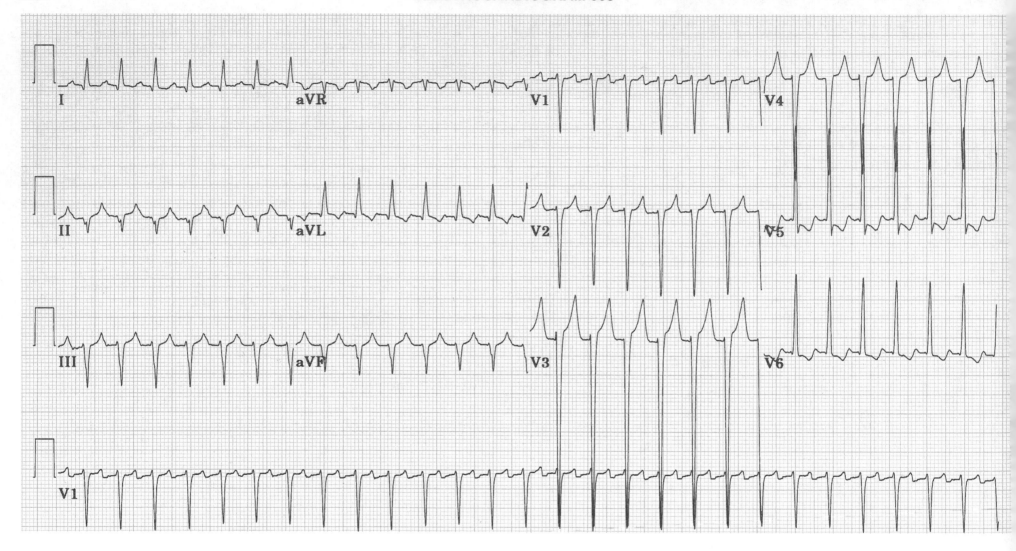

Interpretation Notes: _____

_____

ECG 608 Thirty-three year old gentleman hospitalized with severe congestive heart failure. He has severe left ventricular systolic dysfunction and a suspected non-ischemic cardiomyopathy. At the time of this electrocardiogram he was receiving intravenous dobutamine.

ELECTROCARDIOGRAM 609

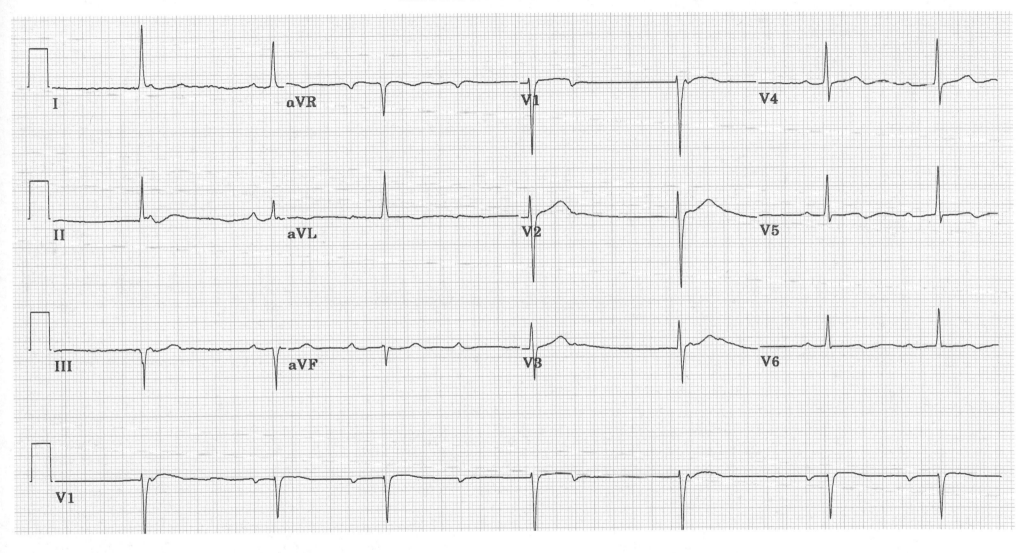

I aVR V1 V4

II aVL V2 V5

III aVF V3 V6

V1

Interpretation Notes: _____

ECG 609 Eighty-nine year old woman with a history of Alzheimer's disease who is admitted to the hospital with mental status changes. Her past medical history includes atherosclerotic heart disease and hypertension.

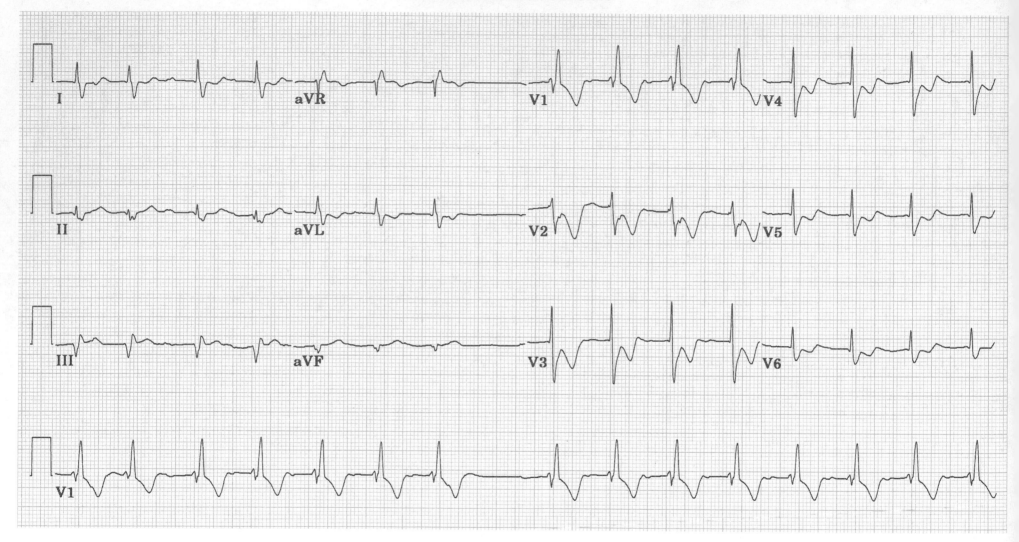

Interpretation Notes: _____

ECG 610 Seventy-four year old gentleman admitted to the hospital acutely for recurrent urinary retention. He underwent successful transurethral resection of the prostate. His past medical history includes peripheral vascular disease and coronary artery disease.

ELECTROCARDIOGRAM 611

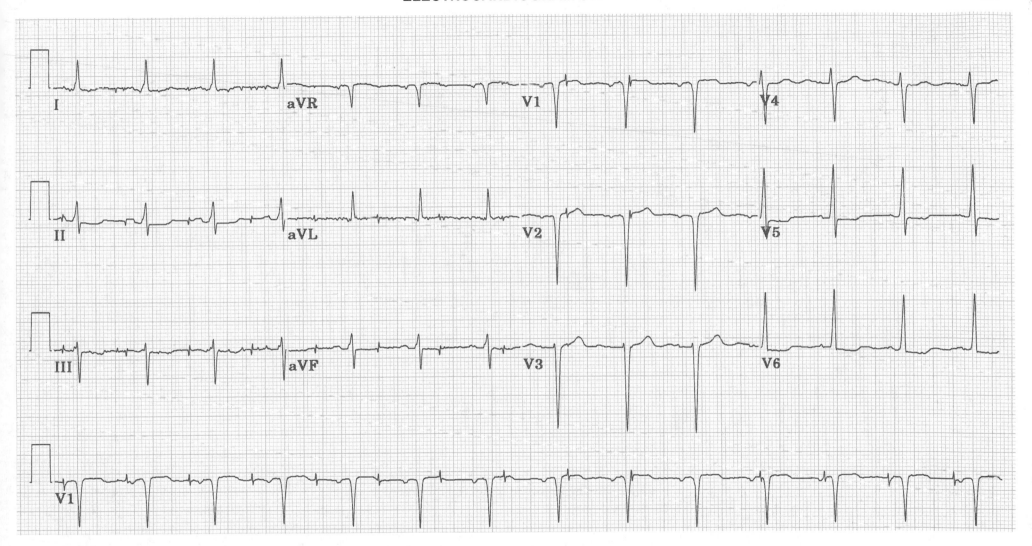

Interpretation Notes: _____

_____

ECG 611 Sixty-two year old gentleman with recurrent congestive heart failure admitted for evaluation and treatment of severe mitral insufficiency. His past cardiac history includes a coronary artery bypass graft operation one year before this electrocardiogram. The patient underwent successful mitral valve reparative surgery.

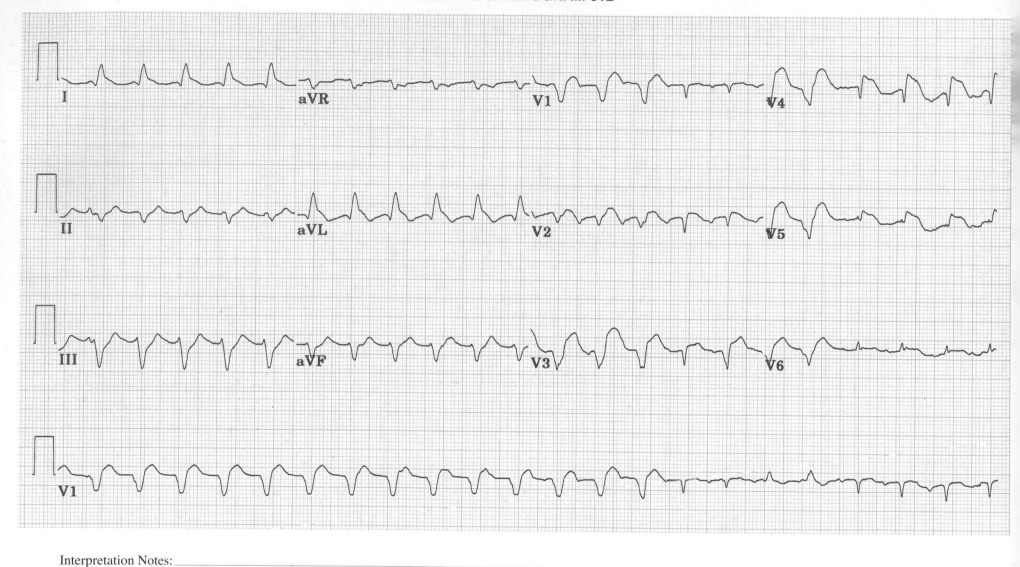

Interpretation Notes: _____

ECG 612 Sixty-eight year old gentleman who underwent a recent diagnostic cardiac catheterization demonstrating severe three vessel coronary artery disease. The patient suffered a cardiac arrest during the procedure. This electrocardiogram was obtained shortly after cardiopulmonary resuscitation. A repeat cardiac catheterization immediately post cardiac arrest demonstrated acute occlusion of the left anterior descending coronary artery. The patient expired shortly after this tracing was obtained.

ELECTROCARDIOGRAM 613

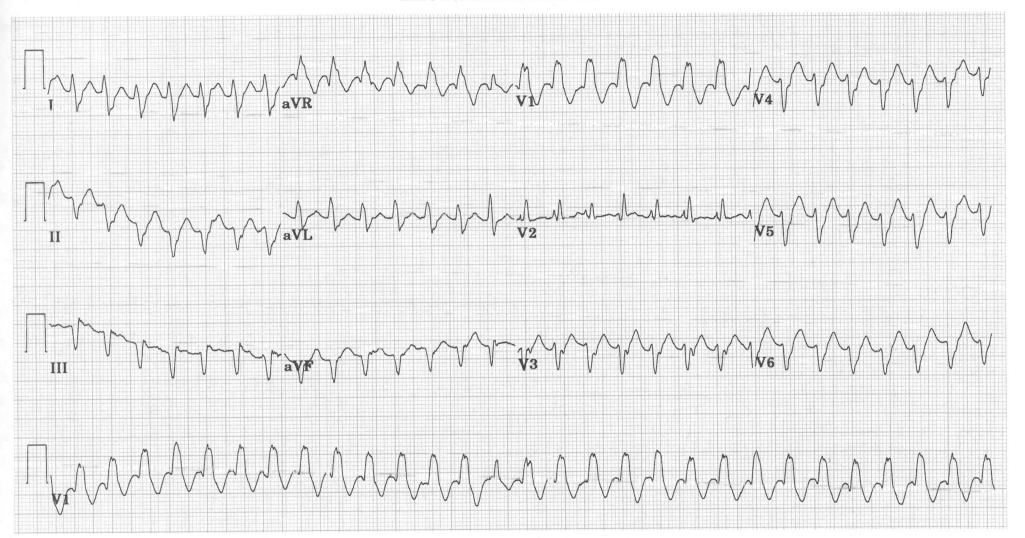

Interpretation Notes: _____

_____

ECG 613 Forty-nine year old gentleman with recurrent idiopathic left ventricular tachycardia referred for radiofrequency ablation. A recent echocardiogram demonstrated normal left ventricular systolic function without evidence of a prior myocardial infarction. His medications included verapamil, sotalol, simvastatin, and aspirin.

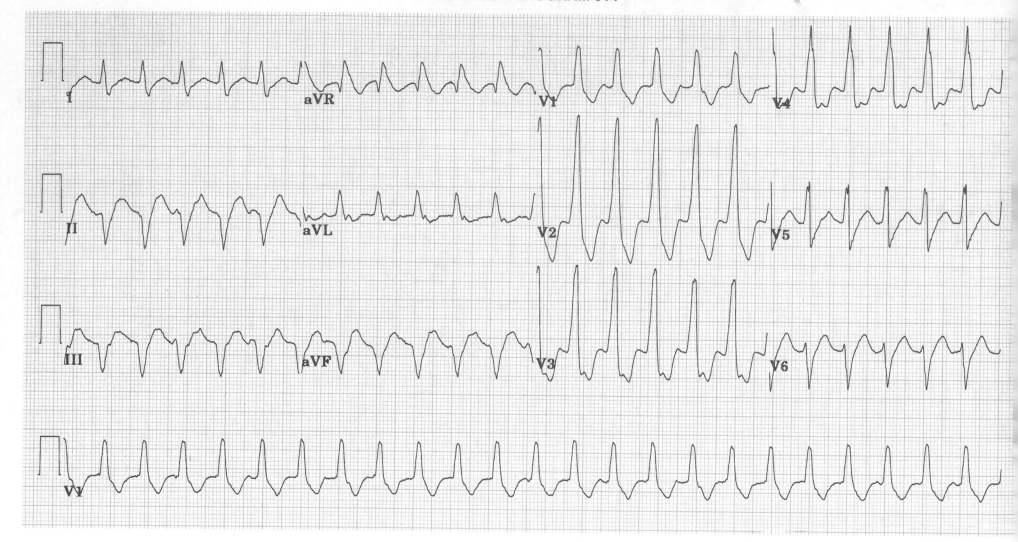

I aVR V1 V4

II aVL V2 V5

III aVF V3 V6

V1

Interpretation Notes: _____

_____

_____

ECG 614 Seventy-three year old gentleman with a history of hypertension, coronary artery disease, and remote coronary artery bypass graft surgery who was admitted for further evaluation and treatment of sustained ventricular tachycardia. He had an implantable cardiac defibrillator placed three months prior to this electrocardiogram. A recent echocardiogram demonstrated moderately severe left ventricular systolic dysfunction. His medications included metoprolol, lisinopril, and aspirin.

ELECTROCARDIOGRAM 615

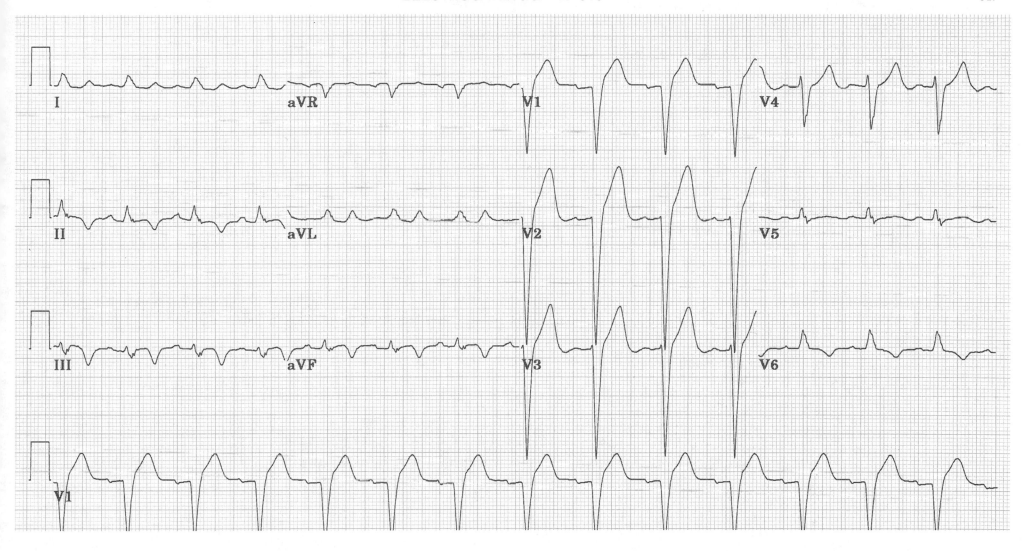

Interpretation Notes: _____

ECG 615 Seventy-two year old gentleman admitted urgently to the hospital with a three hour history of severe central chest pressure. A cardiac catheterization confirmed an acute occlusion of the right coronary artery with superimposed thrombus.

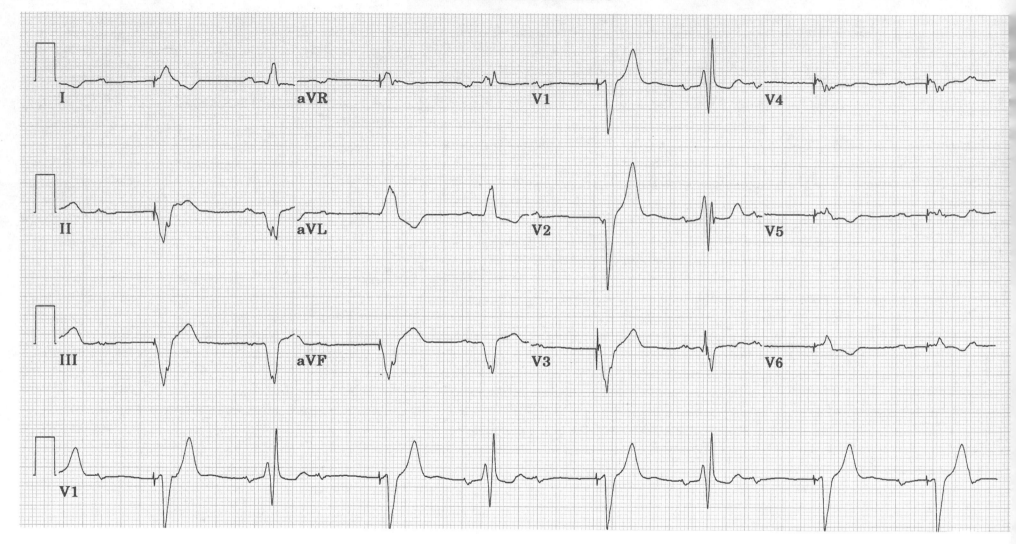

Interpretation Notes: _____

_____

_____

ECG 616 Seventy-six year old gentleman with recent syncope admitted for evaluation. He has a history of a remote inferior myocardial infarction.

ELECTROCARDIOGRAM 617

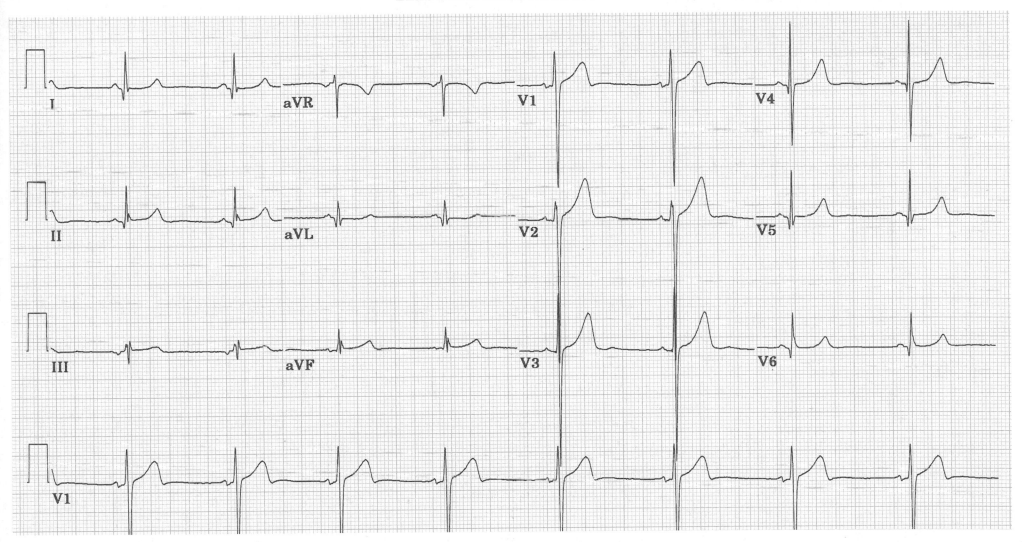

I   aVR   V1   V4

II   aVL   V2   V5

III   aVF   V3   V6

V1

Interpretation Notes: _____

_____

ECG 617 Twenty-five year old gentleman with a history of exertional lightheadedness and a recent echocardiogram documenting advanced hypertrophic obstructive cardiomyopathy.

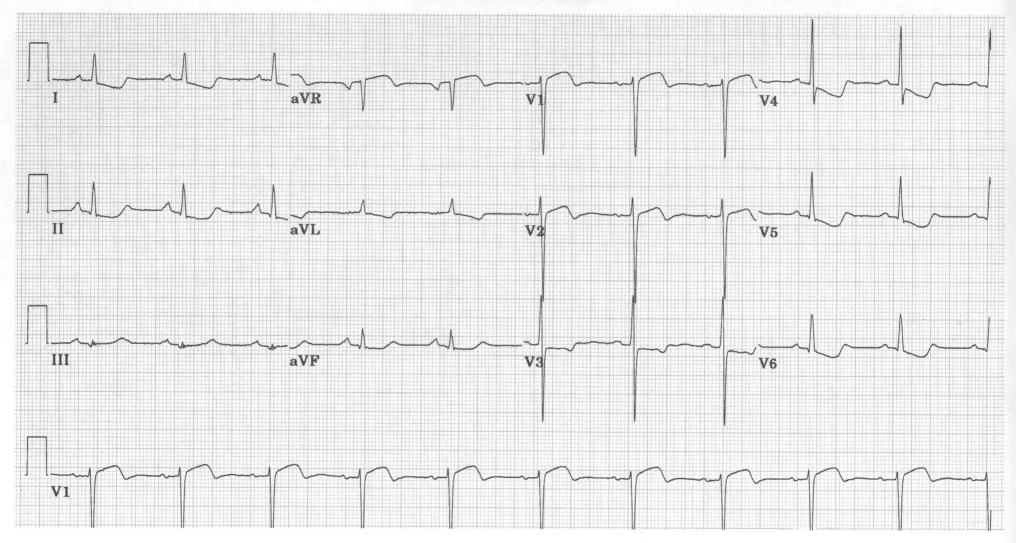

Interpretation Notes: _____

_____

ECG 618 Forty-eight year old woman with severe hypertrophic obstructive cardiomyopathy and pronounced symptoms of exertional dyspnea and pre-syncope immediately status post percutaneous alcohol ablation of her first septal perforator branch of the left anterior descending coronary artery. The patient was resting comfortably in the intensive care unit.

ELECTROCARDIOGRAM 619

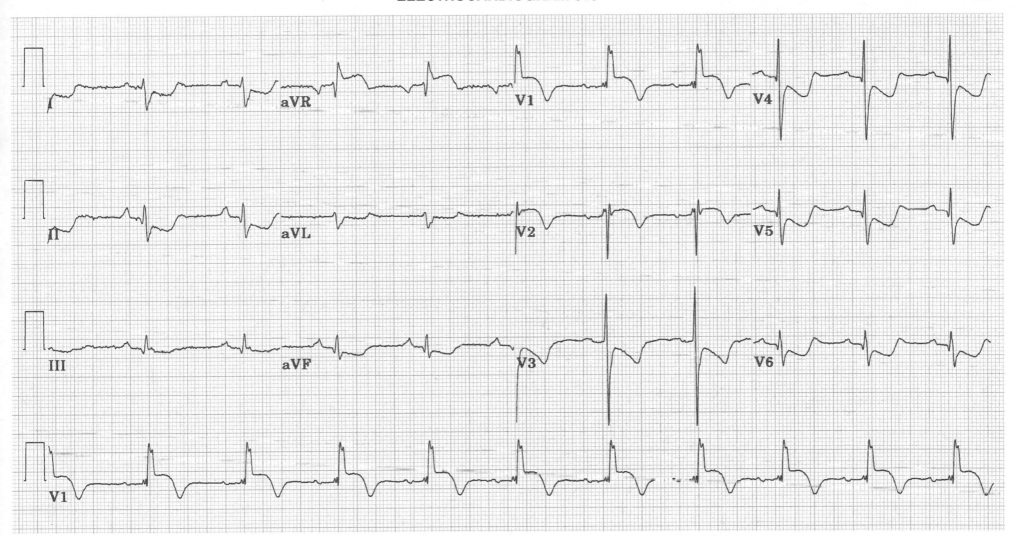

Interpretation Notes: _____

ECG 619 Forty-eight year old woman with severe hypertrophic obstructive cardiomyopathy and pronounced symptoms of exertional dyspnea and pre-syncope immediately status post percutaneous alcohol ablation of her first septal perforator branch of the left anterior descending coronary artery. The patient was resting comfortably in the intensive care unit.

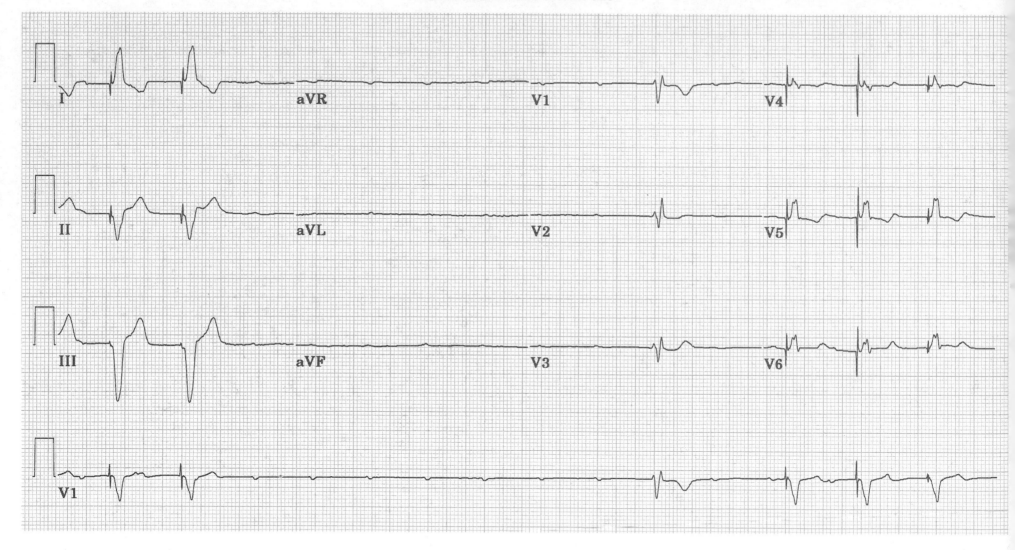

Interpretation Notes: _____

_____

ECG 620 Seventy-eight year old gentleman who is immediately postoperative aortic valve replacement and multi-vessel coronary artery bypass graft surgery. The patient had been pacemaker dependent for several days. The patient eventually underwent permanent pacemaker placement.

ELECTROCARDIOGRAM 621

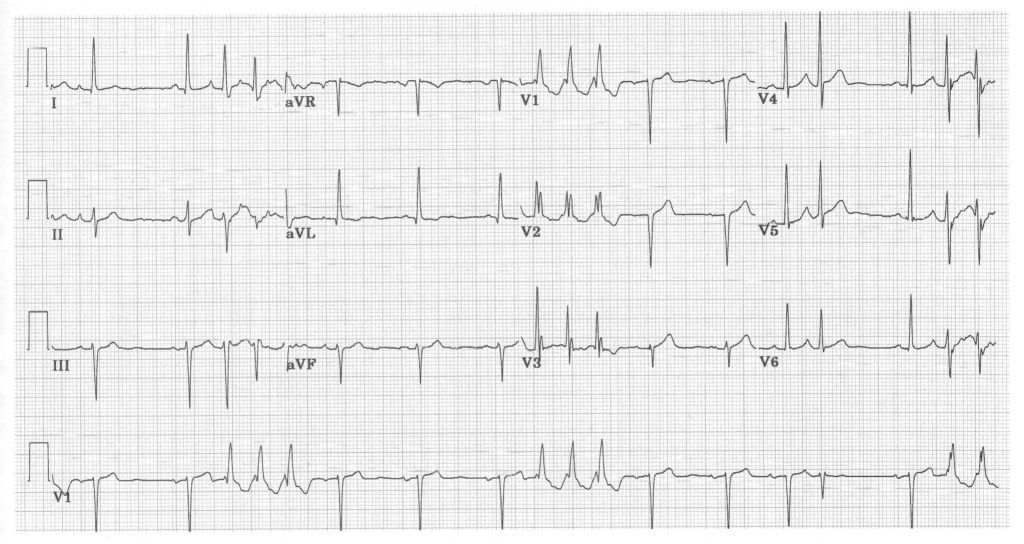

Interpretation Notes: _____

_____

_____

ECG 621 Eighty-four year old woman with severe degenerative osteoarthritis being seen in the outpatient rheumatology clinic. She has no known cardiac disease. She does suffer from long-standing hypertension.

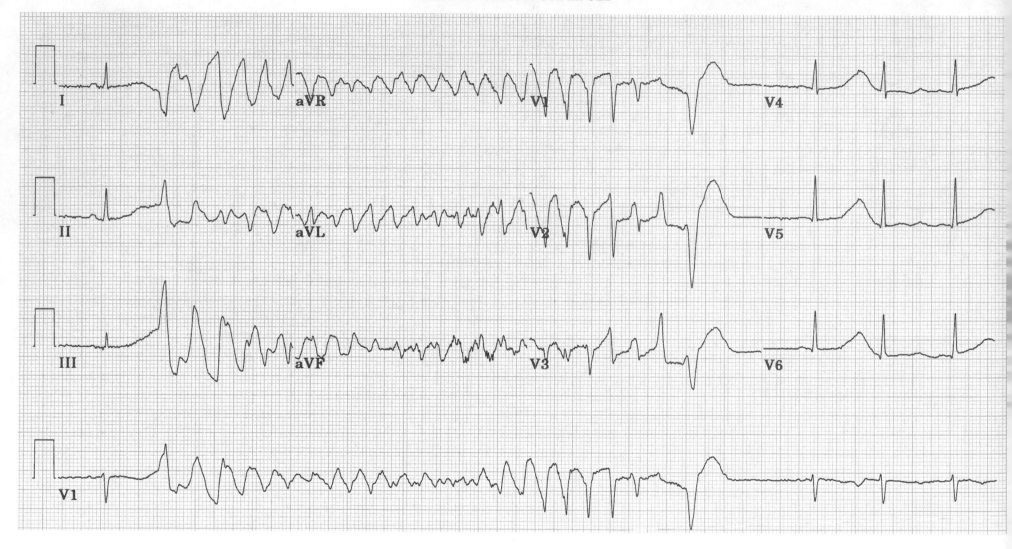

I   aVR   V1   V4

II   aVL   V2   V5

III   aVF   V3   V6

V1

Interpretation Notes: _____

_____

ECG 622 Fifty-one year old woman with metastatic breast carcinoma who is undergoing a bone marrow transplantation. Her serum potassium level at the time of this electrocardiogram was 2.9 mmol/L.

ELECTROCARDIOGRAM 623

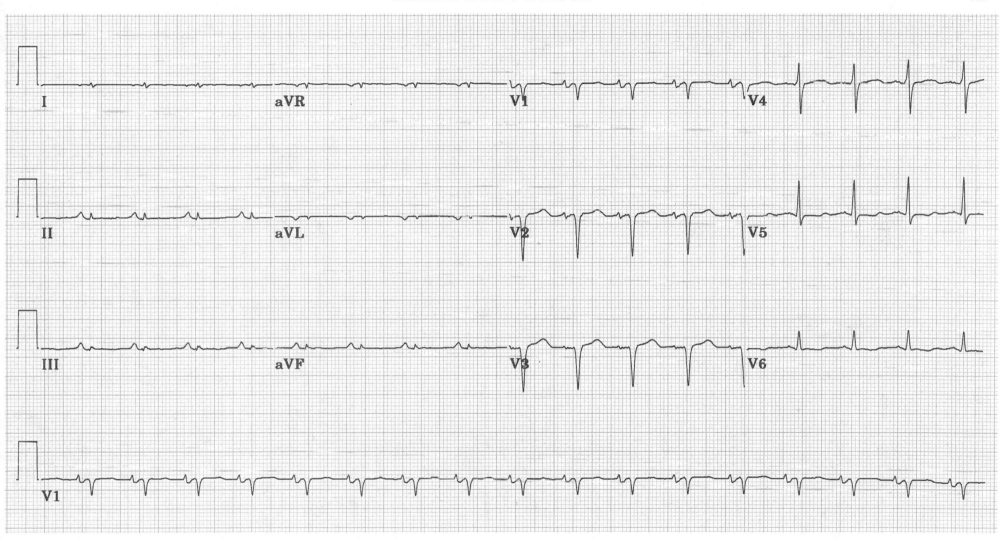

Interpretation Notes: _____

_____

_____

ECG 623 Sixty-eight year old gentleman with biopsy proven amyloidosis who is being seen in the congestive heart failure clinic. On echocardiography the patient has severe left ventricular systolic dysfunction. He currently suffers from intractable congestive heart failure.

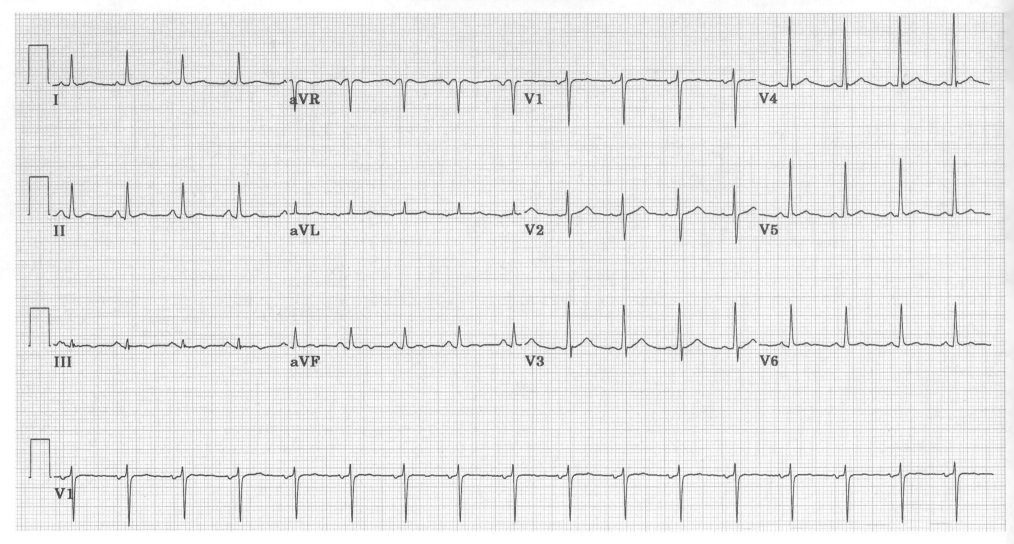

I aVR V1 V4

II aVL V2 V5

III aVF V3 V6

V1

Interpretation Notes: _____

_____

_____

ECG 624 Sixty-eight year old gentleman with advanced multiple myeloma who returns for an outpatient evaluation and medication reassessment. His serum calcium at the time of this electrocardiogram was 13.5 mg/dl.

ELECTROCARDIOGRAM 625

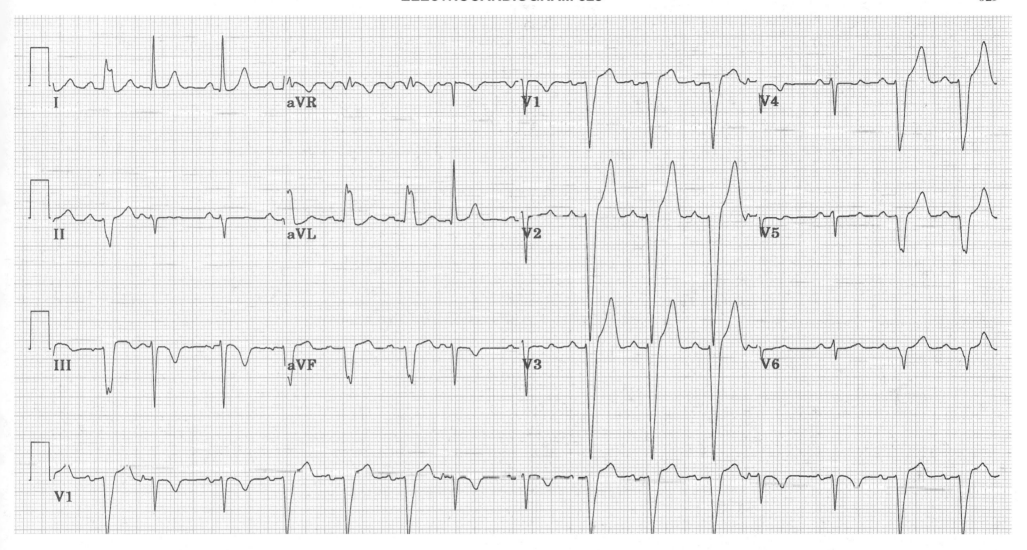

Interpretation Notes: _____

_____

ECG 625 Seventy-two year old woman admitted for evaluation of acute onset diverticulitis. Her past medical history includes hypertension and degenerative joint disease. Her medications at the time of this electrocardiogram included atenolol, amlodipine, and lovastatin.

ELECTROCARDIOGRAM 626

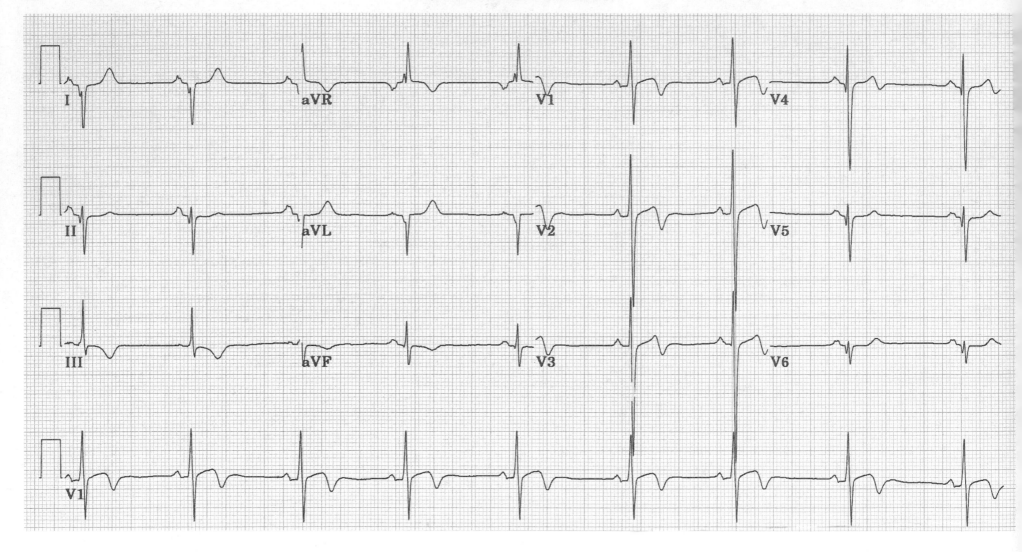

Interpretation Notes: _____

_____

_____

ECG 626 Twenty-eight year old gentleman being seen in the outpatient clinic for a follow-up hypertrophic obstructive cardiomyopathy evaluation. His medications included metoprolol and verapamil. A recent echocardiogram demonstrated hypertrophic obstructive cardiomyopathy and hyperdynamic left ventricular systolic function without evidence of a prior myocardial infarction.

ELECTROCARDIOGRAM 627

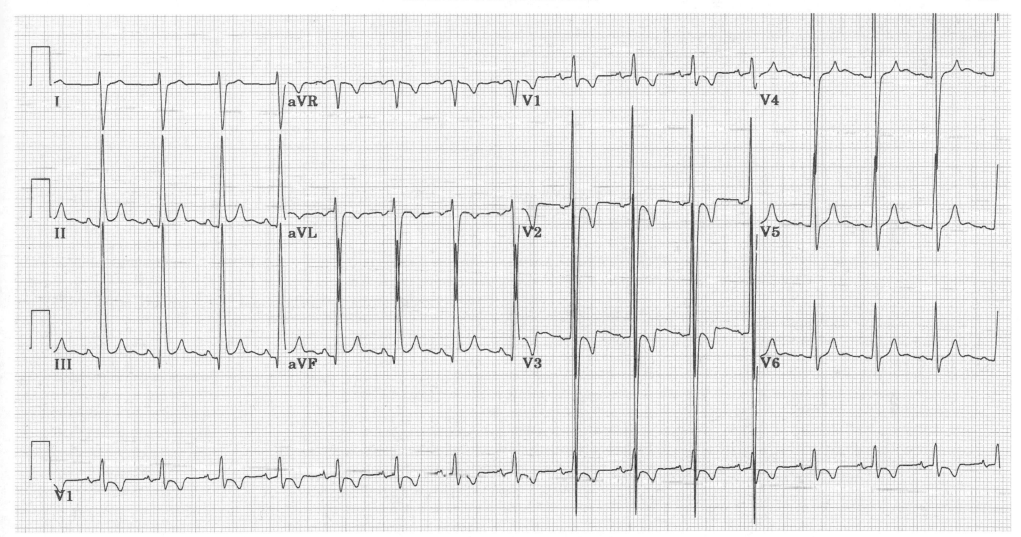

Interpretation Notes: _____
_____

ECG 627 Thirty year old gentleman with a history of a ventricular septal defect, transposition of the great vessels, and a double inlet left ventricle who is recently status post the Fontan procedure.

628

ELECTROCARDIOGRAM 628

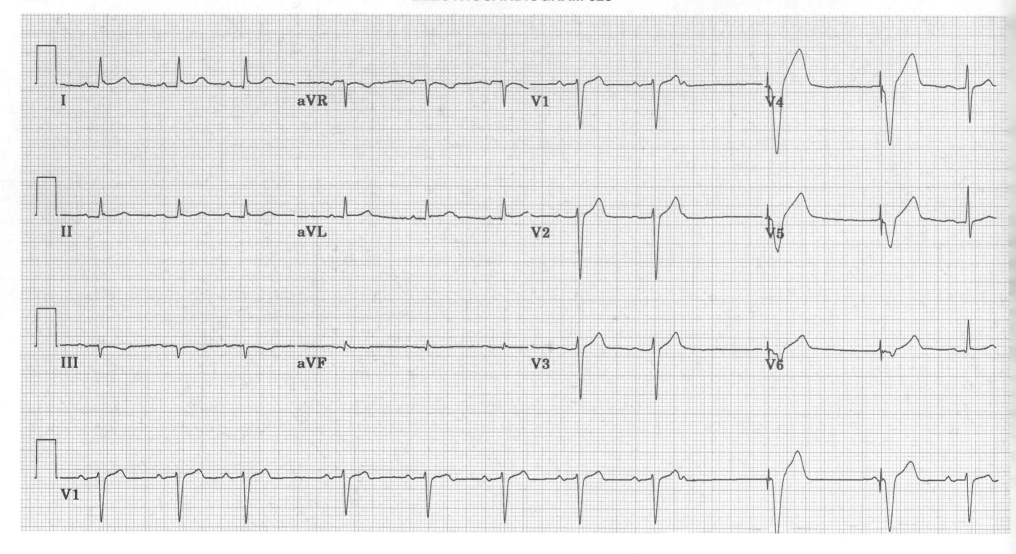

Interpretation Notes: _____

_____

_____

ECG 628 Seventy-four year old gentleman admitted to the hospital with unstable angina who is recently status post coronary artery bypass graft surgery. His medications included metoprolol, aspirin, and atorvastatin. A temporary epicardial pacemaker was placed at the time of his bypass surgery.

ELECTROCARDIOGRAM 629

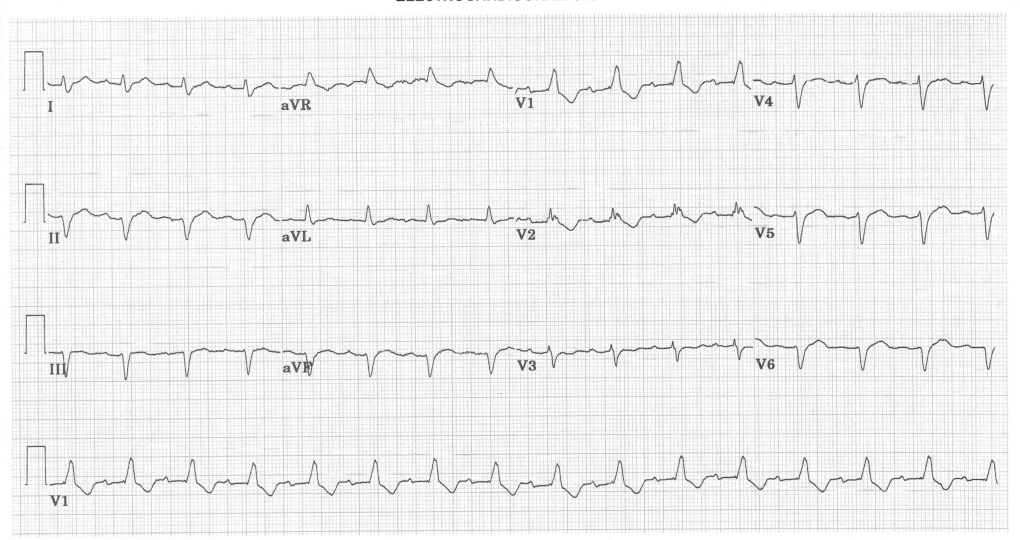

Interpretation Notes: _____

_____

ECG 629 Seventy-four year old gentleman admitted for revision of a prior colostomy. His past medical history includes ischemic heart disease and ischemic left ventricular systolic dysfunction.

630

ELECTROCARDIOGRAM 630

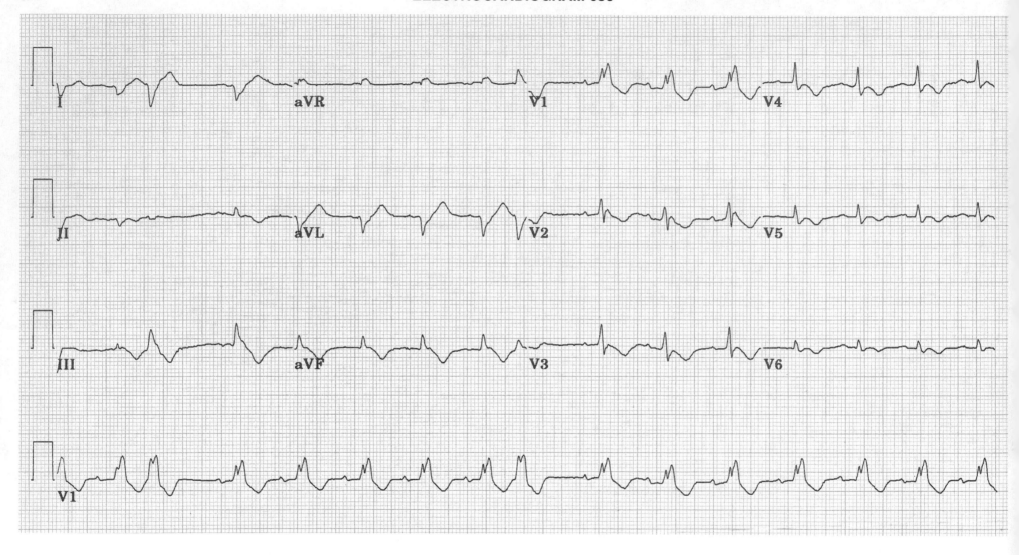

Interpretation Notes: _____

_____

_____

ECG 630 Seventy-four year old gentleman admitted for revision of a prior colostomy for rectal cancer. His past medical history includes ischemic heart disease and ischemic left ventricular systolic dysfunction.

ELECTROCARDIOGRAM 631

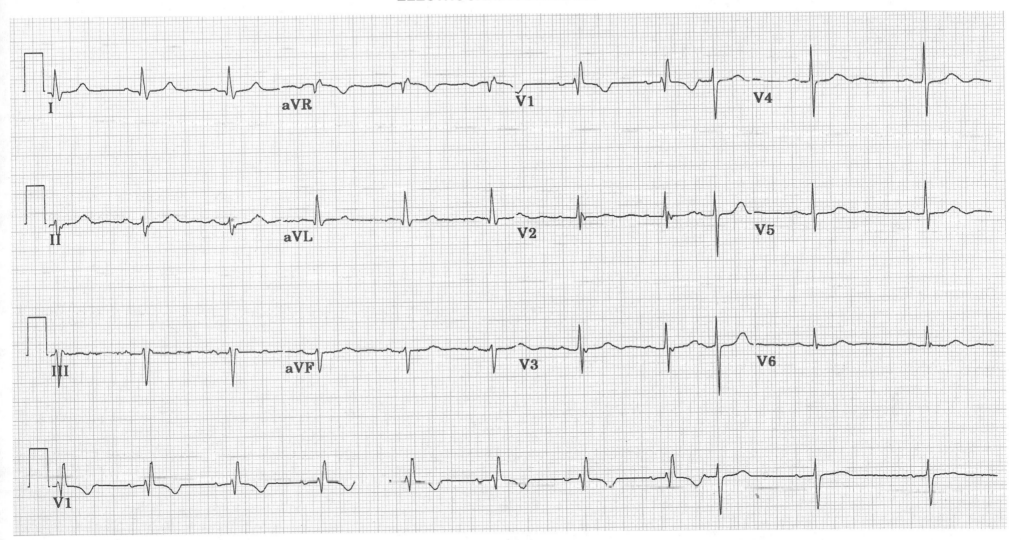

Interpretation Notes: _____

_____

ECG 631 Eighty-seven year old woman with severe osteoarthritis who seeks a second opinion secondary to progressive shortness of breath. Her medications included multivitamins and lisinopril.

A P P E N D I C E S

ELECTROCARDIOGRAM CD-ROM DIAGNOSTIC KEY WORD LIST

1:1 atrioventricular conduction
2:1 atrioventricular block
2:1 atrioventricular conduction
3:1 atrioventricular block
3:1 atrioventricular conduction
4:1 atrioventricular conduction

A
aberrant conduction
accelerated idioventricular rhythm
accelerated junctional rhythm
acceleration-dependent complete left bundle
    branch block
acceleration-dependent complete right bundle
    branch block
acceleration-dependent incomplete right bundle
    branch block
acute myocardial injury
advanced atrioventricular block
amyloidosis
anterior myocardial infarction, acute
anterior myocardial infarction, age-indeterminate
anterolateral myocardial infarction, acute
anterolateral myocardial infarction,
    age-indeterminate
anterolateral apical myocardial infarction, acute
Ashman's phenomenon
asystole
atrial arrest
atrial bigeminy
atrial escape complex
atrial fibrillation

atrial flutter
atrial pacemaker
atrioventricular dissociation
atrioventricular nodal reentrant tachycardia
atrioventricular paccmaker

B
baseline artifact
bifascicular block
biventricular hypertrophy

C
cardiac tamponade
cardiac transplant
cardiomyoplasty
cardiopulmonary resuscitation
central nervous system event
complete heart block
complete left bundle branch block
complete left bundle branch block
    aberrancy
complete right bundle branch block
complete right bundle branch block
    aberrancy
concealed conduction
constrictive pericarditis

D
dextrocardia
digitalis effect
dual atrioventricular nodal physiology

E
early repolarization
Ebstein's anomaly
echo complex
ectopic atrial bradycardia
ectopic atrial complex
ectopic atrial rhythm
ectopic atrial tachycardia
electrical alternans

F
first degree atrioventricular block
fusion complex

H
half standardization
high degree atrioventricular block
high lateral myocardial infarction, acute
high lateral myocardial infarction,
    age-indeterminate
hypercalcemia
hyperkalemia

I
idioventricular rhythm
incomplete right bundle branch block
incomplete right bundle branch block aberrancy
indeterminate axis
inferior myocardial infarction, acute
inferior myocardial infarction,
    age-indeterminate
inferior myocardial infarction, recent

inferolateral myocardial infarction, acute

inferolateral myocardial infarction, age-indeterminate

inferoposterior myocardial infarction, age-indeterminate

inferoposterior myocardial infarction, recent

inferoposterolateral myocardial infarction, acute

inferoposterolateral myocardial infarction, age-indeterminate

inferoposterolateral myocardial infarction, recent

interpolated premature atrial complex

interpolated premature junctional complex

interpolated premature ventricular complex

ischemia

J

junctional bigeminy

junctional bradycardia

junctional escape complex

junctional escape rhythm

junctional rhythm

junctional tachycardia

juvenile T-wave pattern

K

Katz-Wachtel phenomenon

L

lateral myocardial infarction, age-indeterminate

left anterior hemiblock

left atrial abnormality

left axis deviation

left posterior hemiblock

left ventricular aneurysm

left ventricular hypertrophy

left ventricular hypertrophy with secondary ST-T changes

M

misplaced limb leads

mitral stenosis

multifocal atrial tachycardia

myectomy

N

negative U waves

nonconducted premature atrial complex

nonconducted QRS complex

non–Q wave myocardial infarction

nonspecific intraventricular conduction delay

nonspecific ST-T changes

nonsustained ventricular tachycardia

normal electrocardiogram

normal sinus rhythm

normal variant

O

ostium primum atrial septal defect

ostium secundum atrial septal defect

P

pacemaker capture failure

pacemaker fusion complex

pacemaker sensing failure

paroxysmal atrial fibrillation

paroxysmal ectopic atrial rhythm

paroxysmal ectopic atrial tachycardia

paroxysmal junctional rhythm

patent foramen ovale

peaked T waves

peri-infarction block

pericardial effusion

pericarditis

post-extrasystolic ST-T changes

posterolateral myocardial infarction, age-indeterminate

premature atrial complex

premature junctional complex

premature ventricular complex

primary pulmonary hypertension

primary T-wave changes

prolonged QT interval

pseudoinfarction pattern

pulmonary embolism

pulmonic stenosis

Q

quinidine effect

R

rapid ventricular response

retrograde P waves

right atrial abnormality

right-axis deviation

right superior axis deviation

right ventricular hypertrophy

right ventricular hypertrophy with secondary ST-T changes

right ventricular myocardial infarction, acute

rightside chest leads

S

second degree Mobitz Type I (Wenckebach) atrioventricular block

second degree Mobitz Type II atrioventricular block

septal myocardial infarction, acute

septal myocardial infarction, age-indeterminate

septal myocardial infarction, recent

short PR interval

short QT interval

sinus arrest

sinus arrhythmia

sinus bradycardia

sinus capture complex

sinus exit block

sinus node reentrant rhythm

sinus pause

sinus tachycardia

slow ventricular response

supraventricular tachycardia

supernormal conduction
supraventricular tachycardia

T
tetralogy of Fallot
torsades de pointes
tricyclic antidepressant effect
trifascicular block

U
U waves

V
variable atrioventricular conduction
ventricular bigeminy
ventricular escape complex
ventricular escape rhythm
ventricular fibrillation
ventricular pacemaker
ventricular parasystole
ventricular tachycardia

W
wandering atrial pacemaker
wide QRS complex tachycardia
Wolff-Parkinson-White syndrome

Y
Yamaguchi's disease

CARDIAC RHYTHMS/ARRHYTHMIAS

accelerated idioventricular rhythm
accelerated junctional rhythm
asystole
atrial arrest
atrial bigeminy
atrial escape complex
atrial fibrillation
atrial flutter
atrioventricular nodal reentrant tachycardia
echo complex
ectopic atrial bradycardia
ectopic atrial complex
ectopic atrial rhythm
ectopic atrial tachycardia
fusion complex
idioventricular rhythm
interpolated premature atrial complex
interpolated premature junctional complex
interpolated premature ventricular complex
junctional bigeminy
junctional bradycardia
junctional escape complex
junctional escape rhythm
junctional rhythm
junctional tachycardia
multifocal atrial tachycardia
nonconducted premature atrial complex
nonconducted QRS complex

nonsustained ventricular tachycardia
normal sinus rhythm
paroxysmal atrial fibrillation
paroxysmal ectopic atrial rhythm
paroxysmal ectopic atrial tachycardia
paroxysmal junctional rhythm
premature atrial complex
premature junctional complex
premature ventricular complex
sinus arrest
sinus arrhythmia
sinus bradycardia
sinus capture complex
sinus exit block
sinus node reentrant rhythm
sinus pause
sinus tachycardia
supraventricular tachycardia
torsades de pointes
ventricular bigeminy
ventricular escape complex
ventricular escape rhythm
ventricular fibrillation
ventricular parasystole
ventricular tachycardia
wandering atrial pacemaker
wide QRS complex tachycardia

EXAMINATION: DIAGNOSTIC CATEGORIES

1:1 atrioventricular conduction
2:1 atrioventricular block
2:1 atrioventricular conduction
3:1 atrioventricular block
3:1 atrioventricular conduction
4:1 atrioventricular conduction
aberrant conduction
acceleration-dependent complete left bundle
    branch block
acceleration-dependent complete right bundle
    branch block
acceleration-dependent incomplete right bundle
    branch block
advanced atrioventricular block
Ashman's phenomenon
atrioventricular dissociation
bifascicular block
complete heart block
complete left bundle branch block
complete left bundle branch block aberrancy
complete right bundle branch block
complete right bundle branch block aberrancy
concealed conduction
dual atrioventricular nodal physiology
first degree atrioventricular block
high degree atrioventricular block
incomplete right bundle branch block
incomplete right bundle branch block aberrancy
left anterior hemiblock
left posterior hemiblock
masquerading bundle branch block
nonspecific intraventricular conduction delay
peri-infarction block
rapid ventricular response
retrograde P waves
second degree Mobitz Type I (Wenckebach)
    atrioventricular block

second degree Mobitz Type II atrioventricular
    block
short PR interval
slow ventricular response
supernormal conduction
trifascicular block
variable atrioventricular conduction
Wolff-Parkinson-White syndrome

ELECTRICAL AXIS/VOLTAGE

electrical alternans
half standardization
indeterminate axis
left anterior hemiblock
left axis deviation
left posterior hemiblock
low-voltage QRS
right axis deviation
right superior axis deviation

CARDIAC CHAMBER FINDINGS

biventricular hypertrophy
biventricular hypertrophy with secondary ST-T
    changes
Katz-Wachtel phenomenon
left atrial abnormality
left ventricular aneurysm
left ventricular hypertrophy
left ventricular hypertrophy with secondary ST-T
    changes
right atrial abnormality
right ventricular hypertrophy
right ventricular hypertrophy with secondary ST-T
    changes

REPOLARIZATION FINDINGS

acute myocardial injury
digitalis effect
early repolarization
hypercalcemia
hyperkalemia
hypocalcemia
hypokalemia
ischemia
juvenile T-wave pattern
negative U waves
nonspecific ST-T changes
peaked T waves
pericarditis
post-extrasystolic ST-T wave changes
primary T-wave changes
prolonged QT interval
quinidine effect
short QT interval
U waves

MYOCARDIAL INFARCTION

anterior myocardial infarction, acute
anterior myocardial infarction, age-indeterminate
anterolateral myocardial infarction, acute
anterolateral myocardial infarction,
    age-indeterminate
anterolateral-apical myocardial infarction, acute
high lateral myocardial infarction, acute
high lateral myocardial infarction,
    age-indeterminate
inferior myocardial infarction, acute
inferior myocardial infarction, age-indeterminate
inferior myocardial infarction, recent
inferolateral myocardial infarction, acute

inferolateral myocardial infarction,
    age-indeterminate
inferoposterior myocardial infarction,
    age-indeterminate
inferoposterior myocardial infarction, recent
inferoposterolateral myocardial infarction, acute
inferoposterolateral myocardial infarction,
    age-indeterminate
inferoposterolateral myocardial infarction, recent
lateral myocardial infarction, age-indeterminate
non–Q wave myocardial infarction
posterolateral myocardial infarction,
    age-indeterminate
pseudoinfarction pattern
right ventricular myocardial infarction, acute
septal myocardial infarction, acute
septal myocardial infarction, age-indeterminate
septal myocardial infarction, recent

PACEMAKER FINDINGS

atrial pacemaker
atrioventricular pacemaker
pacemaker capture failure
pacemaker fusion complex

pacemaker sensing failure
ventricular pacemaker

TECHNICAL FINDINGS

baseline artifact
misplaced limb leads
right-side chest leads

NORMAL ELECTROCARDIOGRAM FINDINGS

juvenile T-wave pattern
normal electrocardiogram
normal variant

CLINICAL DIAGNOSES

amyloidosis
cardiac tamponade
cardiac transplant
cardiomyoplasty
cardiopulmonary resuscitation

central nervous system event
constrictive pericarditis
dextrocardia
digitalis effect
Ebstein's anomaly
hypercalcemia
hyperkalemia
hypertrophic obstructive cardiomyopathy
hypocalcemia
hypokalemia
ischemia
left ventricular aneurysm
mitral stenosis
myectomy
ostium primum atrial septal defect
ostium secundum atrial septal defect
patent foramen ovale
pericardial effusion
pericarditis
primary pulmonary hypertension
pulmonary embolism
pulmonic stenosis
quinidine effect
tetralogy of Fallot
tricyclic antidepressant effect
Yamaguchi's disease

SUBJECT INDEX